Psychosoci
Foundation of Nursing

Psychosocial Foundation of Nursing

I Clement

MA (Sociology), MA (Child Care and Education)
MSc (Nursing), MPhil (Education)

Principal
VSS College of Nursing, Bengaluru
Karnataka, India

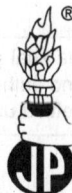

JAYPEE BROTHERS MEDICAL PUBLISHERS (P) LTD

Bengaluru • St Louis (USA) • Panama City (Panama) • London (UK) • New Delhi
Ahmedabad • Chennai • Hyderabad • Kochi • Kolkata • Lucknow • Mumbai • Nagpur

Published by
Jitendar P Vij
Jaypee Brothers Medical Publishers (P) Ltd

Corporate Office
4838/24 Ansari Road, Daryaganj, **New Delhi** - 110002, India, Phone: +91-11-43574357, Fax: +91-11-43574314

Registered Office
B-3 EMCA House, 23/23B Ansari Road, Daryaganj, **New Delhi** - 110 002, India
Phones: +91-11-23272143, +91-11-23272703, +91-11-23282021
+91-11-23245672, Rel: +91-11-32558559, Fax: +91-11-23276490, +91-11-23245683
e-mail: jaypee@jaypeebrothers.com, Website: www.jaypeebrothers.com

Offices in India

- **Ahmedabad**, Phone: Rel: +91-79-32988717, e-mail: ahmedabad@jaypeebrothers.com
- **Bengaluru**, Phone: Rel: +91-80-32714073, e-mail: bangalore@jaypeebrothers.com
- **Chennai**, Phone: Rel: +91-44-32972089, e-mail: chennai@jaypeebrothers.com
- **Hyderabad**, Phone: Rel:+91-40-32940929, e-mail: hyderabad@jaypeebrothers.com
- **Kochi**, Phone: +91-484-2395740, e-mail: kochi@jaypeebrothers.com
- **Kolkata**, Phone: +91-33-22276415, e-mail: kolkata@jaypeebrothers.com
- **Lucknow**, Phone: +91-522-3040554, e-mail: lucknow@jaypeebrothers.com
- **Mumbai**, Phone: Rel: +91-22-32926896, e-mail: mumbai@jaypeebrothers.com
- **Nagpur**, Phone: Rel: +91-712-3245220, e-mail: nagpur@jaypeebrothers.com

Overseas Offices

- **North America Office, USA,** Ph: 001-636-6279734,
  e-mail: jaypee@jaypeebrothers.com, anjulav@jaypeebrothers.com
- **Central America Office, Panama City, Panama,** Ph: 001-507-317-0160
  e-mail: cservice@jphmedical.com; Website: www.jphmedical.com
- **Europe Office, UK,** Ph: +44 (0) 2031708910, e-mail: dholman@jpmedical.biz

Psychosocial Foundation of Nursing

This book has been published in good faith that the material provided by author is original. Every effort is made to ensure accuracy of material, but the publisher, printer and author will not be held responsible for any inadvertent error (s). In case of any dispute, all legal matters are to be settled under Delhi jurisdiction only.

First Edition: **2010**

ISBN 978-81-8448-923-1

Typeset at JPBMP typesetting unit

Printed at Rajkamal Electric Press, Plot No. 2, Phase-IV, Kundli, Haryana.

Preface

Psychosocial nursing deals with patient care, bridges the gap between the information contained at large. This book presents with basic concepts about psychology, sociology and psychosocial-related issues. This book consists of 5 chapters (1-5) of General Concepts, 17 chapters (6-22) of Psychology, 20 chapters (23-42) of Sociology and 8 chapters (43-50) of Psychosocial Issues.

Psychosocial care emphasizes interventions to assist individuals who are having difficulty in coping with the emotional aspects of illness, with life crisis that affect health and health care. In psychosocial care, the nurse focuses on the effects of stress in psychological or physiological illness and on intrapsychic and social functioning of individuals responding to stress.

Psychology is one of the very important subjects in the training of every nurse today. It will enable the nurse to understand herself/himself. This implies an understanding of motives, desires, emotions and ambitions of her/him and his/her patients.

Physical, social, cultural and psychological factors interact dynamically and have an important influence on patient care needs. There are needs common to everyone, no matter their sociocultural background, so-called human needs. These needs when they are not met create tensions and these tensions may give rise to anxiety that can hamper recovery if not relieved.

Culturally, competent nursing care is defined as being sensitive to issues related to culture, race, religion, gender, sexual orientation, and social or economic class. Cultural competence implies not only awareness of cultural differentiation but also the ability to assess and intervene appropriately and effectively.

Psychosocial Foundation of Nursing textbook will prove to be extremely useful for basic nursing students in facing their examinations and also enable them to equip themselves better for their future endeavors.

I Clement

Acknowledgments

I am thankful to the Lord Almighty, who always strengthens me and showers blessings on me to complete my task in time.

My heartfelt thanks to Shri V Sommanna, MLA, Chairman of VSS Group of Institutions, for his constant support and encouragement.

My sincere thanks to my guide and guru BT Basavanthappa, who is a great philosopher, leader in nursing a wonderful person who showers fatherly love, who helps me to discover the world of knowledge.

I am thankful to our Board of Directors of VSS Group of Institutions, Dr BS Arun and Dr Naveen, for their support and encouragement.

I am grateful and extend my thanks to Dr Aswathnarayan, MLA, Chairman of Padmashree Group of Institutions, for his support and encouragement.

I convey my sincere thanks to my beloved wife Mrs Nisha Clement, MSc (N), for her continuous and constant support and encouragement in each step of my life, also I take this opportunity to thank my little ones Cibin and Cynthia.

It is my honor and privilege to thank my parents Mr Irudthyanathan and Arokiamary, my sisters Elizabeth Rani, Mary Saraswathi, and Glory, my brothers, Amalan and Felix for their support in the form of finance, their powerful prayers and encouraging words to complete the task.

This is the time that I should thank my best friend Mr Regi T Kurien (New York) and family, who was with me in my dark times and my hurdle days. I thank him for his love and affection and constant support. I extend sincere thanks to my seniors, classmates and co-workers.

My sincere thanks to Shri Jitendar P Vij (Chairman and Managing Director), Mr Tarun Duneja (Director-Publishing), Mr KK Raman (Production Manager), Mr Akhilesh Kumar Dubey, Mrs Uma Adhikari, Mr V Venugopal (Manager, Bengaluru Branch), Mr H Vasudev (Author coordinator, Bengaluru Branch) and all staff of M/s Jaypee Brothers Medical Publishers (P) Ltd, for bringing this excellent quality textbook.

Contents

Section 4: Psychosocial Issues

Appendices

Abbreviations

A

ABER	Annual Blood Examination Rate
ACHAN	Asian Community Health Action Network
ADS	Antidiphtheri Serum
AFP	Acute Flaccid Paralysis
AGR	Annual Growth Rate
AIDS	Acquired Immunodeficiency Syndrome
AIWS	All India Women's Conference
ALR	Adult Literacy Rate
ANC	Antenatal Clinic/Antenatal Care
ANM	Auxiliary Nurse Midwife (FHW)
ANP	Applied Nutrition Program
APH	Antepartum Hemorrhage
API	Annual Parasite Incidence
AR	Attributable Risk/ Abortion Rate
ARC	Aids Related Complex
ARI	Acute Respiratory Infections
ASHA	Accredited Social Health Activists American Speech and Hearing Association
ASV	Anti-snake Venom
ATS	Anti-tetanus Serum
AYUSH	Ayurveda, Yoga-naturopathy, Unani, Siddha, Homeopathy
AHW	Auxiliary Health Worker
AW	Auxiliary Worker
AWW	Anganwadi Worker

B

BBT	Basal Body Temperature
BCG	Bacille Calmette-Guérin
BDO	Block Development Officer/Office
BHC	Benzene Hexachloride
BHL	Bore Hole Latrine
BHS	Basic Health Services
BMI	Body Mass Index
BMR	Basal Metabolic Rate
BOR	Bed Occupancy Rate
BP	Blood Pressure
BSE	Breast Self Examination
BTU	British Thermal Unit

C

CAL	Calorte
CARE	Cooperative for American Relief Everywhere
CAT	Computer Axial Tomography
CBR	Crude Birth Rate
CCH	Central Council of Health
CCS	Case Control Study
CCV	Cell Culture Vaccine
CCU	Critical Care Unit/ Cardiac Care Unit
CD	Communicable Disease
CDP	Community Development Program/ Project
CDPO	Child Development Project Officer
CDR	Crude Death Rate/ Child Death Rate
CGHS	Central Government Health Scheme
CHAI	Catholic Hospital Association of India
CHC	Community Health Center
CHD	Coronary Heart Disease
CHEB	Central Health Education Bureau
CHN	Community Health Nursing/ Community Health Nurse
CHO	Community Health Officer
CHW	Community Health Worker
CHAI	Catholic Hospital Association of India
CNAA	Community Need Assessment Approach
CMAI	Christian Medical Association of India
CMI	Cell Medicated Immunity
CMR	Child Mortality Rate
CPA	Consumer Protection Act
CPCB	Central Pollution Control Board
CPR	Couple Protection Rate
CSS	Cross-sectional Studies
CSIR	Council of Scientific and Industrial Research
CSSM	Child Survival and Safe Motherhood (Program)
CSF	Cerebrospinal Fluid

D

dB	Decibels (Sound Intensity Unit)
DDCP	Diarrheal Disease Control Program
DDT	Dichlorodiphenyltrichloroethane
DEV	Duck Embryo Vaccine
DLF	Day Light Factor
DGHS	Director General of Health Services
DHF	Dengue Hemorrhagic Fever
DHS	Director of Health Services
DM	Diabetes Mellitus
DMPA	Depot Medroxy Progesterone Acetate
DNA	Deoxyribonucleic Acid
DNR	Doctor Nurse Ratio
DPHN	District Public Health Nurse/Nursing
DPR	Doctor Population Ratio
DPT	Diphtheria, Pertussis, Tetanus (Vaccine)
DPTP	Diphtheria, Pertussis, and Tetanus Plus Inactivated Polio
DR	Death Rate
DSS	Dengue Shock Syndrome
DTC	District Training Center
DTO	District Tuberculosis Officer
DV	Defective Vision
DWL	Dug Well Latrine

E

EAA	Essential Amino Acids
EC	Eligible Couple
ECG	Electrocardiogram
EDD	Expected Date of Delivery
EEG	Electroencephalogram
EFA	Essential Fatty Acid
EL	Expectation of Life
ELISA	Enzyme-linked Immuno-sorbent Assay
EPI	Expanded Program of Immunization
ESI	Employee State Insurance

F

FAP	Food and Agriculture Organization
FBD	Food Both Diseases
FHA	Female Health Assistant
FHW	Female Health Worker
FLR	Fine Needle Aspiration Cytology
FP	Family Planning
FPAI	Family Planning Association of India
FRU	First Referral Unit
FW	Family Welfare
FWS	Family Welfare Service

G

GD	Growth and Development
GFR	General Fertility Rate
GMFR	General Marital Fertility Rate
GRR	Gross Reproduction Rate

H

HAF	Health Assistant Female
Hb	Homoglobin
HBIG	Hepatitis B Imunoglobulin
HCH	Hexachlorocyclohexane (Lindane)
HDCV	Human Diploid Cell Vaccine
HE	Health Education/Educator
HFA	Health for All
HIV	Human Immunodeficiency Virus
HT	Hypertension
HW	Health Worker

I

IBD	Insect Borne Disease
ICD	International Classification of Disease
ICDS	Integrated Children of Medical Research
ICMR	Indian Council of Medical Research
ICN	Internatioal Council of Nurses
IDD	Iodine Deficiency Disorders
IDDM	Insulin Dependent Diabetes Mellitus
IEC	Information Education Communication
IG	Immunoglobulin
ICU	Intensive Care Unit/ Intensive Cardiac Unit
IDC	International Death Certificate
IHD	Ischemic Heart Disease
ILO	International Labor Organization
ILR	Ice Lined Refrigerator
IMA	Indian Medical Association
IMR	Infant Mortality Rate
INC	Indian Nursing Council
IPP	Indian Population Project
IPV	Inactivated Polio Vaccine
IQ	Intelligence Quotient
IRDP	Integrated Rural Development Program
IS	Immune Serum
IU	International Units
IUCD	Intrauterine Contraceptive Devices
IUD	Intrauterine Devices

J

J	Joule
JE	Japanese Encephalitis
JD	Juvenile Delinquency

K

kCal	Kilocalorie
kJ	Kilo Joule
KUB	Kidney Ureters and Bladder

L

LBW	Low Birth Weight (Baby)
LEP	Leprosy Eradication Program
LFT	Liver Function Test
LGVD	Lymphogranuloma Venereal Disease
LHV	Lady Health Visitor
LR	Literacy Rate
LT	Lepromin Test

M

MBD	Mosquito Borne Disease
MBO	Management by Objectives
MC	Menstrual Cycle
MCH	Maternal and Child Health
MDMP	Mid-day Meal Program
MDRB	Multidrug Resistance Bacilli
MDSM	Mid-day School Meal
MFC	Membrane Filter Concentration (Method)
MHS	Maternal Health Services
Minilap	Minilaparotomy
MLC	Medicolegal Case
MLO	Medicolegal Office/Mosquito Larvicidal Oil
MOHFW	Ministry of Health and Family Welfare
MMR	Maternal Mortality Rate
MNP	Minimum Need Program
MPW	Multipurpose Worker
MR	Mental Retardation/ Morbidity Rate/Ratio
MT	Mantoux Test
MTP	Medical Termination of Pregnancy

N

NAB	National Association for the Blind
NACO	National Aids Control Organization
NEERI	National Engineering and Environmental Research Institute
NET En	Nor Ethisterone Enantate

NFCP	National Filaria Control Program
NFHS	National Family Health Survey
NIHFW	National Institute of Health and Family Welfare
NGCP	National Goiter Control Program
NGO	Non-Governmental Organization
NHP	National Health Policy
NHS	National Health Services
NID	National Immunization Day
NLEP	National Leprosy Eradication Program
NMCP	National Malaria Control Program
NMEP	National Malaria Eradication Program
NMHP	National Mental Health Program
NMR	Neonatal Mortality Rate
NPP	National Population Policy
NPR	Net Production Rate/ Nurse Population Ratio
NSS	National Sample Survey
NSV	Non Scalpel Vasectomy
NTCP	National Tuberculosis Control Program
NTV	Nervous Tissue Vaccine
NVBDCP	National Vector Brone Diseases Control Program
NWSP	National Water Sanitation Program

O

OPV	Oral Polio Vaccine
ORS	Oral Rehydration Solution
ORT	Oral Rehydration Therapy

P

PBR	Population Bed Ratio
PCI	Per Capita Income
PCM	Protein Calorie Malnutrition
PEM	Protein Energy Malnutrition
PER	Protein Energy Ratio
PFA	Prevention of Food Adulteration (Act)
PHC	Primary Health Care/ Primary Health Center
PHN	Public Health Nursing/ Public Health Nurse
PID	Pelvic Inflammatory Diseases
PMR	Prenatal Mortality Rate/ Proportional Mortality Rate
PNC	Postnatal Clinic/Care Prenatal Clinic/Care
PNMR	Postnatal Mortality Rate

POP	Progestogen Only Pill
PPH	Postpartum Hemorrhage
PPP	Postpartum Period/ Public Private Partnership
PPS	Postpartum Services/Scheme
PSM	Preventive and Social Medicine
PTAP	Purified Toxoid Aluminium Phosphate
PV	Per-Vaginum

R

RAHA	Raigarh Ambikapur Health Association (MP)
RBR	Rural Birth Rate
RCA	Research cum Action (Latrine)
RCH	Reproductive and Child Health
RF	Rheumatic Fever
RFWC	Rural Family Welfare Center
Rh Factor	Rhesus Factor
RHD	Rheumatic Heart Disease
RhIG	Rhesus Immune Globulin
RHS	Rural Health Scheme/Services
RIG	Rabies Immunoglobulin
RMP	Registered Medical Practitioner
RUSHA	Rural Health & Social Afairs (Vellore-TN)

S

SARS	Severe Acute Respiratory Syndrome
SAR	Secondary Attack Rate
SC	Subcenter/Subcutaneous
SDR	Specific Death Rate
SEWA	Self Employed Women's Association (Gujarat)
SFN	Small Family Norm
SFP	Supplementary Feeding Program
SHC	Secondary Health Care
SIDA	Swedish International Development Agency
SIHFW	State Institute of Health and Family Welfare
SNA	Student Nurses Association
SOS	Save Our Soul
SVV	Split Virus Vaccine
SRS	Sample Registration System
SSF	Slow Sand Filter
STD	Sexually Transmitted Diseases
STI	Sexually Transmitted Infections

T

| TB | Tuberculosis |
| TFA | Target Free Approach |

TBA	Traditional Birth Attendant
TFR	Total Fertility Rate
TIG	Tetanus Immune Globulin
TMFR	Total Marital Fertility Rate
TPP	Twenty Point Program
TT	Tetanus Toxoid
TNAI	Trained Nurses Association of India

U

UCI	Universal Child Immunization
UFWC	Urban Family Welfare Center
UIP	Unlversal Immunization Program
UNDP	United Nations Development Program
UNFPA	United Nations Fund for Population Activities
UNICEF	United Nations International Children's Emergency Fund (Now United Nations Children's Fund)
UNRRA	United Nations Relief and Rehabilitation Administration
USAID	United States Agency for International Development

V

VBT	Vector Borne Transmission
VD	Venereal Diseases
VDRL	Venereal Disease Research Laboratory
VGKK	Vivekananda Girtjana Kalyana Kendra (Karnataka)
VHA	Voluntary Health Association/ Voluntary Health Agencies
VHAI	Voluntary Health Association of India
VHG	Village Health Guide
VHGS	Village Health Guide Scheme
VHW	Voluntary Health Worker
VVM	Vaccine Vial Monitor
VZIG	Varicella Zoster Immune Globulin

W

WBC	Well Baby Clinic
WBD	Waterborne Diseases
WC	Water Closets
WER	Weekly Epidemiological Record/Reports
WHO	World Health Organization
WHD	World Health Day
WSL	Water Seal Latrine
WWF	World Wide Fund (for Nature)

SECTION 1: GENERAL CONCEPTS

Health and Illness

1

DEFINITIONS

1. **Acute illness:** Illness characterized by symptoms that are of relatively short duration, are usually severe and affect the functioning of the clients in all dimensions.
2. **Adaptation:** Process by which changes occur in any of a person's dimensions in response to stress.
3. **Etiology:** Identification of the cause of a problem. The cause may be direct or a contributing factor in the development of client problem or need.
4. **Health:** Dynamic state in which an individual adapts to internal and external environments so that there is a state of physical, emotional, intellectual, social and spiritual well-being.
5. **Health behavior:** Activities through which a person maintain, attains or regains behavior as an expression of personal health beliefs.
6. **Health- belief model:** Conceptual framework that predicts a person's health behavior as an expression of personal beliefs.
7. **Health- illness continuum:** Scale by means of which a personnel's level of health can be described, ranging from high level wellness to severe illness. The scales take in to account the presence of risk factors.
8. **Health promotion:** Activities directed toward maintain or enhancing the health and well-being of clients.
9. **Health promoting behavior:** Considered a third subcategory of health behavior and through assessment, reveal needs for vehicular safety, home safety, domestic violence recognition, recreational safety, occupational safety and health.
10. **Holistic health:** A system of compressive or total care that considers the physical, emotional, social, economical and spiritual needs of the person the response to the illness, and the effect of the illness on the person's ability to meet self care needs.
11. **Models:** Models are graphic or symbolic representations of phenomena that objectify and present certain perspectives or points of view about nature or function or both.
12. **Concept:** Concepts are the elements or components of a phenomenon necessary to understand the phenomenon and derived from impressions the human mind receives about phenomena through sensing the human environment.
13. **Philosophy:** A philosophy is statement of belief and values about human being and their world.
14. **Theory:** Theory refers to a set of logically inter-related concepts, statement, proposition and definitions which have been derived from philosophical beliefs of scientific data and from which questions or hypothesis an be deduced, tested and verified.

15. **Health:** A state of physical, mental and social well-being and the absence of disease or other disorders. It involves constant change and adaptation to stress.
16. **Community:** Community as a group of inhabitants living together in a somewhat localized area under the same general regulations and having common interests, functions, needs and organizations.
17. **Nursing:** Nursing is an art, science and profession by which we render, serve to human being to help him to regain or to keep a normal state of body and mind and when it cannot accomplish this, it help him for the relief from physical pain, mental anxiety or spiritual discomfort.
18. **Community health:** Community (public) health is a science and art of preventing disease, prolonging life and promoting health and efficiency through organized effort.
19. **Community health nursing:** Community health nursing is a synthesis of nursing and public health practice applied of promoting and preserving the health of people. The practice is general and compressive. It is not limited to a particular age group or diagnosis, and continuing, not episodic.
20. **Profession:** A profession is an occupation with moral principles that are devoted to the human and social welfare. The service is based on specialized knowledge and skill developed in a scientific and learned manner.
21. **Quality care:** The degree of which health services for individuals and populations increase the likelihood of desired health outcomes and are consistent with current professional knowledge.
22. **Health care team:** Health care team refers to all of the personal in all of the departments of a health care facility, who provides health care services. They are doctors, nurses, technicians and paramedical staffs.
23. **Primary nursing:** In primary nursing, a professional nurse has total responsibility for a particular patient or group of patients. The model's purpose is to provide continuity and coordination of care.
24. **Primary health care:** It is a essential health care based on practical, scientifically sound and socially accepted methods and technology, made universally acceptable to individuals and families in the community involving their full participation and at a cost that the community and country can afford to maintain at every stage of their development.
25. **Health center:** It is defined as an institution for the promotion of health and welfare of the people in a given area, which seeks to achieve health work through coordination with welfare and relive organization.
26. **Comprehensive health care:** Comprehensive health care is the combined (integrated) curative, preventive, promotive and restorative care made available to the people without distinctions of caste, creed or economic status from birth to death (from womb to tomb).
27. **Primary health center:** Primary health center is an institution for providing comprehensives health care, e.g. preventive, promotive and curative services, to the people living in a defined geographical area. It seeks to achieve its purpose by grouping under one roof or coordinate all the health work of that area.
28. **Health for all:** Health for all has been defined as attainment of a level of health that will enable every individual to lead a socially and economically productive life.
29. **Community development block:** Community development is a process which is designed to promote better living of the whole community, with the active participation by the community itself along with governmental efforts.

30. **Community health nurse:** Community health nurse is person plays important role in helping people learn to care themselves and to work with other community residents to develop the capacity or infrastructure needed to ensure essential health care for every one.
31. **Disease:** Any deviation from or interruption of the normal structure or function of any part, organ or system of the body, manifesting with a characteristic set of sign and symptoms.

CONCEPT OF HEALTH

Health is considered by many as the opposite of illness or disease. For some, it means a well developed or adequately nourished body, capable of various activities and able to withstand physical stress. All communities have their concepts of health integrated as a part of their culture. Widely differing culture groups share the concept of health as a state of balance and harmony.

The WHO has defined health as a State of complete physical, mental, social, spiritual well-being, and not merely absence of disease or infirmity. The concept of positive wholeness or completeness is emphasized and health is seen as more than a physical state. An individual's health is never static and is always in a dynamic equilibrium with his environment.

Physical well-being is measurable although it is of varying ranges and validity. As regards mental well-being, measurable standards vary from culture to culture and hence the criteria for mental well-being may differ from one country to another or from place to place within the same country. There is also difference of opinion as to what is precisely meant by social well-being. Social well-being may be regarded as a state of predisposing condition of health.

Traditionally health has been defined in terms of the presence or absence of disease. Nightingale defined health as a state of being well and using every power the individual possess to the fullest extent. It reflects concern for the individual as a total person functioning physically, psychologically and socially. Mental processes determine people's relationship with their physical and social surrounding their attitudes about life and their interaction with others.

MULTIPLE FACTS OF HEALTH—WHO

1. **Health a three-dimensional state:** "Health is a state of complete physical, mental and social well being and not merely the absence of disease or infirmity."
2. **Health a fundamental right:** "The enjoyment of the highest attainable standards of health is one of the fundamental rights of every human being, without distinction of race, religion, and political belief, economic and social condition."
3. **Health for peace and security:** "The health for all peoples is fundamental to the attainment of peace and security and is dependent upon the fullest cooperation of individuals."
4. **Health a government responsibility:** "Government have a responsibility for the health of their peoples, which can be fulfilled only by the provision of adequate health and social measures."
5. **Health and health information:** "The extension to all people of the benefits of medical, psychological, and related knowledge is essential to be fullest attainment of health."
6. **Health and people cooperation:** "Informed opinion and active cooperation on the part of the public, are of the utmost importance in the improvement of health of the people."
7. **Health and health care:** "Unequal development in different countries in the promotion of health and control of disease, especially communicable disease is a common danger."
8. **Health and child development:** "Healthy development of the child is of basic importance. The ability to live harmonically in changing total environment is essential to such development."
9. **Health "gain for all":** The achievement of any state in the promotion and protection of health is of value to all.

CONCEPTIONS OF HEALTH MODELS

Smith (1983) describes the various conceptions of health in four models. These are the clinical, role—performance, adaptive and eudemonistic models. Each of these models can be defined by the characterization of the extremes of health-illness continuum.

1. **Clinical model:**
   Health extreme: Absence of signs or symptoms of disease or disability as identified by Medical science.
   Illness extreme: Conspicuous presence of these signs and symptoms.
2. **Role performance model:**
   Health extreme: Performance of social roles with maximal expected output.
   Illness extreme: Failure in performance role.
3. **Adoptive model:**
   Health extreme: Flexible adaptation of the person to the environment and interaction with it to the maximal advantage.
   Illness extreme: Alienation of the person from the environment and failure of self-corrective responses.
4. **Eudemonistic model:**
   Health extreme: Exuberant well-being.
   Illness extreme: Enervation, languishing debility.

CONCEPT OF DISEASE

Disease can be considered as something more than mere deviation from health, each disease being a distinct entity, with distinguishing qualities in its pathologic process, its typical clinical appearance and often its characteristic epidemiologic pattern of distribution in terms of time, place and person. The concept of disease also may vary from one society to another society. There will be no difficulty in distinguishing an illness which is severe enough to necessitate bed rest and treatment.

But milder condition of disease and in apparent or subclinical conditions which do not make these individual take to bed are likely to be missed or ignored. Just like the border-line health conditions, diseases of mild nature and in apparent or subclinical conditions are supposed to lie in the middle of a spectrum.

At one end of this spectrum is "optimal health" and at the other end "serious disease" and in between those two ends, various grades of health and disease are located. The milder the disease or the more border-line the health, the more difficult it is to differentiate between health and disease.

FACTORS INFLUENCING HEALTH

Health influenced by various factors which interact with each other and determine the health status of many individual, family and community at large at any given point of time. These factors known as determinants of health. According to WHO expert committee on community health nursing – Technical report series 558 (1974) and Blum, theses factors are categorized as human biology, environment, lifestyle, health and health allied resources.

Human Biology

1. **Genetic inheritance:** Hereditary or genetic predisposition to specific illness is a major physical risk factor. For example, a person with a family history of diabetes mellitus is at risk for developing the disease later in life. Other documented genetic risk factors include family his histories of cancer, coronary disease and renal disease.

2. **Age:** Age increases susceptibility to certain illness. For example, the risk of cardiovascular disease increases with age for both sexes. The risk of birth defects and complications of pregnancy increase in women-bearing children after age 35. Age risk factors are often closely associated with other risk factors such as family history and personal habits.
3. **Race:** Race increases susceptibility to certain illness. For example, the risk of sickle cell anemia is more common in Africans and Mediterranean people.
4. **Self concept:** Self concept implies individual's perception of his or physical, intellectual and social abilities.

Environment

1. **The physical environment:** The physical environment includes atmospheric pressures, gravity, light and sound waves, temperature, humidity, wind velocity, solar radiation, electromagnetic fields and seasonal variations, etc. The variety of pollutants are found to pollute air, water, food and soil and are the cause of various acute and chronic diseases, e.g. gastrointestinal, respiratory, skin cancer, cardiovascular diseases, etc.
2. **The biological environment:** Most of the plants and animals are useful to human being to promote health but are the same time, they human being to promote health but are the same time, the produce diseases like malaria, insect bits and allergic reactions.
3. **The social environment:** The social environments include other people and social institutions, sociocultural events, religious beliefs, moral and ethical values and social rules and regulations, pertaining to living society, socioeconomic support system.

Life Style

Many activities, habits and practices involve risk factors, the stresses of life crises and frequent life changes also risk factors. Health practices and behaviors can have positive or negative effects in health. Practices with potential negative effects are risk factor these include overeating or poor nutrition, insufficient rest and sleep and poor personal hygiene.

Other habits that put a person at risk for illness include smoking alcohol or drug abuse, and activities involving a threat of injury such as skydiving or mountain climbing. Some habits are risk factors for specific diseases. For example, excessive sunbathing increases the risk of skin cancer, and being overweight increases the risk of cardiovascular disease.

Prolonged emotional stress may increase the chance of illness. Emotional stress may occur with events such as divorce, pregnancy and arguments. Job-related stresses, for example, many overtax a person's cognitive skills and decision making ability leading to mental overload or burnout.

Health and Health Allied Resources

1. **Health services:** Health services are directly concerned with improvement of health status of people. Health services can also contribute on socioeconomic development of people because sound health can improve and increase the physical, intellectual and emotional capacity of people to get educated, work and earn for their livelihood improve their life style which will further reinforce their health.
2. **Socioeconomic conditions:** Socioeconomic conditions have significant influence on community health. In developed countries like America, UK and Canada, there has been significant reduction in the morbidity and mortality rates and increases in longevity at birth because of socioeconomic, developments. Socioeconomic conditions include economic status, education, occupation and living standards.

3. **Political system:** The political system has a very strong role in health promotion of people in the country. The health care delivery system is determined by the political system though there is constitutional control. Decisions pertaining to health policy, allocation of funds, programs, manpower development, infrastructure, health technology and delivery of health services are made by the ruling party within the parliament system.

4. **Health related services:** The health related services include education governmental policies; social welfare developmental programs food and agriculture, industry, communication and broadcasting rural and urban development and transportation facilities. The health related services needs to have balanced approach between National Health Policy and Voluntary Health Promotes Active Participation.

CULTURAL FACTORS IN HEALTH AND DISEASE

The member of a particular society quite unconsciously agrees upon a common pattern of living. It includes basic rules for living together. These rules could be understood as the culture of the society. The behavior pattern of a particular culture are not biologically inherited but socially acquired through learning.

Concept of etiology and cure: Supernatural causes like wrath of god and goodness, breach of taboo, past sins, evil eye and spirit or ghost intrusion. Physical causes include the effects of weather, water and impure blood.

1. **Environmental sanitation:** Sanitation is the science of safeguarding health. It is the quality of living that is exposed in the clean home, the clean farm, the clean business, the clean neighborhood and the clean community. Environmental sanitation is nothing but the introduction of such methods which bring about control of all the factors in the physical environment.

2. **Food habits:** Food habits have deep psychological roots and are associated with love, affection, warmth, self-image and social prestige. The diet of the people is influenced by local conditions, religious customs and beliefs. Vegetarianism and hindus beliefs—these food habits have a religious sanction from early days.

3. **Mother and child health:** Mother and child health is surrounded by a wide range of customs and beliefs all over the world. MCH care and good customs such as prolonged breastfeeding, oil bath, massage and exposure to sun. MCH care and bad customs are the child is not put to breast during the first 3 days of birth because of the belief that colostrums might be harmful.

4. **Personal hygiene:** Hygiene is the science of health and includes all factors which contribute to healthful living. Personal hygiene includes all those personal factors which influence the health and well being of an individual. The practice of an oil bath is a good Indian custom. Circumcision is a prevalent custom among muslims which has a religious sanction.

5. **Sex and marriage:** Sexual customs vary among different social, religious and ethnic groups. Orthodox Jews are forbidden to have intercourse for seven days after the menstruation ceases, these custom have an important bearing in family planning. Marriage is sacred. It is the usual social custom in India to perform marriages early at about the age of puberty. Child marriages are fortunately disappearing. The high rate of venereal diseases in Himachal Pradesh is attributed to the local marriage customs.

CONCEPT OF NURSING

Nurses provide care for three types of clients: Individuals, families and communities. Nursing practice involves four areas: Promoting health and wellness, preventing illness, restoring health and care of dying.

1. **Promoting health and wellness:** Wellness is a state of well-being. It means engaging in attitudes and behavior that enhance the quality of life and maximize personal potential. Nurses promote wellness in clients who are both healthy and ill. This may involve individual and community activities to enhance healthy lifestyles such as improving nutrition and physical fitness, preventing drug and alcohol misuse, restricting smoking and preventing accidents and injury in home and work place.
2. **Preventing illness:** The goal of illness prevention programs is to maintain optimal health by preventing disease. Nursing activities that prevent illness include immunizations, prenatal and infant care and prevention of sexually transmitted disease.
3. **Restoring health:** Restoring health focuses on the ill client and it extends from early detection of disease through helping the client during the recovery period. Nursing activities such as providing direct care to the ill person, performing diagnostic and assessment procedures, teaching clients about recovery activities and rehabilitating client to their optimal functional level following physical or mental injury.
4. **Care of dying:** This area of nursing practice involves comforting and caring for people of all ages who are dying. It includes helping clients live as comfortably as possible until death and helping support persons cope with death. Nurses carry out these activities work in homes, hospitals and extended care facilities.

DEFINITIONS OF HEALTH AND NURSING

Health

Health is recognized as a "fundamental right of every human being. The widely accepted definition of health is that given by the World Health Organization (WHO) which states:

"Health is a state of complete physical, mental, social, spiritual well-being, and not merely an absence of disease or infirmity" —*WHO.*

"Health is a quality of life resulting from total functioning of the individual that empower him to achieve personally satisfying and socially useful life"—*Webster.*

"Health is quality of life that enables individuals to live, and serve best"—*William.*

"Health is defined as dynamic state of wellness which exists on a continuum and ranges from a high level of wellness to high level of illness"—*Dunn.*

Nursing

Nursing is a service which includes ministration to the sick, care of the whole patient (his mind as well as body), the care of the patient's environment (physical as well as social), health education and health services to the individual family and society for the prevention of disease and promotion of health.

Nursing is the unique function of the nurse that is to assist the individual (sick or well) in the performance of those activities contributing to health or its recovery (or to a peaceful death) that he would perform unaided if he had the necessary strength, will or knowledge (Virginia Henderson).

Nursing practice is a direct service, goal directed and adaptable to the needs of the individual, the family and community during their health and illness"—*American Nurses Association.*

INTRODUCTION TO HEALTH AND ILLNESS

1. Health in its broadest sense is a dynamic state in which the individual adapts to changes in internal and external environments to maintain a state of wellbeing. The internal environment includes many factors that influence health, including genetic and psychological variables, intellectual and spiritual dimensions and disease processes.
2. The external environment includes factors outside the person that may influence health, including factors outside the person that may influence health, including the physical environment, social relationships, and economic variables because both environments continuously change, the person must maintain a state of well being.
3. Health and illness therefore must be defined in terms of individual. Health can include conditions that the client or nurse may have previously considered to be illness. Health is also closely related to an individual's work place and home life and stressors can be the result of those environments.

CONCEPTS OF HEALTH, ILLNESS AND SICK BEHAVIORS

1. It is useful for the nurse to be aware of the behavioral components of health, illness and sick role behavior.
2. Every person develops a system of health beliefs and attitudes, and these tend to fall within the framework provided by society or cultural heritage.
3. Health behavior activities a person engages in, when feeling well, to take measures to prevent disease and illness or to detect them before symptom occur.
4. Illness behavior activities a person engages in, when feeling ill, that will lead to the defining of the state of health and that will gain help.
5. Sick-role behavior, activities a person engages in believing himself ill. For any individual the level of health behavior is determined by the significance of symptoms—danger value, visibility, ambiguity, fear of unknown, the expectations of those from whom help is sought, feeling about dependence and fear of loss of control, the expectations of the illness position, including past experiences with illness.

ILLNESS -ILLNESS BEHAVIOR

1. Illness is not merely the presence of disease process. Illness is a state in which a person's physical, emotional, intellectual, social, developmental or spiritual functioning is diminished or impaired compared with that person's previous experiences.
2. Illness behavior involves the ways persons monitor their bodies, definite and interpret their symptoms, take remedial actions, and use their health care system.
3. The important internal values influencing the way clients behave when they are ill are their perceptions of symptoms and the nature of the illness. A client's illness behavior can also be affected by the nature of the illness.
4. Acute illness involves symptoms of relatively short duration that are usually severe and may affect functioning in any dimension.

5. Chronic illnesses persist, usually longer than 6 months, and can affect functioning in any dimension.
6. External variables influencing a client's illness behavior include the visibility of symptoms, social groups, cultural background, economic variables, accessibility of the health care system and social support.

STAGES OF ILLNESS BEHAVIOR

Symptom Experience

1. During the initial stage, a person is aware that some thing is wrong. A person usually recognizes a physical sensation or a limitation in functioning but does not suspect a specific diagnosis.
2. The person's perception of symptoms includes awareness of a physical change such as pain, a rash, or a lump.

Assumption of the Sick Role

1. The assumption of the sick role results in emotional changes, such as withdrawal or depression, and physical changes.
2. Emotional changes may be simple or complex, depending on the severity of the illness, the degree of disability and anticipated length of the illness.

Medical Care Contact

1. If symptoms persist despite home remedies, become severe or require emergency care, the person is motivated to seek professional health services.
2. In this stage the client seeks/expect acknowledgement of the illness, as well as treatment. In addition, the client seeks an explanation of the symptoms, the cause of the symptoms, the course of the illness for future health.
3. Client's illness can be validated at any point on the health illness continuum. A health professional may determine that they do not have an illness or that illnesses are present and may be life threatening.

Dependent Client Role

1. After accepting the illness and seeking treatment, the client enters the fourth stage of illness behavior.
2. In this stage, the client depends on health care professionals for relief of symptoms. The client accepts care, sympathy and protection from the demands and stresses of life.
3. It is socially permissible for clients in the dependent role to be relieved of normal obligations and tasks.

Recovery Stage

1. The final stage of illness behavior—recovery and rehabilitation—can arrive suddenly, such as when a fever subsides.
2. The recovery is not prompt; long-term care may be required before the client is able to resume an optimal level of functioning.
3. In the case of chronic illness, the final stage may involve an adjustment to a prolonged reduction in health and functioning.

IMPACT OF ILLNESS ON FAMILY

Behavioral and Emotional Changes

1. People react differently to illness. Individual behavioral and emotional reactions depend on the nature of the illness, the client's attitude toward it, the reaction of others to it, and the variables of illness behavior.
2. Severe illness, particularly one that is life threatening, can lead to more extensive emotional and behavioral change, such as anxiety, shock, dental, anger and withdrawal.

Impact of Family Roles

1. When an illness occurs, the roles of client and family may change. Such a change may be subtle and short term or drastic and long term.
2. An individual and family generally adjust more easily to subtle, short-term changes. In most cases they know that the role change is only temporary.
3. Long term changes, however, require an adjustment process similar to the grief process. The client and family often require specific counseling and guidance to assist them in coping with role changes.

Impact on Body Changes

1. Some illnesses result in changes in physical appearance, and clients and families react differently to these changes.
2. When changes in body image occur, such as results from a leg amputation, the client generally adjusts in the following phases: shock, withdrawal, acknowledgment, acceptance and rehabilitation.
3. Withdrawal is an adaptive coping mechanism that can assist the client in making the adjustments.

Impact of Self-concepts

1. Self-concept is individual's mental image of themselves, including how they view their strengths and weaknesses in all aspects of their personalities.
2. Self-concepts depend in part of body image and roles but also include other aspects of the psychological and spiritual self.
3. Self-concept changes because of illness may no longer meet the expectations of the family, leading to tension or conflict.

Impact of Family Dynamics

1. Family dynamics is the process by which the family functions, makes decisions, give support to individual members, and copes with everyday changes and challenges.
2. If a parent in a family becomes ill, family activities and decision making often come to a habit as the other family members wait for the illness to pass, or they delay action because they are reluctant to assume the ill person's roles or responsibilities.

HEALTH-ILLNESS CONTINUUM (FIG. 1.1)

1. According to Neuman (1990), health on a continuum is the degree of client wellness that exist at any point in time ranging from an optimal wellness condition, with available energy at its maximum, to death, which represents total energy depletion.

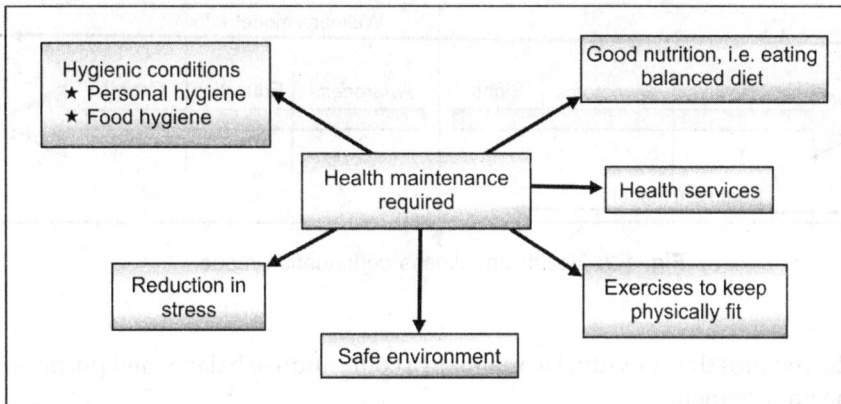

Fig. 1.1: Health maintainee-strategies

2. According to health-illness continuum model, health is a dynamic state that continuously alters as a person adapts to changes in the internal and external environments to maintain a state of physical, emotional, intellectual, social, developmental and spiritual well-being.
3. The continuum is thought of a complex, dynamic process that includes physical, psychological and social components. There are adoptive or maladaptive behavioral responses to internal and external stimuli.
4. Health and illness tend to merge but may represent patterns of adoptive change along the continuum. The direction of change may be reversible, depending on the quality of the individual's adoptive efforts.
5. The individual at the illness end of the continuum is characterized by feeling of uncertainty, helplessness, loss of control, loss of identity and incapacity for problem solving.
6. As the patient is in the sick role, there is incapacity to meet other social roles, the person has sought diagnosis and get treatment.
7. Less far along the illness end of the continuum, as illness behavior are brought in to play, the person may be tired, rundown and irritable with complaints of loss of sleep, appetite, dependence, self-absorption, minor illnesses such as colds, infections, headaches and backaches.
8. Between illness and wellness there is the ambiguous area where no symptoms are present and the person is neither especially well nor especially ill.
9. At the health end of the continuum, as health behaviors are utilized, the person is not only unaware of disease and with out pain, fatigue or somatic complications but also tends to be resistant to infections, industrious, vigorous and physically agile, with a strong sense of identity and autonomy, carring out usual social roles and needing no health care.
10. The goal in preventive health care is to maintain equilibrium between health and illness, with balance in favor of maximum wellness for the individual.

MODELS OF HEALTH AND ILLNESS (FIG. 1.2)

Health-wellness Model

1. It was developed by Dunn (1997), the high level wellness model is oriented toward maximizing the health potential of an individual.

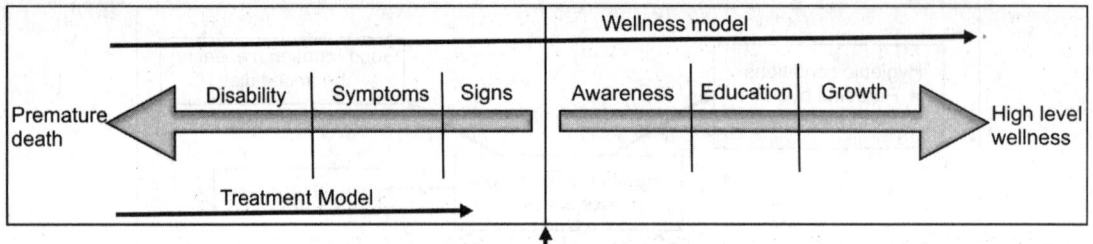

Fig. 1.2: Health and illness continuation model

2. This model requires the individual to maintain a continuum of balance and purposeful direction within the environment.
3. It involves progress toward a higher level of functioning open-ended and expanding challenges to live at the fullest potential.

Agent-host-environmental Model

1. The agent-host-environmental model of health and illness originated in the community health work of Level et al.
2. According to this approach the health or illness of an individual or group depends on the dynamic relationship of the agent, host and environment.
3. The agent is any internal or external factors that its presence or absence can lead to disease or illness.
4. The host is the person or persons who may be susceptible to a particular illness or diseases.
5. The environment consists of all factors outside of the host. It includes physical environment, social environment and biological environment.

Health Belief Model

1. Rosenstoch's (1794) and Bakerand Maiman's (1975) health belief model addresses the relationship between a person's belief and behavior.
2. It provides a way of understanding and predicating how clients will behave in relations to their health and how they will comply with health care therapies.
3. The first component in this model involves the individual's perception of susceptibility to an illness.
4. The second component is the individual's perception of the seriousness of the illness. This perception is influenced and modified by demographic and sociopsychological variables, perceived threats of the illnesses, and focus to action.
5. The third component—the likelihood that a person will take preventive action—is the person's perception of the benefits of taking action.

Health Promotion Model

1. The health promotion model proposed by Pender (1996). It was designed to be a complementary counterpart to models of health protection.
2. Health promotion is directed at increasing a client's level of well-being. The model focuses on three functions.

3. The model also organizes cues into a pattern to explain the likelihood of a client's participation in health-promotion behavior.
4. The focus of this model is to explain the reasons that individuals engage in health activities. It is not designed for use with families or communities.

BIOPSYCHOSOCIAL ASPECT OF HEALTH AND ILLNESS

Introduction

Physical, social, cultural and psychological factors interact dynamically and have an important influence on patient care needs. There are needs common to everyone, no matter their sociocultural background, so-called human needs. These needs when they are not met create tensions and these tensions may give rise to anxiety that can hamper recovery if not relieved (Figs 1.3A and B).

Developmental Needs

1. **Prenatal:** This stage determines many characteristics of the person and to some extend the requirements for use of adaptive resources throughout life.
2. **Neonatal:** Developmental tasks are mostly physical, foundations are begun at this time for later personality responses.
3. **Infancy:** This is a time of much physical, but foundations are begun at this time for later personality responses.
4. **Childhood:** Marked physical growth continues during this time. There is the beginning of role identification and moving out from the family to the peer group and community.
5. **Adolescence:** Many physical and emotional changes occur as growth and maturation continues, changing hormonal activity and search for identity are major stresses for the adolescent.
6. **Young adulthood:** Physical maturation is completed. There are many psychosocial stresses related to family and community roles during this stage.
7. **Middle adulthood:** Developmental tasks are mostly psychosocial, relating to reassessment of goals, physical stamina and hormone output beginning to decline.
8. **Older years:** Physical conditioning is generally declining, and decreased sensory acuity may be noticeable. Developmental tasks are related to sharing accumulated experiences and evaluating achievements.

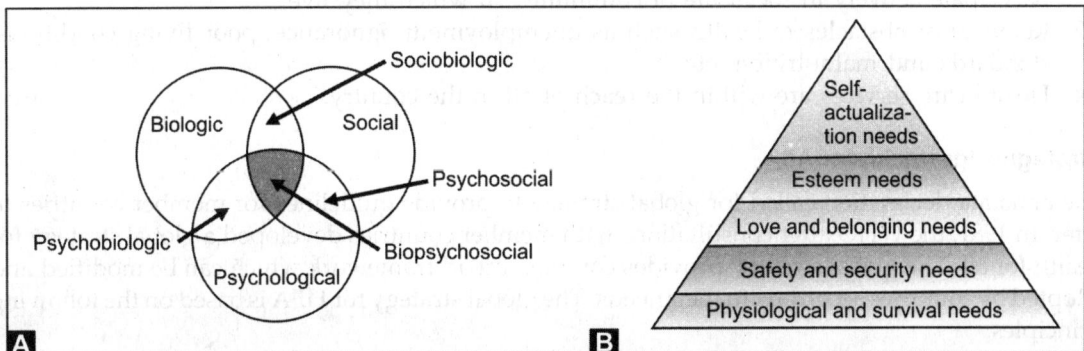

Figs 1.3A and B: (A) Biopsychosocial model, (B) Maslow's hierarchy of needs

Cultural Influences

1. Culture may be thought of as the total way of life of a people, the social legacy the individuals acquire from his or her groups.
2. The culture concept is cardial to an understanding of ourselves and our world.
3. Custom and group habits are referred to as folkways and mores. Folkways are the accustomed and time-honored ways of doing things, the social habits that become routine and that are often performed without thinking.
4. The patient's cultural background helps to determine the way the relationship with the physician or nurse is perceived and facilitates or impedes interaction or communication.

Religious Aspects

1. Religion traditionally has focused on a god beyond the individual and has concentrated it self with relating the individual and has concerned itself with relating the individual to that god.
2. Religious beliefs are seldom held to oneself but are part of group processes, so that there is immediate family or group support for the patient.
3. It helps the patent's own attitude or belief that recovery is possible and that there are forces available to facilitate the healing process.
4. It is important if the nurse is to be of help, to understand not only the spiritual needs of the patient but also the means and methods that organized religion has for meeting those needs.

HEALTH FOR ALL

1. The world health assembly in its 30th meeting in 1977 decided the goal of health for all (HFA) and defined that "Main Social Targets of Governments and WHO" in the coming decades should be the attainment of all citizens of the world by the year 2000 of a level of health that will permit them to lead socially and economically productive life.
2. Attainment of a level of health that will enable every individual to lead a socially and economically productive life.

Health for All Goals

1. Realization of highest possible of health which includes physical, mental and social well-being.
2. Attainment of minimum level of health that would enable to the economically productive and participate actively in social life of community in which they live.
3. Removal of obstacles to health such as unemployment, ignorance, poor living conditions, standards and malnutrition, etc.
4. Health care services are within the reach of all in the country.

Strategies for Health for All

The alma ata declaration called for global strategy to provide guidelines for member countries to refer. In 1981, the WHO after consultations with member countries developed a global strategy for health for all. The global strategy provides common broad framework which can be modified and adopted by countries according to their needs. The global strategy for HFA is based on the following principles.

1. Health is a fundamental human right and a world wide social goal and an integral part of social and economic development of the communities.

2. People have right and the duty of participate individually and collectively in the planning and implementation of their health care.
3. The existing gross inequality in the health strategies is of common concern of all countries and must be drastically reduced.
4. Government has responsibility for the health of their people.
5. Countries and people must become self reliant in health matters.
6. Governments and health professionals have the responsibility of providing health information to people.
7. There should be equitable distribution of resources within and among the countries but should be allocated most to those who need most.
8. Primary health care would be the key to the success of HPA and it has to be the integral part of the country's health system.
9. Development and application of appropriate technology according to health care system of the nation.
10. Research in the field of biomedical and health services must be conducted and findings should be applied soon.

The National Health Policy echoes the WHO a call for HFA and the alma ata declaration. It had laid down specific goals in respect of various health indicators by different dates such as 1990 and 2000 AD.

1. Reduction of infant mortality from the level of 125 (1978) to below 60.
2. To raise the expectation of life at birth from the level of 523 years to 64.
3. To reduce the crude death rate from the level of 14 per 1000 population to 21.
4. To reduce the crude birth rate from the level of 33 per 1000 population to 21.
5. To achieve a net reproduction rate of one rural population.

PRIMARY HEALTH CARE

Definition

Primary health care is essential health care made universally accessible to individuals and families in the community, by means acceptable to them, through their full participation and at a cost that the community and country can afford. It forms an integral part both of the country's health system of which it is the nucleus and the overall social and economic development of the community (alma ata, 1978).

Highlights of this Definition

This definition highlights several attributes of primary health care. It stresses on:
1. Its **essentiality** by observing that primary health is essential health care.
2. Its **accessibility** by observing "made universally accessible to individuals and families in the community.
3. Its **acceptability** by observing by means acceptable to them.
4. Its **patricianly** by observing "acts a cost that the community and country can afford".
5. Its **affordability** by observing "it forms an integral part both of the country's health system of which it is the nucleus and the overall social and economic development of the community".
6. Its **integrality** by observing "it forms an integral part both of the country's health system of which it is the nucleus and the overall social and economic development of the community.

Attributes of Primary Health Care

1. **Accessibility:** Primary health care permeates uniformly to reach equitably to all segments of population.
2. **Acceptability:** Primary health care achieves acceptability through cultural assimilation of its policies and programs.
3. **Adaptability:** Primary health care system is highly flexible and adaptable. It believes in "adaptation" rather than "adaptation".
4. **Affordability:** Primary health care is affordable to consumer as well as providers.
5. **Availability:** Primary health care is always ready to respond to any demand at any time.
6. **Appropriateness:** Primary health care system evolves from the socioeconomic conditions, social values and health situation of a community, it is quite appropriate from all angles.
7. **Closeness:** Primary health center is close at hand to people at their door steps.
8. **Continuity:** Primary health service is a continuous service which extends from "womb to tomb" and addresses the changing needs of an individual in all situations of health and disease.
9. **Comprehensiveness:** Primary health care is comprehensive and the curative needs of the community.
10. **Coordinativeness:** Primary health care is dependent on innersectoral coordination and community participation.

Elements of Primary Health Care

As per Alma Ata declaration primary health care includes:
1. Educration concerning prevailing health problems and methods of identifying, preventing and controlling them.
2. Promotion of food supply and proper nutrition.
3. An adequate supply of water and basic sanitation.
4. Maternal and child health care including family planning.
5. Immunization against the major infectious disease.
6. Prevention and control of locally endemic diseases.
7. Appropriate treatment of common diseases and injuries.
8. Promotion of mental health.
9. Provision of essential drugs.

Principles of Primary Health Care

1. **Equitable distribution:** Primary health care services must be shared equally by all people irrespective of their ability to pay (rich, poor, urban or rural).
2. **Community participation:** Primary health care must be a continuing effort to secure meaningful involvement of the community in the planning, implementation and maintenance of health services.
3. **Coverage and accessibility:** Primary health care implies providing health care services to all which are required by them. The care has to be appropriate and adequate in content and in amount to satisfy the essential health needs of the people and has to be provided by methods acceptable to them.
4. **Inter sectoral coordination:** Primary health care requires joint efforts of other health related sectors such as agriculture, animal husbandry, food, industry, housing, social welfare, public works, communication and other sectors.

5. **Appropriate health technology:** The technology that is scientific, adaptable to local need and socially acceptable instead of costly methods, equipment and technology.
6. **Human resource:** Health resource is very essential to make full use of all the available resources including the human potential of the entire community.
7. **Referral system:** Referral system would be desirable to develop referring from one level to another with laid down procedures and policies.
8. **Logistics of supply:** The logistic of supply include planning and budgeting for the supplies required procurement or manufacture, storage distribution and control.
9. **The physical facilities:** The physical facilities for primary health care need to be simple and clean. It should have a specious waiting area with toilet facility.
10. **Control and evaluation:** A process of evaluation has to be built into assess the relevance, progress, efficiency, effectiveness and impact of the services.

Role of Nurse in Primary Health Care

An extent committee on community health nursing was concerned by WHO Executive Board in July 1974 to recommend way in which nursing could have critical impact on the urgent health problems throughout the world. The committee made specific recommendations.

1. The development of community health nursing services, responsive to community health needs that would assure primary health care coverage for all.
2. The reformulation of basic and postbasic nursing education as to prepare all nurses for community health nursing.
3. The inclusion of nursing in national development plans in a way that would ensure the rational distribution and the appropriate utilization and support of nursing personnel.

Role of Nurse in Primary Health Care

1. Community health nurse work with population, community, family, individual. The focus is multiple or promoting health maintaining a degree of balance toward health.
2. Community health nurse focus on assessment of the impact of the socioeconomical and cultural factors affecting health measures the must constantly be dealt with and take priority in order to make family assume health measures.
3. The community health nurse works with entire spectrum of health and illness conditions from optimal health to minor or severe conditions from acute to chronic illness.
4. The community health nurse works in all kinds of setting such as home, school, clinic, industry, etc.
5. The community health nurse works in school where primary goal is health education and disease prevention.
6. The community health nurse works in industry is to improve the production and employees safety.
7. The community health nurse is responsible for assisting patients and families to coordinate health care, which necessitates contact with personnel from health, welfare and other significant community agencies.
8. Community health nurse has responsibilities in education an training of individuals, auxiliaries and others.
9. The community health nurse involves in provision of direct services to patients both preventive and curative at the out-patient, in-patient clinics and community.

Major Role of Child Health Nursing in Primary Health Care

1. Facilitative role
2. Developmental role
3. Supportive role
   a. Training
   b. Management
   c. Supervision
   d. Program implementation
   e. Program evaluation
   f. Policy making
   g. Program planning
4. Clinical role.

LEVELS OF DISEASE PREVENTION

The disease process, in many instances is susceptible to interruption in order to limit its further progress or the speed of its progression. As disease involves interaction of host, agent and environment prevention can be achieved by altering one or more of these three elements so that interaction does not take place or is interrupted in favor of the host. Effective preventive measure requires that the disease process be interrupted as early in its course as possible.

The interaction between the agent and the host can be avoided either by the elimination of the agent in the environment or by converting the human host susceptible or immune to the attack of the agent. Those attempts to bring about changes in the three elements before the disease stimulus is produced are grouped under one type of prevention namely primary prevention. When the disease stimulus has already been practiced and the disease process has crossed over to the period of pathogenesis, two types of prevention—secondary and tertiary prevention.

Primary Prevention

Primary prevention can be defined as "action taken prior to the onset of disease which removes the possibility that a disease will ever occur". It signifies intervention in the prepathogenesis phase of a disease or health problem or other departure from health.

Primary prevention is applied at the prepathogenic period; it includes health promotion and specific protection

1. **Health promotion:** The first level of prevention is by promoting and maintaining the health of the host by nutrition, health education, good heredity and other health promotion activities.
2. **Specific protection:** It may be directed towards the agent like disinfection of contaminated particles, materials, water, food, and other particles on the assumption that the agent has escaped into these vehicles or environment. Specific protection can also be achieved by immunizations to increase the resistance of the host so that the host will be able to withstand the onslaught of the agent. This is done by the active and passive immunizations.

Secondary Prevention

Secondary prevention can be defined as "action" which halts the progress of a disease at its incipient stage and prevents complications. The specific interventions are early diagnosis, e.g. screening tests, case finding programs) and adequate treatment. The secondary prevention done by early diagnosis and treatment.

Early diagnosis and prompt treatment comes under secondary prevention. If primary prevention fails or when suitable measures are not available (as in cancer) the disease stimulus is bound to be produced. Early detection of the disease is possible by periodic examinations of population groups who are at special risks like antenatal mothers, growing children, industrial worker, etc.

Monitoring of persons middle age and above is one of the modern methods of early detection of cancer. In many instances, this detection of the diseases condition is possible only after the onset of the signs and symptoms. Early detection of the disease ensures prompt treatment so that the disease will not progress further.

Tertiary Prevention

When the disease process has advance beyond its early stages, it is still possible to accomplish prevention by what might be called "Tertiary prevention". It signifies intervention in the late pathogenesis phase. Tertiary prevention can be defined as "all measures available to reduce or limit impairment and disabilities, minimize suffering caused by existing departures and disabilities, minimize suffering caused by existing departures from good health and to promote the patient's adjustments to irremediable conditions". Tertiary prevention includes disability limitation and rehabilitation.

a. **Disability limitation:** It is necessary that the disability that is caused by limited by active medical or surgical treatment so that there is no further deterioration of the disease process.

b. **Rehabilitation:** Those with permanent disability as in the case of leprosy, tuberculosis, polio, mental retardation, etc. will not be able to lead an independent life unless they are rehabilitated. This level will be needed only when have failed in the application of previous levels of prevention.

BIBLIOGRAPHY

1. Balzer Riley J. Communications in nursing, 4th edn, St. Louis 2000, Mosby.
2. Basvanthappa BT. Nursing Administration (1st edn), Jaypee Brothers Medical Publishers: New Delhi, 2000.
3. Buckman R. How to break bad news: A guide for health care professionals. Baltimore, MD: Johns Hopkins University Press, 1992.
4. Craven F Ruth, Hirnle J Constance. Fundamentals of Nursing (4th edition), Lippincott Williams and Wilkins Publications, 2003.
5. Crouch R. Communication is the key, Emerg Nurse 10(3):1,2002.
6. Gabor D. First contact body language. In: how to start a conversation and make friends. Revised edn. Rockefeller center, Fireside Publications, New York 2001:21.
7. Hybels S, Weaver R. Communicating effectively, 5th edn, Boston, 1998, McGraw-Hill.
8. Jayee M. Black and Esther Matassasion- Jacobs, Luckmann and Sorcesens. Medical surgical nursing, 4th edn, WB Saunders Company.
9. Kelly Anita, McKillop, Kevin J. "Consequences of Revealing Personal Secrets." Psychological Bulletin, 1996, v120 (3), 450.
10. Kurtz SM, Silverman J, Draper J. The Calgary-Cambridge referenced observation guides: An aid to defining the curriculum and organizing the teaching in communication training programs. Med Educ, 1996,30:83-89.
11. Leninger M. Cultural care theory, research and practice. Nursing Science Quarterly, 9:2, and summer 73;991.
12. Luft Joseph. "Of Human Interaction," Palo Alto, CA: National Press, 177 pages.;1969.
13. Mandel E, Shulman M, Begany T. Overcoming communication disorders in the elderly, Patient care 31(2): 55,1997.
14. Park. K Preventive and Social Medicine (18th edition), Banarsidas Publishers, 2002.
15. Potter A Patricia, Perry Anne Griffin, Fundamentals of Nursing, Volume-I, 5th edition, Mosby, 2001.
16. Sr. Nancy. Stephanie's principles and practice of nursing, volume one, NR Brothers, 1996.
17. White Lois. Basic Nursing: Foundation of skills and concepts, 1st edition, Delmar, UK, 2002.
18. Wood J. Interpersonal communication, 2nd edn, Cincinnati, 1999, Wadsworth.

2 *Therapeutic Nurse-Patient Relationship*

DEFINITIONS

1. **Communication:** Communication is a two ways or reciprocal process involving exchange of ideas, facts and opinions. The process is not complete unless the receiver has understood the message and his response is known to the sender. Communication involves both informational and understanding. It provides for a feedback mechanism. It is a meeting of minds.

2. **Attention:** The receiver of communication must be attentive and should have open mind. Adherence to the principle of attention will gradually overcome many barriers to communication.

3. **Therapeutic communication:** Therapeutic relationships are goal oriented and goal directed at learning and growth promotion in an effort to bring about some type of change in clients life.

4. **Nurse-client relationship:** Helping relationship is the foundation of clinical nursing practice, the essential element of care with every client in every situation. In such relationship, the nurse assumes the role of professional helper and comes to known the client as an individual who has unique health needs, human responses, and patterns of living. The relationship is therapeutic, promoting a psychological climate that facilitates positive change of growth.

   A therapeutic nurse-client relationship is established and maintained by the nurse through the use of professional nursing knowledge, skills and caring attitudes and behaviors in order to provide nursing services that contribute to the client's health and well-being.

5. **Rapport:** Getting acquainted and establishing rapport is the primary task in relationship development. Rapport implies special feeling on the part of both the client and the nurse based on acceptance, warmth, friendliness, common interest, sense of trust and non-judgmental attitude.

6. **Social relationship:** It is a most common kind of relationship; both individuals are equally involved in this relationship and are concerned with meeting their own needs through the relationship.

7. **Liaison:** Any agency official who work with individual agencies or agency official to coordinate interagency communications.

8. **Feedback:** Communication should be a two-way process. The communicator should try to know the reactions of the receiver. The use of feedback mechanism invokes effective participation of subordinates and it help to make future communications more effective. There should be continuous evaluation of the flow of communication in different directions.

9. **Perception:** When people with different perceptions communicate, they have trouble in getting the meaning across. Every one perceives the message from his own angle or viewpoint.

Perceptions of people differ due to differences in their needs, education, social background, interest, etc. In the absence of an open mind and willingness to see things through the eyes of others; people perceive the same information differently. When the communicator does not enjoy trust and credibility, he fails to convey his ideas to others. Differences in value judgments and references frames also inhibit communication.

10. **Listening skills:** Listening skills means ability to listen others. It is an aural skill, and it requires alertness, attentiveness, inquisitiveness, etc. as essential qualities. One must listen well, what is being said to him and recognize what tone connotes, what is the meaning of accompanying gestures, movements of the body, etc. listening is not simply hearing. A good listener has to be a good observer.

INTRODUCTION

In any nurse-client relationship it is the responsibility of the nurse to establish and maintain appropriate boundaries. Maintaining professional boundaries is an essential component in the provision of safe, competent and ethical nursing care. Nurses must exercise professional judgment when establishing a therapeutic relationship with the client taking into consideration the clients cultural, spiritual, mental and biophysical needs.

The nurse-client relationship is the foundation upon which nursing is established. It is the relationship in which both the participation must recognize each other as unique and important human being.

DEFINITIONS OF NURSE-PATIENT RELATIONSHIP

1. Nurse-client relationship is a helping relationship that is therapeutic in nature, is established to meet the needs of clients and is based up on trust and respect.
2. A therapeutic nurse-client relationship is established and maintained by the nurse through the use of professional nursing knowledge, skills and caring attitudes and behaviors in order to provide nursing services that contribute to the client's health and well-being.
3. The therapeutic nurse-patient relationship is the process by which nurses provide care for clients in need psychological intervention.
4. Interpersonal communication techniques—both verbal and nonverbal are the tools of psychological intervention.
5. Therapeutic relationships are goal oriented and goal directed at learning and growth promotion in an effort to bring about some type of change in clients life.

GOALS OF A THERAPEUTIC RELATIONSHIP

1. Facilitate communication of distressing thoughts and feelings.
2. To assist client with problem solving to help daily living.
3. Help client examine self-defeating behaviors and test alternatives.
4. Promote self care and independence.

NURSES ROLE AND THERAPEUTIC COMMUNICATION

Nurse helps the client to cope-up with strategies dealing with specific situation such as:
1. Helping the client to identify what is troubling the client.
2. Encourage to discuss about the changes needed to make in the client.

3. Explore the feeling about the aspects that cannot be charged, alternative modes of coping.
4. Discuss alternative strategies for creating changes the client desires to make.
5. Discuss the benefits and consequences of each alternative.
6. Assist the client to select an alternative.
7. Encourage the client to implement the change.
8. Provide positive feedback for the client's attempts to create change.
9. Assist the client to evaluate outcomes of the change and make modifications as required.

Conditions essential to development of therapeutic relationships:
Several theorists have identified characteristics that enhance the achievement of therapeutic relationship Roger-1967, Travelbee-1971, Peplau-1969, and Carkhuff-1968.

The above mentioned people stressed the importance of using the therapeutic use of self as a therapeutic tool in the interpersonal relationship development.

Travelbee-1971, described the instrument for delivery of the process of interpersonal.

Nursing as therapeutic use of self, Travelbee defined it as the ability to use ones personality consciously and in full awareness in an attempt to establish relatedness and to structure nursing interventions.

Use of self therapeutic manner requires that nurse have a great deal of self awareness and self understanding, nurses must understand that the ability and extent to which one can effectively help others in time of the need is strongly influenced by this internal value system.

CONDITIONS USED IN THERAPEUTIC RELATIONSHIP

Rapport

Getting acquainted and establishing rapport is the primary task in relationship development. Rapport implies special feeling on the part of both the client and the nurse based on acceptance, warmth, friendliness, common interest, sense of trust and non-judgmental attitude.

Trust

Trust is the basis of a therapeutic relationship, trust cannot be presumed, it must be earned, and trustworthiness is demonstrated through the nursing interventions that convey a sense of warmth and caring of client. Without establishing trust, helping relationship will not progress beyond; it will be a kind of mechanical relationship only to meet the superficial needs of a client.

For example, to establish trust, nurse can do:
1. Provide blanket when the client feels cold.
2. Keeping promises.
3. Provide food when the client is hungry.
4. Being honest.
5. Ensuring confidentiality.

Respect

To show respect is to believe in the dignity and worth of an individual, nurse should be able to attempt, the client and respect him and should consider him/ her worthwhile and treat as human being. The nurse can convey respect by:

1. Calling by name.
2. Spending time with client.
3. Allowing sufficient time for the client to answer the questions.
4. Promoting an atmosphere of privacy during therapeutic interventions without client.

Genuineness

The concept of genuineness refers to the nurses ability to be open, honest and real in interactions with the client. The nurse who possesses the quality of genuineness responds to the client with truth and honesty, client feel more comfortable revealing personal information to the nurse.

Empathy

Empathy is a process where in an individual is able to see beyond outward behavior and sense accuracy another inner experience at a given time. With empathy, the nurse can accurately perceive and understand the meaning and relevance of the client's thoughts and feelings. A relationship is defined as a state of being related or state of affinity between two individuals.

Power

The power of the nurse comes from the authority of own position in the health care system, specialized knowledge, influence with other health care providers and the client's significant others, and access to privileged information.

Intimacy

Intimacy related to the kind of activities nurses perform for and with the client which create personal and private closeness on many levels. This can involve physical emotional and spiritual elements.

TYPES OF RELATIONSHIP

Social Relationship

It is a most common kind of relationship; both individuals are equally involved in this relationship and are concerned with meeting their own needs through the relationship.

Intimate Relationship

It is a relationship between two individuals committed to one another, caring for and responding each other.

Therapeutic Relationship

The nurse and client work together toward the goal of assisting the client to regain the inner resources to meet the life challenges and facilitate the growth.

THERAPEUTIC COMMUNICATION TECHNIQUES

Sl. No.	Technique	Description
1.	Using silence	Accepting pauses or silences that may extend for several seconds or minutes without interjecting any verbal response.
2.	Proving general leads	Using statements or questions that (a) encourage the client to verbalize, (b) choose a topic of conversation, and (c) facilitate continued verbalization.
3.	Being specific and tentative	Making statements that are specific rather than general, and tentative rather than absolute.
4.	Using open-ended questions	Asking broad questions that lead or invite the client to explore (elaborative, clarify, describe, compare, or illustrate) thoughts or feeling. Open-ended questions specify only the topic to be discussed and invite answers that are longer than one or two words.
5.	Using touch	Proving appropriate forms of touch to reinforce caring feelings. Because tactile contacts vary considerably among individuals, families and cultures, the nurse must be sensitive to the differences in attitudes and practices of clients and self.
6.	Restarting or paraphrasing	Actively listening for the client's basic message and then repeating those thoughts and/or feelings in similar words. This conveys that the nurse has listened and understands the client's basic message and also offers clients a clear idea of what they have said.
7.	Seeking clarification	A method of making the client's broad overall meaning of the message more understandable. It is used when paraphrasing is difficult or when the communication is rambling or garbled. To clarify the message, the nurse can restate the basic message or conflicts confusion and ask the client to repeat or restate the message.
8.	Perception checking or seeking consensual validation	A method similar to clarifying verifies the meaning of specific words rather than overall meaning of a message.
9.	Offering self	Suggesting one's presence, interest, or wish to understand the client without making any demands or attaching conditions that the client must comply with to receive the nurse's attention.
10.	Giving information	Providing in a simple and direct manner, specific factual information the client may or may not request. When information is not known, the nurse states this and indicates who has it or when the nurse will obtain it.
11.	Acknowledging	Giving recognition, in a nonjudgmental way, of a change in behavior, an effort the client has made, or a contribution to a communication. Acknowledgment may be with or without understanding, verbal or nonverbal.
12.	Clarifying time or sequence	Helping the client clarify an event, situation, or happening in relationship to time.
13.	Presenting reality	Helping the client to differentiate the real from the unreal.

Contd...

Contd...

Sl. No	Technique	Description
14.	Focusing	Helping the client expand on and develop a topic of importance. It is important for the nurse to wait until the client finishes stating the main concerns before attempting to focus. The focus may be an idea or a feeling; however, the nurse often emphasizes a feeling to help the client recognize an emotion disguised behind words.
15.	Reflecting	Directing ideas, feelings, questions, or content back to clients to enable them to explore their own ideas and feelings about a situation.
16.	Summarizing and planning	Stating the main points of a discussion to clarify the relevant points discussed. This technique is useful at the end of an interview or to review a health teaching session. It often acts as an introduction to future care planning.
17.	Stereotyping	Offering generalized and oversimplified beliefs about groups of people that are based on experiences too limited to be valid. These responses categorize clients and negate their uniqueness as individuals.
18.	Agreeing and disagreeing	Akin to judgment response, agreeing and disagreeing imply that the client is either right or wrong and that the nurse is in a position to judge this. These responses deter clients from thinking through their position and may cause a client to become defensive.
19.	Being defensive	Attempting to protect a person or health care services from negative comments. These responses prevent the client from expressing the true concerns. The nurse is saying you have no right to complain. Defensive responses protect the nurse from admitting weaknesses in the health care services, including personal weaknesses.
20.	Challenging	Giving responses that make clients prove their statement or point of view. These responses indicate the nurse is failing to consider the client's feelings, making the client feel it necessary to defend a position.
21.	Probing	Asking for information chiefly out of curiosity rather than with the intent to assist the client. These responses are considered prying and violate the client's privacy. Asking why is often probing and places the client in a defensive position.
22.	Testing	Asking questions that make the client admit to something. These responses permit the client only limited answers and often meet the nurse's need rather than the client's.
23.	Rejecting	Refusing to discuss certain topics with the client. These responses often make clients feel that the nurse is rejecting not only their communication but also the clients themselves.
24.	Changing topics and subjects	Directing the communication into areas of self-interest rather than considering the client's concerns is often a self-protective response to a topic that causes anxiety. The responses imply that the nurse considers important will be discussed and that clients should not discuss certain topics.

Contd...

Contd...

Sl. No	Technique	Description
25.	Unwarranted reassurance	Using clichés or comforting statements of advice as a means to reassure the client. These responses block the fear, feelings and other thoughts of the client.
26.	Passing judgments	Giving opinions and approving or disapproving responses, moralizing or implying one's own values. The responses imply that the client must think as the nurse thinks, fostering client dependence.
27.	Giving common advice	Telling the client what to do. These responses deny the client's right to be an equal partner. Note that giving expert rather than common advice is therapeutic.

TASK AND SKILLS FOR EACH PHASE OF HELPING RELATIONSHIP

Phase	Tasks	Skills
Preinteraction phase	The nurse reviews pertinent assessment data and knowledge, considers potential areas of concern and develops plan for interaction.	Organized data gathering: Limitations and seeking assistance as required.
Introductory phase 1. Opining the relationship	Both client and nurse identify each other by name. When the nurse initiates the relationship, it is important to explain the nurse's role to give the client an idea of what to expect. When the client initiates the relationship, the nurse needs to help the client express concerns and reasons for seeking help, vague, open-ended questions, such as what's on your mind today? Are helpful at this stage.	A relaxed, attending, attitude to put the client at ease. It is not easy for all clients to receive help.
2. Clarifying the problem	Because the client initially may not see the problem clearly, the nurse's major task is to help clarify the problems.	Attending listening, paraphrasing, clarifying, and other effective communication techniques discussed in this chapter. A common error at this stage is to ask too many questions of the client. Instead focus on priorities.
3. Structuring and formulating the contract (obligation to be met by both the nurse and client)	Nurse and client develop a degree of trust and verbally agree about (a) location, frequency and length of meeting, (b) overall purpose of the relationship, (c) how confidential material will be handled, (d) takes to be accomplished, and (e) duration and indications for termination of the relationship.	Communication skills listed above and ability to overcome resistive behaviors if they occur.

Contd...

Contd...

Phase	Tasks	Skills
Working phase	Nurse and client accomplish the tasks outlined in the introductory phase, enhance trust and rapport, and develop caring.	Listening and attending skills, empathy, respect, genuineness, concreteness, self-disclosure, and confrontation. Skills acquired by the client are non-defensive listening and self-understanding.
1. Exploring and understanding thoughts and feelings	The nurse assisting the client to explore thoughts and feelings and acquires and understanding of the client. The client explores thoughts and feelings associated with problems, develop the skill of listening and gains insight into personal behavior.	
2. Facilitating and taking action	The nurse plans programs within the client's capabilities are considers long- and short-term goals. The client needs to learn to take risks (i.e. accept that either failure or success may be the outcome). The nurse needs to reinforce successes and help the client recognize failures realistically.	Decision-making and goal setting skills. Also, for the nurse: reinforcement skills; for the client: risk taking.
Terminal phase	Nurse and client accept feedings of loss. The client accepts the end of the relationship without feelings of anxiety or dependence.	For the nurse: Summarizing skills; for the client: Ability to handle problems independently.

THE IMPACT OF PRE-EXISTING CONDITIONS

1. **Values attitudes and beliefs:** They are learned way of thinking. Value system may be communicated with behaviors that are more symbolic in nature.
2. **Culture or religion:** They are learned and differ from society to society. Religion can influence communication as well.
3. **Social status:** Studies reported that high-status persons are associated with gestures that communicate their higher-power position.
4. **Gender:** It influences the manner in which individuals communicate. Each culture has gender signals that are recognized as either masculine or feminine and provide a basis for distinguishing between members of each sex.
5. **Age or development level:** Age influences communication and this is never more evident than during adolescence. Developmental influences on communication may relate to physiological alterations.
6. **Environment:** Environment in which the transaction takes place. The place where the communication occurs influences the outcomes of the interaction. Some individuals who feel uncomfortable and refuse to speak during group therapy session may be open and willing to discuss problems privately on a one-to-one basis with the nurse.

NONVERBAL COMMUNICATION

1. **Physical appearance and dress:** Physical appearance and dress are of the total nonverbal stimuli that influence interpersonal responses and under some conditions; they are the primary determinants of such responses.
2. **Body movements and posture:** The way in which and individual positions his or her body communicates messages regarding self-esteem, gender identity, status and interpersonal warmth or coldness.
3. **Touch:** Touch is a powerful communication tool. It is a very basic and primitive form of communication and the appropriateness of its use is culturally determined.
4. **Facial expressions:** Facial expressions primarily reveal an individual's emotional state, such as happiness, sadness, anger, surprise or fear.
5. **Eye behavior:** Eyes have been called the window of the soul. Eye contact conveys a personal interest in the other person. Eye contact indicates that the communication channel is open, and it is often the initiating factor in verbal interaction between two people.
6. **Vocal cues or paralanguage:** Paralanguage is the gesture component of the spoken word. It consists of pitch, tone and loudness of spoken messages, the rate of speaking, expressively placed pauses and emphasis assigned to certain words.

INTERPERSONAL RELATIONSHIP IN NURSING

1. The patient in the hospital experience new and unfamiliar surroundings. It is uptown the nurse to see that the patient feels at ease and adjusts to the hospital routine and the new environment, to help, to cooperate and accept treatment necessary for regaining health.
2. The patient is an important person in the hospital. Treat him as an individual, call him by his name. Help him to overcome fear and anxiety. The nurse should be dignified, cheerful and courteous. Be pleasant with patients but not too familiar. Treat them with sympathy and firmness to gain respect and admiration. Personal appearance is very important in establishing a good nurse-patient relationship. The nurse should not talk or discuss personal affairs or about other patients or hospitals. The nurse-patient relationship must be professional and one of absolute trust, irrespective of caste, creed, or social status. She should not accept any personal gift from patients.
3. The nurse is an important member of a team that must work in cooperation and harmony for the care of patients. She should be familiar with the plan of organization of the hospital and of the nursing department.
4. The nurse must feel accountable to the organization should be honest, dependable and willing to carry out the prescribed treatment and care for the patient. She should maintain her position and dignity. She should not accept verbal orders from the physician (medical personnel). There should be a team spirit.
5. The nurse should have respect for the senior and concern and caring attitude towards fellow nurses, juniors and other supporting staff. She should maintain a healthy and good relationship with various departments.

INTERPERSONAL RELATIONSHIP SYSTEM IN NURSING

Interpersonal relationship is the main concept in professional field. In nursing interpersonal relationship system is explained by many theorists. Imogene King explains the interpersonal relationship system in detail. Interpersonal relationship system is enhancing the nurses to promote herself and clients well-being.

Interpersonal Relationship System (Imogene King)

King (1981) stated human being is the focus for nursing. The primary concerns of nursing are human behavior, social interaction, and social movements (1976), thus, within the context of the paradigm concept of person.

King (1981) included three dynamic interacting open systems:
1. Personal system.
2. Interpersonal system.
3. Social system.

The interpersonal system is composed of two, three or more individuals interacting in a given situation. King (1996) explained that, at the interpersonal system level, individuals increase consciousness and are open to interpersonal perceptions in communication and interactions with persons and things in the environment.

The interpersonal system moves the focus from the individual alone to individuals interacting in dyads, triads, small and large groups. The major concept of the interpersonal system is interaction; subconcepts are communication, role, stress and coping.

King noted that interaction is comprehensive concept in interpersonal systems and that knowledge of interaction is essential for nurses to understand a fundamental process for gathering in formation about human being.

King pointed out the perception, judgments, actions and reactions of the individuals cannot directly observed but must be inferred from the directly observable interaction. Elaborating, she stated, first, the informational component of interactions can be observed as communication. Second, the valuation component of interactions can be observed as transaction because one obviously values a goal, identifies means to achieve it, and takes action to attain it.

King viewed communication as the vehicle by which human relations are developed and maintained, she went to say that all behavior is communication. The general systems framework focuses on intrapersonal and interpersonal communication as well as verbal and nonverbal communication.

Communication is involved in transaction, which is defined as a process of interactions in which human being communicate with environment to achieve goals that are valued. Transactions are goal-directed human behaviors. In general systems frameworks, the concepts of roles was derived from the work of Bennis and Bennis. Three elements of role are intersected.
1. Role is a set of behaviors expected when occupying a position in a social system.
2. Rules or procedures define rights and obligations in a position in an organization.
3. Role is a relationship with one or more individuals interacting in specific situations for a purpose.

King developed her definitions of stress from the writing of Jamis, Monat and Lazarus and Selye. She stated stress is a dynamic state whereby a human being interacts with the environment to maintain balance. For growth, development and performance, this involves an exchange of energy and information between the person and the environment for regulation and control of stressors. Stress is viewed as negative and positive as well as constructive and destructive. King (1981) explained that stress is reduced when transaction are made.

Interpersonal relationship system in nursing, the nurse is an important member of the health care team that must work in cooperation and harmony for the care of the patient. This cooperation and harmony depends upon the interpersonal relationship that is maintained among the members of the health team.

PRINCIPLES OF INTERPERSONAL RELATIONSHIP

1. Learn everyone's name and never address anyone by any nick name.
2. Respect everyone's individuality. Each member of a team is as important as the other.
3. Do not impose anything on anybody.
4. Keep emotion under control.
5. Do not be afraid to admit ignorance.
6. Do not give and take any personal favor.
7. The team leader should not make any excuse regarding his or her responsibility.
8. Develop habits of listening and focus attention on the problems.
9. Do not do or say anything that will disturb other's faith.
10. Be impartial to others and practice justice.
11. The members of team should be loyal, honest, dependable and willing to carry out the directions of the team leader.
12. There should be team spirit or we feeling among the members. The members should work for the interest of the group.
13. There should be mutual understanding between the members; they should be willing to give and take corrections.

PROFESSIONAL NURSING RELATIONSHIPS

It is created through the nurse's application of knowledge, understanding of human behavior and communication, and commitment to ethical behavior. Having a philosophy based on caring and respect for other will help the nurse be more successful in establishing relationships of this nature.

NURSE-CLIENT HELPING RELATIONSHIP

Helping relationship is the foundation of clinical nursing practice, the essential element of care with every client in every situation. In such relationship, the nurse assumes the role of professional helper and comes to known the client as an individual who has unique health needs, human responses, and patterns of living. The relationship is therapeutic, promoting a psychological climate that facilitates positive change of growth.

The nurse establishes, directs and takes responsibility for the interaction and the clients need take priority over the nurse's needs. A helping relationship between nurse and client does not just happen; it is created with care and skill and is built on the clients trust in the nurse. Nursing theorist Imogene King (1971) calls the nurse-client relationship, learning experiences whereby two people interact to face immediate health problems, to share, if possible, in resolving it, and to discover ways to adapt to the situation.

Clients are helped to clarify needs and goals, problem solve, cope with situational or maturational crises, clarify, clarify and strengthen valves, reduce stress and anxiety and gain insight and self-understanding. The nurse-client relationship is character used by a natural progression of four goal-directed phases that often began before the nurse meets the client and continue until the care giving relationship ends.

Socializing is often an important initial component of interpersonal communication. It helps people get to know one another and relax. It is easy, superficial and not deeply personal, whereas therapeutic interactions are often more intense, difficult and uncomfortable. A nurse often uses social conversations to help the client feel comfortable and lay foundation for a closer relationship. During social conversation, clients may ask personal questions about the nurse's family, place of residence and so fourth. The skillful nurse uses judgment about what to share and provides minimal information or deflects such questions with gentle. Humor and refocuses conversation back to the client.

Creating a therapeutic environment depends on the nurse's ability to communicate, and to help clients meet their needs. The nurse provided information, supported client's active decision making, and offered opportunities for clients to engage in social exchange. Nurses often encourage clients to share personal stories, which are called narrative interaction. Through narrative interactions, nurses may begin to understand the context of others lives and learn what is meaningful for them from their perspectives.

Nurses also provide information and use strategies that help clients understanding and change behavior. The nurse uses contracts with clients to establish mutually agreed upon health goals and expectations for behavioral change. The nurse and client work as a team. The nurse offers others the opportunity to make choices, even as simple as choosing a bath time or which time medication to take.

A good way to encourage autonomy is to collaborate with others. Research has show that successful collaboration requires an active and committed involvement by both client and nurse and a joint effort to ward problem solving. Such a relationship will enhance the clients well-being and the nurse's feeling of success.

NURSE-FAMILY RELATIONSHIP

Many situations, especially those in community and home health settings, require the nurse to form helping relationships with entire families. The same principles that guide one to one helping relationship also apply when the client is a family unit, although communication within families requires additional understanding of the complexities of family dynamics, needs and relationships. Collaboration among nurse, client and family care givers is especially important.

NURSE-HEALTH TEAM RELATIONSHIP

Nurses are members of a larger health care community and often function in roles the require interaction with multiple health team members. Many elements of the nurse-client helping relationship are also applied in these collegial relationships, which are focused on accompling the work and goals of clinical setting communication in such relationships may be geared toward team building, facilitating group process collaboration, delegation, supervision, leadership and management.

Both social and therapeutic interactions are needed between the nurse and health team members to build morale and strengthen relationships within the work setting. Every one has interpersonal needs for acceptance inclusion, identity, privacy, power and control and affection.

NURSE-COMMUNITY RELATIONSHIP

Many nurses form relationships with community groups by participating in local organizations, volunteering for community services or becoming politically active. Nurses in a community based practice must be able to establish relationships with their community to be effective change agents. Communication within the community occurs through channels such as neighborhood newsletters, public bulletin boards, newspapers, radio, television and electronic information sites.

ELEMENTS OF PROFESSIONAL COMMUNICATION

Professional appearance, demeanor and behavior are important in establishing the nurse's trust worthiness and competence. They communicate that the nurse has assumed the professional helping role, is clinically skilled and is focused on the client.

1. Being on time.
2. Organized, well-prepared and equipped for the responsibilities of the nursing role also communicate one's professionalism.
3. Courtesy.
4. Use of names.
5. Privacy and confidentiality.
6. Trust worthiness.
7. Autonomy and responsibility.
8. Assertiveness.

COMMUNICATION WITHIN NURSING PROCESS

Nursing Assessment

Assessment of client's ability to communicate includes gathering data about the many contextual factors that influence communication. The context refers to all the parts of something that help determine its meaning. Situations have several aspects that influence the nature of communication, interpersonal relationships and client needs. These include that participant's internal factors and characteristics, the nature of their relationship, the situation prompting communication, the environment and sociocultural elements present.

Nursing Diagnosis

Most individuals experience difficulty with some aspect of communication, most often, the nurse care is directed toward those individuals who experience more serious impairments in communication. The primary nursing diagnostic label used to describe the client who has limited or no ability to communicate verbally is impaired verbal communication.

The related factor for impaired verbal communication focus on the causes of communication disorder. These can be physiological, mechanical, anatomical, psychological, cultural or developmental in nature. For example, deaf older adult with untreated cataracts who has the following nursing diagnosis: Impaired verbal communication related to limited vision, absent hearing and inability to articulate works.

Planning

Once the nurse has identified the nature of the clients communication dysfunction, several factors must be considered is the care plan is designed. Motivation is a factor in improving communication, and clients often require encouragement to try different approaches that involve significant change.

Expected outcomes for the client with impaired communication are important to identify. In general, effective nursing interventions will result in the client experiencing a sense of trust in the nurse and health team.

At times nurses care for well-clients whose difficulty in sending, receiving and interpreting messages interferes with healthy interpersonal relationships. Nurses can plan interventions to help such clients improve their communication skills.

Implementation

It carry out plan of care, nurses need to use communication techniques that are appropriate for the client's individual needs. The most basic nursing interventions used in communication are therapeutic communication techniques. Therapeutic communication techniques are specific responses that encourage the expression of feelings and ideas and convey the nurse's acceptance and respect.

Evaluation

The nurse and client determine whether the plan of care has been successful by evaluating the client communication outcomes established during planning. Nurses can evaluate the effectiveness of their own communication by making process recording, written records of their verbal and nonverbal interactions with clients.

Unacceptable Behavior in the Nurse-client Relationship

According to standard for therapeutic nurse and client relationship Nurses Association of New Brunswick, 2000.

I	Emotion/verbal abuse	1. Sarcasm 2. Intimidation 3. Teasing or taunting 4. Manipulation
II	Physical abuse	1. Using forces 2. Hitting 3. Pushing 4. Slapping 5. Shaking
III	Sexual abuse	1. Sexual intercourse or others forms of physical sexual relations between nurse and the client. 2. Touching of an abusive nature, etc. 3. Touching of a sexual nature. 4. Neglect: Occurs when nurse fail to meet the basic needs of clients who are unable to meet them themselves.
IV	Financial abuse	1. Borrowing money or property from a client. 2. Soliciting gift from a client. 3. Withholding of finances through theft. 4. Influence or pressure to obtain the client's money. 5. Insensitivity to religious and cultural beliefs and values.

MAJOR RECOMMENDATION FOR ESTABLISHING THERAPEUTIC RELATIONSHIP

1. The nurse must acquire the necessary knowledge to participate effectively in therapeutic relationship.
2. Establishment of a therapeutic relationship requires reflective practice. The concept includes the required capacities of: Self-awareness, self-knowledge, and empathy, awareness of ethics, boundaries and limits of the professional role.
3. The nurse needs to understand the process of a therapeutic relationship and be able to recognize the current phase of his/her relationship with the client.

4. The entry-level nursing programs must including both theoretical content and supervised practice.
5. Organizations will consider the therapeutic relationship as the basis of nursing practice and overtime will integrate a variety of professional development opportunities to support nurses in effectively developing these relationships. Opportunities must include nursing consultation, clinical supervision and coaching.
6. Health care agencies will implement a model of care that promotes consistency of the nurse-client assignment, such as primary nursing.
7. Agencies will ensure that at minimum, 70% of their nurses are working on a permanent full-time basis.
8. Agencies will ensure that nurses worked are maintained at levels conductive to developing therapeutic relationship.
9. Staff decisions must consider client acuity, complexity level, complexity of work environment, and availability of expert resources.
10. Organizations will consider the nurse's well-being as vital to the development of therapeutic nurse-client relationship and support the nurse as necessary.
11. Organization will assist in advancing knowledge about therapeutic relationship by disseminating nursing research supporting the nurse in using these findings, and supporting his/her participation in the research process.
12. Agencies will have a highly visible nursing leadership and establishes and maintains mechanisms to promote open conversation between nurse and all levels of management, including senior management.
13. Resources must be allocated to support clinical supervision and coaching processes to ensure that all nurses have clinical supervision and coaching on a regular basis.
14. Organization are encouraged to include the development of nursing best practice guidelines in their annual review of performance indicators/ quality improvement, and accreditation bodies are also encouraged to incorporate nursing best practice guidelines into their standards.

INTERPERSONAL RELATIONSHIP IN NURSING

The relationship that is established between nurse and patient is of great help and is the basis of nursing practice. The relationship has to be established between the nurse, the patient, his family and other members of health team.

Helping relationship is the foundation of clinical nursing practice, the essential element of care with every client in every situation. In such relationship, the nurse assumes the role of professional helper and comes to known the client as an individual who has unique health needs, human responses, and patterns of living. The relationship is therapeutic, promoting a psychological climate that facilitates positive change of growth. A therapeutic nurse-client relationship is established and maintained by the nurse through the use of professional nursing knowledge, skills and caring attitudes and behaviors in order to provide nursing services that contribute to the client's health and well-being.

The six qualities of a nurse, which help her in making good interpersonal relationship, are:
1. Behaving sincerely towards people.
2. Allowing people to express their thoughts and feeling.
3. Having adequate verbal expressions.
4. Attending to understand what people are really communicating (accurate empathy).

5. Attending to interpersonal process occurring whining the therapeutic relationship.
6. Pointing out discrepancies in behavior.

BIBLIOGRAPHY

1. Balzer Riley J. Communications in nursing, 4th edn, St. Louis, 2000, Mosby.
2. Buckman R. How to break bad news: A guide for health care professionals. Baltimore, MD: Johns Hopkins University Press, 1992.
3. Crouch R. Communication is the key, Emerg Nurse 10(3):1, 2002.
4. Gabor D. First contact body language. In: How to start a conversation and make friends. Revised edn. Rockefeller center, Fireside Publications, New York 2001:21.
5. Grant. Child development in India, 3rd edn, Ashish Publishing House, New Delhi, 1992.
6. Hybels S, Weaver R. Communicating effectively, 5th edn, McGraw-Hill, Boston, 1998.
7. Jayee M Black, Esther Matassasion-Jacobs. Luckmann and Sorcesens medical surgical nursing, 4th edition, WB Saunders company.
8. Kelly Anita E, McKillop Kevin J. "Consequences of Revealing Personal Secrets." Psychological Bulletin, v120 (3), 450, 1996.
9. Kurtz SM, Silverman J, Draper J. The Calgary-Cambridge referenced observation guides: An aid to defining the curriculum and organizing the teaching in communication training programmes. Med Educ, 30:83-9, 1996.
10. Leninger M. cultural care theory, research and practice. Nursing Science quarterly, 9:2, and summer 73, 1991.
11. Luft, Joseph. "Of Human Interaction," Palo Alto, National Press, 177 pages, CA (1969).
12. Mandel E, Shulman M, Begany T. Overcoming communication disorders in the elderly, Patient care 31(2): 55, 1997.
13. Potter A Patricia, Perry Anny Griffin. Fundamentals of nursing, 5th edn, Mosby Publication.
14. Santrock JW. Child Development, 7th edn, Brown and Bench Mark Publishers, Sydney, 1996.
15. Sr Nancy. Stephanie's Principles and practice of nursing, volume one, NR Brothers, 1996.
16. Tendon BN, et al. Management of severely malnourished children by village workers through ICDS in India, Journal of Tropical Pediatrics, Vol. 30, 1984,274-79.
17. Wood J. Interpersonal communication, 2nd edn, Cincinnati, 1999, Wadsworth.

3 Growth and Development

DEFINITIONS

1. **Growth:** Refers to an increase in physical size of the whole or any of its parts and can be measured in inches or centimeters and in pounds or kilograms. The term growth denotes a net increase in the size or mass of tissues. It is largely attributed to multiplication of cells and increase in the intracellular substance.

   Hypertrophy or expansion of cell size contributes to a lesser extent to the process of growth.

2. **Development:** Refers to a progressive increase in skill and capacity to function. Development specifies maturation of functions. It is related to the maturation and myelination of the nervous system and indicates acquisition of a variety of skills for optimal functioning of the individual.

3. **Pediatrics:** Branch of medicine concern with growth, development and care of children and treatment of their diseases.

4. **Live born:** A live born neonate is the product of conception irrespective of weight or gestational age that after separation from mother shows any evidence of life such as breathing, heart rate, pulsation of umbilical cord or definitive movement of voluntary muscles.

5. **Growth:** Net increase in the size or mass of tissues, due to multiplication of cells and increase in the intracellular substances.

6. **Development:** Increase in capacity or maturation of function. It is related to the maturation and myelination of the nervous system and indicates acquisition of a variety of skills for optimal functioning of individual.

7. **Therapeutic play:** The process of incorporating play activities in the routine care of pediatric patients to decrease hospital/disease associated stress.

8. **Pathogen:** A microorganism capable of causing disease is a pathogen.

9. **Maturation:** Maturation produces an increase in competence, an ability to function at a higher level depending on the child's heredity.

10. **Heredity:** The heredity of a man and woman determines that their children. Heredity decides the size and shape of the body, hence family member bear resemblance. The characteristics are transmitted through genes, which are responsible for family illness, e.g. diabetes.

11. **Sex:** Sex is determined at conception, after birth the male infant is both longer and heavier than female infant. Boys maintain this superiority unit about 11 years of age. Girls mature earlier, reach the period of accelerated growth earlier than boys and are than taller on the average.

12. **Race:** Distinguishing characteristics called racial or subracial developed in prehistoric humans. Similar physical characteristics are seen in people belonging to the same race. As too height,

tall and short examples exist among all races and subraces. Among civilized groups, inter-marriage has produced mixed racial types.

INTRODUCTION TO GROWTH AND DEVELOPMENT

Introduction

The period of growth and development extends throughout the life cycle. However, the period in which the principal changes occur is from conception to the end of adolescence. The most important period of growth and development is a complex one, in which two cells joined as one normally because a thinking, felling person, who eventually takes a responsible place in society.

Definitions

Growth: It refers to an increase in physical size of the whole or any of its parts and can be measured in inches or centimeters and pounds or kilograms.

Development: It refers to a progressive increase in skill and capacity to function. It causes a qualitative change in the child's functioning.

MEANING OF GROWTH AND DEVELOPMENT

Growth and development are used interchangeably and taken as synonymous terms. Both related to the measurement of changes occurred in the individual after conception in the womb of the mother. Change is the law of nature. An individual starting from a fertilized egg turns in to a full fledged human adult.

In this turn over process he/she undergoes a cycle of change brought about by the process of growth and development in various dimensions physical, mental, emotional, social, etc. Therefore, in the wider sense both the terms growth and development can be used for any change brought by maturation and learning and essentially is the product of both heredity and development.

CONCEPT OF GROWTH AND DEVELOPMENT

1. Growth is one of the parts of developmental process; in strict sense development in its quantitative aspect is termed as growth.
2. Growth may be referred to describe the changes, which take place in particular aspect of the body and behavior of an organism.
3. Growth does not continue throughout life. It stop, when maturity has been attained.
4. The changes produced by growth are the subject of measurement. They may be quantified and are observable in nature.
5. Growth may or may not bring development. A child may grow by becoming that fat but this growth may not bring any functional improvement or development.
6. The term growth refers to an increase in physical size of the whole body or any of its parts.
7. Development refers to progressive increase in physical skill and capacity to function. It causes qualitative change in the childs functioning.
8. Growth is an essential features of life of a child that distinguishes him or her from an adult.
9. The maximum increase in the number of cells occur in the fetal life as evidenced by an increase in the DNA content of tissues.
10. Children are influenced by genetic factors, home, environment and parental attitudes.

11. Development is closely related to maturation of the nervous system, as primitive reflexes disappear, they are replaced by a voluntary activity.
12. Play is a natural medium for expression, communication and growth in children.
13. Both rate and pattern of growth can be modified most obviously by nutrition.
14. Growth is complex; it is measured both qualitatively and quantitatively over a period of time.

BIOLOGICAL PRINCIPLES OF GROWTH AND DEVELOPMENT

Introduction

The biological changes brought about in the individual by the process of growth and development; tend to follow some well-defined principles. There are known as principles of growth and development. These principles are being described below.

Principles of Growth and Development

1. **Principle of continuity:** Development follows continuity, it goes from womb to tomb and never ceases. An individual staring his life from a tiny cell develops his body, mind and other aspects of his personality through a continuous stream of development in these various dimensions.
2. **Rate of growth and development is not in uniform:** The rate of growth and development is not steady and uniform at all times. It proceeds more rapidly in the early years of life but shows down in to later years of infancy. Therefore, at no stage that rate of growth and development show steadiness.
3. **Principle of individual difference:** According to this principle there exist wide individual differences among children with respect to their growth and development in various dimensions; each child grows at his own unique rate.
4. **Uniformity of pattern:** Although development does not proceed at a uniform rate and show marked individual differences, yet it follows a definite sequence of pattern and some what uniform in the offspring. For example, all off springs of human beings begin to grow from head wards.
5. **Development proceeds from general to specific responses:** In all the phrases of childs development, general activity proceeds specific activity, the responses are of a general sort before they become specific.
6. **Principle of integration:** The integration refers to the whole and its parts as well as of the specific and general responses that make a child developed satisfactory in the various dimensions of his growth and development.
7. **Principle of inter-relation:** The growth and development in various dimensions like physical, mental, social, etc. are inter-related and interdependent. Growth and development in any one dimension affects the growth and development of the child in other dimensions.
8. **Development is predictable:** With the help of the rate of growth and development of a child it is possible for us to predict the range with in, which his nature of development is going to fall.
9. **Principle of development direction:** By cephalocaudal development proceeds in the direction of the longitudinal axis (head to foot). First the child gains control over his head and arm and them his legs so that he can stand.

10. **Development is spiral and not linear:** The child does not precede straightly on the path of development with a constant or a steady pace. Actually he makes advancement during a particular period but takes rest in the next following period to consolidate his development.

11. **Growth and development as a joint product of both heredity and environment:** Child at any stage of his growth and development is a joint product of both heredity and environment. His growth and development in any indirectly influenced.

12. **Growth and development proceeds in an orderly sequence:** Growth insight occurs in only one sequence from smaller to longer. Development also proceeds in a predictable order.

13. **There is an optimum time for initiation of experiences or learning:** A child cannot learn task until his or her nervous system is mature enough to allow that particular learning.

14. **Neonatal reflexes must be lost before development can proceed:** An infant cannot grasp with skill until the grasp reflex has faded not stand steadily until the walking reflex has faded.

15. **A great deal of skill and behavior is learned by practice:** An infant practices over and over taking a first step before he or she accomplishers this securely.

16. **Development involves change:** As the development process the child undergoes change in all aspects such as physical, psychological, social, spiritual, etc.

17. **Early development is more critical than later development:** In the early stage the child learns all skills form their parents. For example, toilet training is not given properly; child in future will have elimination problems.

18. **Every area of development has potential hazards:** Each stage of growth and development has own risks, which can be avoided if proper care is given.

19. **Happiness varies at different period in development:** Infant will be very happy once it receives all the needs required for toddler. If the child see the toy, which is pleasing. He tries to get in hand by shoeing the temper tantrum. He never adjusts to the situation but in case of school-age child, he tries to adjust to the situation.

20. **There are social expectations for every development in mental period:** In every period the society expects certain levels of development for an individual.

21. **Children are competent:** A child wants to be accepted. Each child has its own ability and they always try to achieve their needs.

FACTOR INFLUENCING GROWTH AND DEVELOPMENT

Introduction

Growth and development depend on not one but combination of many factors, all interdependent. The relatively typical pattern of growth and development is influenced by heredity and environment. Also genetic inheritance and environmental influences are two primary factors in determining a childs pattern of growth and development.

Genetic Factors

1. **Heredity:** The heredity of a man and women determines that their children. Heredity decides the size and shape of the body, hence family member bear resemblance. The characteristics are transmitted through genes, which are responsible for family illness, e.g. diabetes.

2. **Sex:** Sex is determined at conception, after birth the male infant is both longer and heavier than female infant. Boys maintain this superiority unit about 11 years of age. Girls mature earlier, reach the period of accelerated growth earlier than boys and are than taller on the average.

3. **Race:** Distinguishing characteristics called racial or subracial developed in prehistoric humans. Similar physical characteristics are seen in people belonging to the same race. As too height, tall and short examples exist among all races and subraces. Among civilized groups, inter-marriage has produced mixed racial types.

Nutritional Factors

1. **Poor nutrition:** Nutrition plays a vital role in the body's susceptibility to disease because poor nutrition limits the body ability to resist infection. Poor nutrition also plays a major role in the development of chronic illnesses. Growth and development suffering from protein-energy malnutrition, anemia and vitamin deficiency states are retarded.
2. **Maternal nutrition:** Intrauterine growth retardation and consequently small size of the fetus occur due to nutritional deficiency in mothers, infection and drugs used during pregnancy.

Environmental Factors

1. **Physical environment:** Environment forces act up on the individual. It is the exploding force of an individual potentially to different stimulating forces. The physical environment includes food, temperature, climate, resources, etc.
2. **Mental environment:** It includes the intellectual atmosphere of the school, the libraries, the recreation rooms, labs, etc.
3. **Social environment:** It includes social association the child gets from the beginning. It also includes cultural atmosphere of the society, e.g. religion, folklore, literature, art, music, social convertions and political organizations. The rich is the environment, better is the scope for developing an individual in to a healthy human being.
4. **Socioeconomic level:** The child born into a family of low socioeconomic means may not receive adequate health supervision could leave a child without immunization against measles or other childhood illnesses, and thus, vulnerable to disease that could cause permanent neurological damage may occur.
5. **Cultural influences:** Groups of human being create their own cultures, whereas each individual is influenced or shaped by the culture of which he or she is a part. The effects of a particular culture on a child begin before birth because of the manner in which culture views and treat the members of the pregnant women's family.
6. **Internal influences:** There is evidence that all the hormones in the body affect growth in some manner. Deficiency of growth hormone retards growth while over production results in gigantism.
7. **Characteristics of parents:** Parents with high intelligence quotient (IQ) are more likely to have children with higher level of inherent intelligence.

Prenatal Environment

Prenatal environment climate in which the child's develops. The influences of the intrauterine environment on the child's future development are great, particularly since the uterus shields the fetus from the full impact of external adverse condition.

Postnatal Environment

An environment that provides satisfying experiences promote growth. Since growth and development are inter-related, growth in one area influences and in turn is influenced by growth in all other areas.

CHARACTERISTICS OF GROWTH AND DEVELOPMENT

Introduction

Growth and development are continuous and orderly processes that have predictable sequences. It is important for the nurse to understand this early period as well as the total life cycle of an individual to better understands the behavior of parents and other adults who provide care for the child.

Characteristics

1. Individual differences each child has an individual rate of growth, but the pattern of growth shows less variability. For example, an infant will be able to sit before standing alone. As noted, the age at which an individual child achieves these skills may occur at any point in a range of time.
2. Readiness for certain task the critical periods-during which the learning of certain behaviors occurs are termed critical periods. These are defined as those points at which the maximal capacity for an aspect of development is first present or at which structures to be developed are undergoing rapid growth.
3. Rate of development during the period of growth and development of the total body and its subsystem, growth is sometimes rapid and at times it slows down. Rapid growth occurs during gestation and during infancy. In the preschool years, growth levels off and slows down during the school years.
4. Sequence of growth and development—growth and development proceeds from the head down to the tail or in a cephalocaudal direction. This is particularly evident during the period of gestation and the first year of life. Before birth the head end of the embryo, and fetus enlarges and develops before the tail end does. Postnatal, the infant can control the movement of the head before being able to stand and control the feet.
5. Inter-relatedness of growth and development although growth and development physical, mental, social, emotional, sexual and spiritual proceed at different rates, they are so inter-related in the majority of children that the result is a progressive development of the whole child, from infancy to adult.

Growth of the Systems

Circulatory System

1. **Heart rate:** It reduces with increasing age, infancy 120 beats per minute, one year: 80 to 120 bpm, childhood: 70 to 110 bpm, adolescence to adulthood: 55 to 90 bpm.
2. **Blood pressure increases with age:** The fiftieth percentile ranges from 55 to 66 mm Hg diastolic to 65 to 112 mm Hg systolic. These levels increase about 2 to 3 mm Hg per year starting at age 7 years. Systolic pressure in adolescence higher in males than in females.
3. **Hemoglobin:** Highest at birth 179 per 100 ml of blood. Then decreases to 10 to 15 g by 1 year. Gradual increase in hemoglobin level to 14.5 g per 100 ml between 1 and 12 years of age. The hemoglobin level higher in males than in females.

Respiratory System

1. Respiratory rate decreases with increase in age. Infancy: 30 to 40 per minute, Childhood 20 to 24 per minute, adolescence and adulthood: 16 to 18 per minute.

2. Vital capacity—gradual increase throughout childhood and adolescent with a later life. Capacity in males exceeds in females.
3. Basal metabolism—highest rate is found in the newborn. Rate declines with increase in age, higher in males than in females.

Urinary System

1. Premature and full-term newborns have some inability to concentrate urine. Specific gravity (newborn): 0.001 to 1.02.
2. Glomerular filtration rate greatly increased by 6 months of age, reaches adult value between 1 and 2 years, gradually decreases after 20 years.

Digestive System

1. Stomach size is small at birth, rapidly increases during infancy and childhood.
2. Peristaltic activity decreases with advancing age.
3. Blood glucose level gradually rises from 75 to 80 mg per 100 ml blood in infancy to 95 to 100 mg during adolescence.
4. Premature infants have lower blood glucose levels than do full-term infants.
5. Enzymes are present at birth to digest proteins and moderate amount of fat, but only simple sugars.
6. Secretion of hydrochloric acid and salivary enzymes increases with age until adolescence then decrease with advancing age.

Nervous System

1. Brain reaches 90% of total size by 2 years of age.
2. All brain cells are **present** by the end of the first year, although their size and complexity will increase.
3. Maturation of the brainstem and spinal cord follows cephalocaudal and proximodistal laws.

PRENATAL DEVELOPMENT

Introduction

The word "pre-natal" refers to the period before birth. It begins from the time of conception and ends when the baby is born. In the various life stage of man, prenatal period is the earliest and the most important stage because the foundations for future development are laid during this stage.

Prenatal Life

1. Fertilization or conception occurs, when a sperm from the male pierces the cell wall of an ovum or egg from the female.
2. Once the ovum is fertilized, it begins to grow.
3. At first, the fertilized ovum, which is also called zygote consists of only one cell.
4. After few hours, the zygote divided into two new cells.
5. Still later, each of these two cells also divides.

Development during Prenatal Period

The Period of Ovum

1. The first two weeks from the time of conception until the zygote is attached within the uterus is the period of ovum.
2. Conception occurs in the fallopian tube and the zygote travels down to uterus.
3. It starts dividing and multiplying in the beginning of this period.
4. By the time, it reaches the uterus it is about the size of pinhead.
5. It develops very small ten drills and with the help of these tendrils the ovum to the uterine wall is called implantation.
6. Implantation occurs approximately around 10 days after fertilization.

The Period of Embryo

1. The period of embryo begins from the time of the zygote attachment to the uterine wall.
2. This period is usually lasts from 2 weeks after fertilization to the eight weeks by the end of the period of ovum, the eggs has two distinct parts, one inner cell mass and the other an outer layer called trophoblast.
3. The inner cell mass differentials into three clear layers, of the three layers, the outer layer is called ectoderm form, which will develop the outer layer of skin the hair the nails, parts of teeth, skin glands, sensory cells and the nervous system.
4. The middle layer is called the mesoderm from, which will develop the inner skin layers, the muscles, skeleton and the circulatory and excretory organs.
5. The inner layer is called endoderm form, which will develop living of the entire gastrointestinal tract, the trachea, bronchi, lungs, liver, pancreas, salivary gland, thyroid gland and thymus.
6. The outer layer, the trophoblast will develop into accessory tissues, which protect and nourish the embryo.
7. As the embryo grows, additional life supporting structure continues to develop. Among these are the umbilical cord and placenta, which maintain the connection with the mother's body through, which the embryo gets nutrients and excrete waste.
8. Umbilical and cord is a flexible cord like structure connection the fetus with the placenta.
9. Placenta is a membranous organ into which mother's bloodstream and fetus bloodstream end.
10. Nutrition from the mother blood passes to the fetus through placenta. Also a sac develops, filled with a watery fluid.
11. The embryo, the spontaneous abortion rate is relatively high. Since all organs have their beginning in this stage, development irregularities might occur if the mother takes medicines without medical advice.

The Period of Fetus

1. This period extends from the end of the second month of pregnancy until birth.
2. During this time the various body system, which had their origin in the earlier stage become will developed and begin to function.
3. By the end of the three inches long. Muscles are becoming well-developed and spontaneous of the arms and legs may be observed.
4. The fetus sex can now be distinguished easily by the end of 16 weeks; the mother can feel the movement.

5. By 24 weeks of age, the fetus is capable of swallowing and sucking. By the time the fetus eyelids have developed and are functional.
6. The fetal age of 28 weeks is an important one. By this age the child's nervous, circulatory and other bodily systems have become sufficiently will structure, so that, if born prematurely it can survive. As the fetus become older, it becomes more active.

THE NEWBORN

Introduction

The birth of an infant is one of the most awe inspiring and emotional events that can occur in one's lifetime. After 9 months of anticipation and preparation, the neonate arrives amid a flurry of excitement. The new human being affects the lives of the parent and also the other family members. The nurse provides family- centered care for neonates and their parents based on an understanding of the effects of heredity and environment and the newborn infant in the first several days of life.

Physical Growth during Infancy

1. According to medical standards, the period of the newborn extends from birth to the end of the second week or until the navel is healed, this also called the period of neonate.
2. The term neonate is derived from the Greek word ' Neo' meaning new and the Latin verb "Nascor" meaning to be born. Hurlock refer to this period as the period of infancy.
3. Before the birth, the baby was inside the mother in a comfortable environment. The entire baby was inside the mother in a comfortable environment. All the needs of the fetus were taken care of by the mother's body.
4. But the baby is born, the baby has to do such functions as breathing, ingestion, digestion, excretion, etc. by himself.
5. Hence, the newborn baby has to make a number of adjustments.
6. The four most important, adjustment to temperature change, adjustment to breathing, taking in nourishment, and adjustment to elimination.
7. Because all babies are not capable of adjustment this period is called a critical period.
8. The most critical time in the first day of life. Babies born fulterm, adjust to those conditions well, but underweight babies and premature babies find it difficult to adjust.

Appearance of the Newborn

1. As soon as the baby is born, he/she cries, this birth cry makes the baby's first breath.
2. All the babies look similar in the newborn stage. A newborn baby's body is coated with a cheese like substance.
3. His chinless head seems too big for his body. There is hair not only on his head, but at other places of the body also.
4. The genitals are the first large and prominent.
5. Newborn babies have enlarged breasts which sometimes secrete milk and girls babies occasionally have a brief menstrual flow.
6. The neonate's skull is not yet completed formed. There are six soft spots on his head.

Characteristics of Newborn (During First Week)

Circulatory

Clamping of cord at birth brings changes in fetal circulation, closure of foramen ovale and ductus, arteriosus and obiteration of umbilical arteries produce an adult like circulation within 1 hour after birth.

1. Heart rate regular 120 to 160, but variable depending on infants activity; soft hearts murmur common for first month of life.
2. Hemoglobin level high 14 to 20 g per 100 ml of blood.
3. White blood count high; 6000 to 22000 mm^3.

Respiratory System

Respirations diaphragmatic, irregular, abdominal, 30 to 50 per minute, quiet with periods of apned.

Temperature

Temperature maintained at 97.8°F or 98°F, environmental factors may affect temperature.

Excretory System

1. The first stool is black-green and tenacious, called meconium, by third day, becomes mixed with light yellow called transitional.
2. Newborn should void during first 24 hours, albumin and urates common during first week because of dehydration.

Integument System

1. Lanugo—fine, downy, hair growth over the entire body.
2. Milia—small, whitish, pinpoint spots over the nose caused by retained sebaceous secretions.
3. Mongolian spots—blue-black discoloration on back, buttocks and sacral region that disappear by first year.

Digestive System

1. The newborn has stores of nutrients from intrauterine existence, therefore, needs very little nourishment first few days.
2. Roots and sucks when anything is brought to mouth.
3. Digests simple carbohydrates, fats and proteins readily.
4. Cardiac sphincter of stomach not well-developed, therefore regurgitates if stomach is over fall.
5. Needs to be bubbled frequently to get rid of air bubbles in stomach.
6. Gastric activity remains low for 2 to 3 months.

Neural

1. CNS and brain not well-developed infant needs constant supply of oxygen.
2. Breathing, sucking and crying are early neural activities necessary for the infant's survival.

Sleep

1. Sleep lowers body metabolism.
2. It helps to restore energy and assimilate nutrition for growth.

Nutrition

1. Initial weight loss of 5 to 10 percent of birth weight is normal and usually regained by tenth day of life.
2. Newborn needs to ingest simple proteins, carbohydrates, fats, vitamins and minerals for continued cell growth.

Immediate needs at the time of birth:

1. Aspiration of mucus to provide an open airway.
2. Evaluation by use of Apgar score 1 and 5 minutes following birth score determined by points for heart rate, respiration, muscle tone, reflex irritability and color.
3. Maintenance of body temperature by drying infant and placing next to mother or under radiant warmer.
4. Promotion of interaction between parents and newborn.
5. Constant observation of physical condition.
6. Identification of infant by applying an identification band to infant and mother
7. Eye care prophylactic installation of ordered medicine (e.g erythromycin) in each eye to prevent ophthalmia neonatorum.
8. Assessment of behavioral characteristics during transition period: First period of reactivity, period of inactivity, second period of reactivity.

APGAR SCORING

1. Apgar scoring system is developed by Vrginia Apgar (USA) in 1952.
2. The score is based on observation of heart rate, respiration, muscle tone, reflex activity and color.
3. Each item is given a score of 0, 1, 2. The assessment of Apgar score is done at one and five minutes after birth.
4. Total score of 8-10 indicates ease in adjusting to the extrautrine life. The body's condition is good.
5. Total score of 5-7 indicates moderate difficulty of newborn babies to adjust to the life. The condition is fair .
6. Total score of 0-4 indicates severe distress.

Transitional Assessment

First Stage

1. It lasts for about 6 hours after birth. First 30 minutes after birth, the neonate is alert, cries and has stronger sucking.
2. This time is the best for breastfeeding and eye to eye contact.
3. After these 30 minutes of active period the newborn sleeps 5-6 hrs.
4. During this reactivity period he may have rapid heart rate, rapid respiration, more secretions and decreased body temperature as extrauterine adjustments adaptation.
5. Exposure needs to be avoided during this period.

Second Period of Reactivity

1. It is the period from 6 to 24 hrs after birth, when the neonate awakes after first sleep period.
2. Neonate again becomes active, alert and responsive, gradually his vital signs stabilize.

Neuromuscular Development

1. **Blink reflex:** It may be elicited by shining a strong light such as flashlight or otoscope light on the eye.
2. **Rooting reflex:** If a newborn's cheek is brushed or stroked near the corner off the mouth, the child will turn the head in that direction: The reflex disappears at about the 6th week of life.
3. **Sucking reflex:** When a newborn's lips are touched the baby makes a sucking motion. The sucking reflex begins to diminish at about 6 months of age.
4. **Swallowing reflex:** The swallowing reflex in the newborn is the same as in the adult. Food that reaches the posterior portion of the tongue is automatically swallowed.
5. **Extrusion reflex:** A newborn will extrude any substance that is placed on the anterior portion of the tongue. This protective reflex prevents the swallowing of inedible substance, disappearing at about 4 months of age.
6. **Palmar grasp reflex:** Newborn will grasp on object placed in their palm by closing their fingers in it. It is a primitive relax apparently from a time newborns clung to their mother for safety. The reflex disappears at about age 6 weeks to 3 months.
7. **Step (walk)** in place reflex-newborn, who are held in a vertical position with their feet touching a hard surface will take a new quick, alternating steps. This reflex disappears by 3 months of age.
8. **Placing reflex:** The placing reflex is similar to the step in place reflex, except is elicited by touching the anterior surface of newborn's legs against the edge of a bassinet or table.
9. **Plantar grasp reflex:** When an object touches the sole of an new born's foot at the base of the toes, the toes grasp in the same manner as the finger do. The reflex disappears at about 8 to 9 months of age in preparation for walking.
10. **Tonic neck reflex:** When newborn lies on this backs, their hands usually turn to one side or the other. The arm and the leg on the side to which the hand turns extend and the opposite arm and leg contract. It is also called a boxer or fencing reflex, because the newborn's position stimulates that of someone preparing to box of fence.
11. **Moro reflex:** A Moro reflex can be initiated by starting the newborn by a loud noise or by jarring the abssinet. The most accurate method of eliciting the reflex is to hold newborns in supine position and allow their heads to drop backward an inch or so.
12. **Babinski's reflex:** When the side of the sole of the foot is stoken is an inverted 'J" curve from the heel upward, the newborn flexes the toes. It remains positive (toes fan) until at least 3 months of age, when it is supplanted by the down-turning or flexing adult response.
13. **Magnet reflex:** It pressure is applied to the soles of the feet of newborn laying in a spine position he/she pushes back against the pressure. This and the two following reflexes are tests of spinal cord integrity.
14. **Crossed extension reflex:** One leg of a newborn laying supine is extended and the sole of that foot is irritated being rubbed with a sharp object, such as a thumbnail.
15. **Trunk uncurvated reflex:** When a newborn lies in a prone position and are touched along the pravertebral area by a probing finger, they will flex their trunk and swing their pelvis toward the touch.
16. **Landau reflex:** A newborn, who is held in a prone position with a hand underneath supporting the trunk should demonstrate some muscle tone. Babies may not be able to lift their head or arch their back in this position, but neither should they sag into an inverted 'V' position.
17. **Deep tendon reflex:** A patellar reflex can be elicited in a newborn by tapping the patellar tendon with the tip of the finger. The lower leg will move perceptibly if the infant has an intact reflex.

Parent-child Relationships

Concept of Basic Parent-infant Relationships

1. Early and frequent parent-infant contact is essential for survival (bonding).
2. Childbearing is a development crisis, parenting abilities can be fostered and developed.
3. Biologic changes that occur at puberty and during pregnancy influence the development of nurturance.
4. Interaction between mother and child begins from the moment of conception and can be shared with the father.
5. Love for the infant grows as the patents interact and give cure.
6. As the parent gives to the infant and infant receives the parent in turn receives satisfaction from parenting tasks.
7. Any disturbance in give and take cycle sets up frustrations in parents and infant.
8. Parental behavior is learned and frequent parent infant contact enhances development of parenting abilities; ambivalence is a natural phenomenon as are feeling of resentment.

Infant's Basic Needs

1. Physiologic—food, clothing, bathing and protection from environment.
2. Emotional—security, comfort, founding, caressing, rocking being spoken to and contact with one person on a consistent basis.

Mothering and Fathering

1. Based on biologic in born desire to reproduce.
2. Role concepts that begin with own childhood experiences.
3. Primitive emotional relationship.
4. Maturing process.
5. Fostered by the parent—Infant interaction that constantly reinforces gratification as needs are met and security develops.
6. Abilities that is learned rather than innate.

Significant Phases of Maternal Adjustments

1. Taking in phase—Mother's needs to have to be met before she can meet infant's needs, talks about self rather than infant, does not seem interested in infant.
2. Transition phase—Characterized by mothers starting to take hold, looking at and reaching for infant, touching with fingertips, talking about infant, etc.
3. Taking-hold phase—Kisses, embraces, give care to infant, eye contact, uses whole hand to make contact, calls the infant by name, etc.

Supportive Care to Promote Bonding/Attachment

1. Give parents ample time to inspect and begin to identity with infant, allow the parents to touch, fondle and hold infant.
2. Encourage given and take between parents and infants support these beginning relationships.
3. Teach the parents about their newborn; showing by example helps parents to learn care necessary to meet infant's and their own.

4. Evaluate parents and infant's response and revise plan as necessary, identify beginning of disturbed relationship.

Problems in Newborn

Preterm or Low Birth Weight Infant

1. Preterm infant born before term (36 weeks or less).
2. Low birth weight infant, weighs 2500 g or less at birth.
3. Less subcutaneous fat, therefore, the skin is wrinkled, blood and bony sutures are visible, lanugo present on birth on face, eyebrows are absent, ears are poorly supported by cartilages.

Asphyxia Neonatorum

1. Asphyxia neonatorum means nonestablishment of satisfactory pulmonary respiration at birth. Clinically, it is defined as failure to initiate and maintain spontaneous respiration with in one minute of birth.
2. The clinical features depend upon the etiology, intensity and duration of oxygen lack, plasma carbon dioxide excess and subsequent acidosis.
3. The basic requirements for initiation and maintenance of pulmonary respiration by airway clearenance, sufficient pulmonary perfusion, oxygen diffusion and dissociation capacity and carbonic anhydrase activity of blood.

Respiratory Distress Syndrome

1. It is a deficiency in surface-active detergent like lipoproteins (Surfactant) results in inadequate lung inflation and ventilation.
2. The respiratory distress syndrome occurs commonly in preterm neonates, babies of diabetic mothers and infants delivered by cesarean section or following breech delivery.
3. Clinically manifested by abrupt appearance of dyspnoed and cyanos attack shortly after birth, X-ray shows ground glass mottling.

Meconium Aspiration Syndrome

1. Meconium aspiration syndrome usually occurs in terms of post-term babies, who are small of gestational age.
2. The meconium stained liquor may be aspirated by the fetus-in-utero or during first breath.
3. The meconium may block the small air passages or produce chemical pneumonitis.
4. Diagnosis is mainly based on aspiration of meconium from the trachea at birth.
5. The therapeutic interventions are suctioning after head is delivered, oxygenation and ventilation, prophylactic antibiotic therapy and bicarbonate for acidosis.

Cranial Birth Injuries

1. **Caput succedaneum:** Edema with extravasations of serum into scalp tissues caused by molding during the birth process crosses the suture lines of the bony plates of the skull: No treatment is necessary; it subsides in a few days.
2. **Cephalhematoma:** Edema of the scalp with effusion of blood between the bone and periosteum, stops at the suture line, no treatment is necessary, it appears within a few weeks to a few months after birth, resolution of hematoma can lead to hyperbilirubinemia.

3. **Intracranial hemorrhage**: Bleeding into cerebellum, pons, medulla oblongata caused by a tearing of the tentrorium cerebelli, occurs in preterm infants and following prolonged labor, difficult forceps birth, precipitate birth, version or breech extraction.

Neuromuscular Birth Injuries

1. Facial paralysis—Asymmetry of face caused by damage to facial nerves from and difficult forceps birth.
2. Erb-Duchenne paralysis (Brachial palsy) caused by difficult forceps or breech extraction birth, manifested by a flaccid arm with elbow extended, treatment depends on severity of paralysis.
3. Dislocation and fracture are diagnosed by crepitation, immobility and variations in range of motion, treatment depend on the site of fracture.

Ophthalmia Neonatorum

1. An eye infection caused by *Neissseria gonorrhea* and *Chlamydia trachomatis*.
2. Organism is transmitted from the genital tract of an infected mother during birth or by infected mother during birth or by infected hands.
3. Chlamydial infection can also cause pneumonia.
4. It can be prevented by ophthalmic antibiotic instilled at birth after providing for initial bounding.

Nursing Management in Neonate

1. Establish and maintain patent airway by oropharynx suction to clear the respiratory passage.
2. Maintain normal body temperature—keep the baby away from fan, breeze or airconditioner, maintain the room temperature around 28-30 centigrade.
3. Protection from infection handwashing should be practiced before and after caring or touching the baby.
4. Provide adequate nutrition—put the baby to the mother's breast as early as possible after birth. Do not offer artificial feeds when baby has sucking and swallowing reflex.
5. Observe the elimination pattern—the infant passes urine very frequently during early period. If he does not pass for 10-12 hours, it should be reported to the doctor. The meconium is passed within 24 hours after birth.
6. Providing psychological bonding and supporting cuddling and warmth with close contact with the mother gives the infant feeding of love, affection and security.
7. Parental teaching-parents should be explained about daily observations, feeding, activity, sleep and elimination.

THE INFANCY

Introduction

Infancy is traditionally designed as the period from 1 month to 1 year of age. This year is one of rapid growth and development, with the infant tripling birth weight and increasing length by 50%. During this period the baby's senses sharpen and with the process of attachment to primary care givers from his or her first social relationships. Infants are seen at health care facilities for health maintenance at least 6 months during the first year.

Stages of Infancy

Rapid Growth and Development

1. Infancy is the period of rapid growth and development, inner as well as outer organs developed rapidly at this stage.

2. There is a rapid growth in terms of height and weight and size.
3. There is rapid growth in terms of height and weight and size.
4. There is rapid development of emotions and almost all the emotions are developed in the child during this stage.
5. This stage is marked by intensive motor activity and restlessness.

Dependence

1. Infant depends up on his mother, father and family members for the satisfaction on his basic needs.
2. The infant is a helpness creature and can move and function with the help of others. Even for the emotional satisfaction, he depends upon others.
3. He expects that everybody around him should love him and give him his entire affection and attention.
4. He wants to love and to be loved and in this exchange he totally depends on the mercy of others.
5. In this way the child at this stage is dependent but as he moves into the later years of his infantile behavior, he slowly proceeds towards independence.

Self-assertion

1. The child is helpless one and depends upon others for the satisfaction of his needs, he is quite self-assertive.
2. He tries to dominate his superior and elder ones, his wishes must be fulfilled.
3. He thinks, he is always right and all-round his should obey him.
4. He is the prince although without crown and tries to assert himself all the time in all situations.

Period of Make-believe and Fantasy

1. Infant live in the world of their own creation, this is a period of rich but baseless imagination.
2. As on this stage, the infant has limited potentialities and aspires more than, what he can actually get in the actual life.
3. He compensates himself in fantasy and makes believe.

Selfish and Unsocial

1. In infancy, the child is almost completely egocentric and selfish.
2. He does not want to share his toys or give any of his possessions to anyone else.
3. He wants to have all the things even love, admiration and affection reserved for him.
4. He does not care for the social and moral codes and principles and places his self interest at the premium.

Emotionally Unstable

1. Infancy is the period of violent emotional experiences.
2. The emotions at this stage are marked by intensity, frequency and instability.
3. There are spontaneous and the infant is hardly able to exercise control over them.
4. He is not able to mind his feelings and in this way, the emotional of the infant is generally in the overt form.

Mental Development during Infancy

Developing Curiosity and Questioning Attitude

1. At this age the child is very much curious about knowing so many things around him. The world and the environment is new for him.
2. He is in the habit of questioning like what is this. Answers do not interest him as much as asking questions.
3. His speed of questioning is so rapid that he does not wait the previous answers.

Intellectually not Developed

1. The child at this initial stage is very immature in intelligence.
2. He lacks in reasoning and abstract understanding.
3. He can think only in concrete terms and is not developed in abstract resoning and thinking.
4. The powers of observation, perception, concentration, etc. re also not developed.

Rate Memory

1. The child through not developed much intellectually has a very good memory. But this memorization is without reasoning.
2. It is purely a role memory; he can cram and reproduce the matter easily.

Creativity

1. The period of infancy is also characterized by the tendency of creative impulse in the child.
2. He develops a creative attitude and often engages himself in making or collecting so many things.
3. He tries to take satisfaction in realizing that he can make, construct and perform the activities as his elders do.

Time Concept is not Developed

Time concept is not developed for the child at this stage, the divisions of time such as yesterday, today, tomorrow; month, year, etc. are meaningless as he not yet developed the concept of time.

Sexual Development

1. Although the sex organs at this stage are not developed, yet the sex tendency is in a continuous stage of development.
2. The findings of psychoanalysis like Freud and others have clearly shown that the sexual life of the infant is an rich as that on an adolescent.
3. An infant passes through the three stages of sexual development stages of self love homosexual and heterosexual.
4. At the initial stage, the child derives pleasure from his own body by sucking his thumb or touching the sex organs.
5. Later on he seeks the satisfaction of his sex impulse outside and develops sentiments of love for the mother and father depending upon his sex.
6. Finally, the child develops heterosexual tendency and in his respect the male gets itself attached to the mother and the female child to the father.

Physical Growth

Weight

1. As a rule, most infant double their weight at 4 to 6 months, they triple it by 1 year.
2. During the first 6 months, infants typically average a weight gain of 2 lb per month.
3. During the second 6 months, weight gain is approximately 1 lb per month.
4. The average 1 year old male weight 10 kg (22 lb), the average female weight 9.5 kg (2 lb).

Height

1. The infant increases in height during the first year by 50 percent or grow from the average birth length of 20 inch to about 30 inch (50.8 to 76.2 cm).
2. Height, like weight is best assessment if it is plotted on a standard growth chart.

Head Circumference

1. Head circumference increase rapidly during the infant period, reflecting rapid brain growth.
2. By the end of the first year, the brain has already reached two-thirds of its adult size.

Body Proportion

1. Body proportion changes during the first year from that of a newborn to a more typical infant appearance.
2. The mandible becomes more prominent as bone grows.
3. The circumference of the chest is generally less than that of the head at birth by about 2 cm. It is even with the head circumference in some infants as early as 6 months and in most by 12 months.
4. The abdomen remains protuberant until the child has been walking well.

Body Systems

1. In the cardiovascular system, heart rate slows from 120 to 160 bpm to 100 to 120 bpm by the end of the first year.
2. Respiratory rate of the infant slows from 30 to 60 breaths/m to 20 to 30 breaths/m by the end of the first year.
3. At birth, the gastrointestinal tract is immature in its ability to digest food and mechanically move it along. These functions mature gradually during the infant year.
4. The immune system becomes functional by at least 2 months of age, the infant is able to produce both Ig G and Ig M antibodies by 1 year of age.
5. Ability to adjust to cold is mature by age 6 months.
6. Kidney, liver and endocrine glands remain immature and not as efficient at eliminating body wastes as in the adult.

Teeth

1. The first baby tooth usually erupts at age 6 months, followed by a new one monthly.
2. Teething pattern can vary greatly among children.

Motor Development

Gross Motor Development

1. Ventral suspension position refers to the infant's appearance when held in midair on a horizontal plane, supported by the hand under the abdomen. The 3 months old child lifts and maintains the head well above the plane of the rest of the body in ventral suspension.
2. A Landau reflex—It develops at 3 months. When the infant held in ventral suspension, the infant's head legs and supine extend. When the head is depressed, the hips, knees and elbows flex. This reflex continues to be present in most infants.
3. Neck righting reflex—Begins at four months old children. The infant turns the head to the side, shoulders, trunk and pelvis turn in that direction. This reflex causes the baby to lose his or her balance and roll sideways when lifting the head-up.
4. Sitting position—A 5 months old child can be seen to straighten his or her back when held or propped in a sitting position. By 6 months, children sit momentarily without support.
5. Standing position—the 9 months old child can stand holding onto the coffee table if he or she is placed in that position. At 12 months, a child stands alone at least momentarily.

Fine Motor Development

1. Thumb position—it an ability to bring the thumb and fingers together. It occurs at 4th month.
2. Pincer grasp—a major milestone occurs at 9th month, it is a perforce for use of one hand over the other.
3. At 12th month the infant can play pat a cake and peekaboo, holds a crayon to make a mark on paper. Helps in dressing, such as putting arm through sleeve.

Developmental Milestones

Language Development

1. A child begins to make small, cooing sounds by the end of the first month.
2. By 4 months, an infant is very "talkative", cooing babbling and gurgling when spoken to. He or she definitely laughs our loud.
3. The infant can imitate vowel sounds well, for example, oh-oh, ah-ah and oo-oo at 7 months.
4. By 9 months, the infant usually speaks a first word dd-da or ba-ba.
5. At 12 months, the infant can generally say two words besides ma-ma and dd-da, they use those two words with meaning.

Play during Infancy (Solitary Play)

1. Safety is chief determinant choosing toys (aspirating small objects is one cause of accidental death).
2. One month old children spend a great deal of time watching the parent's face, appearing to enjoy this activity so much that the face may become their favorite "toy".
3. Three months old children can handle small blocks or small rattles.
4. A 6 months old child can sit steadily enough to be ready for bathtub toys such as rubber ducks or plastic boats.
5. Many 9 months old children begin to enjoy toys that go inside one another.
6. The 12 months old child enjoying putting things in and taking things out of container, they like little boxes that fit inside one another or dropping objects such as blocks into cardboard box.

Sensory Development

Vision
1. At one month old child regards an object in the midline of vision.
2. Eye movement coordinated most of the time, follows a light to midline. Visual acuity 20/100 to 20/50 at 1 month.
3. Follows a light to the periphery and has binocular coordination (vertical and horizontal vision) at 3 months.
4. Recognizes familiar object and people at 5 months
5. Seven months old children pat their image in a mirror. Their depth perception has matured to the extent that they can perform such tasks as transferring toys from hand to hand.
6. By 10 months, the infant looks under a towel or around a corner for a concealed object (beginning of object performance).

Hearing
1. Hearing is demonstrated by the 1 month old child who quiets momentarily at a distinctive sound such as a bell or a squeaky rubber toy.
2. Many 3 months old children will turn their heads to attempt to locate a sound.
3. At 5 months of age, the infant demonstrate that he or she can localize a sound downward and to the side, by turning the head and looking down.
4. By 10 months, the infant can recognize his or her name and listen acutely when spoken to.
5. By 12 months, the infant can easily locate a sound in any direction and turn toward it.

Emotional Development

1. At 1 month, watches face intently while being spoken to.
2. Smiles in response to person or object occur in 3 months.
3. Coos and gurgles when talked to; enjoy social interaction at 5 months.
4. At 6 months, infants are increasingly aware of the difference between people, who regularly care for them and strangers.
5. At 7 months children show obvious fear of strangers, they may cry, when taken from their parent, attempt to cling to him or her, and reach out to be taken back.
6. Fear of strangers appears to reach its height during the 8 months, so much so that this phenomenon is often termed 8 months anxiety or stranger anxiety.
7. By 12 months, most children have overcome their fear of strangers and are alert and responsive again when approached. They like to play interactive nursery rhymes and rhythm games, and dance with others.

Cognitive Development

1. Primary circular reaction—During this time, he or she explores objects by grasping them with the hands or by mouthing them. At this stage the infant appears to be unaware of what actions he or she can cause or what actions occur independently. It occurs in third month of life.
2. Secondary circular reaction—It occurs at 6 months of age, during this time, the infant is able to realize that his or her actions can initiate pleasurable sensations.
3. Piaget describes the cognitive process of infant as sensorimotor intelligence for until an individual is about two years old, he concentrates on regularizing his sensation and controlling his motor activity.

Nursing Role in Health Promotion of the Infant

1. **Promoting infant safety:** Accidents are a leading cause of death in children. Most accidents in infancy occur because parents either underestimate or over estimate the child's ability. Nursing intervention is to establish sound parent-child relationship and provide anticipatory guidance for the child's safety.
2. **Preventing aspirations:** The accident that leads to the greatest number of infant deaths in aspiration. Round, cylindrical objects are more dangerous than square or flexible object in regard.
3. **Preventing falls:** Falls are a second major cause of infant accidents. No infant, beginning with the newborn should be left unattended on a raised surface. Normal wiggling can bring a baby to the edge of a bed, couch or table top, resulting in a fall. Teach parents to be prepared for their infant to roll over by 2 months of age.
4. **Nutritional health:** The best food for the infant during the first 12 months of life is breast milk. Breast milk is the most complete diet for the first 6 months but requires supplements of fluoride, iron by 6 months. Iron-fortified commercial formula is an acceptable alternative to breastfeeding. Solids can be introduced by about 6 months.
5. **Activities of daily living:** In the first year, caring for the infant-feeding, bathing, dressing and so forth-occupies what may seem like nearly all of parents waking hours. All these basic care related activities provide important opportunities for caregivers and infants to get to know one another and to become used to each other's personalities and patterns. Nurses play a key role in teaching parents about these activities, stressing their importance.
6. **Vaccinations:** DTP (diphtheria, pertussis and tetanus) given at 2, 4, 6 months, boosters given at 15 months and 5 years of age. MMR (measles, mumps and rubella- Live attenuated vaccine) generally given at 12 months of age because of the presence of natural immunity from mother, a second dose should be administered at 4 or 5 years of age. Polio, trivalent oral polio vaccine infant receive at 2, 4, 6 months. Homophiles influenza type B should be given at 2, 4, 6 and 15 months of age. Chickenpox vaccine (varivax) 1 dose should be given before 12 months.

Social, Emotional and Behavior Problems of Infant

1. Teething most infants have little difficulty with teething. Generally, gums are sore and tender before a new tooth breaks the surface. Because of this pain, a baby might be resistant to chewing for a day to two.
2. **Thumb sucking:** The need is so intense that may infants begin to suck a thumb or finer at about 3 months of age and continue the habit through the first few years of life.
3. **Head banging:** Some infants rhythmically bang their heads against the bars of crib for a period of time before falling asleep. Excessive head banging done to the exclusion of normal development or activity or head banging past the preschool period, suggests a pathological basis. Such children need a referral for counseling and further evaluation.
4. **Sleeping problems:** Sleep problems develop in early infancy because of colic or an otherwise healthy infant takes longer than usual to adjust to sleeping through the night. Breastfeed babies tend to wake more often than those who are formula fed because breast milk is more easily digested. In late infancy, the problem of waking at night the remaining awake for an hour or more becomes common.

THE TODDLER

Introduction

The todder period is usually considered from age 1 to 3 years, enormous changes takes place in the child and consequently in the family. During the toddler period, the child accomplishes a wide array of developmental tasks. Promoting toddler health and maintaining wellness involves knowledge of normal growth and development processes, an understanding of common significant milestones and the ability to anticipate deviations.

Physical Development

1. A child gains only about 5 to 6 Ib (2.5 kg) and 5 inch (12 cm) a year during toddler.
2. Physical growth is slow during toddlerhood; this is because of the toddler's decline in appetite and erratic eating habits.
3. Head circumference equals chest circumferences at 6 months to 1 year of age. At 2 years, chest circumferences are greater than of the head.
4. Toddler tend to have a prominent abdomen—A pouchy belly-because, although they are walking, their abdominal muscles are not yet strong enough to support abdominal contents as well as they will later.
5. They also have a forward curve of the spine at the sacral area (lordosis). As they walk longer, this will correct it self naturally.
6. The toddler waddles or walks with a wide stance, this stance seems to increase the lordotic curve, but it keeps the child on his or her feet.

Physiological Development

1. Brain growth continues slowly, corresponding to advancing intellectual skills and fine motor development.
2. Improved coordination and equilibrium parallels the most complete (by 2 years) myelination of the spinal cord as evidenced by refined walking, jumping and climbing.
3. Respirations slow slightly but continue to be mainly abdominal.
4. The heart rate slows from 110 to 90 bpm; blood pressure increases to about 99/64 mm Hg.
5. In the respiratory system, the lumen of vessels increases progressively so that threat of lower respiratory infection is less.
6. Stomach capacity increases to the point that the child can eat three meals a day.
7. Stomach secretions become more acid, therefore, gastrointestinal infections also become less common.
8. Urinary and anal sphincter control becomes possible with complete myelination of the spinal cord.
9. In the immune system, Ig G and Ig M antibody production become mature at 2 years of age, the passive immunity effects from intrauterine life are no longer operative.
10. The sense of hearing, smell, taste, touch and vision develop and begin to connect, since toddler utilize all five senses to explore the world and exert autonomy and independence.
11. Bladder and bowel control is typically achieving during this time period and children are able to retain urine up to 4 hours before needing to void.

Common Problem

1. **Sibling rivalry:** Sibling rivalry defined as intense feeling of jealousy between siblings, often is seen when an infant is born into a family with a toddler.
2. **Temper tantrum:** It is a outward explosive reaction to inward stressful or frustrating situations that are a normal part of toddler life.

Psychosexual Development

1. According to Freud, toddlers are in the anal stage off development. Freud first pointed out the tension resolving around toddler, bladder training and viewed toilet training as a possible way of resolving conflict and handling stress.
2. Freud believed, improperly managed toilet training could lead to life long psychological trauma with accompanying physical bowel/bladder responses.
3. Toddler is generally able to recognize gender differences by 2 years of age and begin to explore and recognize body parts during toilet training.

Psychosocial Development

1. The three major psychosocial tasks of toddlerhood are gaining self control, developing autonomy and increasing independence.
2. Fifteen months old children are still enthusiastic about interacting with people, providing those people are willing to follow the toddlers where they want to go.
3. By 18 months, toddler imitate the things they see a parent doing , such as study or sweep, so they seek out parents to observe and initiate reactions.
4. By 2 or more years, children become aware of gender differences and may point to other children and identify them as "boy" or "girl".

Emotional Development

1. Toddler who does not develop a sense of autonomy may manifest feeling of shame or doubt.
2. Children who learned to trust themselves and others during the infant year are better prepared to do this than those who cannot trust themselves or others.

Cognitive Development

1. The toddler enters the fifth and sixth stages of sensorimotor thought.
2. During the toddler years, language ability develops rapidly.
3. In tertiary circular reaction stage (12 and 18 months) – describes the toddler as "a little scientist" because of the child's interest in trying to discover new ways to handle objects or new results different actions can achieve.
4. At the end of the toddler period, children enter a second major period of cognitive development–preoperational thought. During this period, children deal much more constructively with symbols then they did while still in the sensorimotor period of cognition.
5. Cognitively toddler are able to recognize and distinguish between shapes of objects, but they are only beginning to classify objects into categories of use.

Play Behavior

1. The toys toddler enjoys most are those they can play with by themselves and that require action.
2. Fifteen months old children are still in a put in, take out stage, so they continue to enjoy stacks of boxes or balls that fit inside each other.

3. They enjoy throwing toys out of a playpen or from a highchair tray as long as someone will pick them up and return them again and again.
4. By age 2 years, toddler began to spend time, imitating adult action in their play, for example, wrapping a doll and putting in to bed, setting the table or driving the car.

Spiritual Development

1. Fowler defined faith as a relational phenomenon, an active relationship with another, a commitment, belief, love and/or hope, which may be directed towards family, religion, god or friends.
2. Attending religious programs similar to a nursery school that emphasize appropriate behavior and positive self-esteem rather than a lesson is important as well.
3. Children at this stage also know that imitating or confirming to rituals results in approval of others who are important to the child.

Major Learning Events

Toilet Training

1. Physical maturation must be reached and attitude of parents play a vital role.
2. Psychological readiness of a child such as able to inform the parent of the need to urinate or defecate.
3. Process of training should begin usually with bowel and bladder.
4. Parental response is to choose a specific word for the act.

Need for Independence without Overprotection

1. Parents should be consistent and set realistic limits.
2. Reinforce desired behavior.
3. Be constructive, geared to teach self-control.

Health Promotion for Toddlers

Childhood Nutrition

1. Provide adequate nutrient intake to meet continuing growth and development needs.
2. Provide a basis for support of psychosocial development in relation to food patterns, eating behavior and attitudes.
3. Provide sufficient calories for increasing physical activities and energy needs.

Injury Prevention

1. Children under 5 years of age account for over half of all accidental deaths during childhood.
2. More than half of accidental child deaths are related to automobiles and fire.
3. Aspirating small objects and putting foreign bodies in ear or nose.
4. Prevention through parent education and child protection is the goal.

Common Health Problems in Toddler

Burns

1. Second and third common causes of death by in individuals less than 15 years of age for boys and girls respectively.

2. Causative agents are thermal, chemical, electrical and radiation.
3. The clinical features are edema formation, fluid loss, circulatory stasis, burn shock and decreased cardiac output.

Poisoning

1. Ingestion of a toxic substances or an excessive amount of a substances.
2. More than 90 percent of poisoning occurs in the home and highest incident occurs in children under 4 years.
3. Improper storage is the major contributing factor of poisoning.

Fracture

1. In children, bones are more easily injured, facture can result without major injury to surrounding tissues.
2. Healing occurs rapidly in children, rapidity of healing is inversely related to the age of the child.
3. The clinical features of facture are generalized swelling, pain or tenderness, diminished function or use of part.

Aspiration of Foreign Objects

1. Obstruction of the airway by a foreign object, can occur any where from larynx to bronchi.
2. It is most common in children 1 to 3 years of age leading cause of fatal injury in children less than 1 year of age.
3. Foods that cause asphyxiation include round candy peanuts, grapes and popcorn.
4. The clinical finding of complete obstruction is substantial retractions, inability to cough or speak, increased pulse rate, respiratory rate and cyanosis.
5. Turn the small child upside down head lower than chest and deliver up to five quick, sharp back blows with the heel of the hand.
6. Abdominal thrust for children aged 1 year and older (Heimlich maneuver).

Child Maltreat

1. One of the most significant social problem affecting children.
2. Majority of abused children are under 4 years of age about 70 to 80 percentage of abuse is by parents or other caregivers.
3. It may be intentional physical abuse or neglect, emotional abuse or neglect and sexual abuse of children.
4. Therapeutic intervention includes treat injury and identifies and protect child from further abuse.

Mental Retardation

1. The DSM-IV defines cognitive impairment on the basis of two criteria; significantly subaverage general intellectual functioning – an intelligence quotient (IQ) of 70 or below.
2. The common causes of cognitive impairment are chromosomal abnormalities, infection *in utero*, and anoxia at birth, fetal alcohol syndrome, and head trauma.
3. Assessment done by using standardized tests notably the Wechsler Intelligence Scale for Children (WISC) or the Stanford-Binet.

Cerebral Palsy

1. Nonspecific term for a neuromuscular disability or difficulty in controlling voluntary muscles.
2. Major causes are anoxia of the brain, congenital or neonatal infection, trauma or prematururity.
3. Clinical findings are delayed motor, speech development, reflex abnormalities and difficulty in sucking and swallowing.
4. Management includes multidisciplinary approach, mobility devices, and surgery to correct spastic muscle imbalance, medication, speech, physio and occupational therapy.

General Nursing Care of Toddlers

1. **Immunization:** Caregivers should be encouraged to complete the initial immunization series in a timely manner to protect their child from infectious diseases.
2. **Nutrition:** Calorie and nutrient requirements increases with age so the caretaker should consider for child's appetite, choices and motor skills.
3. **Elimination:** The nurse should educate parents about the signs of readiness for toilet training, which include the ability to demonstrate cognitive awareness of elimination.
4. **Hygiene:** Toddlers are usually bathed either everyday or every other day, depending on their activity and state of cleanliness. It is always important check the temperature of the bath, water with a thermometer if possible.
5. **Dental health:** An important aspect of the visit is assessment of oral health, education of caretaker regarding correct methods of dental hygiene and counseling on strategies to prevent caries.
6. **Rest and sleep:** Most 2 years old requires 12-14 hours of sleep each day with one or two naps a day. Nightmare is also common in toddlerhood since their dreams seem very real.
7. **Safety and injury prevention:** Prevent can be done through parent education and child protection.

THE PRESCHOOLERS

Introduction

The preschool years span 3 to 6. Although physical growth slows, this is a time characterized by reinforcement of the cognitive, cognitive and social skill begun during the toddler years. The preschooler establishes control of body systems as indicated by the ability to toilet, dress, and feed self and is also able to tolerate longer periods of separation from caregivers and interact cooperatively with adult and other children.

Characteristics of Preschooler

1. **Period of slow and steady growth:** Where the preschooler is the period of rapid and intensive growth the stage of childhood is characterized as the period of slow, steady and uniform growth occurs.
2. **Independence:** Infact at this stage he feels more at home with the world and takes satisfaction by doing his work with his own efforts. By acquiring experiences and developing physically and socially he tries to adjust himself in his environment.
3. **Emotional stability and control:** The preschoolers exercise control over his emotions and express them in appropriate and socially approved ways. His emotional behavior is not guided by instinctive causes but has an appropriate national behind it.

4. **Developing social tendency:** He likes to play in group and share his toys with others. Feeling of mutual cooperation, team spirit and group loyalties are developed among children of their age.
5. **Realistic attitude:** Child at the stage begins to accept and appreciate the hard realities in place of imaginative idealist. He begins to take close interest in the world of realities and tries to adapt himself in real environment.
6. **Formation of sentiments and complexes:** The child at this stage in not in the habit of hiding the feelings and checking his emotions. Therefore, no complexes and formed at this stage whereas childhood stage. At this stage of preschooler's emotional behavior get itself structured into sentiments. Various sentiments like religious, moral, patriotic and esthetic sentiments begin to develop at this stage.

Physical Development

1. **Biological growth:** Children in preschooler grow relatively slowly; they become taller and thinner without gaining much weight.
2. **Weight and height:** The preschooler gains approximately 1.8 kg per year. At age of three years, the child weighs an average of 14.4 kg and at five years, the average weight is 18.3 kg.
3. **Baby proportions:** The typical preschooler looks more like adult than does the toddler because of skeletal maturation. The head and neck continue to decrease in proportion to the size of the rest of the body. The lower extremities grow faster than the head, trunk and arms.
4. **Cardiovascular system:** By age 4 years, heart size is four times birth size and is now similar to that of the adult heart. Murmurs may be discovered during the late preschooler period.
5. **Blood values:** During the preschooler years, fat replaces the red marrow of the long bones. The total leukocyte count is slight higher: 5000 to 13000 from 4 to 6 years of age.
6. **Respiratory system:** With growth, the length of structures in the respiratory tract has increased and the incidence of infections decreases.
7. **Gastrointestinal system:** The process of digestion is mature at this time, but the gastrointestinal system is vulnerable to stress, which may be manifested by mild to moderate dysfunction.
8. **Genitourinary system:** The urinary system is nearly mature by age 5 years. The urine output in the age group is 600 to 750 ml for a 24 hours period. Daytime bladder control is achieved by the end of the preschooler period, with nightmare control still variable.
9. **Immune system:** Adult level of immunoglobulin A [Iq A] are reached during the preschool years. Also children develop antibodies to the agents they are exposed to and to the normal flora in their body.
10. **Nervous system:** By 5 years of age, the nervous system comprises one-twentieth of the total body weight. Cerebral dominance is achieved, as demonstrated by the acquisition of handedness.
11. **Motor development:** As children use their muscles, muscle fibers increase in strength and size. Coordination and the ability to voluntary control movements are increases significantly, allowing them to refine their skills.

Emotional Development

1. The preschooler watches adults and attempt to imitate their behavior.
2. Imagination and creativity allow them to fantasize, trying-out roles and behaviors.
3. Preschool children look forward to becoming like their father and mother. They learn adult roles from their parents, who serve as role models for behavior.

4. A feeling of conflict may also arise from thoughts the child realizes actions were not appropriate. Feeling of guild may also arise from thoughts the child has that are different from expected behaviors.
5. The goal of caregivers during period is to assist children to learn about the world and other people. With this help, preschooler gradually modifies their egocentricity.

Sexual Development

1. Sexual energy, generally, at this stage remains dominant but merges with great forces at the end of the stage.
2. The sexual behavior of the children at this stage is characterized by the development of an attitude of antagonism and indifference towards opposite sex.
3. While this stages the boys and girls play together, they wish to play with the members of their own sex.
4. Due to their varied interests they gradually develop a general attitude of antagonism towards the sexes naturally draws apart. Even when brought together in family gathering boys and girls of this age are barely civil to one another.
5. Sex antagonism enmore pronounced in boys than in the case of girls, the attitude of antagonism, generally takes the form of indifference.

Cognitive Development

1. During Piaget's preoperational stage, between the ages of 2 and 6 years, the child develops the ability to perform mental operations governed by personal perceptions and linkage to events previously experienced.
2. At this stage the child acquires new experiences and tries to adopt himself in his environment and prepares himself to solve the problems.
3. The preschooler gains power of reasoning, thinking observation, concentration, perception, imagination, etc. are developed.
4. He develops the concept of length, time and distance and learns to express himself in various ways.
5. The preschooler uses a personal system for organizing objects and events in his or her mind and reasons from one particular to another, often by unrelated events, when in reality the particulars are not linked at all.

Moral Development

1. The child's moral development is at the most basic level and right and wrong are determined through from rules parents have established.
2. Preschoolers conform to rules strictly for the purpose self-interest that is, to avoid punishment and to have favors returned.
3. According to Kohlberg, moral growth occurs in specific sequences of developmental stages that are preconventional or premoral stage.

Spiritual Development

1. Preschool children continue in fowlers stage of intuitive—projective faith.
2. The preschooler has a concrete conception of god, who has physical characteristics and can understand simple religious stories.

3. The preschool children accept the religion of their parents because for them, parents are omnipotent and powerful.
4. Preschool children are old enough to go to Sunday school. Any discussion of religion should be shared experience between parents and their children.

Language and Speech Development

1. Preschool children use language in a symbolic way. They not only imitate sounds at this stage but also use words to represent things.
2. Language is used by preschoolers to communicate their feelings and ideas. They consistently ask questions and learn about the outside world by seeking the meaning of what they experience through sensory stimulates.
3. Preschool children use progressively longer and more complex sentences and their vocabulary grows rapidly.
4. An analysis of child's questions shows a need for information, for relief from anxiety and for attention.
5. Preschoolers delight in trying out a variety of words. They are unconcerned about the consequences of language and are prone to pick-up words that parents may prefer, they not to have their vocabulary.

Play Activities

1. Play facilitates the development of an optional self-identity by establishment of an imaginary friend, which helps a child work through a particular different time.
2. Activities that promote small muscle development encourage a child's creativity and fine motor skills.
3. Preschool children play actively, they climb, run, hammer, open doors with a bang; and slam them shut.
4. The repetitive play of preschool children is an imitation of the life about them. Many play themes stem from a confusion in children's minds about experiences they have had a real life.
5. The children need to be encouraged to express their own creativity rather than fitting them within a mold of adult expectation. They should be allowed and encouraged to play with toys of their choice independent of gender—role designation.

Nurses Role in Health Promotion

1. **Nutrition:** Preschooler need to eat only one-half as much as adult. The daily requirements ranges from 1300 to 1700 calories, including 30 g proteins. The preschoolers enjoy five meals a day to keep up with energy demand. Food should be selected from the basic four food groups, with a limit of 16 ounces of milk daily.
2. **Accident prevention:** During the preschool years the child begins to explore outside the home and into the neighborhood. It is also important to remember that the preschool-aged child is less reckless, will listen more to rules, and is aware of potential dangers such as hot objects, sharp instruments, or dangerous heights.
3. **Hygiene:** Many preschoolers enjoy their bath time, but the parental assistance may be needed for hair washing, and cleaning finger nails and ears.
4. **Dental health:** The number one dental problem during this time is dental caries, which may cause the premature loss of teeth and a consequent alteration of dental arch, compromising development of the permanent teeth. The preschool child should visit a dentist at least 6 months.

5. **Rest and sleep:** The preschooler sleep a total of 12 hours a day. Preschoolers may have difficulty sleeping in a dark, a proper parental support and guidance is essential during time.

THE SCHOOL CHILD

Introduction

1. The phase of development from 6 to 12 years, the school-age years, is crucial to establishing positive self-esteems, a sense of belonging and feeling of competence. The school children gain new ideas from adults outside the family : Teacher, parents of their friends, policemen and women, television performers, newspaper writers and authors of textbooks with those of their parents.
2. School children learn to think of themselves as person in their own right may resent limits that parents continue to improve on their behavior. Parents need help in understanding the normal growth and development of their child when conflicts areises.Today, child can experience the world beyond the classroom with the help of the internet, electronic mail, educational video tapes and cable television.

Physical Growth and Development

Biological Growth

1. Weight and height during the school years show a sex related difference. Boys tend to gain slightly more weight through 12 years.
2. The yearly height gain is similar in boys and girls, although boys tend to be taller.

Cardiovascular System

1. The heart assumes a more vertical position in the chest because of left ventricular development and downward placement of the diaphragm.
2. Heart murmur peak during 6 to 9 years of age.

Immune System

1. The immune system continues to develop; response to infection is specific and localized.
2. Normal adult levels of the immunoglobulin are reached during the school years.
3. The increased amount of lymphatic tissue in the nasopharynx continues to cause blockage of the Eustachian tube.
4. As the child reaches puberty and the amount of lymphatic tissue decreases, ear infection decreases in direct proportion.

Nervous System

1. By 10 years of age, the nervous system is essentially mature.
2. The maturity is evident in the sensory and motor functions as well as in the cognitive process.

Sensory Development

1. By the time the child reaches the age of 6 years, central visual acuity is established.
2. At age 7 years, visual acuity should be 20/20, which is the adult level.
3. The accommodative and refractive powers of the eye also reach stability.
4. The sense of taste and smell fully mature prior to the school years, allows for greater discrimination.

Skeletomuscular Development

1. Skeletal growth is particularly noticeable in the long bones of the extremities. Growing pain, which occur because the long bone grows faster than the attached muscles.
2. Muscle strength and size also increase at a gradual rate during school age years and six basic gross motor skills such as balancing, catching, throwing, and running; jumping, climbing, continue to be refined.
3. At the same time, improved balance and coordination enable the school-aged child to explore new physical activities, such as bike riding and roller lading.
4. Boys have a greater number of muscle cells than girls, so it is common to find they do well gross motor activities such as throwing and running.

Motor Development

1. Motor development progress in a cephalocaudal and proximal to distal direction, with reinforcement of both gross motor and fine motor skills occurring as the central nervous system matures.
2. The developmental theory of Erik H Erikson identified the major task of the school-age period as identity versus inferiority.
3. During this time, energy is channeled into activities such as school projects, sports and bobbies. The school-age child also develops the ability to work with others on school projects and athletic terms in preparation for becoming a citizen of the world.
4. School children must grow out of the dependency on their family and must find satisfaction in the company of peer groups and adults outside the home environment.
5. During the school years the child develops whole some attitudes towards set as a person and learns the appropriate masculine or feminine social role.

Psychosexual Development

1. Freud believed that, starting at age 6 years and throughout school-age, the child enters a calm period in the development of their sexuality called latency.
2. Freud theorized the school-aged child identified with the same sex parent by modeling the behaviors and emotional of this parent and learned about sex-role behavior and identify by observing caregiver instructions. The media and friendship with children of the same gender.
3. School-age children become much less egocentric and direct their energies beyond themselves. During the early latency period children associate with same sex peers and tend to ignore members of the same age and tend to draw apart from them.
4. Boys and girls should be informed about the reproductive cycle and their respective roles as they approach puberty.

Spiritual Development

1. In school years, fowler identified school children as being in the mythicliteral faith stage.
2. During these years, children are learning many specifics about their children that will develop into a religious philosophy to be used in their interpretation of the world.
3. As children reach pubescence, they begin to be less mythical in their thinking and their beliefs are more controlled by reason.
4. As the child enters preadolescence, he or she realizes self-centered prayers are not always answered and there is no magic involved in religious beliefs, blind faith that previously existed in the younger child is replaced by reason.

Cognitive Development

1. Piaget suggested that around 6 years of age children start to move from the egocentric view of the preschool-age to the more open and flexible thought of the school-aged child.
2. By 7 to 11 years during concrete operational stage characterized by considerable growth in thinking, imagination and language, which allows school-age children to expand and understand their world.
3. School-age children are increasingly able to classify objects in a more complex manner then they could during the preschool years.
4. The school children mental ability permits them to carry on converse and reverse process. They can solve problems because they can manipulate symbols.
5. During the school-age periods, children think not only of the present but also the past and future. Since children can recall events that happened in the past, they become aware that exist over a period of time.

Moral Development

1. The school-aged child is at the conventional level of moral development, when the conscience develops an internal set of "rules" that must be followed in order to "be good".
2. During third stage of moral development, the child's morality is based on avoiding the disapproval of others and maintaining a positive relationship with friends, family and teachers.
3. Children at this level can also demonstrate rigid behavior in an effort to obey the law. These children can take into account circumstances surrounding and incident rather than just looking at the result.

Language and Speech Development

1. During this period of development, children show tremendous growth in their ability to use words.
2. They extend their vocabulary by 20,000 to 30,000 words.
3. Their sentence structure and use of grammar continue to improve and the use if adjectives and pronouns increases.
4. Speech proceeds from egocentric to social. The unique culture of their children is reflects in language acquisition and speech patterns.

Play Activities

1. Plays activities vary with age, number of play activities decreases, whereas the amount of time spent in one particular activity increases.
2. Likes games with rules because of increased mental abilities.
3. Likes games of athletic competition because of increased motor ability.
4. Play serves as a learning tool for children and their play changes with developmental needs.
5. Play becomes more formal, more organized, more competitive and to a degreeless physical active.
6. Parent can assist their school children with learning the rules of organized sports. Although parents may not attending sports events and others activities in which their children participate.

Mental Abilities of School Children

1. Readiness for learning, especially in perceptual organization: Names, months of year, knows right from left, can tell time, can follow several directions at once.

2. Acquires use of reason and understanding of rules, needs consistency.
3. Trial-and-error problem solving become more conceptual rather than action oriented.
4. Reasoning ability allows greater understanding and use of language.

Role of Nurse in Health Promotion

Nutrition

1. Children aged 7 to 10 years require 80 calories per kilogram of body weight.
2. After age in years through adolescence, boys require more protein and iron.
3. Careful meal and physical activity are crucial for the physical and emotional health of the school-aged child.

Accident Prevention

1. Factors contributing to the high incidence of accidents for this group are their increased independence, desire to have peer approach and increased involvement in physically challenging activities.
2. Most accidents are related to motor vehicles, but firearm injuries continue to increase in incidence. The second most frequent cause of accidental death is drowning.
3. Accidents also occur when children are skating, skateboarding or riding a bicycle or minibike.

Elimination

1. School children are old enough to attend school all day, they have learned to control and independently care for their own elimination patterns.
2. Usually stools are well-formed and school-aged children have one to two stools per day. The amount of urine passed is depended on intake, temperature, time of the day and childs emotional state.

Hygiene

1. Children older than 6 or 7 years of age are capable of carrying out their own personal hygiene practices daily and by the time they are 8 or 9 can be held responsible for independently bathing, grooming, dressing and properly discarding their sold clothing.
2. As children become more aware of changes in their bodies are they reach late school-age, they begin to take more interest in and are more reliable in their own grooming and cleanliness.

Dental Health

1. Dental caries resulting from poor nutrition is still a significant problem in the school-age population. Raw sugars and candies are common contributors to the development of dental caries.
2. Dental checkups are recommended every 6 months the school system should incorporate a dental health educational program into the curriculum.

Sleep and Rest

1. The 6 years old child may need 11 to 12 hours of sleep, whereas the 12 years old generally needs only 10 hours.

2. Sleep is essential during the school-age years to foster physical growth and academic performance and failure to receive adequate rest can lead to irritability and lack of attention span at school.
3. Nightmares and night-terrors are less common during the school-age years.

Sex Education

1. It is important and that school-age children be educated about pubertal changes and responsible sexual practices.
2. Sex education should be incorporated into health education throughout the school years in a manner that is appropriate to age and development.

Common Problems Associated with School Children

School Phobia

1. School phobia is fear of attending school. It is a type of "social phobia" similar to agoraphobia (fear of going outside the home).
2. Children who resist attending school this way may develop physical signs of illness, such as vomiting, diarrhea, headache or abdominal pain on school days.
3. The causes of resistance to school, the child may be over dependent on the parents or may be reluctant to leave home because he or she feels that younger siblings will usurp the parent affection while he or she is at school.
4. Handling school phobia requires coordination among the school, school nurse and health care providers who diagnoses the problem.
5. The nurse is the ideal person to coordinate such efforts and to help the parents allow the child some independence not only in going to school but in other activities.

Stealing

1. During early school-age, most children go through a period in which they steal loose change from their mother's purse of father's dresser.
2. This usually happens at around 7 years of age, when they are learning how to make change and discovering the importance of money.
3. Youngsters, who continue to steal, may require counseling, because they should have progressed beyond this normal development step by this age.

Recreational Drug Use

1. Recreational drug use was once considered a college or high school problem is now a problem of school-age. Illegal drugs are available to children as early as elementary school and certainly by the time they reach the seventh or eight grades.
2. Alcohol is available in so many homes and often can be purchased in small stores without proof of age; it is a commonly abused drug of this age group. Cocaine is becoming increasingly easy for children to obtain.
3. Parents should suspect of recreational drug use if their child regularly appears irritable, inattentive or drowsy. School health personnel should be aware of the increase in this practice among students and look for warning signs.

4. Children need to be counseled against this because the recreational drug use leads to cardiovascular irregularities, uncontrollable aggressiveness and possible cancer in later life.
5. Both nurses and parents should be role models of excellent health behaviors when earning for school-age children.

Obesity

1. Many perteenagers, particularly boys, become overweight. Some have been overweight since infancy their propubertal neutral weight gain makes them obese.
2. Obese children begin to develop many of the same health problems as obsess adults, such as hypertension, and elevated total cholesterol level with possible atherosclerosis.
3. A weight reduction program for school-age children that emphasis long-term life changes such as intake about 1200 calories low in fat and designed to reduce weight, active exercise program and counseling program.

THE ADOLESCENT

Introduction

Adolescent is the time period between 13 years and 18 to 20 years, which serves as a transition period between childhood and adulthood. It is a time of explosion, excitement and discovery and sometimes confusion and despair. Adolescent consist of early, middle and late stages. Each is distinguishing by several aspects of adolescent lives and constitute the ages 12-14, 15-17 and 18-21years.

Physical Growth and Development

Weight and Height

Most of the girls are 1 to 2 inches taller than boys coming in to adolescence and generally stop growing with in 3 years from menarche. Thus, those girls who start menstruating at 10 years of age may reach their adult height by age 13.

Musculoskeletal Development

1. Significant changes occur in skeletal size, muscle mass, skin and adipose tissue. Full bone length is first reached in the extremities and moves inwards.
2. The skeletal system grows faster than the muscles and muscle mass increases more rapidly than the hear size.

Teeth

1. Adolescent gains their molars (wisdom teeth) between 18 and 21 years of age. The jaw reaches about size only toward the end of adolescence.
2. Adolescent, whose third molars erupt before the lengthening of the jaw is complete may experience pain and may need these molars extracted because they do not fit their jaw line.

Central Nervous System

1. Brain growth continuous during adolescence, the cell that support and nourish the nervous proliferate even though the number of neurons does not increase.

2. Continued growth of myelin sheath allows faster neural processing and is reflected in the adolescent's increasing ability to think abstractly and hypothesize.

Cardiorespiratory Development

1. The heart almost doubles in weight and increase in the size by about one-half during adolescence.
2. The lung increases in length and diameter during adolescence, and the respiratory rate averages 16-20 breaths per minute.
3. Males have greater capacity, volume and rate because their great shoulder width and chest size.
4. The slower of respiratory system growth relatives to the growth of other body system may be another cause of the inadequate oxygenation and fatigue sometimes experienced by adolescents.

Gastrointestinal System

1. Rapid maturation of the gastrointestinal system occurs during adolescence, and by the 21st birthday, all 32 teeth have erupted.
2. Gastric acidity and capacity increase up to 1500 ml to accommodate and facilitate digestion of the increased food intake that occurs in response to rapid growth.

Genitourinary System Development

1. Secretion of neurohormonal releasing factors by the hypothalamus stimulates the anterior pituitary gland to release follicle-stimulating hormone and luteinizing hormone.
2. In females, FSH stimulates growth ovarian follicle growth and estrogen production. Estrogen causes breast changes, including enlargement and darkening of the reproductive organs such as vagina, uterus, ovaries and growth and darkening of pubic and axillaries hair.
3. In males, FSH is responsible for sperm production and maturation of the seminiferous tubules. LH promotes testicular maturation and testosterone production. Testosterone causes the musculoskeletal system and development of the male reproductive system.

Sexual Development

1. Adolescence is the physiologic period between the beginning of puberty and cessation of bodily growth.
2. Puberty is the stage of life at which secondary sex changes begin. Girls begin dramatic development and maturation of reproductive organs at approximately and maturation of reproductive organs at approximately age of 10 to 13 years; for boys 12 to 14 years.
3. Androgenic hormones are responsible for muscular development, physical growth and increase in sebaceous gland secretions that cause typical acne in both boys and girls.
4. In girls pubertal changes typically occurs, such as growth spurt, increase in the transverse diameter of the pelvis, breast development, growth of pubic hair, onset of maturation, growth of axillary hair and vaginal secretions.
5. The average age at which menarche (the first menstrual period) occurs is 12.5 years. It may occur as early as age as 9 or as late as age 17 years, however, still be within a normal age range.
6. A menstrual cycle can be defined as periodic uterine bleeding in response to cyclic hormonal changes. It is the process that allows for conception and implantation of a new life.
7. Education regarding menstruation is an important aspect of comprehensive sexuality education.

Psychosexual Development

1. According to Freud, the physical changes of puberty reawaken the sexual and aggressive energies felt toward parents during latency a late childhood.
2. Freud argued many psychological issues adolescents face are attributable to physiological changes.

Psychosocial Development

1. According to Erikson, the development task of youngsters in early and midadolescence is to form a sense of identity. If the young persons do not achieve a sense of identity, they develop a sense of role confusion.
2. Body image—adolescents, who developed a strong sense of industry during their school-age have learned to solve problems and are best equipped to adjust to their new body image.
3. Value system—adolescents need to be able to take to peers to develop values. They dress identically with other members of the group.
4. An important part of adolescents self understanding is the value they place on their definition of who they are, which involves self-competency and self-worth.
5. According to Erikson, the youth who is not sure of his identity, shies away from inter personal intimacy or throw himself into acts of intimacy which may involved in intimate relations.

Cognitive Development

1. The final stage of cognitive development, the state of formal operations, begins at age 12 or 13 years and grows in depth over the adolescent years.
2. This step involves the ability to think in abstract terms and use the scientific method to arrive at conclusions. Problem solving in any situation depends on the ability to think abstractly and logically.
3. They can create a hypothesis and think through the probable consequences. Thinking abstractly is what allows adolescent to project themselves into the minds of others and imagine how others view them or their actions.
4. Another significant change is cognitive development. Adolescence generally becomes more sophisticated in their ability to understand words and their related concepts.
5. Another important aspect of adolescent's cognitive development is their broadening ability to assume another perspective.

Moral Development

1. Kohlberg's conventional level of moral reasoning, which has been shown to emerge during adolescence and to persist as the predominant stage of moral functioning thought adulthood.
2. Adolescent male would likely reflect judgment-based reasoning of fourth stage thinking, whereas female adolescents would more likely reflect the relationship based on the third stage.
3. Abstract thinking-new level of social communication and understanding can comprehend satire and double meanings. They can say one thing and mean another.

Spiritual Development

1. Almost all adolescent's question the existence of God and any religious practices they can taught.
2. This questioning is a part of forming a sense of identity and establishing a value system at a time in life when they draw away from their families.

3. Religious and scientific views are often compared as teens decide what is true. More emphasis is placed on internal aspects of religious commitment rather than on attending church.
4. Adolescent's become more oriented towards spiritual and ideological matters and less oriented towards practice, rituals, and strictly observing religious costumes.
5. The late adolescent tends to re-examine and re-evaluate the beliefs and values of childhood and become more personalizes less bound to the traditional religious practices expressed to when younger.

Health Promotion during Adolescent

Nutrition

1. The nutrional objective is to provide nutritional support for demand of rapid growth and high energy expenditure.
2. Support development of appropriate eating habits through verity of foods, regular pattern, and good quality snakes.
3. Nutrition education may be made through association with teenagers concerns about physical appearance, finger control, complexion, physical fitness, athletic ability.

Safety Measures

1. Accidents, most common those involving motor vehicles, are the leading cause of death among adolescents.
2. Drowning is one of the chief accident and athletic injuries tend to occur during adolescence because of the vigorous level of competition that occur.
3. Appropriate education regarding sexual maturity, reproduction, sexual behavior, driver education, hazards associated with smoking, alcohol and drug abuse.

Elimination

1. The elimination patterns for adolescents are similar to adults. They should void an average of 700 to 1400 ml per day and have stool everyday .
2. Constipation in adolescents may be due to a physiological disorder, eating disorder or improper nutritional patterns.

Hygiene

1. Skin care is especially important during this age because of the increased activity of the sebaceous gland, which contributes to acne, increased sweat gland activity requires careful cleansing as well as the use of deodorant and body powders.
2. For female, menstrual hygiene is especially important and may require extra attention.
3. It is important to remind parents and other adult as well as the adolescent that these physical changes that may require more attention to hygiene are normal.

Dental Hygiene

1. Adolescents are generally very conscious about toothbrushing because of fear of developing bad breath.
2. During adolescents, malocclusion, gingivitis and dental trauma may occur, malocclution occurs due to dental crowding or mandibular/facial bone growth changes.

3. The dental teaching should include brushing the teeth at twice a day using a soft- bristled brush and fluoride toothpaste, flossing daily, eating a well-balanced diet and regular dental visits.

Rest and Sleep

1. Protein synthesis occurs most readily during sleep. Because of this, adolescents need proportionately more sleep than school-age children to support the growth spurt during this time which demands the formation of so many new cells.
2. Nurses need to educate both parents and adolescents on the importance of adequate rest and sleep and encourage teens to have realistic activity schedules that do not overextend their time.
3. An adolescent's excessive anxiety and fatigue may also result in sleep disturbances, which can continue into adulthood since adult sleep cycles and habits are formed during adolescent.

Health Problems during Adolescents

Alcohol Abuse

1. Alcoholism and alcohol abuse in adolescence are increasing. Many adolescents who, do drink use it as a mind altering device since it allows participation in risk taking activities they might otherwise avoid.
2. There are numerous hazards of alcohol ingestion. Some may be seen in adolescents, including hepatitis, pancreatitis, gastritis, and neuritis, and cirrhosis, ulcer of gastrointestinal tract, cerebellar degeneration and delirium tremors.
3. Parents and nurses with adolescents who abuse or other mind altering drugs and their family members need to explain about detrimental effects.

Homosexuality

1. Nurses need to recognize that even though many young people explore their own sexual; orientation or homosexual attractions, few who engage in homosexual behavior during adolescents, continue the practice in to adulthood.
2. Nurses and caregivers recognize that homosexual experimentation is not the same as establishing homosexual orientations, acknowledge same bisexual relationships and attractions, and phrase questions about sexuality and sexual activity carefully.

Suicide

1. The number of adolescents committing suicide has increased dramatically over the last few decades.
2. Stresses related to physiosocial, psychosexual or physiological issues have been identified as cause for the increasing number of adolescent suicides.
3. Risk factors of adolescents are previous history od suicide, family history of psychiatric disorders, living without home, history of physical or sexual abuse, unable to meet scholastic expectations of parents and teachers.
4. Suicide programs for teens should be directed at school staff, community agency personnel and students themselves by providing information relative to warning signs, fact, and programs which can enhance self-esteem and social competence.

ADULTHOOD

Introduction

The young and middle adulthood is a period of challenges, rewards and crises. Challenges may include the demand of work and raising families, although adult can also be rewarded by successes in their carrier endeavors and in their personal lives. Adult development involves orderly changes in characteristics and attitudes. Developmental changes are based on earlier characteristics help to shape subsequent behavior and characteristics.

Concepts of Young Adulthood

1. Young adulthood is the period between the late teens and the mid to late thirties.
2. During young adulthood, individuals increasingly separate from their families of origin, establishing carrier goals and decide whether to many and begin families or remain single.
3. Young adults are active and must adopt to new experiences. The transition into middle age occurs when young persons become aware that changes in reproductive and physical abilities signify the beginning of another stage in life.
4. Middle age is a time of continuing transitions when individuals may reassess their goals in life and add new goals.
5. The adult face such crises as caring for their aging parents, possibilities of job loss in a changing economic environment and dealing with their own developmental needs as well as these of their family members.

Maturity Developmental Task

1. People are said to have reached maturity when they have reached a balance of growth in physiological, psychological and cognitive areas.
2. Matured individual feels comfortable with abilities, knowledge and responses that they have developed over the years.
3. They look at the world with a broad view, based on a blend of insight, emotion and imagination. They take problems that can solve but recognize and learn to live with unsolvable problems.
4. Mature people are open to suggestion and can accept constructive criticism without a major loss of self esteem.
5. They weigh other person's input and recommendations what making decisions but are not overly influenced or intimated by others, above all, mature people develop by learning from their one and other experiences.
6. Other characteristics of maturity are related to interpersonal communication and behavior.
7. Mature person acknowledge accomplishments and shortcoming. The mature adults confront tasks openly, use decision making techniques to solve problems and are accountable and responsible for their actions.

Theories of Young Adulthood

Levinson's Phases of Young and Middle Adult Development

1. Early adult transition (ages 18 to 20 years) when the person separates from the family and desires independence.
2. Entrance in to the adult world (ages 21 to 27 years) when the persons prepares for and tries out career and lifestyles.

3. Transition (ages 28 to 32 years) when the person may greatly modify life activities and thinks amount future goals.
4. Setting down (ages 33 to 39 years), when the person experiences grater stability.
5. The payoff years (ages 40 to 65 years), a time for maximal influence, self direction and appraisal.

Gilligan's (1993) Intellectual and Moral Development

1. Gilligan's theory proposes that intellectual and moral development differ between men and women.
2. Women struggle with the issues of care and responsibility and in turn their relationships progress toward a maturity of interdependence.
3. As women progress toward adulthood the moral dilemma changes from how to exercise their right without interfering in the right of others to how to lead a normal life, which includes obligations to themselves and their families and people in general.

Gordon (1991)

1. As women entered professional areas, they hoped to develop the caring and nurturing roles in their male colleagues.
2. Women have long recognized that, without caring, the perceived quality of life is changed. As a result women maintained carrying in the home and educational frustrated in their development.
3. However, women become frustrated in their development because the responsibility of caring was not shared and frequently nurturing become a gender—specific responsibilities.

Diekelmann's Developmental Tasks

1. They active independence from parental controls.
2. They begin to develop strong friendship and intimate relationships out side the family.
3. They establish personal set values.
4. They develop a sense of personal identity.
5. They prepare for life work and develop the capacity for intimacy.

Physiological Development

1. The young adult has completed physical growth by the age of 20. The young adult usually quite active, experience severe illnesses less commonly than older adults.
2. A personal life assessment of the young adult includes assessment of general life satisfaction, hobbies and interests.

Cognitive Development

1. Rational thinking habits increase steadily through the young and middle adult years. Formal and informal educational experiences, general life experiences and occupational opportunities dramatically increase the individual's conceptual, problem solving and motor skills.
2. Identifying preferred occupational areas is a major task of young adults. When people known their educational preparation, skills, talents and personality characteristics, occupational choices are easier and they generally more satisfied with their choices.
3. The young adults are continually evolving and adjusting to changes in the home, work place, and personal lives their decision-making processes should be flexible.

Psychosocial Development

1. The young adult is usually caught between wanting to prolong the irresponsibility of adolescence and wanting to assume adult commitments.
2. The years from 35 to 43 are a time of vigorous examination of life goals, relationships; alterations are made in personal, social and occupational lives.
3. During young adults, people generally give more attention to occupational and social pursuits. During this period individuals attempt top improve their socioeconomic status.
4. During young adults, they take major decisions concerning career, marriage and parenthood.

Health Promotion during Young Adult

1. Young adult lifestyles may putty them at risk for illnesses or disabilities during their middle or older adult tears. Young adults may also be genetically susceptible to certain chronic disease such as diabetes mellitus and familial hyperchostermia.
2. Violence is the greater cause of mortality and morbidity in the young adult population. Death and injury can occur from physical assault, motor vehicle or other accidents and suicidal attempts.
3. Intoxicated young adults may be severely injured in motor vehicle accidents that may result in death or permanent disability to other young adults as well.
4. Sexually transmitted diseases have immediate effects such as discharge, discomfort and infection. They may also lead to chronic disorders, which can result from genital herpes, infertility, gonorrhea or even death.

THE FAMILY

Introduction

The family is an open system, exchanging information and energy within itself and with its environment. Because of its nature and dynamic interaction, the family can change. Families develop their individuals' repetitive ways of functioning. For events that necessitate change within a family, the members will either support or inhibit the factors that permit the change.

Definitions

1. Family is a group defined by a sex relationship sufficiently precise and enduring to provide for the procreation and upbringing of children.
2. Family is a group of persons whose relatives to one another are based upon consanguinity and who are therefore kin to another.
3. Family is a socially recognized unit of people related to each other by kinship, marital and legal ties.

Characteristics of Family

1. **A mating relationship:** A family comes into existence when a man and women establish mating relation between them. This relation may be of a shorter duration of life-long.
2. **A form of marriage:** Mating relationship is established through the institution of marriage. The partners may be selected by parents or by the elders or the choice may be left to the wishes of the individuals concerned.
3. **A system of nomenclature:** Every family is known by a name and has its own system of reckoning decent.

4. **An economic provision:** Every family needs an economic provision to satisfy the economic needs. The head of the family carriers on certain profession and earns money to maintain family.
5. **A common habitation:** A family requires a home or house hold for its living. Without a dwelling place the task of childbearing and childrearing cannot be adequately performed.
6. **Structure of the family:**
   - The basic unit of a society.
   - Composition varies, although one member is usually recognized as head.
   - Usually shares common goals and beliefs.
   - Role change within the group and reflect both individuals and group's needs.
   - Status of members determined by position in family in conjunction with views of society.

Functions of the Family

1. **Reproduction:** Group developed to reproduce and rear members of a society.
2. **Maintenance to provide:**
   - Clothing, housing, food and medical care.
   - Social, psychological and emotional support for family members.
   - Protection because immaturity of young children necessitates that care be given by adults.
   - Status—child is a member of family that is also apart of the larger community.
3. **Socialization:**
   - Child is "acculturated" by introduction to social situations and instruction in appropriate social behaviors.
   - Self identity develops through relationships with other family members.
   - Child learns appropriate sex roles and responsibilities.

Growth of Individual Members Towards Maturity and Independence

Family Life Cycle

Families like individuals, passthrough predictable developmental stages. To predict the likelihood of family using health promotion activities, therefore, it is helpful to assess its developmental stage.

Stages of Life Cycle
1. *Marriage and family*
   - During this stage of family development, members work to achieve the separate identifiable tasks.
   - Establish a mutually satisfying relationship.
   - Learn to relate well to their families of orientation.
   - Establishing a mutually satisfying relationship from the families of orientation.
   - This first stage of family development is a tenuous one, as evidenced by the high rate of diverse or separation of partners at this stage.
2. *The early childbearing family*
   - The birth or adoption of a first baby is usually an exciting yet stressful event, which requires economic and social role changes.
   - An important nursing role during this period is health education about well-child care and how to integrate new members into a family.
   - It is further developmental step to change from being able care for a well baby to caring for an ill baby.
   - The parents, who have difficulty with this step need a great deal of support and counseling from health care providers.

3. *The family with preschool children*
   - A family with preschool children is a busy family because children at this stage demand a great deal of time related to growth and developmental needs and safety considerations as accidents because a major health concern.
   - If a child is hospitalized because of an accident, parents may have difficulty facing the injury because they feel they should have done more to prevent the accident.
4. *The family with school-age children*
   - Parents of school-age, children have the important responsibility of preparing their children to be able to function in a complex world while at the same time maintaining their own satisfying.
   - Important nursing concerns during this family stage are monitoring children's health in terms of immunization, dental care and health care assessment; monitoring child's safety related to electrical and automobile accidents.
5. *The family with adolescent children*
   - The primary goal for a family with teenagers differs considerable from the goal of the family in previous stages, which was to strengthen family ties and maintain family unity.
   - The nurse working with families at this stage, she needs to spend time for counseling on safety, proper care and respect for firearms, the danger of drug abuse and safe sex practices.
6. *The launching center family*
   - The parental roles change from those of mother or father to once removed support people or guideposts.
   - The stage may represent a loss of self-esteem for parents, who feel themselves being replaced by other people in their children's lives.
7. *The family of middle years*
   - When a family returns to a two-partner nuclear unit, as it was before childbearing, the partner may view this stage either as the prime time of their lives.
   - Having a baby at this point in life may be viewed as exciting or worrisome, depending individual circumstances.

THE OLDER ADULT

Introduction

Geriatrics, the care of aged, aging is a normal process of time-related change that occurs thought life. It involves all aspects of the organism and is largely characterized by decline in functional efficiency and decreased capacity to compensate and recover from stress. It dose not necessarily occur in an inter-related or synchronous manner, but it does involve physiological, psychological and social changes that interact to influence behavior and adaptation.

Concepts of Old Age

1. Old age is a normal part of human development and is the final phase of the life cycle.
2. Aging is not something that happens to the other person but is a unique and highly personal experience that affects everyone who lives long enough.
3. Successful adaptation to the aging process probably correlates with the person's previous ability to cope and adopt to change.
4. Other influences include environmental factors, education and sociocultural determinants as well as the health status of the entire body.

5. Gerontology, the study of the aging process and its effects on older persons, become more important with each passing day.

Developmental Theories of Old Age

1. Certain theoretical models of human development help to point out impotent turning points during the late years of the cycle.
2. The theories concerning the life cycle incorporate the social, psychological and biological factors of developmental growth and relate them to age to identity milestones and time development.
3. The theories of Buhler, Jung and Erikson, which are considered to be three of the most prominent theories of adult development, have as a common theme the goal of personal resolution in the second half of life.
4. Buhler's theories perceived that the period from 65 on is one of awareness of the experience of fulfillment or failure, and the remaining years are spend in either a continuance of previous activities or a return to the need satisfying orientations of childhood.
5. Jung suggested that in the second half of life the individual direct his attention inward, so that through an intensive inner exploration he may find a meaning and totality in life that makes the acceptance of death possible.
6. Erikson's theory explains that the years between 40 and 50 challenge those values that a person places on physical power in favor of the value placed on wisdom. People who cling to their waning physical powers becoming more and more depressed, but persons who shift to using their mental abilities as a primary resource appear to age more successfully.
7. The theorists view the first part of life as growth and expansion and the later pat of life as inner withdrawal and contraction.
8. The task of later life involves finding meaning and wholeness in life and considerations about oncoming death.

Kinds of Age

Biological Aging

1. Aging occurs with such changes as whitening of the hair, wrinkling of the skin, decline in eye focus and high-register hearing.
2. Biological aging depends on a combination of factors, including genetic inheritance, finances and good health.
3. The most serious change for most people is their heightened vulnerability to and lessened ability to recuperate from various illnesses.

Psychological Aging

1. Psychological aging refers to a role the individual assigns to himself as he reaches a certain chronological age.
2. The two major threat felt by the older persons are the deterioration of his concept of self, which results in loss of self-esteem and extensive and continual grief over frequently occurring losses.
3. The plight of the aged in the youth oriented society continues to receive attention, and the process of Gerontological counseling is now recognized as a specialized form of helping.
4. The older person should encourage seeing himself as in a dynamic period of growth rather than in a period of rapid deterioration. The older person, for the most part, wishes to be treated as a person on worth and dignity.

Sociogenic Aging

1. Society imposes role on people as they reach a certain chronological age. Older persons are seen by many people in our society as either no people or expendable people, merely because they lived longer.
2. Older people have been told by our society that they are supposed to be physically, socially, sexually and intellectually infirm-slow in comprehending events going on around them and rigid in their ways of thinking and behaving.
3. Society also seems to take the attitude that older people should run away and hide until they die. It is important to note the combination of psychological than biological aging for many people.

Physiological Changes during Old Age

Changes in Homeostasis

1. Homeostasis is the body's ability to maintain a stable internal environment. The complex mechanism of homeostasis regulates fluid and electrolyte balance, blood pressure, temperature and food intake.
2. Man is dependent upon the functional integrity of the cell and the stability of the internal environment. If the homeostatic mechanisms are functioning properly, the body is able to adopt or react stress.
3. However, with aging these mechanisms become less efficient and reserve power is lost. This in turn makes the person more vulnerable to disease. Recovery is also affected since more time is required for the body return to normal after illness.

Changes in the Nervous System

1. The nervous system is extremely vulnerable to the aging process, as in seen in the progressive loss of cells that occurs with advancing years.
2. There are approximately half as many brain cells in the frontal area at age 80 as at 40, with resulting decrease in brain weight.
3. The steady loss of neurons begins surprisingly early in life and affects both brain and spinal cord. There is also a decrease in the blood flow to the brain.
4. Both physiologic changes in the brain and the reduced blood supply may be related to personality changes sometimes encountered elderly.

Changes in Special Senses

1. The aging process produces varying degree of impairment in hearing, vision, smell, taste and pain perception as well as diminished sensation of touch and slowing reflexes.
2. A decreased in the sense of smell and in the number of taste buds at times contributes to a loss of appetite.
3. Diminished sensitivity to thirst needs can lead to dehydration and confused behavior as a result of fluid balance.
4. Hearing impairment, which usually is first noticed in the higher frequencies, can result in impairment of speech discrimination and loss of the full sense of background noises.
5. Vision is affected by a decrease in visual acuity and accommodation to glare and by a marked diminution of night vision and peripheral field of vision.
6. Perception of some types of pain decreases and referral of pain from one part of the body to another seems to become more common with advancing age.
7. The temperature-regulating mechanisms are less reliable and heat-generating activities are reduced.

Cardiovascular Changes

1. In older people, the heart is able to pump effectively under normal circumstances, but because it lacks much of its physiological reserve, it reaches poorly to sudden stress such as blood loss, excessive parenteral fluids or sudden effort.
2. When normal homeostasis is upset, congestive heart failure, arrhythmias and myocardial ischemia may develop.
3. The signs of arteriosclerosis become clinically recognizable when it has reached and advanced stage in the elderly.

Respiratory Changes

1. Most of the changes that occur in pulmonary function in the aged result from loss of elastic tissue surrounding the alveoli and alveolar ducts and from changes in the anteroposterior of the chest owing to rib and vertebral calcification.
2. There is also changes in the tissues of the lungs and decline in its functional capacity, size and structure as well as weakening of the respiratory muscles.
3. Vital capacity becomes reduced while there is a concurrent increase in residual volume. A change in the pulmonary vasculature also occurs.

Changes in the Kidney Function

1. Kidney function decline with age because of a reduction in the number of glomerulus and diminished filtration and tubular function.
2. The blood flow to the kidney is reduced as a result of decreased cardiac output and increased peripheral resistance.

Metabolic Changes

1. As the body ages, the basal metabolic rate slows and the quantity of oxygen used by the tissue is reduced.
2. As metabolic processes change, the glucose tolerance curve tends toward that of the diabetic. If normal standards for glucose tolerance tests were applied to the aged, 50 percent of this population would be classified as diabetes.

Musculoskeletal Changes

1. Generally, there is a slow and steady atrophy of muscles that result in muscle wasting, particularly of the trunk and extremities.
2. With loss of muscle power there is a decrease in strength, endurance and agility.
3. Bones gradually lose calcium and bone porous and lighter, because bone become more brittle, falls are especially dangerous in the elderly.
4. Ligaments calcify and ossify and joints become stiffened from erosions of cartilaginous joint surfaces. Changes in the lining of joint cavities can produce degenerative changes.

Skin and Connective Tissue Changes

1. The skin is among the first structures to show the most obvious associated with aging.
2. As the person ages, there is loss of subcutaneous supporting tissue and resultant thinning of the skin. With the loss of subcutaneous fat, the skin assumes the characteristic appearance of aging-folds, lines, wrinkles and slackness.

3. The dermis become relatively dehydrated and loses strength and elasticity. The skin in general is prone to excess dryness and itching.
4. As a preventive measure, older people should avoid overexposure to the sun, which tends to accelerate aging of the skin and increases the tendency to skin cancer.

Reproductive Changes

1. Physiologic changes occurring with menopause can affect sexual function and activity in older women. Atrophy of the vaginal canal and diminished vaginal secretions can lead to local irritation, bleeding, and pain with sexual activity.
2. In older male, there may be diminished and delayed ability to achieve a full penile erection and a reduction in the frequency associated with psychological changes.

Health Promotion Measures for Elderly

Health Appraisal

1. Varied health assessment techniques can be implemented to help detect and identify elderly people at risk.
2. Many authorities believe that a comprehensive physical examination, including blood examinations, urinalysis and stool test should be carried out annually.
3. Assessment of health habits is necessary as a basis for health counseling. Positive measures for maintaining health include weight control, exercise, proper nutrition, avoidance of cigarette smoking, and protection of accident prevention.

Nutritional Support

1. Dietary inadequacies in the elderly results from such factors as poor nutritional habits, economic constrains and underlying disease condition.
2. Nutrition can have a tremendous impact on health maintenance and disease prevention as well as on the treatment of disease.
3. Older people are vulnerable to low nutrient intake. Dietary studies show that calcium, thiamine, ascorbic acid, and vitamin. Aware the nutrients most commonly lacking in the diets of the aged.
4. The addition of moderate amount of fiber to the diet may alleviate constipation and flatulence. The high incidence of osteoporosis in older women seems to be age-related.
5. Other factors contributing to nutritional deficiencies are social isolation, lack of interest in cooking and eating, and problems in food shopping.

Exercise

1. Activity is one key to the prevention of premature aging. Many of the health problems of the aged arise from a lack of conditioning and diminished response to stress.
2. Exercise maintains muscular tone throughout the body and is effective in the prevention of and rehabilitation following cardiovascular diseases.
3. Exercise training improves functional capabilities, increase vitality and has psychological benefits.

Temperature Regulation

1. Older people cannot tolerate a cold environment and are very susceptible to hyperthermia. The nursing approach is to provide extra blankets may be added for warmth.

2. Efforts are directed to maintain heat and humidity at comfortable levels by fans, airconditioning and humidifiers or dehumidifiers during hot whether.

Hygienic Care

1. With aging, the skin becomes thin and inelastic, predisposing the elderly patient to prevent pressure sores.
2. For elderly people, foot care is essential in order to maintain mobility, physical well-being, and independence. A common foot disorder of this age group includes calluses, bunions, toenail problems, corns and fungus infections.
3. The components of dental care for the aging patients include eating a proper diet, maintaining health oral and denture-bearing structure, being motivated to speak proper care and having adequate dental services available.
4. Problems of constipation and bowel incontinence often can be reduced through systematic habit training. Constipation occurs because of altered mobility, decreased mucus secretion and changes in muscle tone and elasticity of the colon, as well as changes in diet.

Recreation

Recreation is more than just having fun; it is fundamental to physical and mental well-being. No matter how old or disabled one becomes, the desire for the dignity that comes only through purposeful activity is never lost.

Common Health Problems of Elderly

Disease and Aging

1. The aged are particularly vulnerable to disease because of such factors as their decreased physiological reserve, a less flexible homeostatic mechanism and lessened defensive mechanism of the body.
2. Chronic diseases have been called the companions of the aged and most persons over 65 are affected by at least on chronic disease.
3. The major disorders of old age include heart disease, malignancy, cerebrovascular disease, influenza and pneumonia.
4. Disease in the aged does not always present with classic signs and symptoms. The usual clinical manifestations may be absent, attenuated or disguised and atypical signs and symptoms may present.

Falls in the Elderly

1. A fall may be a frightening experience that can lead to immobilization and possibly to pneumonia and complete loss of the ability to walk.
2. Falls by the elderly result from age-related physiologic decline in postural control and detoriation of the central nervous system or from lightheadedness, postural hypotension, heart block and arrhythmias.
3. Special danger arises from osteoporosis, a condition in which the bones lose calcium and thus become thin and brittle. This condition renders an elderly person susceptible to major fractures.

Depression

1. Depression is the most common emotional disorder in the aged. Depression and grief are common with aged since losses are inevitable.
2. Depression resulting from losses can easily be overlooked and may be mistaken for physical or organic mental illness. The patient may exhibit anger, denial, withdrawal, or other maladoptive responses that move him further away from reality.
3. Depression in the aged is usually manifested by feelings of apathy, quietness and emptiness, which may be mistaken for senile changes.
4. Treatment in elderly, usually referred to community health resources, such as the community mental health services can be very beneficial.

Chronic Organic Brain Syndrome (Senile dementia)

1. The term dementia refers to signs and symptoms of intellectual dysfunction owing to differing etiologies and varying pathophysiologic mechanisms that can occur alone and in combination.
2. It is believed to result from diffuse impairment of brain tissue. The most common long-term disorders of cognitive functions (attention, learning, memory) in the elderly are seen in senile dementia (often called Alzheimer's disease).
3. Senile dementia generally refers to a disturbance of mental status or mental deterioration occurring after the age of 65. There are neuropathological changes associated with changes in the patient's cognitive function, which may include loss of neurons, neuro fibrillary tangles, granulovascular changes and neuritic (senile) plaques in the brain.
4. Senile dementia is devasting to the human personality and is a source of anguish and frustration to the patient and loved ones.
5. Senile dementia and related disorders are associated with a high motility rate and significantly shortened life expectancy.

Acute Brain Syndrome

1. Acute brain syndrome is a temporary psychiatric state caused by a physiologic or an anatomical insult to brain tissue.
2. The disorder have a relatively sudden onset and potentially reversible. They associated with acute physical illness of physiologic disturbances, cardiac and circulatory problems, neurological conditions, cerebrovascular disorders, dehydration, electrolyte imbalance, alcohol or drug toxicity and wide variety of infections.
3. In management of acute brain syndrome, the basic disease must be treated or the etiologic toxic agent must be removed.
4. Specific treatment is aimed at alleviating or curing the condition that underlies the confusion: Antimicrobials for infection, removal of drugs, removal of fecal impaction, correction of heart failure, treatment of stroke.
5. Appropriate medications, such as the phenothiazines, which exert much of their calmining action on the lower brain centers, may be administered.

BIBLIOGRAPHY

1. Bennett R, Linda KB. Myles Textbook for Midwives (13th edn). Churchill Livingstone, Edinburgh, 1999.
2. Clement I. 'Paediatric Nursing', AP Jam and Co, New Delhi, 2006.
3. Cold Chain, Management for Vaccine Handlers' Ministry of Health and Family Welfare, New Delhi.
4. Datta AK. 'Essential of Human Embryology', Mumbal. Current Books International Company, 2000.
5. Datta AK. 'Essentials of Neuroanatomy', Current Books International Agency, Mumbai, 2000.
6. Datta DC. 'Textbook of Obstetrics Including Perinatology and Contraception', New Central Book Agency (P) Ltd, Kolkata, 2004.
7. Dennis Rainey. 'Family Life Today, Making those Early Marriage Adjustments' Boston, 2005.
8. Department of Health and Human Services, Centre for Disease Control and Prevention. 'Youth Risk Behaviour Suveillance', USA.
9. Diane M Eraser, Margaret A Cooper. 'Myles Textbook for Midwives', Churchill Livingstone Company, 1991.
10. Dorothy R Marlow, Barbara A Redding. Textbook of Pediatric Nursing, Elsevier Company, New Delhi, 2005.
11. EB Wentell, et al. 'Physical Education Program Improvement and Self-study Guide', High School, Reston, VA. National Association for Sport and Physical Education, 1998.
12. Fogel CI, Woods NF. Health Care of Women A Nursing Perspective, The CV Mosby Company, St. Louis, 1981.
13. Rutishauser S. Physiology and Anatomy; A Basis for Nursing and Health Care, Churchill Livingstone, Edinburgh, 1994.
14. Smith A. The Body, Penguin Books, Harmondsworth, 1985.
15. Thibodeaux GA. Anatomy and Physiology, Mosby, St. Louis, 1987.

4

Theories of Growth and Development

DEFINITIONS

1. **Theories:** Theories are set of inter-related concepts provide direction for research. They are tested and validated through research. Theories are logically inter-related concepts, statements, propositions and definitions, which have been directed from philosophical beliefs of scientific data and from which questions or hypothesis can deduced, tested and verified.

2. **Psychoanalysis:** Psychoanalysis was founded during the late 1800's and early 1900's by the Austrian doctor, Sigmund Freud. Psychoanalysis was based on the theory that behavior is determined by powerful inner forces, most of which are burned in the unconscious mind. According to Freud and other psychoanalysts, from early childhood people repress (force out of conscious awareness) any desires or needs that are unacceptable to themselves or to society. The repressed feelings can cause personality disturbances, self-destructive behavior, or even physical symptoms.

3. Cognitive psychology has its roots in the cognitive outlook of the gestalts. The names of psychologists like Edward Tolman and Jean Piaget are associated with the further propagation of the ideas of this psychology. They believe there is more to human nature than a series of stimulus-response connections. These psychologists concentrate on such mental processes as thinking, reasoning, and self-awareness. They investigate how a person gathers information about the world, processes the information, and plans responses.

4. Humanist psychology advocated by the contemporary psychologists like Maslow, Rogers, Arthur Combs, Gordon Allport reflects the recent human trends in psychology. A school called humanistic psychology developed as an alternative to behaviorism and psychoanalysis. Humanistic psychologists believe individuals are controlled by their own values and choices and not entirely by the environment as behaviorists think, or by unconscious drives as psychoanalysts believe. The goal of humanistic psychology is to help people function effectively and fulfill their own unique potential. The supporters of this approach include the American psychologists, Abraham H Maslow and Carl R Rogers.

5. **Personality theories:** There is same relationship between personality and mental illness. A particular kind of person is likely to develop a particular kind of illness. The schizoid personality is believed to predispose to schizophrenia. Similarly, obsessive, cyclothymiacs and histrionic personalities predispose to obsessive compulsive disorder, manic-depressive psychosis and hysteria.

6. **Monistic theories:** These suggest that mind and body are not separate substances. Thinkers like Aristotle, Hobbs, Hegel and the Behaviorists, collectively thought of as the materialists, postulated that the mind was nothing more than a bodily function. A mind is generally thought to be of a substance other than a physical substance.

7. **Dualistic theories:** According to the dualist view, mind is thought to be of a substance other than a physical substance. Popular dualists were Descartes, Locke and James, who collectively belong to the school of ought known as internationalism. Sometimes, the mind affects the body, and sometimes the body affects the mind. The body and the mind are separate, and they affect one another. We are physical beings because we are extended in space. We are mental beings because we think. But, the mind is not physical in any ways and it exists separately from the body. It is assumed that this interaction occurred in the pineal gland.

8. **Trust:** To trust another, one must feel confidence in that person's presence, reliability, integrity, veracity and sincere desire to provide assistance when requested. Trust is the initial development task described by Erickson. Trust is the base of a therapeutic relationship.

9. **Respect:** Rogers (1951) called this unconditional positive regard. To show respect is to believe in the dignity and worth of an individual regardless of his or here unacceptable behavior.

10. **Genuineness:** Genuineness is the ability to be open, honest, and "real" in interactions with others the awareness of what one is experiencing internally and the ability to project the quality of this inner experiencing in a relationship.

11. **Empathy:** Empathy is to see beyond outward behavior, and sense accurately another's inner experience. With empathy, one can accurately perceive and understand the meaning and relevance in the thought and feeling of another.

A number of scholars have developed theories that can be used in understanding, explaining and predicting behavior in children and adults. No one theory covers the whole spectrum of behavior, thus consider each person from a combination of viewpoints.

THEORIES OF HUMAN DEVELOPMENT

Theories of growth and development are often considered from the perspective of seven following issues, it help to answers several questions that arise regarding growth and development whether development of children occur gradually or abruptly or similarly or differently.

Nature versus Nurture

Nature development is predetermined by genetic factors and not altered by the environment (eye colors, body type).

Nurture development can take different pathways depending on the experience an individual has over the lifetime (Both nature and nurture factors interact to procedure developmental difference).

Continuity versus Discontinuity

Continuity: Charge is orderly and built upon earlier experience, development is gradual, early and late development is connected.

Discontinuity: Development is a series of discrete steps that help the child to perform higher levels of functioning.

Passivity versus Activity

- *Passive:* Child-rearing belief, practices and behaviors cause the children to be either shy or assertive.
- *Active:* Children creatively and actively seek experience to control, direct and shape their development.

Critical versus Sensitive Period

Critical: A limited time span when a child is biologically prepared to acquire certain behavior.

Sensitive period: A time span that is optimal for certain capacities to emerge when the individual is receptive to environmental influence.

Universality versus Context Specificity

Human follow similar development pathways regardless of their culture.

Context specificity: Children are different because of their cultural values, beliefs and experience.

Assumptions of Human Nature

- **Innate purity**: Children are inherently good and born without an initiative sense of what is right or wrong.
- **Original sin**: Children enter the word as a lank state without inborn tendencies and are molded by life experience.

Behavioral Consistency

- **Consistency**: Individual personality characteristics and predispositions cause the children to behave similarly no matter setting.
- **Inconsistency**: Children behavior changes from our setting to another.

THEORIES OF GROWTH AND DEVELOPMENT

The following theoretical views present ways of examining human development during childhood and adolescence.

Age period	Freud	Erikson	Sullivan	Piaget	Kohlberg
Infancy (Birth to 1 year)	Oral (Birth to 1 year)	Trust/Mistrust (Birth to 1 year)	Infant (Birth to 1 year)	Sensorimotor (Birth to 2 years)	Preconventional (Birth to 7 years)
Toddler (1 to 3 years)	Anal (1 to 3 years)	Trust/Mistrust (Continued)	Infant (Continued)	Sensorimotor (Continued)	Preconventional (Continued)
Preschool (3 to 6 years)	Phallic (3 to 6 years)	Initiative/Guilt (3 to 6 years)	Early childhood (Continued)	Preoperational (2 to 7 years)	
School-age (6 to 12 years)	Latency (6 to 12 years)	Industry/ Inferiority (6 to 12 years)	Late childhood (6 to 9 years)	Concrete operations (7 to 11 years)	Conventional (7 to12 years)
Adolescence (12 to 19 years)	Genital (12 years and older)	Identity/ role confusion (12 to 18 years)	Early adolescence (12 to 15 years) Late adolescence (15 to 19 years)	Formal operations (12 years and older)	Post-conventional (12 years and older)

FREUD AND PSYCHOSEXUAL DEVELOPMENT

Introduction

The psychosexual theory emphasizes the importance of unconscious motivation and early childhood experiences in influencing behavior and describes concepts related to personality and stages of development, central to Freudian theory is the notion that two basic biological instincts motivate behavior, must be satisfied and complete for supremacy.

Instinct

1. The life instinct is responsible for such activities as eating, breathing and behavior that express self preservation, love and constructive conduct.
2. The death instinct is a destructive force expressed by self centered and cruel behavior, hate, aggression and destructive components.

Components of Instincts

The ID

1. The ID is the oldest and most central aspect of the human psyche. It is unconscious in its entirety, the individual is not aware of it.
2. The ID contains everything about the individual including drives, needs and wishes all that is inherited, present at birth and found in psychological constitution of the individual.
3. The ID has a biological basis, that is, the nature of our biological makeup necessitates an emphasis upon certain ID impulses.
4. The basic principle that governs the function of the ID termed the pleasure principle. The pleasure is ensured when levels of psychic energy remain low, tension is decreased.

Ego

1. The ego operates according to the "reality principle" allows individuals to be successful and includes memory, cognition, intelligence, problem solving, compromising, separating reality from fantasy and incorporating experiences and learning in to future behavior.
2. The ego development continues during childhood and throughout the life span.
3. The ego is a part of the ID and it has undergone special development resulting in differentiation from the ID.
4. The egoes rationalizes the interaction between individual and the society and acts as a chain in dealing with ID and the external world.
5. The ID functions according to the pleasure principle but the ego functions according to the reality principle.

Superego

1. Superego is an internalized sense of conscience that imposes the moralistic value of society upon the individual. Whereas the ID hedonistic and the ego realistic, the superego is idealistic.
2. The superego determines the moral appropriateness of given activity and insists that the individual act in accordance with its standards.

3. The superego emerges when the child internalizes caregiver or societal values, roles and morals.
4. Superego development becomes apparent in the preschool-aged years, when the child learns socially acceptable behavior.
5. The superego strives for perfection rather than for pleasure or reality.
6. The superego also serves as a disciplinarian by creating feeling of remorse and guilt for transgressing rules and self praise and pride for adhering to rules.

STAGES OF PSYCHOSEXUAL DEVELOPMENT

Basic Concepts of Psychosexual Development

1. Freud believes that the first five years of life were the most critical in the development of the personality.
2. During this period, the child passes through a series of psychosexual stages of development in which particular body region serves as a source of extreme pleasure for the child.
3. Freud also believed that the nature of the flow of the individual's psychic energy during the childhood and adolescent years is also critical, particularly during the first five years of life.
4. Freud has identified different stages of psychosexual development and described in detail their stages and their attributes.
5. The stages are ordered in sequence and include oral stage, anal stage, phallic stage, latency stage and genital stage.

Oral Stage

1. Freud holds that during the first 12 to 18 months, the infant is in the oral stage of its development.
2. This stage is time of extreme pleasure seeking with the mouth, including the lips and tongue and regarding oral activities as the source of pleasure.
3. The primary source of pleasure for the child in the first 6 to 8 months of life could be identified with the sucking and swallowing.
4. During this stage, the child drives pleasure from oral stimulation arising from food and the fondling of the mouth by other people; this is referred to as oral incorporative behavior.
5. When a child gets fixated at the oral stage may as an adult, in future would become obsessed with activities such as eating, drinking or smoking.

Anal Stage

1. The anal stage occurs during the twenty-fourth and thirty-sixth months of life.
2. At this stage, the pleasure of the child centers on the anal or buttocks region.
3. In this stage, the child derives immense pleasure in elimination of faces.
4. Freud suggested that methods of caregivers use to toilet train children during this period may have long lasting effects on personality.
5. Problems arising due to enforcing the toilet training during this stage can result in excessive repulsion of faces, i.e. soiling the pants or retention of faces or constipation.

Phallic Stage

1. During the fourth and fifth years of life the genital region of the child serves as the source of deriving pleasure.

2. Freud holds that the child at this stage of development is concerned with the manipulation of the genitals and become sexually interested in the opposite sex parent.
3. This process is termed the Oedipus complex in the case of the boys and the Electra complex in the case of girls.
4. During these years, children also develop a strong incestuous desire for the caregiver of the opposite gender.
5. Resolution and control allows children to identify with the caregiver of the same gender and fosters male and female identify.

The Latency Stage

1. Freud held that 6 to 12 years of life represented a quite time in which sexual instincts were sublimated into more acceptable activity such as school work and extracurricular endeavors.
2. Since by now the superego has developed sufficiently to keep the ID under control, children in this period rapidly learn about society and themselves while developing useful skills.
3. They increasingly identity with the same gender caregiver and become intensely involved with their same gender peers.

Genital Stage

1. The final stage of psychosexual development is labeled genital stage.
2. This stage begins with puberty, during this period of time the pleasure seeking child is transformed into a reality oriented adolescent.
3. The genital sexual organ in the process of development starts assuming its place in serving as a source of sexual pleasure.
4. The adolescent vacillates between dependence/independence from parents; learn how to form loving relationships and mages sexual urges in socially appropriate ways.
5. These psychic conflicts are necessary for fully functioning and mature adult personality development.

ERIKSON AND PSYCHOSOCIAL DEVELOPMENT

Introduction

Erik Erikson (1902-1994) acknowledged the contribution of biological factors to development, but felt that the environment, culture and society were also important. Erikson's psychosocial theory of development stresses the complexity of inter-relationship existing between emotional and physical variables during one's lifetime.

Concepts of Psychosocial Development

1. Erickson's lifespan development consisted of eight sequential stages.
2. Five of these stages describe infants through adolescents.
3. Each stage is dominated by major developmental conflicts or crises related societal demands and expectations that must be addressed or resolved before the individual can progress to the next stage.
4. The resolution of each conflict or crisis might be positive (favorable and growth enhancing) or negative (unfavorable, frustrating and making later development difficult).
5. Erikson believed that major conflicts occurring during each stage are rarely completely resolved.

The main points of Erikson's theory are:

1. Each stage of development contains a psychological challenge or critical period, during which the person must deal with a major life change. If the person fails to meet the challenge, he or she faces certain difficulty in achieving the next level of development. For example, infants who do not achieve a sense of trust that their needs will be met will have difficulty in achieving autonomy as toddlers.
2. In each stage of development, a significant person or group exerts a lasting influence on the ongoing development of the child. For example, the person who acts as family caregiver is most significant to the infant whereas the peer group has greater influence on the adolescent.
3. Similar to Havighurst's theory, the individual must accomplish certain tasks related to the psychological challenge of each particular stage. Children are able to perform these tasks with help from parents, siblings and other important people.
4. Certain virtues are appropriate for each developmental stage. Virtues are beneficial, challenging and exciting characteristics that emerge as individuals successfully accomplish the tasks of that developmental stage and thus successfully resolve the psychological challenge.

Erikson's theory of psychological development—Childhood

Concept	Infancy (1-12 months)	Toddlerhood (1-3 years)	Preschool (3-6 years)	School-age (6-12 years)
Challenge	Trust vs. mistrust	Autonomy vs. shame and doubt	Initiative vs. guilt	Industry vs. inferiority
Significant	Family caregivers	Family	Family	School and neighborhood
Necessary accomplishment	Development	Learn appropriate behaviors, learn right from wrong	Learn rules and regulations, establish independence	Learn to get along with others; learn school subjects
Virtues	Hope	Self-control, will power	Direction, purpose	Self-esteem, competence
Ways to help the child succeed	Establish routines, satisfy basic needs	Set limits let child make simple choices encourage curiosity give gentle guidance	Consistent discipline, explain things praise	Manage sibling rivalry give responsibility, recognize accomplishments away from home.

Stages of Psychosocial Development

Trust versus Mistrust

1. The first stage of trust versus mistrust occurs during infancy (1 month to 1½ years).
2. The baby becomes familiar with growing number of sensual experiences that coincide feeling good as the baby spends more and more time awake.
3. The mother of the baby becomes a familiar presence and the baby learns that it can trust her to care for its needs.
4. The baby's beginning ability to trust itself and the correlation of its inner belief with outer reality provide the baby with the first, rudimentary sense of ego identity.
5. The baby learns hope, which is the first virtue to arise is something that can be realized.

Autonomy versus Shame

1. During the toddler years (1½ to 3 years) autonomy versus shame and doubt occurs.
2. Autonomy develops as children discover their new abilities while improving language and motor skills and learning competencies related to bathing, eating, toileting and dressing.
3. Shame occurs if assertiveness and independence are considered unacceptable or ineffective by caregivers.
4. Doubt occurs if children learn to mistrust not only themselves, but also others in the immediate environment.
5. The virtue will develops out of the child's earliest efforts at self-control and its observations of the superior will of others.

Initiative versus Guilt

1. During the fourth and fifth year of life from the third stage, now the ego quality of initiative enables the child to plan and set about tasks.
2. The child becomes eager to learn and learns quickly, it begins to master skills and tries hard to perform well.
3. The danger during this stage of development is the development of guild; guilt may arouse by sexual fantasies in particular.
4. Guilt occurs, when caregivers frequently reprimand behaviors reflecting initiative, children experiencing guilt may become passive, reluctant or refuse to participate in activities.
5. While playing the child learns how to master reality by repeating difficult situations and tasks and by finding out what things may be useful for experimenting with.

Industry versus Inferiority

1. The major developmental task of the school-age years 6 to 11 years is industry versus inferiority.
2. Industry involves mastery of social, physical and intellectual skills and operation towards and competition with peers.
3. Inferiority develops when school-aged children are ridiculed by peers, do not measure up to adult or their own expectations, or lack certain skills so they are not always the best, first fastest or smartest.
4. Through the child's application to work and its development of a sense of industry, the virtue of competence, the exercise of dexterity and intelligence in the completion of tasks emerges.
5. Instruction and methodology is necessary but it is important that it apply its intelligence and abounding energy to some undertaking such a school, chores at home, manual skills, art, sports, lest it develops the feeling of being less able than others.

Identity verses Identity Confusion

1. At the onset of the teens, Erickson's model of psychosocial development greatly expands and depends the Freudian Portrayal of the life cycle.
2. In this fifth stage of the cycle that the young person, according to Erickson is just beginning to form and identity.
3. They become aware that they have the strength to control their own destinies and feel the need to define themselves and their goals.

4. Adolescents want to take their place in society, whether in more or less conventional roles or in roles that challenge established ways.
5. Adolescents often experience "identity confusion" they are conflicted enormously about whether and how to give expression to their strong sexual urges.
6. Role confusion occurs, when the adolescent is unable to acquire a sense of direction, self or place within the world.

Intimacy versus Isolation

1. The young adult makes commitment to another, moves from the relative security of self-identify to the relative in security of self-identify to the relative insecurity involved in establishing intimacy with another.
2. Isolation and self-absorption occurs if unsuccessful. The psychosocial strength during young adult is love.

Generativity versus Stagnation

1. This is the seventh stage and it encompasses the years of adulthood from about 30 to 65, it sees the development of generatively the "concern for establishing and guiding the next generation".
2. This means that adult wants to have children to whom they can transmit their values.
3. In a broader sense, generativity includes productivity and creativity.
4. Some people fulfill the "parental drive" by generating products and ideas rather by giving children.
5. Erikson is 1964, says that care is the "widening concern for what has been generated". It refers to the need to look after others and to teach them.
6. The person seeks to guide the next generation of risks feelings of personal in completeness.

Integrity versus Despair

1. Older adult seeks a sense of personal accomplishment, adapts to triumphs and disappointments with certain ego integrity and accepts death or fall into despair.
2. They perceive that their lives have had an order and a meaning with a larger order.
3. Erickson (1963) says that integrity is the patrimony of soul. In other words, we inherit our integrity from overselves, our integrity reflects all that we have been and done and achieved.
4. The danger is that one may feel "despair" in contemplating the ups and downs of one's life and the nearness of death.
5. The older people function somewhat more slowly they may remain playful and retain a curiosity that they can use to sortout and integrate their experiences.

SULLIVAN AND INTERPERSONAL DEVELOPMENT

Introduction

Harry Stack Sullivan (1982-1949) focused on interpersonal relations as important motivators and the source of psychological health. His interpersonal theory posits that self concepts are the key to personality development. He acknowledged the importance of the environment (especially the home) and also emphasized the role of social approval and disapproval in forming a child's self concept.

Concept of Interpersonal Development

1. Sullivan believed personality development was largely the result of childhood experiences, interpersonal encounters and the mother-child relationship.
2. The development results from interpersonal relationships with others in maximizing satisfaction of needs while minimizing insecurity.
3. Sullivan believed that development results from interpersonal relationships in the infancy, childhood, juvenile, preadolescent, adolescent and late adolescent eras.

Stages of Sullivan's Interpersonal Theory of Development

Stage	Age	Characteristics
Infant	Birth to 18 months	Learns to rely on others especially mother "good me/bad me" emerges
Early childhood	18 months to 6 years	Learns to clarify communication recognize approval/ disapproval delays gratification
Late childhood	6 to 8 years	Increasing intellectual abilities learns to control behavior and own place in the world
Preadolescence	9 to 12 years	Vulnerable to tasting "chum" important
Early adolescence	12 to 15 years	Mastering independence develops relationships with persons of opposite gender
Late adolescence	15 to 19 years	Masters expression of sexual impulses forms responsible and satisfying relationship with other.

Stages of Interpersonal Development

Infancy Era (0 -2 years)

1. It encompasses birth to when the child is able to use words that convey the same meaning to the child as they do to others (18 months).
2. The primary task reveals around learning to rely on others, especially the primary caregiver, to gratify physiological needs and achieve satisfaction.
3. Infants are sensitive to others attitudes and emotions, while these needs are being met.
4. The infant learns to differentiate self from others, through trial and error.
5. The infant learns from parental interactions to rely on others to gratify needs and satisfy wishes.
6. The infant develops a sense of basic trust, security and self-worth, when this occurs: Ends with language development.

Childhood Era (2-6 years)

1. Language development allows for education, development of body image and self-perception.
2. The children are able to communicate better with others, thereby facilitating interpersonal relationships.
3. The children develops self-esteem with sublimation child learns to communicate needs through the use of words and the acceptance of delayed gratification and interference with wish fulfillment.

4. Excessive parental disapproval during this time may cause children to view themselves and the world as negative and or hostile.

Juvenile Era (6-10 years)

1. It is characterized by increasing intellectual ability and developing internal control over behavior.
2. Children learn to pay attention to other's wishes, from satisfying relations with peers of both genders and sometimes oppose rules.
3. Relation with peers allow child to see self objectively develops conscience.
4. The child behavior is connected to others opinions, organizes and uses experiences in terms of approval and disapproval received.
5. The child begins using selective inattention and disassociates these experiences that cause physical or emotional discomfort and pain.

Preadolescent Era (10-13 years)

1. Children participate in an expanding world that provides confrontation with rules and knowledge about themselves.
2. They realize their status within the peer group is based on performance or vulnerable to teasing and become interested in relating closely to a peer of the same gender, which Sullivan calls the chum.
3. The children develop same sex friends, moves from egocentrism to love. They able to form satisfying relationships and work with peers.
4. The children use competition, compromise and cooperation.

Early Adolescence (13-17 years)

1. They are interested in sexual activity and learn how to establish satisfactory relationship with other members of opposite sex.
2. Early adolescents may demonstrate a variety of behaviors including rebellion, dependence, cooperation and collaboration as they become independent.

Late Adolescence (17-19 years)

1. Sullivan believes initial feelings of love for the opposite gender emerge here, as the individual learns to master expression of sexual impulses, from responsible and satisfying relationship and use communication skill in interactions.
2. They develop personality integration able to integrate the needs of society, without becoming overwhelmed with anxiety.

Young Adulthood

Becomes economically, intellectually and economically self-sufficient.

Old Adulthood

Older adulthood learns to be interdependent and assumes responsibility for others.

Senescence develops an acceptance of responsibility for what life is and was and of its place in the flow of history.

Theory Application

1. Sullivan emphasizes the significance of interpersonal relations with others on personality development, and meeting the child's basic needs in a timely and appropriate fashion.
2. Nurses need to teach caregivers about Sullivan's theory so they may help their child develop a healthy personality and realize the importance that they, the caregivers have a child's life.

PIAGET AND COGNITIVE DEVELOPMENT

Introduction

Jean Piaget (1896-1980) began studying children's intellectual development during 1920s. Piaget was a famous psychologist; he studied the intellectual development in children in great deals. He says that the child is born with the ability to organize his experience. Piaget's theory of intellectual development in children is known as cognitive theory of development. He has predicted different stages in cognitive theory.

Stages of Piaget's Theory of Cognitive Development

Stage	Age	Characteristics
Sensorimotor reflex	Birth to 1 month	Predictable, innate, survival reflexes
Primary circular reactions	1 to 14 months	Responds purposefully to stimuli, initiates, repeats satisfying behavior
Secondary circular reactions	4 to 8 months	Learns from intentional behavior motor skills/vision coordinated recognize familiar/objects
Coordination of secondary schemes	8 to 12 months	Develops object permanence anticipates others action, differentiates familiar/unfamiliar
Tertiary circular reactions	12 to 18 months	Interested in novelty, repetition, understands casualty, solicits help from others
Mental combinations	18 to 24 months	Simple problem solving, imitates
Preoperational Preconception	2 to 7 years 2 to 4 years	Egocentric thought, mental imagery, increasing language
Initiative	4 to 7 years	Sophisticated language decreased egocentric, thought reality – based play
Concrete operations	7 to 11 years	Understands relationships, classification conservation, seriation, reversibility, logical reasoning limited, less egocentric thought
Formal operations	11 years and older	Capable of systematic abstract thought.

Concepts of Cognitive Theory

1. According to Piaget, the baby is in the sensorimotor stage between birth and two years.
2. During the sensorimotor stage, the child understands his world through sensory organs and through his motor abilities.
3. Piaget believed intellectual growth followed an orderly progression based on the child's maturational level, experiences with physical objects, interactions with caregiver, other

adults and peers, and an internal self-regulating mechanism that responded to environmental stimuli.

4. He used several terms schema, assimilation, accommodation, equilibrium to describe cognitive development.
5. This sensorimotor stage has six substages.

Stages of Sensorimotor

Stage I: Reflex Activity (0-1 years)

1. Reflexes are voluntary responses to certain stimuli. A large number of relaxes are present in the infant at the time of birth.
2. These include responses like breathing, swallowing, digestion, etc. and the first month off life of the baby is a time for exercising these reflex activities.

Stage II: Reflex Activity (1 to 4 months)

1. Between the first and the fourth months, the baby indulges in investigating his parts of the body.
2. The investigation includes sucking his own thumb and gasping his foot.
3. These activities are done in a repetitive way and Piaget calls them circular reaction, because they are repeated to become habitual behavior. These are all referred to as primary circular reaction.

Stage III: Coordination and Reaching Out (4 to 8 Months)

1. During this stage, the baby reaches out for objects other than his own body.
2. This reaching out involves a number of coordination like eye-hand coordination and coordination between large, muscles and finger muscles of the body. These reaching out responses are called secondary circular reactions.
3. A phenomenon called object permanence begins to appear in this stage. Piaget meant the ability to represent an object, whether or not it is actually present.
4. For example, when a baby searches for a toy when it is hidden, it shows that he has object permanence. The toy remains in his mind even when it is not present before his eyes.

Stage IV: Goal Directed Behavior (8 to 12 months)

1. The child exhibits purposeful behavior between 8 and 12 months.
2. For example, the child may remove things for the purpose of obtaining another or may open something to get what is inside.
3. By goal-directed behavior, we mean purposeful behavior. Goal directed behavior can be observed clearly only in this period.

Stage V: Experimentation (12 to 18 months)

1. In this stage, he begins to experiment actively with things to discover how various actions will affect an object.
2. Breaking a play thing to see what is inside, inserting objects in to his nostrils; ears, etc. are examples of his experimentation. These reactions are called tertiary circular reaction.

Cognitive-structural Perspective

1. Cognitive-structural theorists are concerned with how children learn to reason, use language, and think, rather than what they learn.
2. These theorists believe cognitive development is the result of the interaction between central venous system maturation and active involvement with the environment.
3. They also believe children constantly adapt to their world by integrating new knowledge with existing knowledge.
4. Jean Pieget was fascinated by the process and steps children took as they discovered, reinvented, understood and acquired knowledge of his world around him.
5. During the sensorimotor stage infants use sight and motor skills to learn about the environment and become familiar with their abilities.
6. The child manipulates toys, mobiles and bright pictures or photographs are helpful since young children in this stage receive comfort from these objects.

Stage VI: Problem Solving and Mental Combination (18 to 24 months)

1. The child is able to solve problems by mental combinations of signs, symbols or images between 18 and 24 months.
2. During this stage, object permanence fully develops.
3. The child is able to remember objects for a brief while when they are removed from sight.
4. The child can solve simple problems like how to wake-up his sleeping parent.
5. The child imitates others and engages in make believe plays.
6. Elementary logic is found is child's responses.

SKINNER AND OPERANT CONDITIONING

Introduction

Operant conditioning, a term originated by BF Skinner (1904-1990), involves behavioral changes due to either negative (Punishment) or positive (reinforcement) consequences rather than just the occurrence of a stimuli, skinner discovered that behavioral change become more permanent, when consequences were provided intermittently rather than continuously acquiring new behaviors or habits due to reinforcing or punishing stimuli.

Concept of Operant Conditioning

1. According to the behaviorists, the responses are learned because they operate on or affect the environment. This is referred to operant conditioning.
2. The label "operant conditioning" emphasizes the operations, movements, involved in the learning which the person or animal perform and that they are followed by some consequence that determines whether or not the organism will repeat the operations in future.
3. The responses emitted by the organism conditioned to the stimuli that preceded them are called "operants" and operant conditioning pertains to conditioning of responses of this kind.

Principles of Reinforcement

1. Any event that increases the frequency of a preceding response is termed a reinforce.
2. A reinforce may be a tangible reward, it may be praise or attention or even by an activity.

3. Getting a chocolate after reciting a poem, just saying good when one proceeds in right direction in an activity, showing some appreciation.
4. Positive reinforce that strengths a response by presenting a positive stimuli after a response and negative reinforce that strengthens a response by reducing or removing an aversive, unpleasant stimulus.
5. Reinforces may be primary or secondary ones, primary reinforces and concerned with those that directly reinforce the succeeding movement or activity.
6. Reinforcement could be scheduled—we can give reward everytime the desired act occurs or we may reward only on certain time when the desired act occurs.

Basic Assumptions Concerning Human Nature

1. Skinner's approach to understanding of basic human nature is exposed in radical behaviorism.
2. He attempts to account for the origin and ongoing dynamics of human personality in terms of operant and respondent conditioning, schedules of reinforcement, response extinction and phenomena such as stimulus generation and emotional reactions to reward and punishment.
3. Skinner considers that the complexity of human behavior, including language and thought, is in no way different one from that of the chain behavior sequence of the rat in terms of behavioral dynamics with regard to its origin and development.

Theory Application

1. Operant conditioning principles are amendable for application in a variety of areas of human behavior.
2. Essentially, these applications involve direct reinforcement of behavior either by presenting a positive reinforce as reward for desirable acts or presenting a negative reinforce as a punishment for undesirable acts.
3. Any behaviors, according to operant principles, that has a high frequency of occurrence.
4. In school setting operant conditioning is applied to improve the instruction through programmed learning but also keep the behavior problems in classroom.
5. In classrooms frequently employed technique of behavioral management is called time-out technique. In this technique the child is placed in an empty barren room, which does not heave any source of pleasurable stimulation for the child, whether it includes in an undesirable behavior.
6. Time-out techniques are effective to eliminate undesirable behavior through extinction due to non-reinforcement. This has been found effective to mange temper tantrums.
7. Biofeedback uses the operant conditioning technique for making individuals learn to control their own physiological functioning.
8. Operant conditioning has been successfully applied to treat the psychosomatic diseases such as backache, headache, asthma and high blood pressure.
9. Desensitization or counter conditioning technique attempt to condition for organism to emit positive responses to aversive stimuli. For example, one it made to learn relax when threatened by mild degree of anxiety.
10. Systematic desensitization has been used to successfully treat "neurotics". Wolfe (1963) treated an adolescent who had a hand washing compulsion using systematic desensitization.
11. Operant reinforce principles are being applied in marriage therapy or marital counseling. Behavior contracting services as a technique to treat partners in these cases.

12. Self-reinforcement, one becoming his/her dispenser of reinforcement is possible and may stand as primary behavior change strategy. This technique of one self providing reinforcement to self has been found to be successful in promoting weight gain.

BRONFENBRENNER AND ECOLOGICAL THEORY

Introduction

1. Urie Bronfenbrenner (1917) offers an organizational framework for examining the environmental framework for examining the environmental influences on human development. According to Bronfenbrenner, the child's world is like a set of nested Russian dolls, with three systems (Microsystems, exosystem, macrosystem) ranging from the most immediate setting or context, to the more remote setting or context.
2. The developing individual, embedded within the center of these system, has a unique heritage (physical appearance, maturation rate, emotionality, innate intelligence, physical health, gender), which is different from any other person. As individual mature, they impact and are impacted by these changing systems and relationships differently.

Stages of Ecological Theory

Macrosystem

1. This system is large, enduring and contains cultural and subcultural ideologies and belief.
2. Although macrosystem effect may not be obviously apparent in the life of any one individual, the macrosystem profoundly affects development.
3. For example, children living in poverty or an inner city ghetto are exposed to beliefs and values that are different than those of children living in an affluent suburb.

Exosystem

1. This system indirectly affects development; it includes social settings the individual never directly experiences even though these experiences provide an importance influence.
2. Example of the exosystem is caregiver settings, social networks or educational levels.

Microsystem

1. The microsystem is the child's immediate environment and includes daily interactions with others (family, peers, teachers, neighbors, religious leaders) other community resources (school, church).
2. The importance of the microsystem changes across development, during infancy, the family and home are of primary importance, whereas in middle childhood and adolescence, the peer group and school become more important.

Ecological Theory Application

1. In ecological theory, the child is viewed holistically, as a member of a unique family, neighborhood and cultural belief system that all impact development.
2. Ecological theory also suggests that important influence parents have on their children.
3. Ecological theory reminds us that home and cultural environment are not the same.
4. Ecological theory helps to understand the human development can proceed along several different pathways depending on the interplay of internal/external forces within the individual.

5. Bronfenbrenner also reminds us that the influence children have on parents and other family members is as important as the effect family members and parents have no children.

KOHLBERG AND MORAL DEVELOPMENT

Introduction

Lawrence Kohlberg (1927-1987) formulated a theory of moral development that described changes in thinking about moral judgments and reflected societal norms and values.

Concept of Moral Development

1. Kohlberg believed moral development was influenced by internal and external factors.
2. The internal factors include empathy, intelligence, impulse control and the ability to judge behavior.
3. The external factors included rewards, punishment, family structure and parent/peer contacts.
4. Kohlberg suggests moral growth progressed through universal and invariant sequences of three broad levels.

Stages of Kohlberg's Theory of Moral Development

Stage	Age	Characteristics
Preconventional	Birth to 1 year	Cannot differentiate right from wrong
Punishment and obedience orientation stage	2 to 3 years	Conforming behavior based on fear of punishment
Instrumental realistic orientation stage	4 to 7 years	Conforming behavior based on rewards
Conventional level	7 to 12 years	
Interpersonal concordance orientational stage	7 to 10 years	Behavior evaluated on intent and others reactions
Authority and social order maintaining orientation stage	10 to 12 years	Obeys out of respect for laws and authority
Pastconventional level	12 years and older	
Social contact/ legalistic orientation stage	12 years through adolescence	Believes laws should further human values and express majority views
Universal ethical principles orientation stage	Adolescence through adulthood	Right/wrong defined on universal, comprehensive

Stages of Moral Development

Stage I: Preconventional Level

1. **Premoral stage:** It is birth of 2 years, the impulses rule behavior, infants and young children are unable to differentiate right from wrong.
2. **Punishment and obedience orientation stage:** It is from 2 to 3 years, during this stage behaviors, decisions and conformity to rules are based on fear of punishment rather than respect for authority.

3. **Instrumental realistic orientation stage:** It is 4 to 7 years, the rules are obeyed to gain rewards or satisfy personnel objectives.

Stage II: Conventional Level

1. **Interpersonal concordance orientation stage:** It is 7 to 10 years, the behaviors and decisions are evaluated on the basis of one's intent and concerns about others reactions.
2. **Authority and social order-maintaining orientation stage:** It is usually 10 to 12 years, the child obeys out of respect of law and authority.

Stage III: Postconventional Level

1. **Social contract/legalistic orientation stage:** It is usually 12 years through adolescence, the child believes laws should further human values and express majority views.
2. **Universal ethical principles orientation stage:** It is usually adolescence through adulthood, the right/wrong defined on universal, comprehensive and consistent, yet personal ethical principles.

BANDURA AND SOCIAL DEVELOPMENT

Introduction

Socialization or social development means training child in the cultural group. The children are prepared for their adult roles through a process of socialization that takes place from birth to adulthood. Children learn to socialize by meeting and communicating with people of various ages and by participating in the activities of family life and in the doing of their peer and community groups.

Concepts of Social Development

1. According to social learning, children learn by imitating and observing others (model) as well as conditioning.
2. Social learning theorists also believe behavior is influenced by the environment and learned through various experiences.
3. Bandura believes modeled behavior can be weakened or strengthened depending on whether it is punished or rewarded.
4. Bandura suggests observational learning, where children acquire a variety of new behaviors.

Social Development

1. Learning to live happily with family and other adults is quite different from making friends in a peer groups.
2. In adult-child relationship the child learns to live within certain restrictions set by adults, even though at times these restrictions may not be consistently imposed.
3. Bandura found children tend to model behavior of children and adults of their same gender more often than not and makes model behavior of others more often than females do.

Theory Application

1. Positive behavior should be reinforced by encouragement, praise and other rewards and behaviors needing to be altered or removed from a child's repertoire can be extinguished by either ignoring or punishing.

2. Some academic and preschool program and parents use behavior modification and time-out activities to modify and change undesirable behavior in children.
3. Conditioning can also help develop new or extinguish undesirable behavior by providing specific guidelines, determining available reinforces, identifying responses acceptable for reinforcement and planning how reinforces will be scheduled so behavior is repeated.

FOWLER'S SPIRITUAL DEVELOPMENT

Introduction

A religious belief is basic to our idealized view; the religion may be based on the theories of atheism or agnosticism. A family's religion may be closely tied to its cultural background. It influences the family's interpersonal relationships and responsibilities. Fowler (1974) has identified seven stages of faith development–five can be associated with child's psychosocial, cognitive and moral development.

Concept of Spiritual Development

1. Fowler has developed a staged theory of faith, which parallels the formal development process proposed by Piaget and Kohlberg although differing in emphasis on emotional and feeling.
2. According to fowler, faith is a human universal that is expressed through beliefs, rituals, and symbols specific to religious traditions.
3. It is multidimensional and way of learning about life. Beginning is a relationship with other being; faith implies trust and reliance upon other.
4. Faith also knows, which allows the individual to construct the point of other persons and groups.

Stages of Faith

Primal Faith (Infancy)

1. Paralinguistic and preconceptual, this stage embodies the trust between parents and infants.
2. Parents and children form a mutual attachment and progress through a period of care-and-take.
3. The primary caregiver provides the infant and the young child with a variety of experiences that encourage the development of mutuality, trust, love and dependence, progressing to autonomy.

Intuitive-Projective Faith (Early Childhood)

1. Most typical from ages 3 to 7 years, this stage is characterized by the child forming long-lasting images and feelings.
2. During the preschool years, the values and beliefs of parents are assimilated and parental attitudes toward religious beliefs and moral codes are conveyed to children.
3. Children tend to follow parental beliefs because they are part of their daily life rather than from an understanding of their basic concepts.
4. Imaginations, perceptions and feelings are the mechanism by which the child explores and learns about the world at large.
5. The cultural beliefs of the family influence the child's concepts of health and sex.

Mythic-Literal Faith (Childhood and Beyond)

1. Beginning at about age 7 years, children's beliefs derive from the perspective of others.
2. Most school-aged children are interested in religion and accept the existence of a deity.

3. Stories become the gateway to learning about life.
4. In valuing the stories, practices and beliefs of the family and the community, the child reaches stage three of faith development.

Synthetic Convention (Adolescent Period and Beyond)

1. In this stage, a person's experience extends beyond the family to peers, teachers and other members of society.
2. As a result of cognitive abilities, the individual is aware of the emotions, personality patterns, ideas, thought and experiences of self and others.
3. Adolescents become increasingly aware of spiritual disappointments and recognize that prayers are not always answered.
4. Some begin to question established parental religious standards and drop or modify some religious practices.

Individuating-Reflexive

1. Adolescents become more skeptical and start comparing religious standards of their parents with others as they determine which to adopt and incorporate into their own set of religious values.
2. Religious standards are compared with scientific viewpoints. Many are uncertain about religious ideas and will not gain insight until late adolescence or early adulthood.

BIBLIOGRAPHY

1. Adele Pilliten. 'Child Health Nursing, Care of the Child and Family', Lippincott Company, Philadelphia, 1999.
2. Adele Pilliten. 'Maternal and Child Health Nursing, Care of the Childbearing and Childrearing Family', Lippincott company, Philadelphia, 1999.
3. Alphonsa Jacob. 'Paediatric Nursing' NR Brothers Publishers, Indore, 2003.
4. Annamalai University, MA. Psychology Study Material. 'Life Span Psychology' Chidambaram, 2000.
5. Arunasree S, et al. 'Play and Children' College Souvenir' Government College of Nursing, Hyderabad, 2005.
6. Arvind Saili. 'Challenges in Neonatology, a Compendium of Management Protocols, Jaypee Brothers Medical Publishers, New Delhi, 1997.
7. Basic Guide to Reproductive Child Health Programme. Department of Family Welfare, Government of India.
8. Behrman, et al. 'Textbook of Pediatrics', Prism Books P Ltd, Bangalore, 1996.
9. Boedecker. 'Women's Life Patterns. Role Involvement and Satisfaction at Midlife', Doctoral dissertation abstract. Pennsylvania State University, 1979.
10. Bullog Vern, Bannie Bullough. The Emergency of Modern Nursing, Macmillan, New York, 1969.
11. Caldwell LL, Smith EA. 'Health Behaviours of Leisure Alienated Youth' Loisir. et. Society and Leisure 1995;18(1).
12. Carlin M. 'Large Group Treatment of Severely Disturbed/Conduct Disordered Adolescents', 'International Journal of Group Psychotherapy', 1996;46(3).
13. Davis Fred. The Nursing Profession, Five Sociological Essays, Wiley, New York, 1966.
14. Fox CO. "Toward a sound historical basis for nurse- midwifery", Bull, American College of Nurse Midwives 1969;14:76.
15. Parulekar V Shashank. Textbook for Midwives (2nd edn). Vora Medical Publishers, Mumbai, 1995.

Epidemiology and Nursing

5

DEFINITIONS

1. **Incidence:** Number of people developing the disease during a defined time period per 1000 population.
2. **Prevalence:** Number of people having disease at a given point of time (point prevalence) or during a defined time period (period prevalence) per 1000 population. The number consists of all cases including new and old ones.
3. **Rate:** Number of occurrences of an event per unit time. It is the time fraction in which all cases contributing to numerator are also counted in denominator. Denominator is the entire population at risk. Rates are generally expressed as per 1000.
4. **Case:** A person identified as having a particular disease, behavior or condition. Cases may be divided in to possible, probable and definite depending on how well a set of specific criteria is satisfied.
5. **Carrier:** Presence of a specific infectious agent in the absence of clinical disease. A carrier serves as potential source for further transmission in the community; temporary carrier state lasts for less than six months. Chronic carrier state may last life long.
6. **Contact:** Exposure to a source of an infection. Transmission due to direct contact may occur when skin or mucous membranes touch, as in body contact, kissing and sexual intercourse. Disease transmitted by contact is also known as contagious disease.
7. **Reservoir of infection:** The natural habit of an infectious agent where the infectious agent may survive or multiply. It may be human, animal or inanimate environment such as soil.
8. **Pathogen:** A microorganism capable of causing disease is a pathogen; those that do not cause disease and are part of the normal flora are known as non-pathogens. Opportunity pathogens are microbes, which are capable of causing disease only when the host resistance is compromised.
9. **Epidemic:** Occurrence of a disease in a community area, clearly in excess of what is expected. This is also referred to as an outbreak. A worldwide epidemic is known as pandemic.
10. **Eradication:** Extermination of an infectious agent resulting in cessation of transmission of infection altogether from given area.

DEFINITIONS OF EPIDEMIOLOGY

1. Epidemiology is a branch of medical science which treats of epidemics (Park, 1873).
2. Epidemiology is the branch of the mass phenomena of infectious diseases (Frost, 1927).

3. Epidemiology is the study of the disease, any disease as a mass phenomenon (Greenwood, 1934).
4. Epidemiology is the study of the distribution and determinants of disease frequency in man (Mac Mahnon, 1960).

Epidemiology is defined as the study of the distribution and determinants of health-related states or events in specified populations, and the population of this study to the control of health problems (John M Last 1988).

Epidemiology has no single definition to which all epidemiologists subscribe; three components are common to most of them. First studies of disease frequency, second studies of the distribution and third studies of the determinants.

Epidemiology is a compound of three Greek words "epi" Meaning upon, "demos" meaning people, and "logos" meaning science. Thus, on etymological basis, epidemiology is a science that deals with mass phenomena. This "definition" though not precise, is sufficiently broad based to suit the expanding scope of epidemiology.

Epidemiology is the study of various factors and conditions that determine the occurrence and distribution of health, disease defect, disability and death among groups of individuals (Clark, 1965)

Epidemiology is the study of the distribution of a disease or a physiological condition in human population and of the factors that influence this distribution (Lilienfeld, 1980)

Epidemiology is the study of distribution and determinants of disease frequency in man (Mohom, 1960).

OBJECTIVES OF EPIDEMIOLOGY

According to the International Epidemiological Association (IEA), epidemiological has three main objects:
1. To describe the distribution and magnitude of health and disease problems in human population.
2. To identify etiological factors (risk factors) in the pathogenesis of disease.
3. To provide the date essential to the planning, implementation and evaluation of services for the prevention control and treatment of disease and to the setting up of priorities among those services.

SCOPE OF EPIDEMIOLOGY

Epidemiology has very wide scope, wider than what is normally conceived. Besides communicable and noncommunicable diseases, the field of epidemiology covers all other health related states and events such as alcoholism drug abuse accidents, divorces, migrations, etc.

Epidemiology studies the distribution of health related states and events. The distribution is viewed in three epidemiological dimensions of time, place, and person.

Epidemiology studies the determinant of health related states and event. These determinants are identified by observing the distribution pattern of diseases and verifying cause effect relationships.

Epidemiology finds application in the control of health problems. Having identified the determinants and their cause effect relationships, epidemiological principles guide the formulation of appropriate interventional strategies for the prevention and control of health problems.

COMPARTMENTS AND SCOPE OF EPIDEMIOLOGY

1. **Descriptive epidemiology:** It deals with the distribution of health states and events in the three epidemiological dimensions of time, place and person.

2. **Analytical epidemiology:** It deals verification of cause effect hypothesis of health related states and events formulated on the basis of their distribution pattern.
3. **Experimental epidemiology:** It deals with experimental confirmation of the cause effect associations upheld by observational studies of analytical epidemiology.
4. **Applied epidemiology:** It deals with the use and application information collected through descriptive, observation and experimental studies.
5. **Constructive epidemiology:** It deals with the application of epidemiological methodology in the investigation of epidemics and their management during epidemic and inter—epidemic phases.

PRINCIPLES OF EPIDEMIOLOGY

1. Epidemiology is the study of occurrence distribution and causes of disease of mankind. It is mainly concerned with the preventive and social science, an important aspect of community medicine. Epidemiology focuses on population or community to measure the distribution and determinants of disease for the purpose of preventing disease and promoting health.
2. Epidemiology approach offers the community health nurses a theoretical basis or framework implementing and evaluating health care at community level.
3. Epidemiology primary purpose is disease prevention and early intervention for the maintenance and promotion of health by which the ultimate aim that is the well-being of the society can be achieved.
4. Epidemiological difference between infectious and noninfectious diseases mainly depends on the element of time. In comparison to infectious disease, noninfectious diseases have long incubation period and a lower frequency of occurrence.
5. Epidemiological process in which the epidemiological investigation tasks place in six steps, 1. Establishing the occurrence of a problem, 2. Verifying the diagnosis, 3. Collecting related data, 4. Describing the occurrence in terms of person, place and time, 5. Formulating a hypothesis and 6. Testing the hypothesis.
6. Epidemiological study methods can be classified in different ways and there is no strict limitation about any classification.
7. Epidemiological measurements are so many criteria or standards are set also used for these measurements. The main measurements have concern with morditiy and morbidity.

NURSING AND EPIDEMIOLOGY

Epidemiology and nursing are important for the attainment of optimal health of the individuals, families and communities. But the approach may be different to achieve this goal. Nursing is as old as mankind. Epidemiology is also an older concept that is found in the health field since 3rd century BC.

Epidemiology aims at describing the occurrence of disease, risk identification and providing data for prevention and control. Community health nursing has the greater concern with the occurrence of disease, health problems and risk factor prevalent in the community. Both epidemiology and nursing need community participation.

The resent nursing is more inclined to communities' health care setting, as it is necessary to raise the health status of the individual and the nation. Thus, both epidemiology and nursing are utmost essential in the field of health science. Nursing and epidemiology are closely related, mutually helpful, and inseparable and have co-existence.

Epidemiology describes the future trends of disease and recommends the specific control measures which are based upon the epidemiological studies. Nursing researches also provide the clues and steps for prevention of the diseases. Community health nurse is a key person in the health information system as well as in health management.

USES OF EPIDEMIOLOGY

Epidemiology process is bound to continue in future adding new challenges to the practice of public health. In these circumstances epidemiology is designed to play an increasingly important role in defining the magnitude of the problems, forecasting their long-term consequences and deriving appropriate strategies for their promotion and control. Presently, the use of epidemiology is mainly confined to following areas.

1. **Disease antecedents:** Epidemiology has always stressed the importance of exploring the natural history of disease in their entirely, with special stress on the identification of disease antecedents rather than disease consequents.
2. **Disease correlates:** Epidemiology has revolutionized the concept of etiology and etiogenesis. Epidemiological studies identified a variety of disease correlates not all of which are casually associated diseases, and some of which behave as risk factors. The risk factors increase the probability of contracting a particular disease.
3. **Disease behavior:** Epidemiological surveillance is applied to disease of international significance. Disease behavior is studied by a process of epidemiological surveillance whereby diseases are kept under constant observation firstly to identify their normal distribution patterns and normal temporal fluctuations, and secondly to detect any deviation in their expected behavior patterns.
4. **Disease and causation:** Epidemiological studies not only establish cause effect association of many noncommunicable diseases, but also estimate the strength of associations in terms of relative and absolute risks. The most notable example are the cause effect associations established by epidemiological studies between smoking and lung cancer and smoking and coronary heart diseases.
5. **Strategy formulation**: Epidemiology plays an important role in strategy formulation for disease control programs and improves program efficiency and effectiveness. Control and eradication of disease is much more complex than their prevention or treatment. A sound control strategy is one that epidemiologically relevant and operationally feasible.
6. **Program evaluation:** Program performance is evaluated by measuring achievements in various operational areas of the program. Evaluation of public health program is both managerial and epidemiological process.

ADVANTAGES OF EPIDEMIOLOGY

1. Epidemiology provides framework within which basic science and behavioral science can be used for community nursing practice.
2. Epidemiology provides an interdisciplinary language to promote interprofessional communication and trust.
3. Public health principle of family is the unit of society prevention and control of disease and health promotion are activated and quantities through epidemiological approach.
4. The epidemiologic model promotes understanding the relationship between environment and agent that expose susceptible populations at risk of impediments to health.

5. The epidemiology helps to plan effective need based health care services on the basis of epidemiological information regarding frequencies and distribution of disease and disabilities their associated factors and causes.
6. The epidemiology helps to determine the effectiveness of health care services planned and implemented on the basis of predetermine criteria regarding its relevance, effectiveness, efficiency and impact on community health. This can help to plan better services in future.
7. Nursing process extended through application of epidemiological methods to describe community needs and evaluate nursing services.
8. An epidemiological perspective provides a method of extending the relationship of family problems to community welfare.
9. The epidemiology helps to identify syndrome by describing the distribution and association of clinical phenomena in the population.
10. The epidemiology helps to determine the usefulness and effectiveness of new innovative techniques, measures and programs.

EPIDEMIOLOGICAL TRIAD

The epidemiology demands a broader concept of disease causation that synthesized the basic factors of agent, host and environment. An individual health is never static and is always in a dynamic equilibrium with environment. The condition of health is seen as the resultant of various ecologic interactions determines the health status in the human organism (Fig. 5.1).

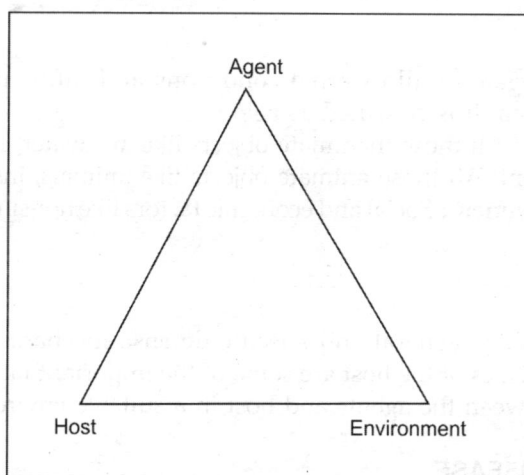

Fig. 5.1: Epidemiological triad

Agent Factors

Disease causing agent in the environment may be classified into the following categories. Inanimate group of agents mainly responsible for noncommunicable disease such as physical agents, chemical agents, nutritional agents and biological agents (Fig. 5.2).
1. **Physical agents:** Heat, light, radiation, etc
2. **Chemical agents:** Acids, alkalies, metals, etc.
3. **Nutritional agents:** Lack or excess nutritional factors.

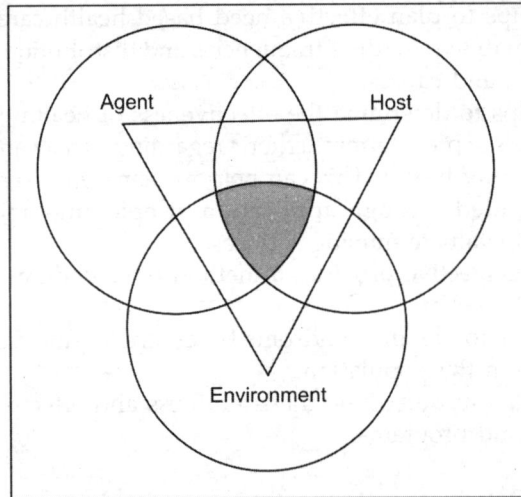

Fig. 5.2: Interaction of agent, host and environment

4. **Biological agents:** The disease caused are always transmissible from one individual to another individual and therefore they are called "communicable diseases". Some of the communicable diseases are transferable only through another medium like insects, where the agents undergo certain changes in their cycles.

Environmental Factors

Environment is the aggregate of all external conditions and influence affecting the life and development of an organism. It is classified as below.
   a. **Physical environment:** All those inanimate objects like air, water, food, etc.
   b. **Biological environment:** All those animate objects like animals, insects and other humans.
   c. **Socioeconomic environment:** Social and economic factors like housing social group, education, etc.

Host Factors

Age, sex, habits and customs, general and specific defense mechanism genetic make-up and psychobiological characteristics of the host are some of the important factors which determine the outcome of interaction between the agents and host in a suitable environment.

NATURAL HISTORY OF DISEASE

Every disease has a period before man is involved and this is called the "period of prepathogenesis" where the inter-relations of the various agent, host and environmental factors which bring the agent and host that follow will take place in the "period of pathogenesis". If the host is able to withstand the stimulus the disease process will not be allowed to progress.

If the agent takes the upper hand the disease progresses with the tissue and physiological changes in the body. During the early part of this period (early pathogenesis) the disease will not be recognized (unless special examinations like the vaginal test—PAP test in the detection of cervical cancer are available) may be missed. Further progression of the disease produces signs and symptoms of the disease. This may progress further, if not recognized and treated early, into disability, defect

PERIOD OF PREPATHOGENESIS		PERIOD OF PREPATHOGENESIS	

Natural history of disease diagram:

Disease process →Before man is involved→ / → The course of the disease in man→

Agent   Host

(inverted triangle)

Environmental Factors
(known and unknown)
Bring agent and host together
or produce a disease
providing stimulus

DEATH

Chronic state

Defect

Disability

Illness

Clinical horizon   Signs and symptoms

Tissue and
physiologic changes

Immunity
and
resistance

Stimulus or agent
becomes established
and increases by muliltiplication

RECOVERY

In the
human   Interaction of host → Host reaction →
host   and stimulus

Early → Discernible → Advanced → Convale-
pathogenesis   early lesions   disease   scence

LEVELS OF PREVENTION	PRIMARY PREVENTION		SECONDARY PREVENTION	TERITARY PREVENTION	
MODES OF INTERVENTION	HEALTH PROMOTION	SPECIFIC PROMOTION	EARLY DIAGNOSIS AND TREATMENT	DISABILITY LIMITATION	REHABILITATION

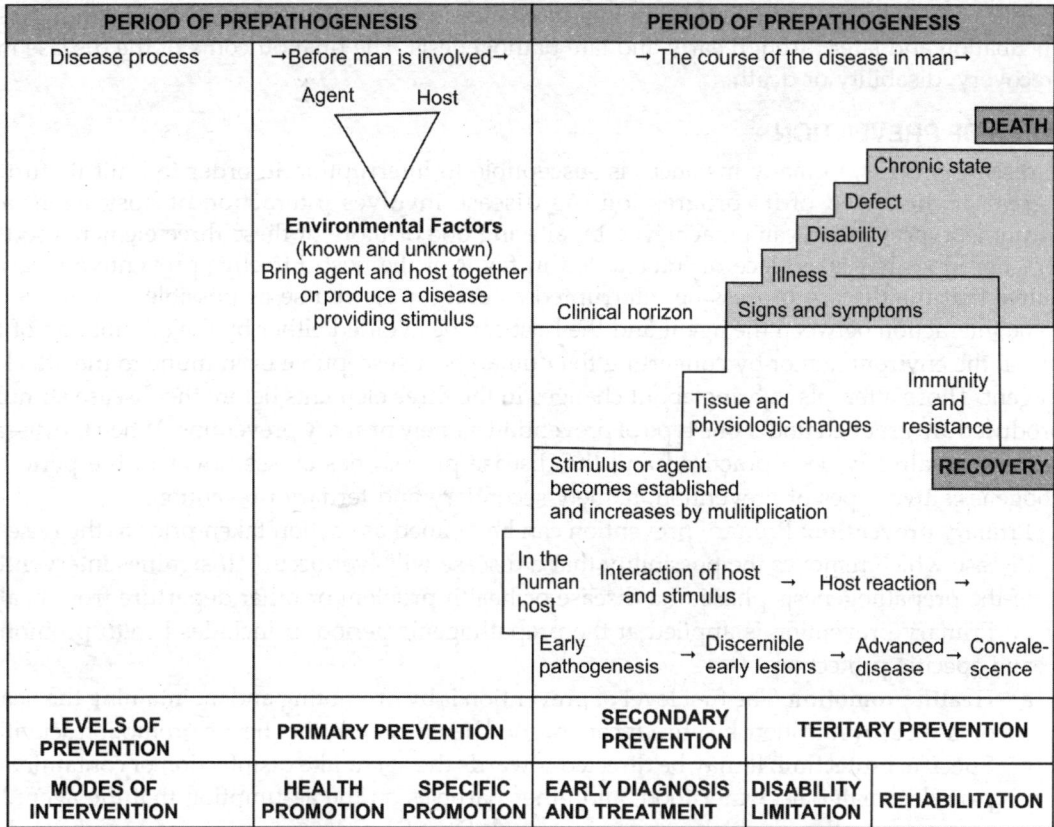

Fig. 5.3: Natural history of disease (from preventive medicine for
the doctor in his community, by Leavell and Clark with permission of McGraw-Hill Book Co)

or death or to a complete recovery without any disability depending on the host factors and effectiveness of treatment taken (Fig. 5.3).

Disease results from a complex interaction between man an agent (or cause of disease) and the environment. The term natural history of disease is a key concept in epidemiology. Each disease has its own unique natural history, which is not necessarily the same in all individuals, so much so, and general formulation of the natural history disease is necessarily arbitrary.

Prepathogenesis Phase

Prepathogenesis phase is a period preliminary to the onset of disease in man. The disease agent has not yet entered man, but the factors which favor its interaction with the human host already exist in the environment. The causative factors of disease may be classified as agent, host and environment. Prepathogenesis period is not sufficient to start disease in man. There is an interaction of these factors to initiate the disease process in man.

Pathogenesis Phase

Pathogenesis phase begins with the entry of the disease agent in the susceptible human host. The further events in the pathogenesis phase are clear cut in infectious disease. The disease agent multiplies and induces tissue and pathological changes the disease progresses through a period of incubation and later through early and late pathogenesis. The final outcome of the disease may be recovery, disability or death.

LEVELS OF PREVENTION

The disease process, in many instances is susceptible to interruption in order to limit its further progress or the speed of its progression. As disease involves interaction of host, agent and environment, prevention can be achieved by altering one or more of these three elements so that interaction does not take place or interrupted in favor of the host. Effective preventive measure requires that the disease process be interrupted as early in its course as possible.

The interaction between the agent and the host can be avoided either by the elimination of the agent in the environment or by converting the human host susceptible or immune to the attack of the agent. Those attempts to bring about changes in the three elements before the disease stimulus is produced are grouped under one type of prevention namely primary prevention. When the disease stimulus has already been practiced and the disease process has crossed over to the period of pathogenesis two types of prevention, namely secondary and tertiary prevention.

1. **Primary prevention**: Primary prevention can be defined as "action taken prior to the onset of disease which removes the possibility that a disease will ever occur". It signifies intervention in the prepathogenesis phase of a disease or health problem or other departure from health.

    Primary prevention is applied at the prepathogenic period; it includes health promotion and specific protection.

    a. **Health promotion:** The first level of prevention is by promoting and maintaining the health of the host by nutrition, health education, good heredity and other health promotion activities.

    b. **Specific protection:** It may be directed towards the agent like disinfection of contaminated particles, materials, water food, and other particles on the assumption that the agent has escaped into these vehicles or environment. Specific protection can also be achieved by immunizations to increase the resistance of the host so that the host will be able to withstand the onslaught of the agent. This is done by the active and passive immunizations.

2. **Secondary prevention:** Secondary prevention can be defined as "action" which halts the progress of a disease at its incipient stage and prevents complications. The specific interventions are early diagnosis, e.g. screening tests, case finding programs) and adequate treatment. The secondary prevention done by early diagnosis and treatment.

    Early diagnosis and prompt treatment comes under secondary prevention. If primary prevention fails or when suitable measures are not available (as in cancer) the disease stimulus is bound to be produced. Early detection of the disease is possible by periodic examinations of population groups who are at special risks like antenatal mothers, growing children, industrial worker, etc.

    Monitoring of persons middle age and above is one of he modern methods of early detection of cancer. In many instances, this detection of the diseases condition is possible only after the onset of the signs and symptoms. Early detection of the disease ensures prompt treatment so that the disease will not progress further.

3. **Tertiary prevention:** When the disease process has advance beyond its early stages, it is still possible to accomplish prevention by what might be called "Tertiary prevention". It signifies intervention in the late pathogenesis phase. Tertiary prevention can be defined as "all measures available to reduce or limit impairment and disabilities, minimize suffering caused by existing

departures and disabilities, minimize suffering caused by existing departures from good health and to promote the patient's adjustments to irremediable conditions". Tertiary prevention includes disability limitation and rehabilitation.

a. **Disability limitation:** It is necessary that the disability, that is caused by limited by active medical or surgical treatment so that there is no further deterioration of the disease process.

b. **Rehabilitation:** Those with permanent disability as in the case of leprosy, tuberculosis, polio, mental retardation, etc. will not be able to lead an independent life unless they are rehabilitated. This level will be needed only when have failed in the application of previous levels of prevention.

APPROACHES AND METHODS OF EPIDEMIOLOGY

Epidemiological Approaches

The epidemiological approach to problems of health and disease is based on two major foundations: 1. Asking questions and 2. Making comparisons. The community health nurse or any health worker need to bear in mind always to use what is known as epidemiological approach in the control of communicable diseases, which includes finding out the source of infection. For this community health nurse needs to have a guide in the following manner of questioning.

1. When did the disease occur?
2. Where did the disease occur?
3. Who were the people affected?
4. Why should it appear?
5. What should be done to prevent the spread?

Asking Questions and Making Observations

Epidemiological studies are done to know the incidence and prevalence of disease in the various subgroups of population by time, place and person. Epidemiologist asks variety of questions and makes observation related to nature and extend (magnitude) of the problem, geographical distribution (where?) time trends (when?) and personal characteristics of people who get the disease (who?). Answer to these questions would help in finding clues to the determinants of disease which are further evaluated.

Making Comparisons

The basic approach in epidemiology is to make comparisons and draw inferences. This may be comparison of two (or more groups)—one group having the disease (or exposed to risk factor) and the other groups not having the disease (or not exposed to risk factors), or comparison between individuals.

Making comparison is another approach which is very important in epidemiological studies, especially analytical and experimental studies to test etiological hypothesis of various disease and evaluate the effectiveness of preventive and therapeutic measures. The similar group for comparison can be obtained either by random selection method or by matching selected characteristics which might affect the results and interpretation.

EPIDEMIOLOGICAL METHODS

Epidemiological methods are applied to know the disease etiology. Various epidemiological studies can be conducted to find out the occurrence of disease in people or persons which may be involved in process of spreading the disease. Epidemiological study methods can be classified in different ways and there are no strict limitations about any complements another.

Descriptive Method

Descriptive epidemiology deals with the distribution of health related states and events by time, place and person. Distribution of cases by time of their appearance gives the time trend of disease. The time trends commonly observed are epidemic, seasonal, cyclical and secular.

Objectives of descriptive method:
1. To provide a data base for planning, providing and evaluating health services.
2. To evaluate the trends in health sector and provide a basis for comparisons among groups.
3. To identify problems for further analysis.

Data collection in descriptive method:
1. Personal characteristics such as age, sex, race, marital status, occupation, education, income, social class, dietary pattern, habits.
2. Place distribution of cases, i.e. areas of high concentration, low concentration and spotting cases in the map.
3. Time distribution trends such as year, season, month, week, day and hour of onset of the disease.

Analytical Method

Analytical method studies comprise two distinct types of observational studies are case control study and cohort study.

Analytical method is carried out to test the hypothesis. These hypotheses are formulated on the information gathered from the descriptive method.

Approaches of analytical method:
I. **Case control study:** It is often called **Retrospective studies** are a common first approach to test casual hypothesis. A case control study is a longitudinal observational enquiry undertaken to verify the existence as well as the strength of cause, effect associations in disease phenomena.

   Case control studies are used for:
   1. Estimating the risk of exposure to various factors associated with disease phenomena.
   2. Identify the modifiable causal factors that can be arrested in the interest of public health.
   3. Evolving risk intervention strategies for prevention and control of public health problems.

II. **Cohort study:** Cohort study is another type of analytical study which is usually undertaken to obtain additional evidence to refute or support the existence of an association between suspected cause and disease. Cohort study is known by variety of names—prospective study, longitudinal study, incidence study and forward—looking study.

   Cohort study is useful for:
   1. Estimating directly the risk of exposure to various factors associated with disease phenomena.
   2. Exploring the natural history of disease in entirely and identifying additional pathological events to complete the natural history.
   3. Identifying appropriate outcome events in the natural history of diseases for appropriate intervention for disability limitation.
   4. Identifying modifiable causal factors for evolving appropriate risk intervention strategies.

Experimental Method

An experimental method is a longitudinal interventional process of trial or verification, undertaken to confirm cause effect relationship of disease phenomena or to evaluate the efficiency of various preventive or curative procedures or programs applicable in hospital or community settings.

Experimental studies used for:

1. Confirming cause effect associations or judging the validity of hypotheses established by observational studies.
2. Evaluating various treatment modalities and interventional procedures applicable in hospital situations.
3. Evaluating the feasibility, efficacy and relevance of various preventive programs of public health significance.
4. Evaluating the feasibility, efficacy and relevance of various risk, intervention approaches of public health importance.

MODE OF DISEASE TRANSMISSION

Communicable disease may be transmitted from the reservoir or source of infection to a susceptible individual in many different ways, depending upon the infections agent, portal entry and the local ecological conditions (Fig. 5.4).

1. **Direct contact:** Infect may be transmitted by direct contact from skin to skin, mucosa to mucosa or mucosa to skin of the same or another person. For example, during touching, kissing, sexual intercourse (STD, AIDS, leprosy, skin infections) and scratching through fingers.

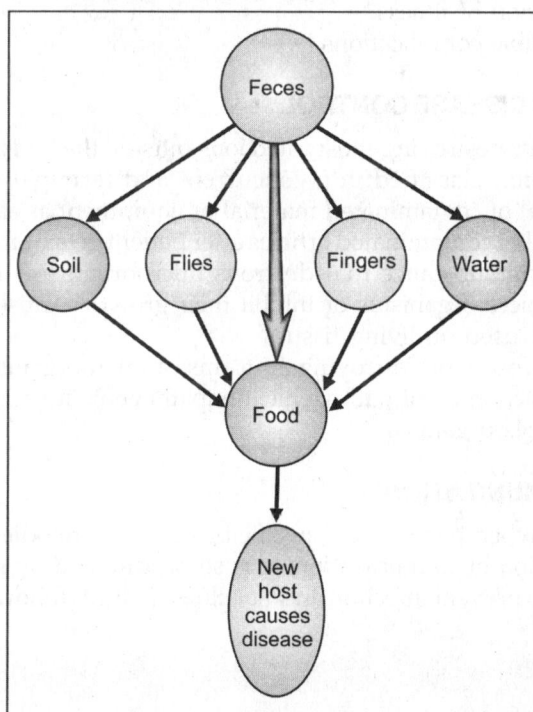

Fig. 5.4: Process of transmission of fecal borne disease

2. **Droplet infection:** Droplet infection occurs due to contact transmission by infections agents contained in most respiratory secretions. The micro organisms from nasopharyngeal secretions during coughing, sneezing or speaking and spitting, talking into the surrounding atmosphere (for example, respiratory infections, TB, meningitis, etc.).
3. **Contact with soil:** Infectious agent (microorganisms) are present in soil can cause disease, when the host comes in the contact with soil (for example, hookworm, tetanus, etc.).
4. **Inoculation into skin or mucosed:** The disease agent may be inoculated directly into the skin or mucosa. Transmission of infection (syringe/needle) as infection after dog bite.
5. **Transplacental (vertical):** Transmission of infectious agent can occur transplacentally.

General Measures of Controlling Communicable Diseases

The control of communicable disease implies mainly the prevention of disease, primary prevention or secondary prevention or combination of both. Tertiary prevention is not so significant in the disease control. The term disease eradication indicates absolute termination of the disease. It implies the cessation of infection and disease. The term disease elimination comes in middle category between the control and eradication.

Objectives of Disease Control

1. To decrease mortality and morbidity.
2. To reduce disease occurrence.
3. To reduce the risk of disease transmission.
4. To reduce the financial burden to the population.
5. To decrease the duration of illness.
6. To prevent from possible complications.

TECHNIQUES USED FOR DISEASE CONTROL

1. **Disinfection:** Killing or destroying most infectious outside the body by physical, chemical or any means. Disinfection classified into concurrent and terminal disinfection. Concurrent disinfection is disposal of contaminated material or equipment as early as possible. Terminal disinfection is disposal of contaminated articles after patient gets transfer or discharge or death.
2. **Antiseptic:** A chemical substance that destroys microorganisms or inhibits their growth. Antiseptics destroy micro organisms or inhibit their growth. Antiseptics are less strong and are safe enough to be used on living tissues.
3. **Sterilization:** It is a process of destroying all forms of microorganisms (including spores). It is the complete destruction of all pathogenic, nonpathogenic microorganisms and viruses or elimination of all viable organisms.

HOST DEFENSES BY IMMUNIZATION

A person is said immune when he possess "specific protective antibodies or cellular immunity as a result of previous infection or immunization or is so conditioned by such previous experience as to respond adequately to prevent infection and /or clinical illness following exposure to a specific infectious agent."

Active Immunity

Active immunity depends upon the humoral and cellular responses of the host. The immunity produced is specific for a particular disease, i.e. the individual in most cases is immune to further infection with the same organism or antigenically related organism for varying periods depending upon the particular disease.

1. **Humoral immunity:** It comes from the B-cells (bone marrow derived lymphocytes) which proliferate and manufacture specific antibodies after antigen presentation by macrophages. The antibodies are localized in the immunoglobulin fraction subpopulations able to help B-lymphocytes.
2. **Cellular immunity:** Cellular immunity plays a fundamental role in resistance to infection. It is mediated by the T-cells which differentiate into subpopulations able to help B-lymphocytes.
3. **Combination of the above:** In addition to the B and T lymphoid cells which are responsible for recognizing self and nonself very often, they macrophages and human K (killer) cells, and their joint functions constitute the complex events of immunity.

Passive Immunization

It is a process of conferring immunity by administrating readymade antibodies of human or animal origin. The immunity offers specific protection for a limited period, lasting for a few months.

1. **Normal human Ig:** It is used to prevent measles in highly susceptible individuals and to provide temporary protection (up to 12 weeks) against hepatitis A infection for travelers to endemic areas and to control institutional and household outbreaks of hepatitis infection.
2. **Specific human Ig:** These preparations are made from the plasma to patients who have recently recovered from an infection or are obtained from individuals who have been immunized against a specific infection and specific human Igs are used for chickenpox prophylaxis of hepatitis B and rabies and tetanus prophylaxis in the wounded.
3. **Antisera or antitoxins:** These are prepared from non-human sources such as hourses. Antitoxins used against tetanus, diphtheria, botulism, gas gangrene and snake bite. Administration of antisera may occasionally give rise to serum sickness and anaphylactic shock due to abnormal sensitivity of the recipient.

ROLE OF NURSE IN EPIDEMICS

Epidemiology and community health nursing are utmost essential in the field of health science. Epidemiology and nursing are closely related for the attainment of optimal health of the individuals, families and communities. Community health nurse take active role to identify and investigates the problem during outbreak of epidemics.

1. Community health nurse has a greater concern with the occurrence of disease, health problems and risk factors prevalent in the community. The community health nurse works for the prevention and control of disease at various levels.
2. Community health nurse participate as one of the team member especially when it is large scale investigation, e.g. occurrence of any epidemic or community level general health survey or specific health survey, surveillance activities and screening, etc.
3. Community health nurse take active participation in prevention and control of communicable disease such as notification of certain specific disease like measles, diphtheria, tetanus, hepatitis rabies, STD to the health authority and also identify sources of infection and methods of spread of infection.
4. Community health nurse provide health education for the community regarding preventive and control measures epidemics, because she plays a key person in the health information system in the community.
5. Community health nurse takes vital role during at any unusual occurrence of any disease, she investigates regarding frequency and distribution and possible determinants analysis of

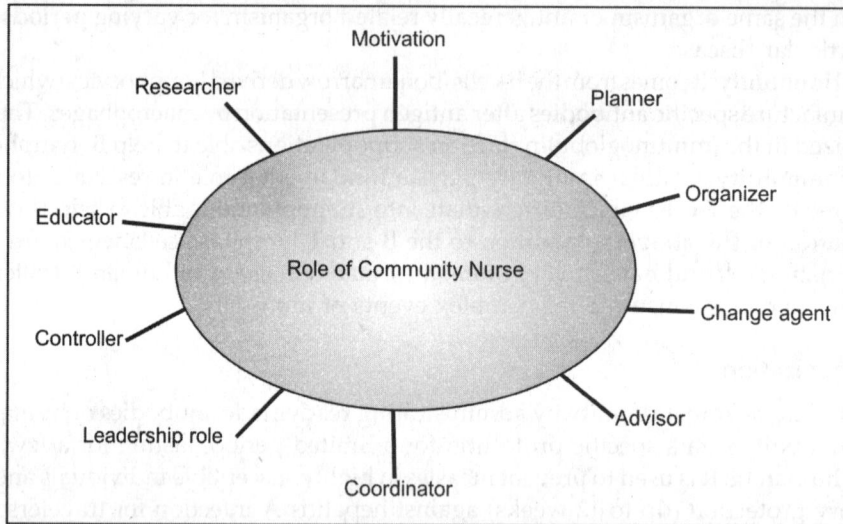

Fig. 5.5: Role of nurse in community participation

information collected, comparison with previous findings and with rates at the national level and planning and implementation of prevention and control program.

ROLE OF NURSE IN COMMUNITY PARTICIPATION

The community health nurse is responsible for maintaining link between the village and the health care delivery system. The community health nurse has to strengthen health care services. In each village, there is a "health house" or a subcenter which covers 5,000 populations with a community health worker or multipurpose health workers and a traditional birth attendant supervised by the community health nurse (Fig. 5.5).

1. **Motivator:** Motivation plays an important role in community participation. Community health nurses working together and motivate people to sharing the management of health care delivery system. Motivation is also to play an important role in filling the gap between health personnel and community people. Encouraging for social mobilization for community participation to enabling communities to be principal partners in health care development.

2. **Planner:** Planner role depends upon the health assessment done by the community people and plan according to their felt need and priorities setting by the participation of community.

3. **Organizer:** She has to organize the structure community participation to perform the task to achieve the common goal. She has to decide and delegate work among with community people. She makes arrangement for community resources.

4. **Change agent:** She serves as a positive change agent. She is able to make others more effective by increasing their capabilities. She encourages the community to develop capabilities and to change in their attitudes and behavior.

5. **Advisor:** She gives suggestions and advices on practical situations which require immediate actions. She shows concern to their problems and helps them to solve the problems.

6. **Coordinator:** She is linkage between communities and health care system. Communities must be linked to health system facilities which will serve as referral centers, as well as source of

technical expertise for correct information provider. The community health nurse coordinates the health services with community participants.

7. **Leadership role:** She leads the group by giving them directions, ensuring byway communication providing supervision and guidance by coordinating their activities. She helps people to identify their health problems and become self-reliance in their health matter.

8. **Controller:** She has to monitor the activities and make sure that it is proceeding in right direction or there are some difficulties. She takes correct action according to the situation.

9. **Educator:** It is one of the important functions of community health nurse to educate communities to promote health and prevent illness, help people to gain knowledge, modify health attitudes, behavior and competence to become self-dependant.

10. **Researcher:** She makes use of investigative approach to identify health problems, gather information, to get the feedback and further plan health intervention by problem solving approach.

BIBLIOGRAPHY

1. Basavanthappa BT. Community Health Nursing, Commence Participation, Jaypee Brothers, 1st edn 97-99.
2. Bonnie K, Taneja R, Nasasi G, K Roy TK. Community Participation to Reducing HI V/AIDS transmission 2001.
3. Clarke PN, Cody WK. Nursing theory-based practice in the home and community: The crux of professional nursing education. Adv Nurs Sci 17;1994:41-53.
4. Gulani KK. Community Health Nursing: Community participation. Kumar Publishing House, 1st edn, 47-53.
5. Hunt R, Zureck EL. Introduction to community based nursing. Philadelphia, Lippincott-Raven 1997.
6. National League for Nursing. A vision for Nursing Education. NLN Press, New York, 1993.
7. Park, K, Textbook of Preventive and social medicine "Community Participation," Banarasidas Publication, 17th edn, l0, 26, 650-56.
8. Patni S. Textbook of Community Health Nursing, Role of nurse, 1st edn, 11-14.
9. Sen Gupta NC, Community participation in tuberculosis programme, bull IUAT 1972, 47,102-06.
10. Steiger NJ, Lipson JG. Self-care nursing and practice. Bowie MD Robert Brady, 1985.
11. Talaja S. NRHM Newsletter, "ASHA", Published by Deptt. of Health and Family Welfare, Government of India, 1st edn.

SECTION 2: PSYCHOLOGY

6

Introduction to Psychology

DEFINITIONS

1. **Psychology:** It is a study of systematic and scientific study of human and animal behavior. It has own special methods, which help us in gathering and organizing its subjective matter or the essential facts about it.
2. **Introspection:** It means looking within, looking into the working of our own minds and reporting, what we find there.
3. **Psychotherapy:** The application of specialized techniques to the treatment of mental disorders or to the problems of everyday adjustment. The major techniques employed by psychotherapists include depth interviews, conditioning, suggestion and interpretation.
4. **Psychotic:** Characterizing a state of psychosis or resembling the behavior of an individual, who has a psychosis.
5. **Psychophysiological:** It is pertaining to processes that have both bodily or material and psychological or mental aspects.
6. **Psychosis:** A severe mental disorder characterized by disorganization of the thought process, disturbances in emotionality, disorganization as to time, space and person and in some cases.
7. **Psychosocial:** It is pertaining to social relationships involving psychological factors.
8. **Psychosomatic disorders:** A disorder caused by a combination of organic and psychological factors. In psychosomatic disorders there may be tissue changes, as with peptic ulcers.
9. **Psycho techniques:** The practical application of psychological principles to the control and management of behavior.
10. **Psychometrics:** The branch of psychology dealing with the development and application of statistical and other mathematical procedures to psychology.

INTRODUCTION

The word 'psychology' is derived from two Greek words, 'psyche and logos'. 'Psyche' means soul and 'logos' means study of psychology, as a scientific discipline in an extremely exciting field of knowledge. It continuous, to grow at an accelerating field pace each year, and continues to provide answer to the question about the human behavior.

Psychology has enormous potential if offers us the hope of both understanding and improving the quality of life. Psychological knowledge has been used in measuring intelligence, designing school curricula, helping troubled marriages, controlling aggression, selling products and treating both the young and old with greater sensitivity and humaneness.

DEFINITIONS OF PSYCHOLOGY

1. Psychology is defined as "a science of human and animal behavior".
2. Psychology is a science, which aims to give us better understanding and control of the behavior of the organism as a whole.
3. Psychology as the scientific study of behavior does not exclude mind and other internal process from the field of psychology; what a person does his or her behavior is the outcome of the internal mental process.
4. Psychology is the science of human and animal behavior; it includes the applications of this science to human problems.
5. Psychology is the study of processes or activities of man in relation to his environment—Woodworth.
6. Psychology related to reaction to any and every situation of life—Skinner.
7. Psychology is the science or study of the mind and how it functions—Oxford dictionary.

NATURE OF PSYCHOLOGY

1. Psychology deals with the mind and its working and that the knowledge of psychology helps in reading other peoples mind.
2. Psychology is concerned with behavior and while dealing with behavior it extends it to animal behavior.
3. Psychology possesses a well organized theory, which is supported by the relevant psychological laws and principles.
4. Psychology has its applied aspects in the form of various branches of applied psychology like industrial, legal, clinical and educational psychology.
5. Psychology has established facts, principles and laws of the behavior in the subject psychology enjoys universal applicability in practical life, other bodies of the knowledge and future researches in its own field.
6. Psychology as a science deals systematically with human behavior, with the motives, feelings, emotions, thoughts and actions of men and women.

PSYCHOLOGY AS A SCIENCE

1. A science is a body of systematized knowledge that is gathered through careful observations and measurements of events in experiments set up by the scientist to produce the events being studied of course, all events studied by a scientist are not necessarily produced experimentally. At times, he has to observe the spontaneous events.
2. The psychologist do experiments and make observations, which others can repeat, they obtain data often in the form of quantitative measurements, which others can verify.
3. As a science, psychology is a systematic data from experiments and observations are essential, but from them to make some sense in helping us, understand events, they must be organized in someway. Scientific theories are important tools for the organization of observed facts.
4. The most three essential requirements for a field of knowledge to be called a science. Firstly, it deals with observable facts, secondly, science is not a mere collection or description of facts, it aims at the explanation of facts, thirdly, every science has its own methods, accordingly to these a scientist has to choose a problem for investigation.
5. Measurement in psychology is often more difficult than it is in science such as physics and chemistry because many of the psychological studies cannot be measured directly by physical scales. For example, emotion, intelligence, and attitudes.

6. Psychology is related to many other sciences such as biological sciences, sociology, philosophy, psychiatry. Its scope is very wide, it has many branches such as general psychology, animal psychology, child psychology, abnormal psychology, clinical psychology and applied psychology.

PSYCHOLOGY AS A BEHAVIORAL SCIENCES

1. Psychology deals with certain aspects of behavior as does anthropology, sociology, economics or political science. All these sciences concern themselves with a specific aspect of behavior.
2. Psychology deals with the general nature of behavior. It does not select a single aspect of behavior like the rest if the behavioral sciences. It pervades the entire range of behavior and the basic principles underlying it.
3. Psychology includes not only the conscious behavior and activities of human mind but also the subconscious and unconscious. Consequently, it covers not only the overt behavior but also the covert behavior involving all the inner experiences and mental processes.
4. An organism like a human being constantly behaves. So also the animals, psychology as a science of behavior deals with these acts of the organism. The environment means the surroundings objects and circumstances. It may be physical or social in nature.
5. Overt behavior is the most obvious and outwardly expressed form of behavior. It is easily observable. Covert behavior is not so easily observable. The initial activities of feeling, thinking and the like are the examples of covert behavior, while the activities like walking, smiling, hitting, etc. are those overt behaviors.
6. Behavioral sciences are concerned with the observation and explanation of human behavior either in single individuals or in groups. Psychology also inter-related with many other biological sciences.

RELATION OF PSYCHOLOGY WITH OTHER FIELDS OF STUDY

1. **Psychology and biological sciences:** These studies gives light on their behavior and are closely related to the study of mental functions.
2. **Psychology and sociology:** It deals with the activities of a group of people taken as a whole. It studies traditions, customs, intuitions and other group of behaviors.
3. **Psychology and philosophy:** There is a close relationship between the two as both philosophy and psychology attempt to interpret human behavior.
4. **Psychology and Psychiatry:** Psychiatry deals with study, diagnosis and treatment of the mentally ill.

SCOPE OF PSYCHOLOGY

Psychology deals with all types of experience in society or private like all phases that emerge in the realism of human life. Psychology discusses the inner dynamics of behavior like motives and emotions. It concerns itself with individual differences in behavior and tries to find out the factors that explain these differences. It also deals with the study of abilities and aptitudes. Psychologists have also devised appropriate tests for measuring these abilities and aptitudes in people. Psychology also consider the working of the sensory and response mechanism. It discusses the impact of the physical stimuli on sense organs. It also discusses and investigates the working of the senses organs, nervous system, muscles and glands. Social and community psychology deals with individual, family and group for the prevention of illness and promotion of health. It includes various types of group phenomena like public opinion, propaganda, attitudes, beliefs and crowd behavior.

HISTORY OF PSYCHOLOGY

Introduction

The subject psychology has a long past but a short history. The meaning of this statement is simply that human kind has given thought to psychological questions for many centuries. The ancient philosophers wrote at length about psychology. However, psychology as an established and recognized science in universities and colleges is less than one hundred years old.

The date, when psychology became a field of study formally detached from philosophy is generally taken as 1879, the date when Wilhelm Wundt, the principal founder of experimental psychology established the first psychological laboratory in Leipzig, Germany.

Brief Historical Background of Psychology

1. **Karen Homey (1885-1952):** Holistic psychology personality attributes are the result of the interaction between the person and environment.
2. **Edith Jacobson (1897-1978):** Object relation theorist. Infants experience of pleasure or unpleasure as the core of the relationships with the mother.
3. **Carl Gustav Jung (1875-1961):** Analytical psychology. Collective unconscious as consisting of all human kinds.
4. **Kern Berg (1928):** Borderline personality organization. Several defense mechanisms responsible for rapid alterations of transference.
5. **Sren Kierkegaard (1813-1855):** Philosophical theory. Behavior on the basis of response to stimuli.
6. **Melanie Klein (1882-1960):** Traditional Psychoanalysis. Gratifying experiences reinforce basic trust.
7. **Heinz Kohut (1913-1981):** Theories of self psychology. Patients become aware of their excessive needs for approval and self gratification.
8. **Jaoques Lacan (1901-1981):** Interpsychic concepts of Freud. Primary process of thought is actually uncontrolled free flowing sequences of meaning.
9. **Kurt Levin (1890-1947):** Field theory. Behavior becomes a function of the person and his environment.
10. **Abraham Maslow (1908-1970):** Self-actulation theory. The need to understand the totality of a person.
11. **Adolph Meyer (1950-1966):** Theory of psychobiology. Introduced the concept of common sense psychiatry disoriented behavior as reaction to genetic, physical, psychological, environmental and social stresses.
12. **Gardner Murphy (1895-1979):** Parapsychology. Explained the essential stages of personality development such as stage of undifferentiated wholeness, stage of differentiation and stage of integration.
13. **Henry Murray (1893-1988):** Personology. It describes the study of human behavior. He focused on motivation, which is a need that is aroused by internal or external stimulation. He developed TAT (thematic apperception test).
14. **Frederick S Perls (1893-1970):** Gestalt theory. Behavior represents more than the sum of its parts.
15. **Sandor Rado (1840-1972):** Theories of adaptational dynamics disordered behavior by interfering with the organism's ability for self-regulation.

16. **Otto Rank (1884-1957):** Theory of birth trauma. The personality is divided into impulses, emotions and will.
17. **Wilhelm Reich (1897-1957):** Character armor. The personality that serve as a resistance to self understanding and change. It is classified into 4 type's hysterical, compulsive, narcissistic and masochistic character.
18. **Carl Rogers (1902-1987):** Person centered theory of personality and psychotherapy. Personality not as a static entity composed of traits and patterns by as a dynamic phenomenon involving every changing communications, relationships and self concepts.
19. **BF Skinner (1904-1990):** Operant Learning. Personality was not different from the other behaviors or sets of behaviors it required maintained and strengthened.
20. **Harry Stack Sullivan (1892-1949):** The total configuration of personality traits is known as the self system.

Structuralism

1. The aim of the school of psychology called structuralism was to analyze conscious experience into its sensory elements.
2. Wilhelm Wunt (1912) had subjects in his laboratory introspect (look in to their own minds) and report the sensory elements experiences such as hearing melodies, seeing paintings and tasting foods.
3. Structuralism did not receive its name from Wundt but from its critics. Critics of Wundt's approach felt that Wundt was too interested in the static structure of the human mind and not its dynamic quality.

Functionalism

1. Functionalism is contrast to structuralism, emphasized the changing and dynamic quality of consciousness.
2. The father of functionalism William James (1890) compared the human mind to a river always flowing and changing.
3. Functionalism as its name implies, asserts that consciousness has a function an aim. Functionalism provided an impetus for psychologists who are interested in applying psychology to industry and education.

Behaviorism

1. Behaviorism came into being in the 1910's with the writings of John B Watson.
2. Watson (1919) claimed that the concept of consciousness was unnecessary for psychology. He thus attacked at once both structuralism and functionalism.
3. The essential idea in behaviorism is that consciousness cannot be observed. It is completely private and personnel.
4. Watson suggested using more specific concepts such as habits or Pavlov's conditioning reflexes. Watson's aim has to transform psychology from quasi philosophical study of the mind into valid "Science of behavior".

Gestalt Psychology

1. Gestalt psychology came into being as a reaction against Wundt's structuralism. It came into prominence in Germany. Simultaneously when behaviorism was gaining attention in America.

2. During 1910's without being aware of one another's development. The father of Gestalt psychology is Max Wertheimer.
3. The essential point of Gestalt psychology is that it is important to explain everything by analyzing it downward, by always reducing it something that is presumably on a more basic level.

Psychoanalysis

1. The father of psychoanalysis is Sigmund Freud. His personal influence in psychology made itself known over a long period of time beginning in the later part of the nineteenth century and ending in the 1930's.
2. Freud argued that motives, ideas and memories often exist in human personality outside of consciousness (awareness).
3. The human mind is like iceberg. The exposed tip represents consciousness. The large region below water level represents the unconscious domain of the mind. Freud argued that the unpleasant or painful ideas are repressed or pushed down into the unconscious.
4. Freud devised a technique called free association for making repressed material available to consciousness. Freud believed that if a neurotic patient could see into the nature of his conflicts than those conflicts would lose most of their power to make the patient suffer.

Neo-Freudian Theories

1. Several contemporary psychoanalysts like Karen Homey, Erich, Formm and Harry Stack Sullivan are all referred to as neo-Freudians.
2. Their theories of personality are essentially revisions of Freuds while they differ from each other in many specific details and they are similar in that they all emphasized the role of culture in the development of personality rather than biological drives or instincts.
3. According to Harry Stack Sullivan, personality does not exist apart from interpersonal relations. In other words, there is no personality, unless one is interacting with others.

Humanistic Psychology

1. A single individual cannot be named as the father of humanistic psychology. The movement known as humanistic psychology did not become a powerful force in psychology until the 1960s.
2. Humanistic psychology is characterized by the belief that man is always struggling to become. Humanistic psychology sees the individual's task in life as the making of a series of conscious choices between constructive and destructive alternatives.
3. The humanistic psychology is also termed existential psychology or existential humanistic psychology.

BRANCHES OF PSYCHOLOGY

Introduction

The science of psychology, since its foundation, has grown into different levels. Its application is widely used. Among the other branches of pure psychology may be included experimental psychology, comparative psychology and physiological psychology. The branch of applied psychology includes clinical psychology, individual psychology, human psychology and educational psychology, etc.

Subfields of Psychology

Physiological Psychology

It is a branch, which experimentally investigates the physiological bases of behavior including the anatomical structure and physiological processes which are related to psychological events, psychological processes and mental functions. It often uses operative technique, investigating the functions of brain for instance, by removing portions of the brain tissue and noting the effect upon behavior.

Experimental Psychology

- Experimental psychology that studies the process of sensing, perceiving, learning and thinking about the mind.
- It is the observation of concomitant variations and interpretation of the concomitance as cause and effects. In this method, a systematic controlled scientific methodology in the investigation of psychological phenomena is used.
- The systematic presentation of the methodology and the results are usually within the context of a laboratory. The work of experimental psychology overlaps with that of the focus of biopsychology as well as that done by other types of psychologist.

Developmental Psychology

- Developmental psychology deals with the changes in behavior that accompanies change in age from conception to death.
- Since behavior and abilities change most rapidly during the early years, child psychology has traditionally received the most attention from developmental psychologist.
- Development psychology has both pure and applied aspects.

Social and Personality Psychology

- Social psychology is the study of the individuals in the growth and relationship of group to one another. Thus, social psychology considers the psychological interrelations of people forming families, crowds, societies and mobs and of the leader with his followers.
- It includes the study of the formation of group attitudes and opinions. It is thus forced into a consideration of social and national conflict, or race prejudice and similar manifestation of the inter-relations of the conflicting needs of many individuals.
- Personality psychology is concerned with individual people and administration of psychological tests extensively. The personality psychologist is interested in understanding the nondeviant or normal cases.

Clinical Psychology

- Clinical psychology is the practical application of dynamic and normal psychology to the problem of human adjustments.
- Clinical psychology is devoted to study, diagnosis and treat behavior disorders. It is the largest subfield of psychology.
- A clinical psychology is well trained in the etiology of causes of the various forms of abnormal behavior such as psychoneuroses, psychoses, etc. and also trained in various methods of diagnosis of abnormal behavior through psychological testing.

Counseling Psychology

- Counseling psychology is related to clinical psychology but different in that the problem it deals with is generally of less serious in nature.
- Personal, vocational and educational guidance are provided. Psychologist who are well versed in the different diagnosis and treatment of such minor behavior problems are known as psychological counselors.
- The counseling psychologist deals with individuals if milder emotional and personal problems. He also practices psychotherapy as well as depending upon the severity of the problems.

School Psychology

- The counseling psychologist who administers tests and guides individual students is generally called as school psychologists.
- The school psychologist is on specializing in problems associated with elementary and secondary an educational system who utilizes psychological concepts and methods in programs or reactions which attempt to improve learning conditions for students.

Industrial-Organizational Psychology

- Industrial-organizational psychology is concerned with the psychology of the workplace. Specifically, it considers issues such as productivity, job satisfaction and decision making.
- The first application of psychology to the problems of industries and organizations was the use of intelligence and aptitude tests in selecting employees.
- Now private and public organizations also apply psychology to problems of management and employee training, to supervision of personnel, to improving communication within the organizations to counseling employees and to alleviating industrial conflict.

Consumer Psychology

- Consumer psychology considers peoples buying habits and the effects of advertising on behavior.
- Consumer psychologist to research on consumer attitude towards the company's product.
- As a subfield of psychology, the psychology principles are applied to practical problems of consumer products.

Health Psychology

- Health psychology explores the relationships between psychological factors and physical ailments or disease.
- For instance, health psychologist are interested in long-term stress can affect physical health.
- They are also concerned with identifying ways of promoting behavior related to good health or discouraging unhealthy behavior such as smoking.

Cross-cultural Psychology

- Cross-cultural psychology investigates the similarities and differences in psychological functioning in various cultural and ethnic groups.
- Psychologist specializing in cross-cultural issues investigates the ways in which people in different culture attribute their academic successes or failures leading to differences in scholastic performance.

Forensic Psychology

- Forensic psychology is another emerging specialty the works hand with the legal, court and connectional system.
- Forensic psychologist assist police in a variety ways, from developing personality profiles of criminal offenders to helping law-enforcement personnel understand problems like family conflict and substance abuse.
- They may also assist judges and parole officers in making decisions about the disposition of convicted offenders.

METHODS OF PSYCHOLOGY

Introduction

The scientific method is emphasized as the basis for investigation. The founding of Wundt's laboratory marked the beginning of the formal application of the scientific method to problems in psychology. This method is neither identified with any particular kind of equipment, nor is it associated exclusively with specific research procedures.

Definition

Method is defined as a systematic procedure involved in the investigation of facts and concepts. It also uses special techniques in psychology such as experimental method or the clinical method used to collect facts.

Methods used in Psychology

1. Descriptive techniques.
2. Introspection.
3. Naturalistic observation.
4. Case history.
5. Survey.
6. Experimental method.
7. Rating scale and check list.
8. Genetic or development method.
9. Psychological and educational tests.

Descriptive Techniques

- Introspective method, naturalistic observations, case history or case studies and survey can be clustered together as descriptive techniques.
- These methods provide different way to describe behavior, without any attempt to interfere with the behavior under study.
- Descriptive techniques can provide useful information about how different techniques can provide useful information about how different events behaviors are related to each other.

Introspection

- Introspection is one of the oldest methods use for investigating consciousness. It is a process of analyzing a conscious experience by reporting the sensory qualities of the stimuli that are expressed.

- The word introspection means "to look within". In introspection subjects were presented with a particular stimulus or task and asked to describe their mental state as thoroughly as possible.
- This method is used to observe the individual, analyze and reports his own feelings, thought or all that passes in his mind during the course of a mental act or experience.
- This method cannot be used by children or animals of mental defectives because, they cannot introspect. By the early 20th century psychologist recognizes the inadequacies of introspection.

Naturalistic Observation

- Naturalistic observation is a method within the descriptive research category on a topic. Just as the name states, phenomena of interest are systematically observed as they occur in nature.
- The researcher observes behavior in its natural setting and systematically. The systematic observation means that from the wide array of ongoing behavioral interaction, the researcher selects the focus and categories of his/her observations.
- The systematic observation the means of the naturalistic observation method is probably the oldest and in some ways most basic form of scientific research.

Case History

- The detailed study of a single individual's behavior over an extended period of time is called a case history or case study.
- In a typical case study, the researcher presents a detailed description of the personality and behavioral characteristics of an individual.
- The goal of this procedure is to provide a detailed description of a person aver time as opposed to the naturalistic observation.

Surveys

- Surveys study large and small population of selecting representative samples chosen from the population to discover the relative incidence, distribution and inter-relation of psychological and sociological variables.
- In survey research, the researcher simply collects data about psychological and sociological variables or characteristics of a sample that represents a known population in natural setting.
- The survey research is concerned with conditions or relationships that exist, opinions that are held processes that are going on, effects are evident or trends that are developing.
- That survey research which involves samples usually is called as "Sample Survey".

Experimental Method

- The experimental method is the technique of discovering information by means of experimentation.
- An experiment is a series of observations carried out under controlled conditions for the purpose of testing a hypothesis.
- In using the experimental method, the researcher systematically manipulates one or more variables to determine hoe those variables affect behavior.
- In an experiment, the variable that is manipulated is called the independent variable while the behavior that is measured is called dependent variable.
- In the experiment method, the experimenter has complete control over the laboratory situation. The extraneous variances are controlled. The measurements in a laboratory are more precise because they are more with precision instruments.

Rating Scale and Checklist

- There are commonly used devices of observing and evaluating personality of behavior traits. In rating scales we rate on individual on the possession or absence of certain traits on a certain scale.
- The measurement scale has five degree of the trait to be rated. This is a five-point scale. Some scales have three or seven degree.
- In a checklist examiners may be provided with a list of traits or qualities and may be asked to point-out or check-up ones that apply to particular persons.

Genetic or Developmental Method

- This method seeks to find out he causes of a complicated behavior in its simple beginning. It assumes that a full appreciation of each behavior patterns of an adult requires, the study of simple behavior patterns more complex gradually as individual grows in age.
- These sample behavior pattern grow more complex gradually as the individual grows in age. For example, if we are interested in understanding the learning behavior of an adult, we should begin with the learning behavior in his preadolescence and in the light of these, arrive at some conclusions about the learning behaviors in adulthood.

Psychology and Educational Tests

Theory and practice no matter related to any field of knowledge, represent idea and action. One is as necessary as the other not only for their own survival but also for rendering some service to the humanity. Therefore, in any scheme of study there should be a close integration of theory with practice. Psychology is not an exception. Here too we must pay due emphasis over the practical work besides theoretical insight with the subject. Being a student of educational psychology you must be well versed in using and employing the theory and contents of psychology in a practical way. You yourself may also have a curiosity to know your intellectual level, your interests and aptitudes, your personality make up, your adjustment to your self and the environment, etc. You can know such things about them through their measurements and this measurement is possible through the relevant psychological tests. Many of these tests have been constructed and standardized by the psychologists and researchers in India as well as abroad. In their test manuals, they have described all about their test, its usability, method of administration, scoring and interpretation, etc. for the benefit of its users.

1. *Standardized tests:* Standardized tests include tests for intelligence, achievement, personality, study skills, aptitude and interest. These have been developed scientifically by psychologists and educators after long experimentation.
2. *Achievement tests:* Generally fall into two categories.
   a. **Level of achievement tests:** Which show at what level a student is able to function in a variety of Subjects and skills. A teacher would use this type of test at the beginning of the year to assess the range of achievement in his class so that he may screen the class in to working groups.
   b. **Qualitative achievement tests:** Once the teacher has determined range of achievement; he will find these tests helpful to show the breadth and depth of each childs understandings and skills in a particular subject.

Characteristics of Psychological Tests

Carefully developed and researched psychological tests have several characteristics:
1. Standardization.
2. Objectivity.
3. Based on sound norms.
4. Reliability.
5. Validity.

   1. *Standardization:* It refers to the consistency or uniformity of the conditions and procedures for administering a test. To achieve standardization, people must be tested under uniform conditions.

   2. *Objectivity:* It refers primarily to the scoring of the test results. The scoring process must be free of subjective judgment or bias on the part of the scores.

   3. *Test norms:* To interpret the results of a psychological test, a frame of reference or point of comparison must be established so that the performance of one person can be compared with the performance of others. This is accomplished by means of test norms. The distribution of test scores of a large group of people is similar in nature to the individual being tested. For example, a science graduate applies for a job that requires mechanical skills and achieves a score of 83 on a test of mechanical ability.

     This score alone tells us nothing about the level of the applicant's skill, but if we compare that score of 83 with the test norms the distribution of scores on the test from a large group of science graduates — then we can ascribe some meaning to the individual score. If the mean of the test norms is 80 and the standard deviation is 10, we know immediately that an applicant who scores 83 has only an average or moderate amount of mechanical ability. With this comparative information, we can evaluate objectively the applicant's chances of succeeding on the job relative to the other applicants tested.

   4. *Reliability:* It refers to the consistency of a person's scores. For example, a boy takes a cognitive ability test and achieves a mean score of 100 and after one week if we repeat the test and he achieves a mean score of 72, we would describe the test as unreliable because it yields inconsistent measurements.

   5. *Validity:* It refers to the test's accuracy in measuring what it is supposed to measure. For example, if a test is a valid measure of intelligence, people's scores on that test should be strongly correlated with their grades in school.

Development of Psychological Tests

Several steps were involved in development of psychological tests. These include:
1. Analysis of the situation in which the tested skills are to be used.
2. Tentative selection of the test items.
3. Development of a standardized method of administration and scoring.
4. Administration of all test items to a large representative group of individuals.
5. Final selection of items.

Evaluation of the Final Test

   1. **Analysis of the situation:** In this test detailed analysis of the psychological processes required for successful performance of the task in question is carried out.

2. **Tentative selection of the test items:** In the second step after the analysis has been made the psychologist selects tests already available or devices tests which he feels will measure the processes.
3. **Development of standardized procedures:** Psychological tests to be administered and scored in the same way for every individual tested in order to obtain consistent results.
4. **Administration of the test to a representative group:** In this step, the psychologist administers the test to a representative group of subjects to see if they score the way expert judgment or other evidence suggests. In these way, psychologists were able to determine the effectiveness of the test.
5. **Final selection of the test items:** In this process many test items are either discarded or revised so that they contribute more directly to the overall purpose of the test. This procedure is called item analysis. The final selection of items is based on empirical findings.
6. **Evaluation of the final test:** Effectiveness of the final test is evaluated in terms of a specified criterion.

Types of Psychological Tests

Psychologists categorize tests in two ways based on how they are constructed and administered and based on skills and abilities they are designed to measure.

Classification of psychological tests based on construction and administration:
- Individual and group tests
- Speed and power tests
- Computer-assisted tests
- Paper-pencil and performance tests

1. **Individual and group tests:** Individual psychological tests are designed to be administered to one person at a time. Group tests are designed to be administered to a large number of people at the same time.
2. **Speed and power tests:** Speed tests have a fixed time limit, at which point everyone taking the test must stop. Power tests have no time limit, applicants are allowed as much time as needed to complete the test.
3. **Computer-assisted tests:** It is a means of administering psychological tests to large groups of applicants in which an applicant's response determines the level of difficulty of succeeding items. For example, in computer-assisted testing individual does not have to waste time answering questions below his level of ability. The computer program begins with a question of average difficulty and if the individual answers correctly, it proceeds to questions of greater difficulty. If not, it asks less difficult questions.
4. **Paper-pencil and performance tests:** Paper-pencil tests are in printed form; answers are recorded on a standard answer sheet. Performance test assess complex skills, such as word processing or mechanical ability for which paper-pencil tests are not appropriate.

Classification of psychological tests based on tests of knowledge, skills and abilities:
1. Achievement tests
2. Aptitude tests
3. Intelligence tests or cognitive ability tests
4. Interest tests
5. Neuropsychological tests

6. Occupational tests
7. Personality tests
8. Specific clinical tests:

Achievement tests: Achievement tests are used in educational or employment settings and they attempt to measure the achieved knowledge such as Mathematics or spelling. For example, term ending exams.

Aptitude tests: These tests measure specific abilities such as mechanical or clerical skills. These include measurement of perceptual speed and accuracy, attention to detail, the capacity to visualize and manipulate objects in space, principles of mechanical operation, ability to operate computers. For example, General Aptitude Test Battery (GATB), Differential Aptitude Test (DAT)

Intelligence tests: These tests attempt to measure intelligence, i.e. basic ability to understand the world around. For example, Stanford-Binet scale, Army Alpha Test, Army General Classification Test.

Interest tests: Psychological tests to assess a person's interests and preferences; used primarily for career counseling.

Neuropsychological tests: These tests measure deficits in cognitive functioning (ability to think, speak, reason, etc.). The deficit in cognitive functioning may result from some sort of brain damage such as strike or a brain injury.

Occupational tests: They attempt to match interests with the interests of persons in known careers.

Personality tests: They attempt to measure basic personality style. Two of the most well-known personality tests are:

The Minnesota Multiphasic Personality Inventory (MMPI)
The Rorschach inkblot test

Specific clinical tests: They attempt to measure specific clinical matters, such as current level of anxiety or depression. For example, Hamilton rating scale for depression, Brief psychiatric rating scale.

Uses of Psychological Tests

1. It is easier to get information from tests than by clinical interview.
2. The information from tests is more scientifically consistent than the information from a clinical interview.
3. They assist in diagnosis. For example, Rorschach inkblot test.
4. They assist in the formulation of psychopathology and identification of areas of stress and conflict. For example, Thematic Apperception Test.
5. They help to determine the nature of deficits present. For example, Cognitive neuropsychological assessments.
6. They help in assessing severity of psychopathology and response to treatment. For example, Hamilton rating scale for depression, Brief psychiatric rating scale.
7. They help in assessing general characteristics of the individual. For example, assessment of intelligence, assessment of personality.
8. These tests are also used for forensic evaluations, regarding litigation, family court issues or criminal charges.
9. These tests assess level of functioning or disability, help direct treatment and assess treatment outcome.

CONCLUSION

Literary meaning of psychology is the science of mind. Some others have accepted it, as the science of consciousness. Both of these meanings are not the appropriates of psychology, as the modern psychology does not recognize mind and gives more importance to the mental processes or modes. According to modern concept, psychology is the study of human behavior. It includes stimulated behavior and internal mechanism. Psychology deals with the mind and its working and that the knowledge of psychology helps in reading other peoples minds. Scope of psychology is very extensive. Behavior is associated with life and psychology with behavior. It studies all normal, abnormal, child, adult, man and animals and also compares them.

BIBLIOGRAPHY

1. A concised textbook on psychiatric nursing (Comprehensive Theoretical and Practical approach) Bhatia MS, l994.
2. Ahuja N. A short textbook of psychiatry, Jaypee Brothers Medical Publishers, 3rd edn, 1995.
3. A Textbook of Psychiatric & Brooking (Julia). London, Mental Health Nursing, 1992.
4. Aggarwal JC. Education Vocational Guidance and Counseling revised and enlarged 8th edn, Doaba House; New Delhi; 1998;Chapter 23:257-71.
5. Basvanthappa BT. Nursing Education, Jaypee Medical Publications, 2nd Edition, New Delhi.
6. Best W John, Kahn V James. Research in Education; 7th edn, Asoke K Ghosh; Prentice Hall of India Pvt Ltd, New Delhi, 2002;25, 26,106-07.
7. Bimla Kapppor. A Textbook of Psychiatric, Kumar Nursing Publishing House, Delhi 1992.
8. Essentials of child psychology, Connell (HM) Blackwell Scientific Publications, 1989.
9. Flippo Edwin B. Principles of personnel management, McGraw Hill, New York, 1975.
10. George K Aleyamma. Principles of curriculum development and evaluation; Vivekananda Press, Nammakkal, Tamil Nadu, 2002; Chapter-5, evaluation, 120-90.
11. Geropsychiatric Nursing 1995. Higstel (Mildrito) Mosby.
12. Gupta CB. Principles and Practice of Management, 4th edn, National Publishing House, New Delhi, 316-30.
13. Heidgerhen H Loretta. Teaching and Learning in School of Nursing: Principles and inc. (HOD; 3rd edn, Konark Publishing Pvt Ltd, Delhi 1994;629-68.
14. Lancaster Jeanette. Nursing Issues and Managing Change, Sally, Schrefer, Mosby Publications 1999, Evaluation Program; 496-502.
15. Manual of psychiatric nursing care plans. Schultz (J M) Scott, 3rd edn, 1989.
16. Mental Health and Mental lllnessed 4. Barry (PD) JB Lipincott, 1990.
17. Mental Health Nursing, A Holistic Approach Pasquali CV Mosby and Co, 1989.
18. Mental Retardation: A manual for multi-rehabilitation. National Institute Work of Mental Health, Bengaluru, 1998.
19. Psychiatric Emergencies. Talley and King, Macmillan, New York, 1994.
20. Psychiatric Mental Health, Townsend (Mary c) Philadelphia Nursing Concepts of Care, 1993.
21. Psychiatric Nursing, Keltnero (Norman) Mosby, 1995.
22. Psychiatric Nursing Care Plans 2. Fortinash K Mosby, 1991.
23. Psychiatric Nursing: Biological and behavioral concepts, Otong (DA). WB Saunders 1995.
24. Wise Yoder. Leading and Managing in Nursing; Coon L. Nancy; Mosby Publications; Missouri; 1995; 200-01.

Biology and Behavior

7

DEFINITIONS

1. **Aggression**: A general term applying to behavior aimed at hurting other people, also applies to feelings of anger or hostility. Aggression functions as a motive, often in response to threats, insults or frustrations.
2. **Alarm reaction**: The first stage of the general adaptation syndrome, consists of prompt responses of the body, many of them mediated by the sympathetic system, which prepare the organism to cope with stressors.
3. **Assimilation**: In Piaget's theory of cognitive development, the modification of one's environment so that it fits into already developed ways of thinking and behavior.
4. **Associated areas**: Regions of the cerebral context involved in such complex physiological functions as the understanding and production of language, thinking, and imagery.
5. **Behaviorism**: The view that human and animal behavior can be understood, predicted and controlled without recourse to explanations involving mental states.
6. **Hormone**: A secretion of a specific organ, often an endocrine gland into the bloodstream, where it is carried to various organs of the body to have an effect, a chemical messengers.
7. **Neurobiology**: The science of the nervous system includes neuroanatomy, neurophysiology, neurochemistry, neuropharmacology, neuroembryology, physiological psychology and other disciplines concerned with the structure, function and development of the nervous system.
8. **Neurotransmitter:** A chemical substance stored in vesicles and released into synaptic clefts or neuromuscular junction, to excite or inhibit neurons or muscle fibers.
9. **Puberty**: The period, during which the capability for sexual reproduction is attained, it is marked by changes in both primary and secondary sexual characteristics and is dated from menarche in girls and the emergence of pigmented pubic hair in boys.
10. **Wernicke's area**: An area in the temporal lobe of cerebrum which is necessary for the recognition of speech sounds and therefore for the comprehension of language, also plays a part in the formulation of meaningful speech.

BEHAVIOR AND NEUROSCIENCE

Introduction

It is the field of study that examines the biological roots of behavior. This interdisciplinary includes the study of genetic factors, hormonal factors, neuroanatomy, drugs, development factors and environmental factors to team about brain—behaviors relations.

The human brain is the most complex of complicated structure in known universe. Scientists have estimated that the about human brain is composed of 180 million nerve cells, 50 million of which are devoted to processing information.

Major Activities of Brain

1. The brain monitors and controls our basic life support system, such as breathing and digesting.
2. It directs our movements and maintains our balance and posture.
3. It receives and interprets information from the world around as.
4. It records significant it records significant and sometimes insignificant event into our memory.
5. It allows us to solve problems, use language and think of new ideas.
6. It enables us to feel materials such as soft cotton and to experience emotions such as happiness and snows.
7. Working together with the glands of the endocrine system and the rest of the nervous system.

Historical Review of Biology and Behavior

1. Early Greek and roman physicians believed that behavioral problems were caused by imbalance of vital fluids that moved through the body and brain. Only after the renaissance did people accept the view that behaviors and thought were reduced by specific structures in the brain.
2. During the nineteenth century, neurologist performed autopsies on former patients and discovered the brain areas responsible for producing and comprehending speech. This work led to other discoveries that should that specific psychological functions were associated with specific brain areas.
3. Early in the twentieth century, research on the physiological basic of behavior showed that when an area of the brain is destroyed sometimes remaining portions can take over its function. This view that different areas of the brain can be equivalent to one anther is called equipotentiality theory.
4. According to integrationist theory, complex psychotically functions are based on number of basic abilities. These basic abilities may be involved in the same psychological function. Our thoughts and actions are a product of the functions of interrelated neural structures.
5. Today, neuropsychologists use a variety of procedures to learn about brain behavior relation. Much of this work is based on studies of laboratory animals. They perform brain operations to se how the removal or destruction of brain tissue in a particular area affects. Now the medical imaging technique makes it possible to examine the living brain.

NEURON

Introduction

The nerve cells called "Neurons" are the basic units of operation in nervous system. By themselves, though they cannot explain the complexities of thought and emotion. It is only when the wires are arranged in to complicated patterns by become of producing action and thought.

Basic Neural Processes

1. The nervous system is basically constellated from only two different types of cells, Nerve cells; the neurons receive and transmit neural signals to other parts of the body.

2. **Glial cells:** The more numerous of the two support and protect the neurons. Glial cells take their name form the French word for glue. The from a connective, network that holds together the brains billions of neurons.
3. The glial cells insulate none neuron from another throughout the nervous system and clear always cellular debris when neurons system and clear away cellular debris when neurons degenerate and die.
4. A continuous layer of glia surround the blood vessels in the brain to establish a blood—brain—barrier a protective shield that prevents many harmful chemical substances from passing the blood to brain.

Structure of Neuron (Figs 7.1 and 7.2)

1. Neurons are of many different shapes and sizes but they share certain anatomical features. Neurons have a cell body, dentists and an axon.
2. The cell body consists of a membrane boundary that surrounds the nucleus and internal contents of the cell. The nucleus in the portion of cell that contains deoxyribonucleic acid (DNA) Strands of protein that holds the genetic blue print for the cells makeup and function. Neuropsychological—field of psychology that represents the convergence of this scientific discipline in called as neuropsychology.
3. The cell also contains protoplasmic material that manufactures chemical substances used to communicate with other neurons.
4. Reaching out from the cell body like the branched of the tree, dendrites receive information form other neurons. The longer and more complex a neurons dendrites, the greater number of connections it can make with other cells.

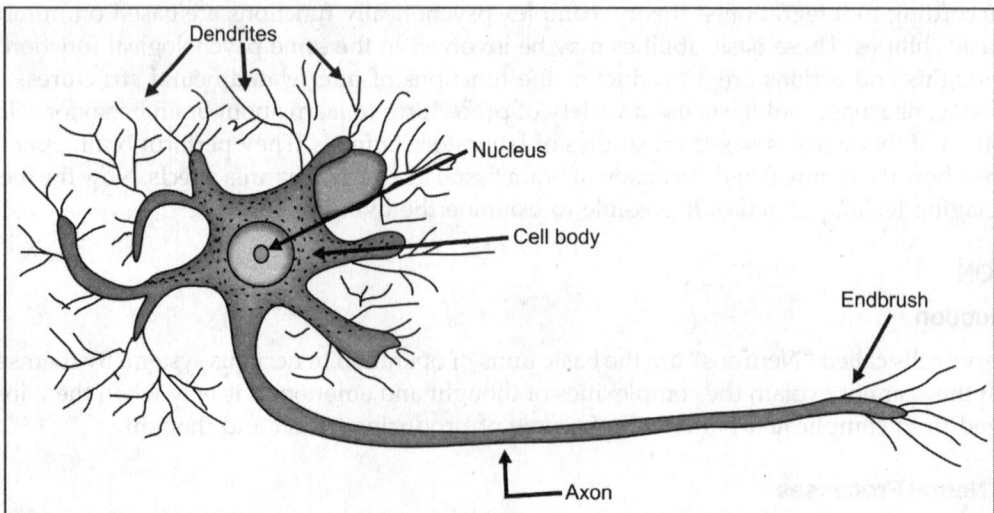

Fig. 7.1: Neuron

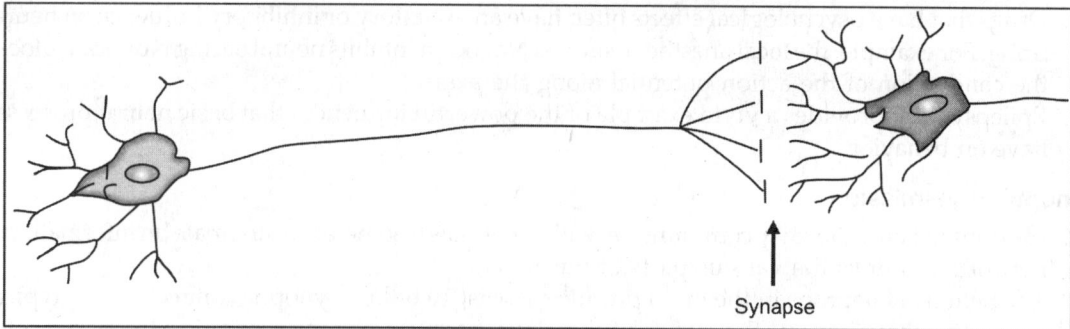

Fig. 7.2: Synapse between two neurons

5. Neural signals are transmitted to other cells by the axon, a single fiber that emerges form the cell body. Axons in the brain are usually less than one millimeter long. But axons from the spinal cord to the big to can reach lengths of three feet or more.
6. The chemical substances can travel in both directions along on axon and more than one type of chemical massage can be passed to the receptors of an adjacent cell.
7. **Myelin sheath:** Axons are usually coated with an insulating material called a myelin sheath that is produced by the glial cells. Myelin also helps prevent the scrabbling of neural messages.
8. Nodes of ranvier periodic proaks in the myelin sheath, which cause than axon to resemble a headed necklace, are called nodes of ranvier. These nodes allow axons with myelin insulation to transmit neural signals faster than uninsulated axon can because the signals can be transmitted along the axon by jumping from one note to the next.

Neural Impulses and their Transmission

1. When a neuron is sufficiently stimulated by another neuron, there is an electrical reaction in the walls of the axon that travels over the entire length of the walls of the axon the terminals.
2. The electrical reaction is called the neural impulse depending upon the diameter of the axon and the thickness of the myelin sheath, a neural impulse travels at a rate of approximately 2 to 2000 miles per hour.

Neural Firing

1. Neural impulses are generated by electrochemical processes involving the cell membrane.
2. When a nerve cell is strongly stimulated by another cell, there is a chemical change in the cell membrane, the membrane becomes permeable causing positively charged ions from the outside to enter and negatively changed ions from the inside to exit.
3. This change quickly reverses the cell membrane's electrical change at the point of stimulation and causes the adjacent portion of the cell membrane to reverse its change as well.
4. For a neuron to generate an impulse, it must receive a certain level of stimulation. This is called the threshold level the neuron fires in a uniform and unchanging way.
5. Neuron can fire even without outside stimulation. There is a baseline level of spontaneous activity in each neuron as it lies waiting for new stimulation. That stimulation can come either in the form of excitatory influences that increases.

6. Drugs that have psychological effects often have an excitatory or inhibitory influence on neural firing. For example, the local anesthetic such as Novocain inhibits neural baring Novocain blocks the conduction of the action potential along the axon.

7. Epilepsy itself provides a vivid example of the powerful influences that basic neural processes have on behavior.

Synoptic Transmission

1. Neurons not only fire, they communicate with other cells to generate on to create on informational network that links the various parts of our body.

2. The billions of neurons in the brain produce at least 10 billion synoptic connections. A typical neuron my have several thousands of these synapses, small gaps separating the nerve cells.

3. The electrical impulse that has traveled down the axon of the transmitting cell must has traveled down of the transmitting cell must be converted into a chemical messenger that stimulates another neuron across the synoptic junction.

4. In neurological terms, the transmitting cell is called the presynaptic neuron, the receiving cell is called the postsynaptic neuron, and the chemical messenger is known as the neurotransmitter. Since neurotransmitter affects other cells chemically, this means the most drugs messengers that are transmitted from one cell to another.

Levels of Integration within the Central Nervous System

The central nervous system, as has already been observed, carries out the important function of integrating behavior. The sensory nerve impulses travel from organs through the peripheral nervous system to the central nervous system and at this level is integrated in the form of a motor nerve impulse which goes to the effectors (muscles and glands) which give response. The integration that is basic to all behavior functions at different levels in central nervous system. The simplest integration of behavior takes place at the level of spinal cord, in the form of reflex action.

In addition to this spinal integration there are numerous other integrations at the subcortical levels. They function within the medulla, thalamus, hypothalamus and cerebellum. Medulla controls the necessary balance of vital, body functions. While undertaking a strenuous activity like running, climbing, etc. the rate of breathing goes up. This is due to medullar control. Similarly, the control of pulse rate and blood pressure takes place by the activity of medulla.

Finally, the most complex and important integrations take place at the cortical level. Cerebrum and its cortex are the most developed and best evolved regions of the brain. Several association area are situated in the cortex. As already discussed, learning of new things and memories of past experience are stored at several cortical centers. It is due to this specialized area that higher mental processes like learning, thinking, and reasoning, problem solving, imagining and remembering are possible for human beings. All complex emotional and motivated responses too are controlled by the cortex.

From the above discussion, however, it will be wrong to conclude that the brain functions in parts. The brain is such an extraordinary. Mechanism that it can function in parts and also as a whole.

NEUROTRANSMITTERS AND BEHAVIOR

Introduction

Neurotransmitters are manufactured in the pragmatic neuron and stored in ting sacs called vesicles located in the axon terminals of the pragmatic neuron, it forces the vesicles to break, like cannon fining a burst of shells, and the vesicles shoot their chemical contents—the molecules of the neuro-transmitter into the synaptic junction.

A receptor site is simply a portion of an adjacent neuron that receives the molecules of a neurotransmitter. Since, there are specific receptor sites different types of neurotransmitters will key into a given receptor site.

Types of Neurotransmitters

Acetylcholine (Ach)

1. **Location:** Brain, neuromuscular junction and in the peripheral nervous system. It may be critical for normal thinking.
2. **Effects:** Deficiency of acetylcholine causes paralysis Alzheimer's disease. Excess may cause violent and muscle contriction. Drugs that increase Ach in cerebral cortex appear to help teaming and retention.

Amino Acids

1. **Location:** Brain used by neurons for fast excitation and inhibition. Glutamic acid aspartic acid – for excitation. Gamma-aminobutric acid and glycine for inhibition.
2. The effects of amino acids are liked to the control of anxiety. The deficiency causes mental deterioration (hunting tons chorea).

Catecholamine

1. **Location:** Brain and peripheral nervous system it includes both and norepinephrine (NE).
2. Dopamine plays major role in the regulation of movement deficiencies causes Parkinson's disease, excess may cause major disturbances of thought, perception, emotion behavior.
3. Norepinephrine (NE) affects arousal and mood deficiency causes depression, excess cause's agitation and manic condition.

Neuropeptides

1. **Location:** Brain-released during painful or stressful situation, end options.
2. Neuropetides causes pain reduction and may be involved in eating, memory, sexual behavior and mood.

Serotonin

1. **Location:** Central nervous system influences sleep and body temperature.
2. Deficiency of serotonin causes depression.

Action of Neurotransmitters

1. The excitatory or inhibitory influence can change a neurons threshold for fining. These excitatory or inhibitory influences are determined by the synaptic cells.
2. Synaptic sites at dendrites tend to be excitatory, while synaptic sites at the cell body tend to be inhibitory.
3. Consequently, a neurotransmitter at an inhibitory synapse will make it less likely to fire. At any given time, a cell receives neurotransmitters from various receptor sites.

4. The postsynaptic neuron analysis the incoming excitatory and inhibitory signals and fires only if the net level of stimulation passes its firing threshold.
5. When this threshold is reached the electrical to chemical, chemical to electrical transmission process is almost complete.
6. All that remains are for the neurotransmitter to be deactivated to that the postsynaptic neuron can be stimulated again.

Deactivation or Re-uptake

1. Deactivation can occur in one of two ways, fist an enzyme at the synapse can break, breakdown the neurotransmitters.
2. Second the neurotransmitter can return to the presynaptic neuron. This process is called re-uptake and it is the most common form deactivation.
3. Deactivation is crucial for without it the nervous system would become, over stimulated, this would lead to tremors and eventually death.
4. Some insecticides and nerve gases produce their deadly effects by blocking the deactivation of neurotransmitters at the neuromuscular, thus victims die of uncontrolled muscle spasms.
5. Neurotransmitters and diseases.

Depression

1. A group of drugs called tricycles among the most successful in reliving depression are believed to increase the availability of both neurotransmitters in certain areas of the brain.
2. The recent research that the antidepressant effects of these drugs may be related to increased sensitivity of the receptors for those two neurotransmitters (norepinephrine, and serotonin) rather than a mere change in the actual levels of these brain chemicals.

Drug-related Behaviors

1. A wide variety of commonly used drugs have the effect of exchanging thought processes emotional states, or behaviors.
2. Extensive research has linked the brain opiates to an array of behavioral and mental processes, including a sense of well-being and euphoria, counteracting the influence of stress, modulating food and liquid intake, facilitating learning and memory and reducing.

ENDOCRINE SYSTEM AND BEHAVIOR

Introduction

The endocrine system is a chemical communication network that sends messages throughout the nervous system and accretes hormone that affect body growth and functioning although the endocrine system is thought of a distinct form the brain, nervous system and sense organs, it has important functional relationships with these statures.

Concepts on Behaviors

1. About three hundred years age, the French philosopher Rene Descartes proposed that the pineal gland is the point of interaction between the soul and the body.
2. The endocrine glands are distinguished from duct glands. Also they are said to be ductless because they secrete their products, chemical messengers called hormones they directly enter in to the bloodstream.

3. The duct glands secrete their substances into body cavities or the surface of the body. Examples of duct glands are the salivary digestive and tear glands.

Pituitary Gland

1. The pituitary gland is located at the base of the skull near the hypothalamus as is about the size of a pea. It is sometimes called the master gland in view of the fact its hormones often play the role of triggering the activity of other endocrine glands.
2. One of the key hormones released by the pituitary is the growth hormone, which controls a number of metabolic functions, including the rate of growth of the bones and soft tissues.
3. The pituitary also produces a number of huge protein molecules called neuropeptides, these substances acts as eating and drinking, sexual behaviors, sleep, temperature refutation, pain reduction, and responses to.

Thyroid Gland

1. The thyroid gland, located within the neck, response to pituitary stimulation by releasing the hormone thyroxin.
2. The principal function associated with the thyroidal gland is the control of body metabolism, the rate at which a person, burns glucose circulating in the bloodstream.
3. The metabolism is in turn closely linked to motivational and mood states the thyroid has important impact on behavior.

Parathyroid Glands

1. The four parathyroid glands are found behind the thyroid gland itself. They are small gland and they secrete a hormone that regulates a metabolism of calcium and phosphorus.
2. Disorders of the parathyroid glands could bring about defective above development during a child's early years of development.

Adrenal Gland

1. The adrenals are pair of glands, located just above each kidney, that influence our emotional state, level of energy and ability to copy with stress.
2. They consist of two parts an inner core called the adrenal medulla and outer layer called the adrenal cortex.
3. The medulla produces epinephrine and norepinephrine making the heart beat faster, diverting blood from the stomach and intestine to the voluntary muscles.
4. At times of stress the hypothalamus causes the pituitary to release ACTH (adrenocorticotropic hormone) which in turn stimulates the adrenal cortex to increase its secretion of a number of hormones the influence metabolism.

Thymus Gland

1. The thymus gland is located below the thyroid gland and under the breast.
2. **Bone:** The thymus gland appears to play its major role in infancy and childhood.
3. Secreting a hormone associated with the body's capacity to resist infection. When a child has an infection, the thymus sends a message to the spleen and the lymph node.

4. The message tells these structures that they should produce lymphocytes, cleaning cells that attack foreign organisms in the bloodstream. Once the body's immune system is developed, the thymus loses some of its functional role.

Pancreas Gland

1. The pancreas gland secretes two important hormones, insulin and glycogen.
2. Insulin is the hormone that induces the oxidation or burning of blood sugar.
3. If a person's pancreas is defective and it is unable to secrete adequate amount of insulin, the person will suffer from diabetes or chronic high blood sugar.

Gonads

1. There are two types of gonads. There are the ovaries in female and testes in the male.
2. The ovaries are located in the vicinity of the uterus, one ovary on either side. In addition to producing egg cells, they also produce hormone. Estrogen is identified as playing a principal role in determining secondary female characteristics such as breast development and lack of facial hair.
3. Progesterone cooperates with estrogen in the regulation of ovulation and in the preparation of the uterus for pregnancy.
4. Testosterone plays an important role in determining secondary male characteristics such as facial hair, voice depth and muscular development.

GENETICS AND BEHAVIOR

Introduction

Genetics is the study of how traits are inherited or passed on from parent to child. The cells from which we started contain genes, which are the basic units of heredity. They determine our sequence of growth into a human baby. Genes determine our blood group, coloration and many other traits. In general, genes determine the resemblance between the newborn and the parents.

General Concepts of Genetics

1. Genetics are located in the nucleus of every cell in the body. They are composed of deoxyribonucleic acid (DNA) which contains blue prints for life.
2. Living organisms are made of protein and DNA controls the way in which protein chains are built.
3. Material for constructing protein surrounds cells and DNA sends out messenger molecules ribonucleic acid (RNA), to control how the material is fashioned into specific kinds of protein chains.
4. Every living cell contains 20,000 and 125,000 genes grouped together in cluster of a thousand or more. They are arranged in thread like chains called chromosomes.
5. The cells in human body have 46 chromosomes, arranged in 23 pairs. We inherit one member of each pair from our father and the other from our mother.
6. Genes are transmitted from generation to generation by means of sex cells. A female gamete is called ovum and a male gamete is called a sperm.

7. Ovum and sperm combine their chromosomes when they unite to form one cell called a zygote. Thus zygotes have 46 chromosomes, half from the father which determine our genotype or genetic inheritance, for the rest of our lives.

Genetic Errors

1. Errors are made occasionally in transmitting genes from one generation to the nest. As a result, children are sometimes born with abnormal chromosome structures, which are called mutations.
2. Two Xs and a Y: People with an XXY mutation of ten have characteristics of both sexes. They might have developed breasts and small testicles.
3. Two Y and an X: Males with an extra Y chromosome (XXY) are often taller than other males. On the other hand XYY males in the general population are no more aggressive than normal males.
4. Another kind of genetic mutation is one in which a persons has 47 chromosomes because of an extra one added to pair 21.
5. Children with chromosomal abnormalities suffer from Down's syndrome, a disorder characterized by mental retardation and unique physical appearances, including folds on the eyelid corners, a round face, a head with a flattened back, a short neck and a small nose.

Causes of Mutation

1. Some people carry mutator genes that increase the rate of mutations in other genes.
2. High temperatures can increase mutation rate. Males generate sperm in their scrotum, a sac that is usually cooler than the rest of the body in mammals.
3. Radiation has been linked to mutation rate, X-rays are one source of radiation and pregnant mothers are advised to avoid them.
4. Radiation before pregnancy may also increase mutation rate. Recent evidence suggests the exposure to radiation may explain the increased risk of having Down's syndrome, babies for older mothers.

Genetic and Behavioral Problems

Genetic Influences and Schizophrenia

1. While research and debate continue over the role of biological factors and life-experience in schizophrenia, a consensus in forming on one major point.
2. One of studies that have convinced many people involves identical and fraternal twins. Identical twin pairs have identical heredity, fraternal – twin pairs do not so if schizophrenia is strongly influenced by genes.

Genetic Factors and Depression

1. The cognitive-learning or life-experience factors may be involved in depression; many investigations believe that biological factors also play a role.
2. Some physiological deficit, either inherited or acquired in other ways, is thought to make some people especially vulnerable to depressive episodes. We have known for sometime that hereditary factors play a role in some depression.

CONCLUSION

The term behavior is usually extensively in psychology. Its scope is not limited to physical activities but includes all sense organs (eyes, ear, tongue, skin, and nose) all activities of brain (concentration, imagination, thought, effort, memory intellect, etc.). Thus human behavior includes all activities and this indicates the concept of Woodworth that psychology is the science of activities. It is very important to study the health behavior of man from the point of community health because human behavior is a result of complex interaction between body and mind. The inter-relation between physical and mental processes affects the total health of individual.

BIBLIOGRAPHY

1. Arnold MB (Ed.). The Nature of Emotion, Penguin, Baltimore, 1968.
2. Baddeley AP. The Psychology of Memory, Basic Books, New York, 1976.
3. Bandura A. Principles of Behaviour Modifications, Rinehart and Winston, New York, Holt, 1969.
4. Carlson NR. Psychology of Behaviour, Boston, Allyn and Bacon, 1977.
5. Furguson ED. Motivation: An Experimental Approach. Rinehart and Winston, New York, Holt, 1976.
6. Goddard FA. The Human Senses, 2nd edn, Wiley, New York, 1972.
7. Hilgard ER, Bower GH. Theories of Learning 4th edn, Prentice-Hall, Englewood Cliff, NJ 1974.
8. Hochberg JE. Perception, 2nd edn, Englewood Cliffs, Prentice Hall, NJ, 1978.
9. Hulse SH, Deese J, Egeth H. The Psychology of Learning, 4th edn, McGraw-Hill, New York, 1975.
10. Johnson PM. Systematic Introduction to the Psychology of Thinking, Harper and Row, New York, 1972.
11. Korman AK. The Psychology of Motivation, Englewood Cliffs, Prentice Hall, NJ, 1974.
12. Lindsay H, Nirman DA. Human Information Processing, 2nd ed, Academic Press, New York, 1977.
13. Morgan CT, King RA. Introduction to Psychology, 6th edn, Tata McGraw-Hill, New Delhi, 1982.
14. Morgan CT. A Brief Introduction to Psychology, Tata McGraw-Hill, New Delhi, 1975.
15. Mueller CG. Sensory Psychology, Englewood Cliffs, Prentice Hall, NJ., 1965.
16. Munn, Norman L. Introduction to Psychology, Oxford and IBH, New Delhi, 1973.
17. Robinson DN. An Intellectual History of Psychology, Macmillan, New York, 1976.
18. Strongman KT. The Psychology of Emotion, Wiley, New York, 1973.
19. Thompson RF. Introduction to Psychological Psychology, Harper and Row, New York, 1975.
20. Vinacke WE. The Psychology of Thinking, 2nd ed, McGraw-Hill, New York 1974.

Educational Psychology

8

DEFINITIONS

1. **Educational psychology:** In this branch of psychology, we try to study the behavior of the learner in relation to educational environment. As a science of education, the subject matter of this branch helps in improving all the processes and products of education. The teachers can teach well and the students can learn well with the help of the knowledge and skills gained through the study of this subject. It also helps the teachers in gaining proper insight for bringing desirable modification in the behavior and seeking an all round harmonious development of the personality of the students.

2. **Social psychology:** This branch of psychology studies the human behavior in relation to his social environment. One's behavior as a member of the group, the process of communication and interpersonal relationship. Group dynamics and social relationship, etc. form the subject matter of this branch.

3. **Learning:** Learning is the process by which an activity originates or is changed through reacting to an encountered situation, provided that the characteristics of the change in activity cannot be explained on the basis of native response, tendencies, maturation, or temporary states of the organism.

4. **Maturation:** Maturation is a developmental process within which a person, from time to time manifests different traits, the 'blueprints 'for which have been carried in his cells from the time of first conception.

5. **Operent conditioning:** Operant conditioning refers to a kind of learning process whereby a response is made more probable or more frequently by reinforcement. It helps in the learning of operant behavior, the behavior that is not necessarily associated with known stimuli.

6. **Intelligence:** Intelligence is the aggregate or global capacity of an individual to act purposefully, to think rationally, and to deal effectively with his environment. Intelligence consists of an individual's those mental or cognitive abilities which help him in solving his actual life problems and leading a happy and well-contented life.

7. **Emotional quotient:** The concept of EQ in understanding and measuring one's level of emotional intelligence in the same way and as we utilize the concept of IQ in understanding, utilizing and measuring one's level of intelligence or intellectual potential. As a result the term emotional quotient represents a relative measure of one's emotional intelligence potential in the same way as intelligence quotient (IQ) does for the measurement of one's intellectual potential.

8. **Creativity:** Creativity is the capacity of a person to produce compositions, products or ideas which are essentially new or novel and previously unknown to the producer.
9. **Creative process:** The creative process is any process by which something new is produced— an idea or an object including a new form or arrangement of old elements. The new creation must contribute to the solution of some problem.
10. **Creative thinking:** Creative thinking means that the predictions and or inferences for the individual are new, original, ingenious, unusual. The creative thinker is one who explores new areas and makes new observation, new predictions, and new inferences.

INTRODUCTION

Educational psychology provides a base to education. It studies the problem which crop up in the education of the children. Educational psychology has it primary concern with a viewpoint, with the organization of information and with group of techniques and activities for a sound education. It is an area of experiment, not a collection of specific subject matter.

Through this subject the contents, techniques and ways of functioning of psychology are applied in the solution of the problems of the class-room. It may be remembered that educational psychology is not, merely general psychology applied to educational problems. The number of researches in various areas connected with educational psychology is increasing at a phenomenal rate.

NATURE OF EDUCATIONAL PSYCHOLOGY

1. Psychology is a science which studies all the aspects of human behavior. It concerned with the reasons of human behavior and with those principles which may predict a behavior and bring modifications in it.
2. Education is mainly a social process. The chief aim of it is to modify behavior. In this sense both education and psychology are similar.
3. From the fusion of psychology and education, we get that branch of psychology which we call as educational psychology.
4. Educational psychology is the study of human behavior as it is influenced by the social process. It also studies those processes, which provide an understanding of the way in which the modifications are brought in the behavior.
5. Educational psychology has its own applied theory. This theory is as basic as the theory underlying the discipline of psychology.

DEFINITIONS OF EDUCATIONAL PSYCHOLOGY

1. Education psychology is that special branch of psychology concerned with the nature, conditions, outcome and evaluation of school learning and retention—*Anusubel.*
2. Educational psychology is that branch of psychology which deals with teaching and learning — *Skinner*
3. Educational psychology describes and explains the learning experiences of an individual from birth through old age—*Crow and Crow*

IMPORTANCE OF EDUCATIONAL PSYCHOLOGY

It helps in the realization of education aims
1. It offers new viewpoints.
2. It ensures proper discipline in the proper manner.

3. It sets forth proper techniques and methods of teaching.
4. It keeps the educator informed about individual differences.
5. It helps in the understanding of group behavior.
6. It asks the teacher to teach according to the stages of development of the child.
7. It emphasizes the role of the learner.

AIMS AND OBJECTIVES OF EDUCATIONAL PSYCHOLOGY

1. Developing proper attitudes in the teacher.
2. Assisting the teacher to setup appropriate educational situations.
3. Helping the teachers in teaching their pupils sympathetically and impartially.
4. Helping them in the organization of the subject-matter.
5. Helping them to have a clear understanding of social relationships.
6. Assisting the teacher to understand his own job.
7. Making the teacher conversant with methods and techniques for the analysis of his and others behavior.
8. Organizing the proper guidance programs.
9. Guiding the administrators.
10. Helping them in planning out the proper evaluation techniques.
11. Furnishing the teacher with proper method.

GENERAL CATEGORIES OF EDUCATIONAL PSYCHOLOGY

1. Learning which is by far the most frequent topic in the field.
2. Readiness of learning—which includes the phenomena of interest, aptitudes and motivation.
3. Mental health and social adjustment, which focus on the noncognitive purposes of the school and correlates of intellectual learning.
4. Measurement and evaluation, which comprises the techniques for assessing the education growth of learners, diagnosing learning problems and clarifying the criteria to be used in an evaluation of the school.

EDUCATION AND EDUCATIONAL PSYCHOLOGY

Education by all means is an attempt to mould and shape the behavior of the pupil. It aims to produce desirable changes in him for the all-round development of his personality.

The essential knowledge and skill to do this job satisfactorily is supplied by educational psychology as Peel puts it in the following words, "Educational psychology helps the teacher to understand the development of his pupils, the range and limits of their capacities, the processes by which they learn and their social relationships".

Scope of Educational Psychology

By mentioning the areas around the above five pivots, the picture of the boundaries and limits of educational psychology cannot be taken as complete. Infact, sketching of such a full picture is quite a difficult task because of the fact that educational psychology is a developing and fast growing science. Like any other developing branch of science it multiplies itself every year. New ideas are coming into picture because of the result of new researches and experiments. The change is the law of nature and education being a dynamic subject is changing very fast. The new problems in the process of education are coining with a faster rate and for their solution, educational psychology is trying harder with the result that new concept, principles, and techniques are taking their birth in the sphere of educational psychology. Therefore, it is unwise to fix the hedge or boundary around the fertile ground of educational psychology by defining its scope. It will not only hamper the progress of this developing subject but also prove an obstacle in the progress of education.

Therefore, the boundaries of educational psychology must be left free for future expansion so as to facilitate the inclusion of all what is created in this field in future to solve the problems of education and help the smoothening of teaching learning process.

Objectives or Needs of Educational Psychology

Educational psychology is best defined as science of education. In its simple meaning, therefore, it should stand for supplying all the essential knowledge, skills and other related art and techniques to all the persons associated with the process of education for exercising their roles as effectively as possible. Therefore, the objectives or needs served by the subject educational psychology in view of its wide scope and fields of application may be broadly identified in the five major heads like below:

1. To help the students in the task of learning and seeking all-round growth and development of their personality.
2. To help the teachers in their task of teaching and performing other duties for the welfare their students.
3. To help the guidance and counseling personnels working in the field of education for providing needed services on their part.
4. To help the educational authorities and administrators like educational planners, policy makers, curriculum framers, evaluators, educational administrators, etc. for exercising their roles as effectively as possible.
5. To help the educational researchers in carrying out their tasks effectively for the improvement of the process and product of education.

Methods of Educational Psychology

Educational psychology is the scientific or systematic study of the behavior of the learner in relation to his educational environment. This behavior can be studied by a simple approach called observation. However, this observation method has to be adjusted depending upon the conditions in which observations have to be made, the procedure and tools adopted.

The following are the various methods of observation under different situations.

1. **Introspection method:** This method which is the oldest method of studying behavior where the learner should make a self observation i.e. looking in word. For example, when a person is angry he may be asked to determine how he felt during that period of anger by his own observation. This method is simple, direct, cheap and reveals one's behavior. But this method lacks reliability and can be used only for adult normal human beings. This method requires the support of other methods which are more reliable.
2. **Observation method:** In this method, the learners behavior is observed under natural conditions by other individuals. Such observation will be interpreted according to the perception of the observer. This helps to find out behavior by observing a persons external behavior. For example, if a person frowns we can say that he is angry. But when we are studying behavior in natural conditions we have to wait for the event to take place. This method is helpful in studying the

behavior of the children. However, this method will explain only observed behavior subjectivity of the investigation may affect the results.

3. **Experimental method:** In this method, behavior is observed and recorded under controlled conditions. This is done in psychological laboratory or in classrooms or outside the classrooms in certain physical or social environment.

These experiments require the creation of artificial environment. Therefore the scope is limited. Human behavior is very dynamic and unpredictable. This method is also costly and time consuming.

4. **Case history method:** This method is one of the steps used in the clinical method of studying behavior. This method is used for those who are suffering from physical or mental disorders. For this the case history has to be made of the earlier experiences of the individual which may be responsible for the present behavior. Information is also collected from his parents, family, relatives, guardians, neighbors friends, teachers, and from reports about the individual's past. This information will enable the clinical psychologists to diagnose and suggest treatment if there is any problem. However, this method will be successful only if the clinical researcher is technically efficient.

CONCEPT OF EDUCATION

1. Education modifies the behavior. It brings such changes in the behavior of a child which is for his good. In the past, the education of a child meant the filling up of the child's mind with stuffed knowledge.
2. The modern education aims at the harmonious development of the personality of the child. The schools and the teachers are to create such situation were the personality can be developed freely and fully.
3. Education is a social process; its main concern is the modification of behavior. Thus educational psychology studies the human behavior as it is influenced by the social process of education.
4. It also studies and investigates those processes that lead to the understanding of the way in which behavior is modified through education.
5. Education psychology constitutes the foundations of education. It provides an approach to educational problems and set of techniques for studying children and problems that arise in their function.

Psychological Basis of Education

1. Psychology deals with response to any and every kind of situation the life presents. Educational psychology deals with the behavior of the human being in educational situations.
2. To make an estimate of the value of educational psychology, it is necessary to understand the modern concept of education.
3. Education provides both, experience to the individual and his adjustment to the environment. It is also a process which is individualistic as well as social in its nature.
4. The bringing of psychological basis in education has resulted in completely overhauling our outlook on education. Now education is a much more pleasant process than what it was. Information and instructions are replaced by the word help and guidance. Love, sympathy and play are considered most important in the educational process.

VALUES OF EDUCATIONAL PSYCHOLOGY

1. The study of educational psychology should develop the student's interest in people both children and adults and help him to understand them.
2. The study on educational psychology should have a favorable effect on the attitudes, behaviors and psychological understanding of students in the both personal and professional relationship.
3. The study of educational psychology should enable the students to use the body of knowledge that is derived from research studies in this field and that helps to explain the way in which learning occurs.
4. The study of educational psychology should improve the effectiveness of the prospective teacher's ability to learn.
5. The study of educational psychology should foster the student's appreciation and understanding of research on education.

Major Subdivisions of Educational Psychology

1. Psychology and education.
2. Human growth and development
3. Learning
4. Personality and adjustments
5. Group psychology
6. Measurement and evaluation
7. Statistical and research methods

ELEMENTS OF EDUCATIONAL PSYCHOLOGY

Learner

1. In educational process the learner occupies the most important place. There can be no teaching without there being a learner. By the learner we mean the pupils who individually or collectively comprise the classroom group.
2. The teaching is the classroom to a great extent depends on the personality's developmental stages and psychological problems of the students.

Learning Process

1. Learning process is the process by which people acquire changes in their behavior, improve performance, recognize their thinking or discover new ways of behaving and new concepts and information.
2. This process may be directly observable as while the pupils learn writing, computing, talking, etc. or may be indirectly observable as in perceiving, thinking and remembering. The concern of the educational psychologist is with the way in which the learning process takes place.

Learning Situations

1. This refers to the environment in which the learner find himself and in which the learning process takes place.
2. The teacher's attitude, the class-room setting, the emotional climate of the school and the interest the community takes in the school affairs may all form the part of the learning situations.

LIMITATIONS OF EDUCATIONAL PSYCHOLOGY

1. The application of educational psychology can be made in a limited manner keeping in view the nature of teaching. In accordance with the nature of teaching, the experience, interest, attitude, etc. are as essential for a teacher as the knowledge of psychology.
2. The educational psychology is limited to the extent that the testing of facts or search of new facts is only helpful in arriving at a decision. They do not lead automatically to ultimate decisions or judgments.
3. The educational psychology is bound by the boundaries of psychology.

CONCLUSION

Educational psychology is nothing but one of the branches of applied psychology. It is an attempt to apply the knowledge of psychology to the field of education. It consists of the application of the psychological principles and techniques to human behavior in educational situations. In other words, educational psychology is the study of the experiences and behavior of the learner in relation to educational environment.

BIBLIOGRAPHY

1. Allport GW. Pattern and Growth in Personality, Holt, New York 1961.
2. American Association on Mental Deficiency as cited by Kisker, 1973 .
3. American Psychiatric Association. Diagnostic and Statistical Mannual of Mental Deficiency 2nd ed, DSM—II, Washington DC, 1968.
4. Andrews TG (Ed). Methods of Psychology, John Wiley, New York, 1960.
5. Atkinson RC, Shiffrin RM. Human memory: A proposed system and its control processes in KW. Spence and JT spence (Eds). The psychology of learning and motivation: Advances in Research and Theory, Vol. 2 Academic Press, New York, 1968.
6. Baron R. Emotional Intelligence Quotient Inventory. A Measure of Emotional Intelligence, 1997.
7. Barton Hall. Psychiatric Examination of the School Child, Edward Arnold, London, 1947.
8. Bhatia HR. Element of Educational Psychological, 3rd edn, Orient Longman, Kolkata, 1968.
9. Bigge Moris L. Learning Theories of Teachers, Universal Book Stall, Delhi (First Indian reprint), 1967.
10. Biggie ML, Hunt MP. 'Psychological Foundations of Education, Harper and Row, New York, 1968.
11. Bingham WVD. Aptitude and Attitude Testing, Harper and Brothers, New York, 1937.
12. Binnet A, Simon T. The Development of Intelligence in children, Williams and Wilkins, Baltimore, 1916.
13. Blair GH, Jones RS, Sirnpsonn RH. Educational Psychology, Macmillan, New York 1954.
14. Boring EC, Lang field HS, Weld HP (Eds). Foundations of Psychology, New York.
15. Brown JF. Educational Sociology, Prentice Hall, New York 1960 (5th printing).
16. Brown JF. The Psychodynamics of Abnormal Behaviour, Asia Publishing House, New Delhi (Indian Reprint), 1969.
17. Brubaeker J. Philosopher of Education. MC Graw Hill, New York, 1939.
18. Burt C. The subnormal mind, Oxford University Press, London, 1955.
19. Burt C. The lung Delinque, 3rd edn, University of London Press, London, 1938.
20. George W. The Disorganized Personality, McGraw Hill (International student edition—Ill), 1964.

Guidance and Counseling

9

DEFINITIONS

1. **Guidance:** Guidance is the assistance made available by qualified and trained person to an individual of any age, to help him to manage his own life activities, develop his own point of view, make his own decision and carry on his own burden. In educational context, guidance means assisting students to select courses of study appropriate to their needs and interests, achieve academic excellence to the best possible extent, derive maximum benefit of the institutional resources and facilities, inculcate proper study habits and satisfactorily participate in curricular and extra-curricular activities.

2. **Educational guidance:** Educational guidance helps the students to get maximum benefit out of education and to solve their problems related to education. The emphasis is on providing assistance to students to perform satisfactorily in their academic work, choose the appropriate course of study, overcome learning difficulties, foster creativity, improve levels of motivation, utilize institutional resources optimally such as library, laboratory, etc.

3. **Vocational guidance:** Vocational guidance is the assistance provided for selection of a vocation and preparation for the same. It is concerned with enabling students to acquire information about career opportunities, career growth and training facilities.

4. **Personal guidance:** Personal guidance refers to the guidance offered to students for enabling them to adjust themselves to their environment so that they become efficient citizens. Adolescent behavior to a great extent depends upon the moods and attitudes of the adolescent. Emotional instability is a characteristic of adolescents and this is often the cause of many of their personal problems. Personal guidance will help them to solve these problems.

5. **Social guidance:** Social guidance enables the student to make substantial contributions to the society, assume leadership, confirm to the social norms, work as team members, develop healthy and positive attitudes, appreciate the problems of society, respect the opinions and sentiments of fellow human beings, acquire traits of patience, perseverance and friendship. Its main purpose is to enable the student to become an efficient citizen.

6. **Health guidance:** Health guidance implies the assistance rendered to students for maintaining sound health. Sound health is a pre-requisite for participating in curricular and cocurricular activities. This type of guidance focuses on enabling students to appreciate conditions for good health and take steps necessary for ensuring good health, maintaining sound, physical and mental health.

7. **Counseling:** Counseling is an accepting, trusting and safe relationship in which clients learn to discuss openly what worries and upsets them, to define precise behavior goals to acquire

essential social skills and to develop the courage and self-confidence to implement the desired new behaviors. Counseling is a process of enabling the individual to know himself and his present and possible future situations in order that he may make substantial contributions to the society and to solve his own problems through a face-to-face personal relationship with the counselor.

8. **Individual counseling:** This is a one-to-one helping relationship between the counselor and the counseled. It is focused upon the individual's need for growth and adjustment, problem solving and decision making. This type of counseling requires counselors with the highest level of training and professional skills. In addition, it also requires that they have a certain personality type as well; counseling will be rendered ineffective unless counselors exhibit such personality traits as understanding, warmth, humaneness and positive attitudes towards the client.

9. **Group counseling:** This form of counseling is sometimes successful with clients who have not responded well to individual counseling. This group interaction helps the individual to gain insight into his problems by listening to others discussing their difficulties. Group counseling often not only helps the individual to change, but also enhances his desire and ability to help others faced with distressing life circumstances.

10. **Eclectic counseling:** In eclectic counseling, the strategy arises out of the appropriate knowledge of individual behavior and a combination of directive and other approaches. Irrespective of the differences, all approaches should have developmental, preventive and remedial values.

GUIDANCE SERVICE

Introduction

The guidance is one of the major applications of psychology. It enables or assists the individual to solve educational, vocational and psychological problems. "To guide" means a sort of help, assistance or suggestions for progress. In the field of psychology and education, the word "guidance" is having a specific meaning. It refers to a process of helping the individual to discover himself which means, his potentialities and propensities, capacities and capabilities, abilities and aptitudes, interests and natural endowments and to help him in achieving maximum advantage of the individual and state.

Concept of Guidance

1. Guidance refers to a process of assisting the individual to develop his body, mind, personality and character and to help him in achieving maximum educational, vocational, and personal or psychological adjustments.

2. Guidance is regarded as a kind of specialized service provided to the individual to solve problems of crucial nature.

3. Guidance is regarded as any form of assistance given to child who makes his best development of personality.

4. Guidance is not confined to a professional setting, since, it is a continuous process starting from early childhood extending up to sometimes old age.

5. Guidance is the educational context, for example, means assisting students to select courses of study appropriate to their needs and interests, achieve academic excellence to the best possible.

6. Guidance is not just providing direction, imposition of one's viewpoint on another, making decision for another individual, carrying burden of another's life.

Definitions of Guidance

1. Jones (1951) holds that 'guidance' involves personal help given by someone, it is designed to assist a person to decide where he wants to go, what he wants to do or how he can best accomplish his purpose; it assists him to solve problems that arise in life.
2. Crow and Crow, fundamental of all guidance is the help or assistance given by a competent person to an individual so that the latter may direct his life by developing his point of view make his own decision and carry out those decisions.
3. Fowler's believes strongly the purpose of guidance is to help the student to make more favorable adjustments.

Principles of Guidance (Hollis and Hollis, 1965)

1. The debility of the individual is supreme.
2. Each individual is different from every other individual.
3. The primary concern of guidance is the individual in one's social setting.
4. The attitudes personal perceptions of the individual provide the basic for action.
5. The individual generally acts to enhance one's perceived self.
6. The individual has the innate ability to learn and therefore can be helped to make choices that will lead to self-direction consistent with reality.
7. The individual needs a continuous guidance process from childhood onwards.
8. Each individual may at times need the information and personalized assistance given by competent professional personal.

Elements of Guidance

1. Guidance focuses our attention on the individual and not the problem.
2. Guidance helps to the discovery of abilities of an individual.
3. Guidance is based on interests, abilities, assets, needs and limitations of the individual.
4. Guidance gives rise to self-development and self-direction.
5. Guidance makes the individual to plan wisely for the present and future.
6. Guidance makes the individual to become adjusted in the new environment.
7. Guidance is helpful in achieving success and happiness.

Characteristics of Guidance

1. The basis of guidance is individual differences, it is a known fact no two individual are alike. Individuals are different in capacities, capabilities, potentialities, propensities, abilities, aptitude and variations within the individual.
2. Guidance is the basis of redid code of ethics, it is important to follow a rigid code of ethics in guidance programmed.
3. The basis of guidance is on educational and vocational objectives, it means that guidance realization of educational and vocational aims and objective.
4. Guidance is able to develop the insight of an individual; the counselor is helpful to the individual in such a way that he gains insight to make his own decisions and choices.

5. Guidance regards most of the individuals as average normal persons; it must be known to all the students that the services of guidance workers are available to all.
6. Guidance is slow but a continuous process; individuals need considerable time to make suitable adjustments and are unable to make wise decisions choices and adjustments in a day or so.
7. Guidance is universal, it is essential for all the pupils of all the stages. It is for those who seek it and also for those who do not seek it.
8. Guidance is planning, guidance personnel attempts to review the entire situation and gives plans for future in educational, vocational and social field.
9. Guidance is developmental as well as comprehensive guidance is developmental because it is dealing with the month-to-month, year to year and stage to stage.
10. Guidance is practical side of education; education sets the goal while guidance makes the realization of that goal.
11. Guidance is mainly child-centered, guidance worker or counselor does not impose anything on individual but he tries to find out the needs of the child and provides him only his suggestions.
12. Guidance is considered as an organized service and not incidental, i.e. it is a service, which is having a specific purpose.
13. Guidance is specialized and generalized service, many persons such as the teacher, the parent, the headmaster; the counselor and the career master play their specific role.

Basic Assumptions of Guidance

1. The differences between individuals in native capacities, abilities and interests are quite significant.
2. Variations within the individual himself are quite significant.
3. Native abilities are not generally specialized.
4. Abilities and aptitudes do not depend upon race, color and sex.
5. There is need for assistance to certain crisis.
6. The school is in a strategic position to provide the needed assistance.
7. Guidance is progressive self-directive but not prescriptive.

Purposes of Guidance

1. **Understanding the individual:** The main purpose of guidance is to discover and understand capacities and potentialities of the individual and to make evaluation of the self in relation to personal and social experience and to use the self more efficiency in every day living.
2. **Help the individual in making adjustments:** Another aim of guidance is to assist the individual so as to be making satisfactory and maximum adjustments to home, to school, to teachers, to pupils and to society.
3. **Develop personal abilities and potentialities:** Another purpose of guidance is to help the individuals to develop their abilities, potentialities and points of view, to develop their body, mind, personality and character.
4. **Improve school activities:** The guidance programmer helps the school staff to solve problems and improve all the activities of the school.
5. **Coordinating home, school and society:** Erikson as correctly said that one of the important purposes of guidance has been coordinating home, school and community influences on the child.

Need for Guidance

1. **Educational need:** Guidance has given to the students to select of subjects of counsel, to select of books, to select of hobbies, to select of co-curricular activities, to develop study habits, to organize time and work, to concentrating on studies, to building social relationship and to make satisfactory progress and adjustments in school.
2. **Psychological need:** Guidance is required from psychological and social point of view. Youth of twentieth century is subjected to much great emotional strain in the home and in the community. The number of problem children, delinquent children, backward children and maladjusted children has been increasing in our schools.
3. **Vocational need:** The vocational guidance is essential for helping the individual to know himself, for knowing the world of work, adequate information about jobs, skills and opportunities for making a right choice in the vocation according to his abilities, interest and aptitudes and to obtain suitable jobs in their chosen fields.
4. **Social need:** Society is becoming complex starting changes have occurred in the entire structure of our economic, social and political system.

Types of Guidance

1. Educational guidance
2. vocational guidance
3. Religious guidance
4. Guidance for home relationship
5. Guidance for citizenship
6. Guidance for leisure and recreation
7. Guidance for personal well-being
8. Guidance in right doing
9. Guidance in thoughtfulness and cooperation
10. Guidance in wholesome and cultural action.

INDIVIDUAL GUIDANCE SERVICE

Introduction

Introduction guidance service is some type of help which is provided to individual to understand his potentialities, develop his potentialities, make the best use of his potentialities and solve his problems. Individual problems are concerned with physical health, home problems, school problems, leisure time problems, sex problems other emotional and psychological problems and vocational problems.

Stages of Individual Guidance Service

At Elementary Stage

1. The childhood period refers to the period of growth and development. During this stage the basic foundations of physical, intellectual, emotional, social and other type of personality development are laid.
2. It is considered to be the most impressionable period of life, when the character traits, attitudes, values and habits get developed.

3. Some of the task or purposes of individual guidance service at this stage are to make a right start in the school, to build good physique and to make emotional adjustments.

At Secondary Stage

This is regarded as the most critical stage of individual's developments because it is the stage of stress and strain, storm and strife, heightened emotionality and hypersuggestibility, anxieties and worries, conflicts and frustrations. The main aims of individual guidance at this stage are as follows.
1. To make the individual to solve problems concerning physical health.
2. To make the individual to solve problems concerning sex, emotionally and mental health.
3. To guide the individual in making family adjustments.
4. To advise the individual in making social adjustments including adjustment with school.
5. To guide the individual in making suitable progress in the school.

At College Stage

The main purpose, aims or functions of individual's guidance at college stage are as follows.
1. Guidance is essential to help the individual in solving all types of his emotional problems, sex problems and other personal problems.
2. Guidance is also need to help the individual in making adjustment with new environment.
3. Guidance is also need to help the individual in developing healthy ideas and building a new philosophy of life.
4. Guidance also essential to help them in participating in social activities.
5. Guidance is also essential to help the individual in making suitable educational progress.
6. Guidance is also essential to help the individual in getting suitable job.

Need for Individual Guidance Service

1. **Problems concerning physical health:** The advice and treatment of an expert may be require by an individual for curing his physical ailment and building up his physique.
2. **Family problems:** There are many family problems such as the strained relationship between child and his parents, between husband and wife, between brothers and sisters, constant quarrels between the father and mother, presence of step-father or step-mother in the house. Jealousy among various siblings in the family may contribute another factor in home environment, which may become a potent cause of maladjustments.
3. **Utilization of leisure time:** In order to utilize the leisure time profitably and individual might require guidance. He might need to be guided in sports, games and hobbies.
4. **Personal problems:** Sometimes, the main cause of maladjustments are personality problems such as bullying, teasing, frightened, anxiety, nail-biting, thumb-sucking, grinding of teeth and inferiority complex, these difficulties require competent guidance.
5. **School problems:** The individual may be unable to make progress in various academic, physical, social and recreational activities of school and thus require guidance.
6. **Vocational problems:** The individual might require guidance for selecting the occupation, for adequate training for particular occupation, or for the change of an occupation.
7. **Religious problems:** The individual might be having certain religious doubts or wrong philosophy of life for which he might require guidance.
8. **Marital problems:** Happy man is one who has got the good life partner. For carrying out the right choice of a partner the person might require guidance.

9. **Sex problems:** Sometimes individuals have sex problems due to menstruation, nightmares, excessive sex curiosity, heterosexual interests and activities. In order to help the individual in solving sex problems and in leading a healthy sexual life, individual guidance becomes essentials.

10. **Old age problems:** Old age brings its own problems. At this age various organs of the body loses their strength and the various senses like eyesight, hearing and smell, etc. will start growing feeble day by day. Such an age group requires guidance regarding proper utilization of time and for keeping the body in strength.

Steps Involved in Individual Guidance Service

Collection of Facts

1. Post of all physical details such as age, sex, physical health and defects like defect in eye-sight, defect in hearing defect in nose, throat, etc. are to be noted.

2. Then family details such as family background, size, education, income of parents, order of birth in the family and other members in the family, discipline in the home, mutual relations between different members of the family are to be noted.

3. Then details regarding attitude towards school, classmates, teachers, subjects, co-curricular activities, achievements in examinations, sports and co-curricular activities. Failure and promotions, positions and distinction in the class and main difficulties in school or college subjects are to be noted.

4. The details concerning vocational choices, special skills vocational interests and ambitions, jobs held in the past, satisfied or dissatisfied during the job, reasons of dissatisfaction, relation with the employer, etc. are to be noted.

5. Then, the details of social development such as individuals relations with parents brothers and sisters, other relatives, playmates, class-fellows, teachers, friends, neighbors, etc. are to be noted.

6. Then, the details concerning mental abilities such as intelligence, aptitudes and other mental abilities should be collected with the help of various tests and examinations intended for the purpose are to be noted.

7. Finally, the details concerning other qualities of personality like individuals emotional maturity, interests, motives, ambitions and ideals are to be noted.

Sources of Collecting Information About the Individual

1. **Parents:** Parents can provide quite useful information about the child. This information can be obtained by inviting parents to school on special occupations or contacting them at their homes.

2. **Teacher:** Teachers are also able to provide much information about the student. This information has been based on observation, individual records, marks secured in examinations, interview and home visits.

3. **Students:** The primary sources of students (individual's) data have been students themselves and other individuals in the schools. Also their friends and companions can also provide much useful information about them.

4. **Guidance worker:** A guidance worker can obtain information about students from many sources. He may able to collect this information from family doctors, social workers and members of the community.

Diagnosis of the Problems

1. After collecting relevant information concerning individual the guidance worker would like to analyze the information so as to find out the ways and means of solving the problem.
2. This process involving the analysis of information and efforts to find out ways and means of solving the problem is called diagnosis of the problem.
3. The guidance worker is unable to impart individual guidance to the individual without proper diagnosis of the problem.

Prognosis

1. It involves the visualizing the extent to which the guidance workers will be successful in solving person's problem.
2. Guidance workers visualize the result to the guidance which he offers to the individual so as to solve his problems.
3. For example, by observing a person's past performance in mathematics and by measuring his mental abilities, it is possible to make some tentative estimate of what he will achieve after the guidance is rendered.

Therapy

1. Here the guidance worker offers a satisfactory solution of the problem. He will make the individual gain an inspirit into his problem.
2. Various techniques used in therapy include suggestion sublimation through substitution, rational persuasion, re-education, play therapy, and change in environment, psychoanalysis, group therapy, occupational therapy and on-directive therapy.

Follow-up Action

1. After providing guidance it becomes essential to know that upto what extent the problem is solved. Hence, follow-up becomes essential. Individual guidance is more or less incomplete without follow-up. The following methods find use in follow-up study.
2. Card file method—In this method, details of interview such as name of the interview his age, sex, address, purpose of interview and details of the problems have been indicated.
3. Questionnaire method—Guidance workers gives questionnaire to counselee. In the questionnaire those items are included which deals with various aspects of the progress of problems concerning which the advice was provided.
4. Contact through letters—In this method, counselee is contacted through letters, which can be used even to provide further guidance to the person.

COUNSELING SERVICE

Introduction

We have quite often heard the term counseling used in newspaper in the context of counseling for engineering, demission computer related admissions and so on. Counseling forms the heart of all guidance programmed. As we know that proper functioning of the heart, similarly the success or failure of the guidance programmed could be determined by counseling service.

Meaning of Counseling

1. Counseling refers to a progress in which the people are made to approach or an individual level. He gets help in educational, vocational or psychological field only at problem points.
2. In counseling the subject matter would be pupil's needs, abilities, aims, aspirations, plans, decisions, actions and limitations.
3. Counseling may be referred to a sort of specialized personalized and individualized service which makes effective use of information gathered about any individual.
4. This information provides self-insight, self-analysis and self-direction. This self-direction helps individual to make maximum education, vocational and psychological adjustments.

Definitions of Counseling

1. Pepinsky (1954) state that counseling is a process involving an interaction between a counselor and a client in a private setting, with the purpose of helping the client change his behavior so that satisfactory resolutions of needs may be obtained.
2. Crow and Crow's view, counseling or assisting an individual in the solution of his problems. The interview has an important place in guidance, but is only one stage in the whole process of counseling.
3. Bernard and Fullmer's views, basically counseling involves understanding and working with the individual to discover his unique needs, motivations and potentialities and to help him appreciate them.

Characteristics of Counseling

1. Counseling is based on person to person relations.
2. It involves two individuals one seeking help and the other, a professionally trained who can help the first.
3. The main aim is to help the counselor to discover and solve his personal problems independently.
4. In order to help and assist properly the counselor must establish a relationship of mutual respect, cooperation and friendliness between the two individuals.
5. The counselor will try to discover the problems of the client and helps him to setup goals and guide him through difficulties and problems.
6. The main emphasis in the role of counseling process is laid on the counselor's self-direction and self-acceptance.
7. Counseling is democratic and the counselor sets up a democratic pattern and allows the counsel to do freely whatever he like while with the consultant and not under the consultant.

The Rules and Roles of Counseling

Remedial Role

1. It entails working with individuals or groups, to assist them in remedying problems of one kind or another.
2. As noted by kagan et al. (1988) remedial interventions may induce personal, social counseling or psychotherapy at an individual, couples (e.g. marital counseling).
3. Crisis intervention and various therapeutic services for students requiring assistance with unresolved life events are additional examples of work at the remedial level.

Preventive Role

1. It is one in which the counseling psychologist seek to "anticipate, circumvent, and if possible, forestall, difficulties that may arise in the future.
2. Preventive interventions may focus on what are called psychoeducational programmers aiming to forestall the development of problems or events.
3. Example: Drug prevention/awareness programmers, suicide prevention programmed for high risk and psychological adoption of orphan children which gives them a feeling of belongingness.

Educational and Developmental Role

1. The purpose which is to help individuals to plan, obtains, and derives maximum benefits from the kinds of experiences which will enable them to discover and develop their potentialities.
2. Examples of this would include various workshops or seminars. Another example might be a study skill class the college students aimed at making good students even more effective.
3. The key features of the developmental role are that when performing it one is going beyond prevention and is involved in enhancement.

Goals of Counseling

1. Facilitating behavioral change
2. Enhancing copying skills
3. Promoting decision-making
4. Improving relationships
5. Facilitating client potential.

Comparision of Counseling with Other Terms

1. **Guidance and counseling:** Guidance and counseling are not synonyms. Counseling forms a part of guidance. Not all of it.
2. **Counseling and interview:** Interview is a part of counseling; it is only a technique which is used in the process of counseling.
3. **Counseling and advising:** Counseling does not give advice, a wise counselor ever provides advice until it becomes absolutely essential.
4. **Counseling and teaching:** Counseling does not mean teaching. Teaching is related to academic and instinctual problems, whereas counseling is related to social and emotional problems.
5. **Counseling and psychotherapy:** Counseling is not considered as psychotherapy although it is used by psychotherapist as one of the technique of treatment. Counselor does work in educational setting, while psychotherapist does work in medical setting.

THEORIES OF COUNSELING

1. E Williamson is the leading architect of this school of thought.
2. It also called prescriptive or counselor centered counseling.
3. It is considered to be problem-centered and paido-centred.
4. It is the counselor, who prepare plans and sees through the process.

Assumptions

1. All the efforts should be done to tackle the problem of the counselee.
2. As counselor is more competent than the counselee, it means that the former plays a more active role than the client.
3. Counseling is more or less an intellectual rather than emotional process and hence an intellectual aspect is assigned more weight age than emotional aspects.

Steps of Directive Counseling

1. **Analysis:** Collection of data is carried out from a variety of sources by using a variety of tools and techniques.
2. **Synthesis:** Summarizing and organizing the data are to be carried out so as to reveal the clients assets, liabilities, adjustments and maladjustments.
3. **Diagnosis:** At this stage an attempt should be made to find out the root cause of the problem exhibited by the client.
4. **Prognosis:** At this stage the future development of the client's problems should be predicted.
5. **Treatment:** It includes establishing report, advice or plan programmers.
6. **Follow-up:** Here the counselor makes an attempt to help the client with new problem or with recurrences of the original problem, and ascertains the effectiveness of counseling provided to him.

Advantages of Directive Counseling

1. It is more economical in time.
2. It emphasis mainly lay on the problem but not on the individual.
3. Directive counseling lays more emphasis on the intellectual rather than the emotional aspects of the personality of the individual but not at the emotional level.
4. The directive counseling methods used have been direct, persuasive and explanatory.

Limitations of Directive Counseling

1. The counselor would never become independent of the counselor.
2. Directive counseling is unable to keep the counselee away from making mistakes in future.

NON-DIRECTIVE COUNSELING

Introduction

1. Carl Rogers is the chief architect of this school of thought.
2. It is also known as permissive counseling or client centered counseling.
3. In this type of counseling if the client—the counselor who forms the pivot or the center. It is the counselee who plays the main role.
4. It is the who actively participates in the process, gets insight into his problem by using the counselor and takes decisions to taken action.

Assumption of Non-directive Counseling

1. Independence and integration of the client have been more important than the client.
2. Emotional aspects have been more significant then intellectual aspects.

3. Creating an atmosphere in which the client can work out his understanding has been more important than cultivating self-understanding in the client.
4. Counseling results in a voluntary choice of goals and a conscious selection of courses of action.

Steps of Non-directive Counseling

1. The client is able to recognize the need of counseling and come for help. Help is sought and not given.
2. The counselor is able to define the situation and creates congenital atmosphere.
3. Attitude of the counselor has been friendship, sympathy and affection. He is interested in the child and encourages free expression of feeling regarding the problem of individuals.
4. The counselor makes an attempt to understand the feelings of the individual.
5. The counselor accepts as well as recognizes the positive and negative feelings.
6. The counselor will pay attention to negatives self-feelings of the client or child and changes him from negative self-feelings to positive self-feelings, from emotional release to gradual insight.
7. The counselor makes the client to translate his insight to action.
8. A decreased need for help is desired and the client is the one who decides to the contact.
9. Positive steps towards the solution of the problem situation begin to start.

Advantages of Non-directive Counseling

1. It is slow but sure process which makes the individual capable of making adjustments.
2. No tests are used in it and therefore avoid all that is laborious and difficult.
3. It is able to remove the emotional block and makes the individual to bring the repressed thoughts in conscious level, thereby reducintension.

Limitations of Non-directive Counseling

1. It is quite slow and time consuming process. In school it is not feasible as counselor has to attend many students.
2. The child, the client or the student or the counselor are unable to make the decisions himself. Hence, we fail to rely up on his resources, judgment and wisdom.
3. There are many individuals who may lead from stages to stage. The counselor's passive attitude might be able to irritate the counselee so much that he might hesitate to express his feelings.

ECLECTIC COUNSELING

Introduction

1. Eclectic counseling may be defined as the synthesis and combinations of directive and non-directive counseling.
2. In this counseling, the counselor has been neither too active as in directive counseling, nor too passive as in non-directive counseling.
3. In elective counseling the counselor first of all consider the personality and needs of the counselee and than selects the directive or non-directive technique that would be serve the purpose best.
4. Throne is the chief architect of eclectic counseling.

Steps of Eclectic Counseling

1. To diagnose the cause.
2. To analyze the problem

3. To prepare a tentative plan for modifying factors.
4. To secure effective conditions for counseling.
5. To interview and stimulate the client to develop his own resources and to assume its responsibility for trying new models of adjustments.
6. To do proper handling of any related problems which may be able to contribute to adjustments.

Generalizations

1. Generally passive methods should be used whenever possible.
2. Passive techniques are preferred in the early stages if the client is telling his story. This allows emotional release.
3. Active methods are to be used with specific indication.
4. Complicated methods should not be tried until simpler methods have failed.
5. All counseling should be client-centered.
6. Every child should be given an opportunity to resolve his problems non-directly.
7. Directive methods are generally involved in situational maladjustment where a solution can not be achieved without involving cooperation of other persons.
8. Some degree of directive ness will be inevitable in all counseling even in reaching the decision to use passive methods.

Limitation of Eclectic Counseling

1. Eclectics are not possible because it is not possible to merge directive and non-directive concepts together.
2. According to some writers, eclectics are vague, superficial and opportunistic.

BASIC PRINCIPLES OF COUNSELING

1. **Acceptance:** The client must be accepted as a whole person as a human being.
2. **Respect for the individual:** Importance is attached to respect for individual.
3. **Permissiveness:** All schools of counseling would accept relative permissiveness of counseling relationship.
4. **Learning:** All schools of counseling should accept the learning element in counseling.
5. **Thinking in rather than for the client:** It is another basic principle of counseling.

FUNCTION OR DUTIES OF COUNCELOR

1. Programmed of guidance and its organization—This includes such as vocational information service, self-inventory service, and personal data collection service, counseling service, vocational preparatory service, placement and employment service, follow-up or adjustment service.
2. Orientation implies a sort of preparation which includes collecting data about sources of jobs, disseminating information to pupils and planning activities.
3. Data collection should be done about the individual, administering the test and analyzing the same.
4. Interviews and individual counseling should be held.
5. Contact should be made outside agencies like parents, guidance, bureaus and employment exchanges.
6. Placement and follow-up work should be done.

CHARACTERISTICS OR QUALIFICATIONS OF COUNSELOR

Personality Traits

1. **Breadth of interest:** A counselor must be interested in various types of people, jobs and organization.
2. **Cooperation:** A counselor should cooperate with all the staff in a cheerful manner.
3. **Refinement:** A counselor should not be over—confident but he should be modest and humble towards the pupils.
4. **Magnetism:** A counselor should create confidence in others and put other at ease.
5. **Considerateness:** A counselor should understand the difficulties a teachers, exhibit human understanding and possess real love for fellowmen.

Training and Preparation

1. Good education which includes knowledge of humanities like sociology, psychology, economics, history and geography, etc.
2. To know principles of guidance.
3. To know of objectives, curriculum and methods of secondary schools.
4. To know vocational activities.
5. To know methods of imparting occupational information.
6. To know psychological tests in guidance services.
7. To know of organization of guidance services.

Experiences

1. Competence as a leader in guidance programmed.
2. Competence as a counselor.
3. Competence in interpreting and using information.
4. Competence in placement and follow up services.
5. Competence in using community resources.
6. Competence in evaluating the counseling service itself.

EDUCATIONAL GUIDANCE

Introduction

Guidance services are meant to help students make proper adjustments with the environment in which they are living and also make the best possible contributions commensurate with one's strengths and limitations. Educational guidance refers to guidance to students in all aspects of education.

The emphasis is on providing assistance to students to perform satisfactory in their academic work, choose the appropriate course of study, overcome learning difficulties foster creativity, improve levels of motivation and utilize institutional resources optimally such as library, laboratory, etc.

Definitions

1. According to author Jone's the educational guidance deals with assistance given to pupils in their choices and adjustments with relation to schools, curriculum, courses and school life.
2. According to Myer, educational guidance refers to a process which is concerned with bringing about an individual pupil which his distinctive characteristics on the one hand and differing group of opportunities and requirements on the other, a favorable setting for the individual's development or education.

Objectives of Educational Guidance

1. To monitor academic Programme of students.
2. To identify special learners such as academically backward, gifted and creative.
3. To assist students in further education.
4. To provide assistance to special learners by catering to their educational needs.
5. To diagnose the learning difficulties of students in different subjects.
6. To help students in their adjustments to curriculum and co curricular demands of the educational programs.
7. To provide career information.

Need of Educational Guidance

1. **Wastage and stagnation:** There occurs a lot of wastage and stagnation in education. The number of failures in the examination is responsible for much wastage to the nation.
2. **Diversified curriculum:** The curriculum is being diversified in the higher secondary and multipurpose schools. Therefore, the need for guidance in the selection of subjects of studies is becoming an almost necessity.
3. **Decision for further education:** Educational guidance is needed in order to help the pupil to make the best use of their potentialities and resources.
4. **Preparation for future vocation:** There is an urgent need is required for preparing and helping the pupils for further vocation while keeping in view their potentialities, interests and aptitudes and the demands of the society.
5. For balanced life simple vocational education is not sufficient, children must be educated to love and help together.

Purposes of Educational Guidance

1. **Wise selection of the curriculum:** It is known that the pupil's success in the field of education depends upon the wise selection of curriculum. Hence, an important purpose of educational assists in selecting a curriculum in accordance with their abilities, aptitudes and interests.
2. **Improvement in methods of study:** Another aim of educational guidance is to improve the methods of study. The methods of study includes such factors as made of reading mode of taking notes, methods of memorizing and summarizing.
3. **Providing special methods of education to backward students:** Guidance is mainly given to evolve special methods of education for pupils who usually fail at examinations, show signs of delinquency indiscipline or runaway from classes. The methods of education for backward children are evolved by keeping in view the causes of backwardness include special schools and specialists and special curriculum and special methods of teaching.
4. **Making special arrangements for gifted students:** Another specific aim of educational guidance is to arrange special educational programs for the gifted students.
5. Taking into account the failures at examination a large number of failures at various examinations is responsible for much wastage and stagnation. Many students lose their mental equilibrium as a result of failure.
6. Educational guidance is to help the students to secure information concerning the possibility and desirability of further schooling.
7. Educational guidance is to help them to know the requirements for entrance into the school of their choice.
8. Educational guidance is to help the students to find the purpose and functions of different types of schools.
9. Educational guidance is to guide them in selection of vocations.

Stages of Educational Guidance

At Elementary Stage

1. To help pupils to develop good habits, right attitudes, and basic skills.
2. To helping pupils to make a good beginning.
3. To help pupils to plan intelligently.
4. To help pupils to obtain the best out of their education.

At Secondary Stage

1. Helping the child to know himself.
2. Helping the child to understand the environment.
3. Helping the child to make the right choice of subjects.
4. Helping the child to know about the college education.

At College Stage

1. Providing library facilities for broadening the mental horizon of the students.
2. Providing special guidance for certain subjects and preparation for examination.
3. Providing special guidance for selection of books and reference books.
4. Guiding the individual to learn how to read books, how to make notes how to summarize and organize the materials and how to make use of quotations.

Factors Involved in Educational Guidance

1. Secondary schools become less selective.
2. Emphasis upon individual difference.
3. Growing complexity of the world of work.
4. Expansion of the school programs.
5. The concept of child-growth and development.
6. Beneficial effects of group-testing.
7. Influences of social and economical conditions.

Basic Principles of Educational Guidance

1. Guidance should be provided to all.
2. Standardized tests should be employed.
3. Selection of curriculum should be done.
4. Remedy should be given in the beginning.
5. Relevant information has to be obtained.
6. Follow-up study must be there.
7. Relationship between school and parents should be set up.

VOCATIONAL GUIDANCE

Introduction

In this scientific and technological age one of the most important aspects of man's life is vocation. Therefore, one has to choose vocation for himself. One of the main aims of education is to give maximum help is one's professional life. If vocational aim of education is not fulfilled then education becomes worthless.

Vocational guidance is fundamentally an effort for conserving the priceless native capacities of youth and the costly training provided for youth in the school. It conserves these riches of all human resources by the individual to invest and use them where will bring greatest satisfaction and success to himself and greatest benefit to society.

Definitions

1. According to international labor organization, vocational guidance as assistance given to an individual in solving problems related to occupational choices and progress with due regard for the individuals characteristics and their relation to occupational opportunity.
2. According to vocational guidance association, vocational guidance is the process of assisting the individual to choose an occupation, prepare for it, and enter up on and progressing in it.

Need of Vocational Guidance

1. To increase the number of occupations.
2. Vocational guidance to maintain the health.
3. To promote personal and social values.
4. To discover and utilize the human potentialities.
5. To meet the needs of an individual and complex nature of the society.
6. To promote financial growth of an individual and society.

Special Aims of Vocational Guidance

1. To assist the student to acquire suck knowledge of the characteristics and functions, the duties and rewards of the group of occupations.
2. To enable him to find what general and specific abilities, skills, etc. are required for the group of occupations.
3. To give opportunity for experiences in school that will give much information about conditions of work as will assist the individual to discover his own abilities help in the development of wider interests.
4. To help the individual develop the point of view that all honest labor is worth and that the most important bases for choice of an occupation.
5. To assist the individual to acquire a technique of analysis of occupation information and to develop the habit of analyzing such information before making a final choice.
6. To assist him to secure such information about himself, his abilities, general and specific, his interest and his powers as he may need for wise choice.
7. To assist economically handicapped children who are above the compulsory attendance age to secure through public or private funds, scholarships or other financial assistance.
8. To assist the student to secure knowledge of the facilities offered by various educational institutions for vocational training and the requirements for admission to them, the length of training offered and the cost of attendance.
9. To keep the worker to adjust himself to the occupation in which, he is engaged; to assist him to understand his relationship to workers in his own related occupations and to society as a whole.
10. To enable the student to secure reliable information about the danger of alluring short cuts to fortune.

Characteristics of Vocational Guidance

1. It helps the child to develop his potentialities to all optimum level.
2. It is a process which helps the person to impart occupational information, broadening his occupational horizon and including his interest in vocational self-help.
3. It is a process which helps individual to select an occupation for life, to prepare for it and to place him against a suitable job. Also his progress in the job is to be watched.
4. It is a process which helps in the persons to develop and accept an integrated and correct picture of himself and his role in the economy of the society to which he belongs.
5. It is a process which helps the individual to evaluate his role in term of reality or practicability.
6. It is a process which helps the individual to achieve the vocational goal. The process of achieving the vocational goal should be useful to society.
7. It is a process which helps the individual to make adjustments in relation to his occupation or job.
8. It is a process which helps the individual to make adjustments in relation to his occupation or job.

Guidance Counseling in the Hospital

The problems created due to illness vary not only with each individual patient but also with the different stages of the illness and at different points of the patient's hospital experience. When dealing with sick people counselor must keep in mind that they are particularly susceptible to strains, stress and conflicts and are often complaining, demanding and fault finding. They may misinterpret what is conveyed to him.

Problems Faced by Sick People

1. **Fear, anxiety and frustration:** Hospitalization brings out fear, anxiety, etc. in the patient. Uncertainty regarding the diagnosis, its implication, strain and tension in facing the unknown future gives rise to feeling of helplessness, bewilderments and insecurity. Counseling helps in reinforcing his feelings of warmth and importance which could help to counteract existing anxiety. This can be done through providing reliable and authoritative answers to the questions. Help the patient to accept the reality of the situation himself so that he neither exaggerates the seriousness of illness nor minimizes its impact on the adjustments, he will be compelled to make.
2. **Reaction to authority:** Feeling of insecurity and helplessness are aggravated by the need to submit to his daily activities. Counseling helps in restoring the patient's sense of self-responsibility and encourages the patient to follow prescribed regimen.
3. **Counseling of families:** Counseling cannot be confined to the patient but must be extended to family members as well. Social, economic and emotional problems which illness creates for the patient have repercussion on the family members as well. Positive values inherent in family living have to be utilized for the members to get adjusted regardless of the degree of incapacity. Help the family members to gear their demands in accordance with the limitations imposed by illness and assist them in utilizing whatever potentialities the patient possesses for active participation in family living.
4. **Problems at discharge:** During discharge if the patient carries incapacitating residue of the illness, it is likely to interfere either temporarily or even permanently with normal functioning. Encouraging the patient in planning for his return to normal living is a helpful device in preparing him to assume a greater degree of self-direction. Such help is given by the counselor by assisting

with living arrangements, adjustment or securing of medical follow-up which is of value not only because these are concrete services, essential for the patients well-being, but also a means of enhancing the patients feeling of importance with the visible proof of interest in his welfare, the patient begins to see himself as a person of worth.

The nurse as a caretaker has a very important role in giving all the psychological support to the patient to solve the problems, cope up with future problems and overcome them. Counseling work in the nursing setting involves using all the skills one has, to make the patient feel at ease and to help him to be healed as much as cured. Counseling is part of the nurse's duty as she carries out total patient care.

Guidance and Counseling in Nursing Educational Institutions

Guidance and counseling will assist nurses in developing proper attitude, commitment, dedication and other qualities required for a successful nursing practice. Moreover, emerging and re-emerging diseases, technological advancements in patient care evolving of new specialties especially in the clinical areas, changing role of nurses in health care sector impact of Consumer Protection Act, etc. underlines the need of a viable guidance and counseling service in all nursing institutes. The need for guidance and counseling in nursing education can be summarized as follows:

1. To help students adjust with new environment in the nursing institute.
2. To help in developing qualities required for a successful nursing practice.
3. To help students in getting adjusted with the clinical environment.
4. To help students keep in touch with the latest trends in nursing and to reap benefits from the trends.
5. To help students in developing positive learning habits, especially in skill learning so that they can retain and transfer the learned lessons in a better way.
6. To help in the development of appropriate coping strategies in order to deal with stress in a productive manner.
7. To help nursing students in establishing a proper identity.
8. To help them develop a positive attitude towards life.
9. To help them overcome periods of turmoil and confusion.
10. To help students in developing their leadership qualities.
11. To motivate them for taking membership in professional organizations after completing their studies.
12. To help them take advantage of the technological advancements in patient care.
13. To help them develop readiness for changes and to face challenges both in the personal as well as professional life.
14. To help them carry out the responsibilities as a worthwhile health team member.
15. To help them in proper selection of careers both in India and abroad.
16. Motivate them to pursue higher education according to their abilities and interest.
17. To assist the needy students in availing financial assistance from appropriate organizations.

Stages of Vocational Guidance

At Elementary Stage

1. It is in this period that habits, skills and attitudes develop.
2. For developing the basic skills and attitudes.
3. For developing the habit of doing the work in a neat and systematic manner.
4. For developing good inter-personal relationships.

At Secondary Stage

1. To help pupil to appraise or know their vocational assists and liabilities.
2. To make pupils to be familiar with various occupations and their requirements.
3. To help pupils to make a right choice.
4. To help pupils to prepare themselves for entering into the occupations of their choices.
5. To help pupils to get suitable jobs in their chosen field.
6. To help pupils to think seriously whether to go to college or not.

At College Stage

1. To help people for making a comprehensive study of the cancer which they would like to pursue.
2. To help pupils to relate their studies to vocations that is open to them.
3. To help pupils for acquainting themselves with different avenues of work.
4. To help pupils to acquainting themselves with avenues for higher studies and various programs for financial assistance, scholarships, stipends, grants, fellowship, etc.
5. To help pupils to make contacts that would help in putting their plans into successful operation.

CONCLUSION

The terms guidance and counseling are often interchangeably used causing confusion to many. Guidance and counseling are so inter-related that in practice, the processes are at times undifferentiated, but at other times clearly differ. Knowledge of guidance and counseling are necessary for a nurse to become a good nonprofessional counselor. She also should have a better personality which will determine her success in counseling.

BIBLIOGRAPHY

1. Anthikad Jacob. Psychology for Graduate Nurses. 4th edn, Jaypee Brothers Medical Publishers, New Delhi, 2007.
2. Bhatia BD, Craig Margaretta. Elements of Psychology and Mental Hygiene for Nurses in India. Orient Longman, Chennai, 2005.
3. Das G. Educational Psychology, Kind Books, New Delhi.
4. Gross Richard, Kinnison Nancy. Psychology for Nurses and Allied Health Professionals, Hodder Arnold, London, 2007.
5. Hilgard RE, Atkinson CR, Atkinson LR. Introduction to Psychology. 6th edn, Oxford and IBH Publishing Co. Pvt. Ltd, New Delhi, 1975.
6. Hurlock B Elizabeth. Developmental Psychology. A Life Span Approach, 5th edn, Tata McGraw-Hill , New Delhi, 2002.
7. Khan MA. Psychology for Nurses. Academa Publishers, Delhi, 2004.
8. Kupuswamy B. An Introduction to Social Psychology. Media Promoters and Publishers Pvt. Ltd, Mumbai, 1994.
9. Mangal SK. Advanced Educational Psychology, 6th edn, Prentice Hall of India Pvt Ltd, New Delhi, 2007.
10. Mangal SK. General Psychology. Sterling Publishers Pvt Ltd, New Delhi, 2006.
11. Matlin W Margaret. Psychology. 3rd edn, Harcourt Brace College Publishers, Philadelphia, 1999.
12. Morgan T Cifford, Kind A Richard, Weisz R John, Schopler Jobn. Introduction to Psychology. 7th edn, Tata McGraw-Hill Publishing Company Limited, New Delhi, 2004.
13. Myers G David. Social Psychology. 6th edn, McGraw-Hill College, Boston, 1991.

14. Nagaraja KR, Begum Shamshad B, Sudarshan CY. MCQs in Psychology for Nursing and Allied Sciences. Jaypee Brothers Medical Publishers Pvt. Ltd, New Delhi, 2006.

15. Ramnath Sharma. Psychology and Mental Hygiene for Nurses. Kedarnath Ram Nath and Co, Meerut.

16. Robert S Feldman. Understanding Psychology. 6th edn, Tata McGraw-Hill Edition, New Delhi, 2004.

17. Sinclair C Helen, Fawcett N Josephine. Altschul's Psychology for Nurses. 7th edn, Bailliere Tindall, London, 1991.

18. Skinner E Charles. Educational Psychology. 4th edn, Prentice-Hall of India Pvt. Ltd., New Delhi, 1996.

19. Taylor E Shelley. Health Psychology, 6th edn, Tata McGraw-Hill Edition, New York, 2006.

20. Zwemer J Ann. Basic Psychology for Nurses in India. BI Publications Pvt. Ltd., Chennai, 2003.

Learning

10

DEFINITIONS

1. **Learning:** Learning is the process by which an activity originates or is changed through reacting of an encountered situation provided that the characteristics of the change in activity cannot be explained on the basis of native responses tenderizers, maturation or temporary states of the organism like fatigue or effect of drugs.

2. **Insight learning:** In a typical in sight situation a problem is passed, a period follows during which no progress is made and then the solution comes suddenly. A learning curve of insight learning would show no evidence of learning for a time, then suddenly learning would be almost complete.

3. **Conditioning:** Conditioning is a form of learning in which a reflex or some aspect of behavior is brought under the control of a stimulus; we will define conditioning in terms of the procedures used to bring it about. These procedures, with examples, are described below. Although conditioning has been investigated in humans and animals, with generally similar findings, the majority of experiments on conditioning have employed animal subjects, in which learning prior to the experiment can be more easily controlled.

4. **Skill learning:** Right from the birth, the child acquires skill. His bodily organs learn to handle the things. He moves his legs and begins to crawl. In course of time, he learns other motor skills, like walking, speaking, drawing, writing, reading, playing music, cycling and swimming, etc.

5. **Perceptual learning:** The child gets sensations through his organs of sense, and he attaches meaning to each sensation. The earliest sensations of the infant are undifferentiated to the extent that he cannot differentiate between one object and another. In course of time, he recognizes specific objects, and perceives these separately.

6. **Conceptual learning:** As concrete thinking leads to abstract thinking, perceptual learning is followed by conceptual learning. A concept is a general idea, universal in character. A child sees a particular cow, and forms some ideas of a cow, with some particular characteristics. Here the ideation is on the basis of one particular cow. This is the particular percept but when the child sees a number of cows, with some common characteristics, he locates certain general qualities in all the cows, and on the basis of these he forms a conception of 'cow'. This is on the basis of percept which is made general.

7. **Associative learning:** Conceptional learning is helped by associative learning in amassing a wealth of knowledge. New concepts are tagged with the past concepts through association.

8. **Appreciational learning:** While conceptual learning is on the affective side, a child from the very beginning utilizes his inborn trait of esthetic sensibility, and acquires concepts colored by appreciation.
9. **Attitudinal learning:** Attitudes are generalized dispositions for certain particular concepts, things, persons or activities. A child develops an attitude of affection towards his mother, an attitude of reverence towards the teacher, and an attitude of belongingness towards the family. His attitude towards play is most favorable. All this he learns and adopts gradually.
10. **Reinforcement:** Reinforcement is a collective term meaning either reward or punishment. It is often used when a principle is stated which applies to both reward and punishment for instance, "Reinforcement is most effective when it occurs immediately after the response."

INTRODUCTION

An individual begins to learn soon after his birth and goes on learning throughout his lifetime. An infant is quite helpless at birth, suit slowly he learns to adapt himself to the environment around him. There are usually two factors involved in his learning this adjustment to the environment; they are maturation and the ability to profit by experience.

Learning occupies an important position in the life of an individual. Most of one's behavior shows evidence of some type of learning or the other. It is learning that makes an adequate adjustment of life situations possible. Learning implies cumulative improvement. The nature of improvement can be clearly gauged by the changes which take place while learning is progress.

MEANINGS OF LEARNING

1. Learning is a change in behavior; it is a change that takes place through practice or experience.
2. Learning is not a reflex action, it means that winking or withdrawal of leg when knee is struck is not learning.
3. Learning may be for conscious purpose or it may be for biological and social adjustments.
4. Through learning, in a person permanent or temporary changes are produced.
5. It can be for adjustment or maladjustment. It can create a socially—adjusted individual or it may give rise to antisocial behavior.
6. Learning is a self-active process which takes place in a social setup or environment.
7. Learning is a process that is purposeful and goal-directed. It also consists in establishing the right stimulus-response connections.
8. Learning is universal and continuous; it is a continuous never ending process that goes from womb to tomb.
9. Learning prepares an individual for the necessary adjustments and adaptation.

DEFINITIONS OF LEARNING

1. Bernhardt defines Learning as "the more or less permanent modification of an individual's activity in a given situation, due to the practice in attempts to achieve some goal or solve some problem."
2. Learning is a change in the individual following upon changes in his environment.—*Peel*
3. Learning is the process by which behavior is originated or changes through practice or training—*Kingsley and Garry.*

4. The term learning covers every modification in behavior to meet environmental requirements—*Gardener Murphy.*

5. Learning is the process by which an activity originates or is changed through reacting to an encountered situation, provided that the characteristics of the changes in activity cannot be explained on the basis of native response, tendencies, maturation or temporary states of organism—*Higard.*

6. Learning defined as an expected and permanent change in the behavior, brought about as a result of practice—*Hillguard and Atkinson.*

7. Learning is acquiring new activities or enhancing or improving the old activities—*Underwood.*

8. Comparatively, learning is the serial or gradual change of the behavior. This is a special process, which takes place as a result of observation or training—*ML Mann.*

DETERMINANTS OF LEARNING

1. **Kind of material:** It is observed that certain type of material is more easily mastered than some other type. The meaningful material is more easily learned than the matters that lacks meaning. Verbal learning takes place at an ideational level. When one tries to understand the concept of specific gravity, he learns with the help of ideas.

2. **Method of learning:** There are certain methods of learning which are found to be effective than certain others. These methods are related to the way he breaks up the learning material and the time spent in learning.

3. **Practice:** Repetition in terms of trials are necessary for all learning activities. All learning is based up on some amount of practice.

4. **Motivation:** Effective learning is directly related to the strength of the motives. Educationist try to utilize different motives to make the pupil's learn better. Out of all the external goals with which motives can be connected, the inner goals like interest and curiosity are bound to be strong motivating forces.

5. **Intelligence:** Learning cannot take place effectively without intelligence. Intelligence enables to understand things, to see relationships between things, to reason and judge correctly and critically.

6. **Maturation:** Learning and maturation contribute to the development of the person. Those two actually are so interlinked that any line of separation is hardly visible. Maturation is growth which takes place regularly in an individual without special condition of stimulation, such as training and practice.

7. **The learner:** Besides these situational factors, the learner himself is the most vital factor in deciding the efficiency of learning. The learner's intelligence, his age and experience make considerable difference in learning effectiveness.

STEPS IN LEARNING PROCESS

1. Motivation within the learner.
2. Goal or goals become related to the motivation.
3. Barriers or difficulties are perceived and experienced and tension arises. Strong barriers may cause excessive tension which may altogether discourage and confuse the learner.
4. The search for an appropriate solution to the problem or an appropriate line of action to reach the goal.

5. The most appropriate line of action is selected and practiced and inappropriate behaviors dropped.

LAWS OF EFFECTIVE LEARNING (THORNDIKE)

Major Laws of Learning

The Law of Readiness

1. Learning takes place best when a person is ready to learn. If a person is ready to act, acting gives him satisfaction.
2. Some sort of preparatory attitude or the mind-set is necessary. The learned should be stimulated to learn new things in such a way that he obtains satisfaction out of learning that.

The Law of Exercise, Use and Disuse or Practice

1. Learning takes place through, exercise and repetition. We learn skills in games, music, craft, typing or in nursing by constant exercise and practice.
2. An activity which is not used or practiced or exercised for sometime, tends to be forgotten by disuse.
3. The learner should be provided with opportunities of practicing and repetition. But repetition should be continual rather then continuous.
4. Most of the nursing skills and procedures are learned through practice on the wards and in the public health field.

The Law of Effect or Satisfaction and Dissatisfaction

1. We learn things and to do things that give us satisfaction and we learn not to do things which annoy us.
2. The connections between stimuli and response become strong when we derive satisfaction from those responses, but remain weak or are unformed when we are annoyed.
3. Activities which are accompanied by a feeling of pleasure or satisfaction are more readily and effectively learnt than activities which are unpleasant or annoying.

Minor Laws of Learning

1. The law of maturation
2. The law of purpose
3. The law of selection
4. The law of association
5. The law of recency
6. The law of multiple learning.

TYPES OF LEARNING

Verbal Learning

1. Learning of this type helps in the acquisition of verbal behavior.
2. The language we speak, the communication devices we use are the result of such learning.
3. Rote learning and rote memorization, which is a type of school learning is also included in verbal learning.

4. Sign, pictures, symbols, words, figures, sounds and voices, etc. are employed by the individual as an essential instrument for engaging him in the process of verbal learning.

Motor Learning

1. The learning of all types of motor skills may be included in such type of learning.
2. Learning how to swim, riding a horse, driving a car, flying a plane, playing piano and handling various instruments are the example of such learning.
3. The art of these skills can be acquired through a systematic and planned way of the acquisition and fixation of a series of organized actions or responses by making use of some appropriate learning methods and devices.

Concept Learning

1. A concept in the form of a mental image denotes a generalized idea about the things, persons or events.
2. The formation of such concepts on accounts of previous experiences, training or cognitive process is called concept learning.
3. Such type of concept learning proves very useful in recognizing, naming and identifying the things. All of our behaviors, verbal, symbolic, motor as well as cognitive is influenced by our concepts.

Problem Solving Learning

1. In the ladder of learning and acquisition of behavior, problem—solving denotes a higher type of learning.
2. Problem solving learning requires the use of the cognitive abilities like reasoning, power of observation, discrimination, generalization, imagination, ability to infer and draw conclusions, trying out novel ways and experimenting, etc.
3. Problem solving learning has essentially caused human being to contribute significantly to the process and improvement of society.

Serial Learning

1. Serial learning consists of such learning in which the learner is presented with such type of learning material that exhibits some sequential or serial order.
2. Children often encounter such a learning situation in schools where they are expected to master lists of material such as the alphabet, multiplication tables, the names of all the states in their country, etc.

Paired-associated Learning

1. In this learning, learning tasks are presented in such a way that they may be learned on account of their associations.
2. The name of a village like Kishnapur is remembered on its association with the name of Lord Krishna or a girl's name Ganga by learning it in the form of making parried association with the river gangs.
3. The practice with such procedure then helps in building what is known as associate learning.

THE GOALS OF LEARNING

1. The goals in learning can be classified in to two broad categories: the acquisition of knowledge and the acquisition of skill.
2. The acquisition of knowledge means the bringing up of intellectual and emotional modification and control in the individual through learning.
3. The acquisition of skill refers to the sensory motor modification and control through learning.

Acquisition of Knowledge

Perception

1. Perception refers to the acquisition of specific knowledge about objects or events directly stimulating the sense at any particular moment.
2. A young child sees a women, in the past, the women has fed her. On the basis of that experience, he comprehends that a women is his nurse or mother. The type of learning at perceptual level is known as perceptual learning.

Conception

1. Conception means the acquisition of organized knowledge in the form of concepts or general ideas, which transcend any particular percept.
2. The child gets the perception of orange, apple, banana, etc. and is able to locate certain general qualities in them.

Associate Learning

1. Associate learning corresponds to memory both as the deliberate recall and recognition, past experience and a habit or automatic memory due to association.
2. Associate learning is fundamental to all other learning.

Appreciation

1. Appreciation is the acquisition of ideas, attitudes or dispositions characterized by an emotional tone.
2. In our knowledge this factor is present as the effective or feeling element. When we talk about an ideal, we are talking about a concept which is colored by appreciation.

Acquisition of Skills

1. Under skill are included the sensory motor process: writing, reading, musical performance, language acquisition in its vocal aspect, drawing and the arts generally.
2. True learning is enrichment of experience it is because of this view of learning process that today we find an emphasis on activity programs, learning by doing the project method, self-activity, etc. rather than on book learning.

THEORIES OF LEARNING
Classical Conditioning (Fig. 10.1)
Introduction

Classical conditioning gets its name from the fact that it is the kind of learning situation that existed in the early "classical" experiments of Ivan P Pavlov (1849-1936). In the late 1890's, this famous Russian physiologist began to establish many of the basic principles of this form of conditioning. Classical conditioning is also called respondent conditioning or Pavolvian conditioning.

```
Bell ─────────────── Looking in the direction

Food ─────────────→ Salivation
```

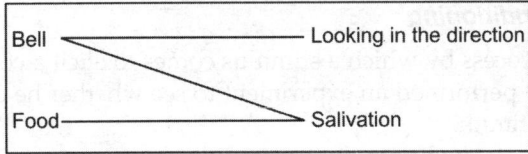

Concept of Classical Conditioning

1. The dog salivated not only upon actual eating but also they saw the food, noticed the man who.
2. In every animal and person, there are a number of innate stimulus—response association—connections wired in at birth, before any learning occurs.
3. Classical conditioning is constructed upon these inborn neurological connections.
4. Through learning, a pervious neutral stimulus can come to acquire some of the same properties as unconditional stimuli. In this case the previously neutral stimulus is called conditioned stimuli (CS) and the response it produces is called a conditioned response (CR).
5. Pavlov described the process by which associations are acquired and become the source for more general behavior or more complex ones, as well as the ways in which the learned responses could be unlearned or extinguished. These processes include acquisition, higher-order conditioning and extinction.

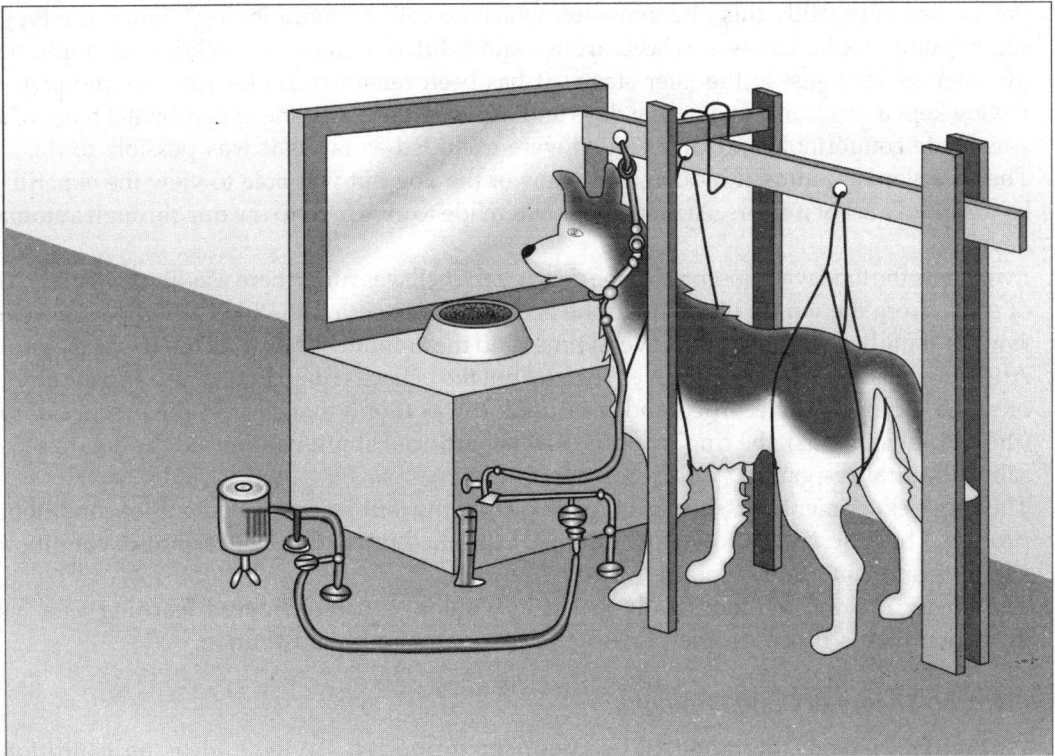

Fig. 10.1: Classical conditioning

Principles of Classical Conditioning

1. **Acquisition:** It is the process by which a stimulus comes to elicit a condition response. To see how this occurs Pavlov performed an experiment to see whether he could produce salivation to previously neutral stimuli.
2. **Extinction:** This process related with the gradual disappearance of the conditioned response on disconnecting the S-R association is called extinction.
3. **Stimulus generalization:** It is referring to a particular state of learning behavior in which and individual once condition to response to a specific stimulus is made to respond in the same in response to other stimuli of similar nature.
4. **Stimulus discrimination:** Stimulus discrimination is the opposite of stimulus generation. Here in sharp contrast to response in a usual fashion the subject learns to react differently in different situations.
5. **Association:** Repetition of the conditioned stimulus, followed by the unconditioned stimuli and consequent response must occur without exception.
6. **Reinforcement:** It is not only the association of two stimuli and a response that is essential but what works in conditioning is the effect of reinforcement. Food in this case, which has a reinforcing effect strengths and bond between the condition stimulus and the unconditioned response changing it ultimately in the form of a conditioned response.

The basic process of classical conditioning as shown in Figs 10.2A to C.

Pavlov's Experimentation

1. Pavlov began to study this phenomenon, which he called "conditioning". Since, the type of conditioning emphasizes was a classical one—quite different from the conditioning emphasized by other psychologist at the later stage—it has been renamed as classical conditioning.
2. Pavlov kept a dog hungry for a few days and the tried him on to the experimental table which was made comfortable and distractions were excluded as far as it was possible to do.
3. The observer kept himself hidden from view of the dog but was able to view the experiment by means of a set of mirrors. Arrangement was made to give food to the dog through automatic devices.
4. Every time the food was presented to the dog and the bell was rung, there was automatic secretion of saliva from the mouth of the dog. The activity of presenting the food accompanied with a ringing of the bell was repeated, several times and the amount of saliva secreted was measured.
5. After several trials, the dog was given no food but the bell was rung. In this case also the amount of saliva secreted was recorded and measured. It was found that even in the absence of food (the natural stimulus), the ringing of the bell (an artificial stimulus), caused the dog to secrete saliva (natural response).
6. The above experiment thus, brings in to the picture the four essential elements of conditioning process. They are natural or unconditioned stimulus, unconditional response, conditioned stimulus and condition response.
7. The theory of conditioning as advocated by Pavlov, thus considered learning as a habit formation and is based on the principle of association and substitution.

John Watson Theory of Conditioning

1. Watson (1878-1958) the father of behaviorism supported Pavlov's ideas on conditioned responses. Watson tried to demonstrate the role of conditioning in producing as well as eliminating the emotional response such as fear.

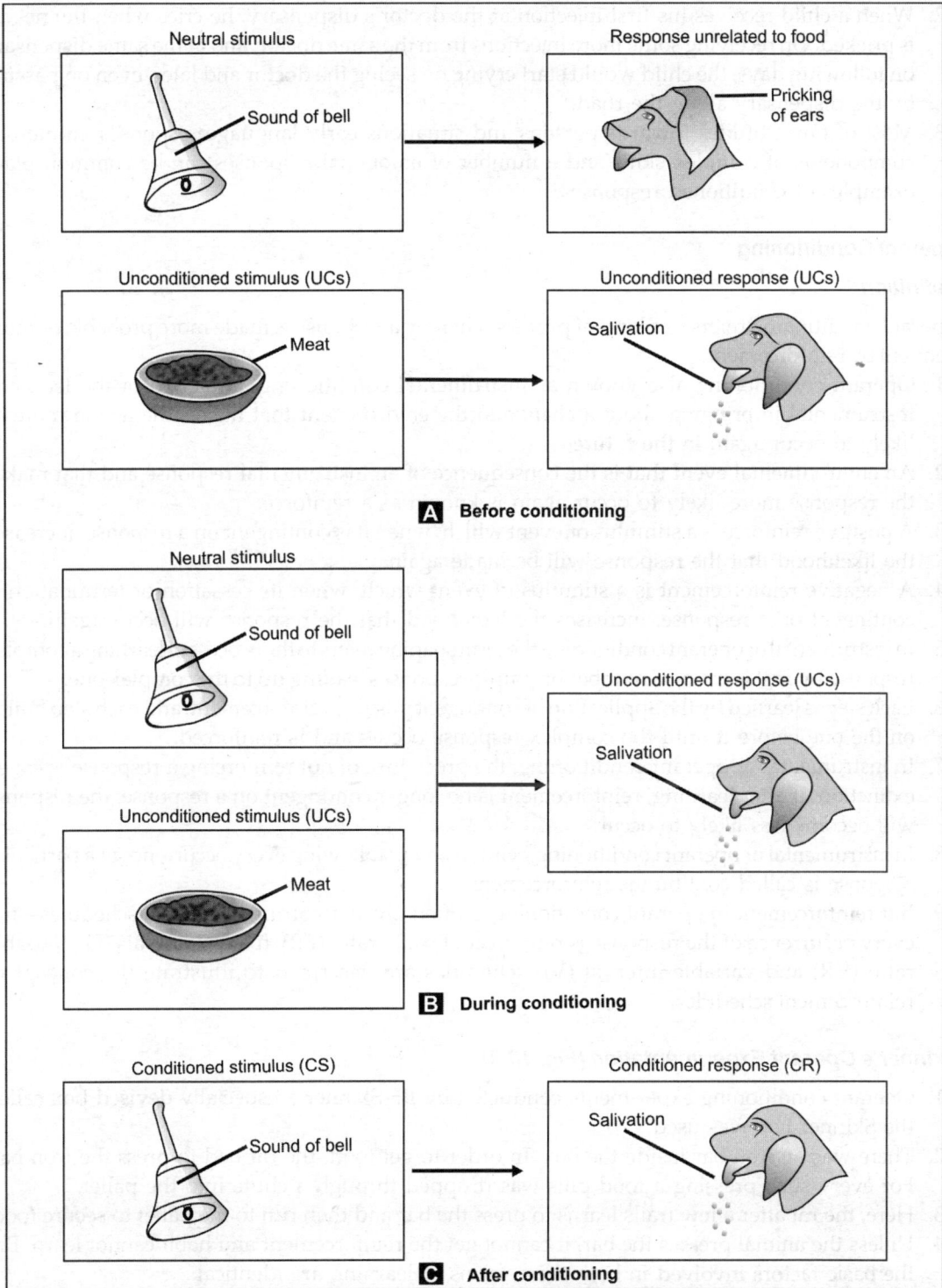

Figs 10.2 A to C: The basic process of classical conditioning

2. When a child receives his first injection at the doctor's dispensary, he cries when the needle is pricked. On receiving some more injections from the same doctor, and at the same dispensary on following days, the child would start crying on seeing the doctor and later, even on passing by the dispensary along the road.

3. Most of our attitudes towards persons and situations early language responses, numerous components of complex skills and a number of emotional responses can be common place examples of conditioned responses.

Operant Conditioning

Definition

Operant conditioning refers to a kind of process whereby a response is made more probable or more frequent by reinforcement.

1. Operant conditioning also known as instrumental conditioning, an action of the learner's instrumental in bringing about a change in the environment that makes the action more or likely to occur again in the future.

2. An environmental event that is the consequence of an instrumental response and that makes the response more likely to occur again is known as a reinforce.

3. A positive reinforce is a stimulus or event which, when it is contingent on a response, increases the likelihood that the response will be made again.

4. A negative reinforcement is a stimulus of event which, when its cessation or termination is contingent on a response, increases the likelihood that the response will occur again.

5. In instrumental or operant conditioning the term shaping refers to the process of learning a complex response by first learning a number of simple responses leading up to the complex one.

6. Each step is learned by the application of contingent positive reinforcement, and each step builds on the one before it until the complex response occurs and is reinforced.

7. In instrumental or operant conditioning, the procedure of not reinforcing a response is called extinction. If after learning, reinforcement is no longer contingent on a response, the response will become less likely to occur.

8. In instrumental or operant conditioning, reinforcement following every occurrence of a particular response is called continuous reinforcement.

9. But reinforcement in operant conditioning is often given according to certain schedules—not every occurrence of the response is reinforced. Fixed –ratio (FR), fixed –intervals (FI), variable ratio (VR) and variable-interval (VI) schedules are described to illustrate the concept of reinforcement schedules.

Skinner's Operant Experimentation (Fig. 10.3)

1. Operant conditioning experiments conducted by BF Skinner a especially devised box called the Skinner box was used.

2. There was an iron bar inside the box. In order to get food, the rat had to press the Iron bar. For every such pressing a food pills was dropped through a chute into the pallet.

3. Here, the rat after a few trails learns to press the bar and then run to the pallet to secure food.

4. Unless the animal presses the bar, it cannot get the reinforcement and habit cannot learn. But the basic factors involved in both these forms of learning are identical.

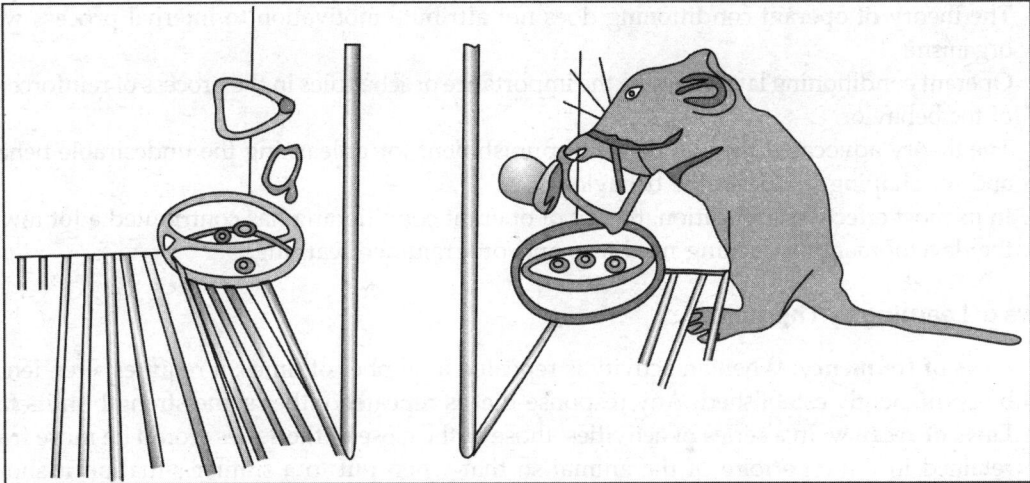

Fig. 10.3: Instrumental conditioning experiment (Skinner)

Schedules of Reinforcement

1. **Continuous reinforcement schedule:** It is hundred percent reinforcement schedules where provision is made to reinforcement or rewards every correct response of the organism during acquisition of learning.
2. **Fixed internal schedule:** In this schedule the reinforcement is given after a fixed number of responses.
3. **Variable reinforcement schedule:** When reinforcement is given at varying individuals of time or after a varying number of responses, it is called a variable reinforcement schedule.

Difference between Classical and Operant Conditioning

Classical conditioning	Operant conditioning
1. It helps in the learning of respondent behavior.	It helps in the learning of operant behavior.
2. It is called type—S conditioning because of the emphasize on the stimulus.	It is called R conditioning because of the emphasis on the response.
3. This beginning is being made with help of specific stimuli that bring certain response.	Here, beginning is made with the responses as they occur naturally or unnaturally, shaping them into existence.
4. Strength of conditioning is usually determined by the magnitude of the condition response.	Here strength of conditioning is shown by the response rate.

Implication of Operant Conditioning

1. The principle of operant conditioning may be successfully applied in the task of behavior modification.
2. The task of the development of human personality can be successfully manipulated through operant conditioning. According to Skinner, "we are what we have been rewarded for being."

3. The theory of operant conditioning does not attribute motivation to internal process within organism.
4. Operant conditioning lays stress on the importance of schedules in the process of reinforcement of the behavior.
5. The theory advocated the avoidance of punishment for unlearning the undesirable behavior and for shaping the desirable behavior.
6. In its most effective application, theory of operant conditioning has contributed a lot towards the development of teaching machines and programmed learning.

Laws of Learning by Thorndike

1. **Laws of frequency:** When an activity is repeated a number of times; it requires a tendency to be permanently established. Any response that is repeated either some strength in its favor.
2. **Laws of recency:** In a series of activities, those at the close of the series would be more freshly retained in the repertoire of the animal so that when put to a similar situation it shows a tendency to respect them.
3. **Law of effect:** This is perhaps the most important among all the laws. It says that the response that gives the organism the satisfaction of success is the one that is most likely to be fixed. On the other hand, when the response does not lead to such a satisfaction is tends to be discarded.

TRIAL AND ERROR LEARNING

Introduction

The theory of trial and error learning propagated by Thorndike emphasizes that we learn through a trial and error mechanism. In trying for a correct behavior, one tries hard in so many ways and may commit so many errors before a chance success. On subsequent trials he may learn to avoid erroneous ways, repeat the correct ones and finally learn the proper way.

Concept of Trial and Error

1. When we are placed in a new situation or face a new problem we have to seek solution, which we are not able to perceive in the beginning.
2. This made of learning is slow, wasteful and unintelligent. It requires more time and greater energy than higher types learning.
3. Learning implies establishment of new connections between the stimulus and response. These new connections are gradually established blind process of trial and error.
4. In this kind of learning which is very common in animals, there is assumed to be at first nothing but random, aimless reaction, but in which there emerges after a time a chance correct response that finally is stamped into the neuromuscular system of the animal.
5. There are random movements in the beginning, gradually the number of random movements is reduced along with error and finally the goal is reached. Thus improvement takes place through repetition.
6. The principles involved in the process as to how the learner stabilizes the new response pattern, gives the clue to the under standing of learning by trial and error.

Thorndike Trial and Error Experiments

1. In the typical experiments of Thorndike, he made use of a puzzle box that could be opened by some mechanical contrivance, e.g. pressing a button on its floor.
2. When a hungry cat was placed inside this puzzle box and food like fish was placed outside the box within the sight of the animal, the cat would struggle hard to come out of the box.
3. In this process she went through a series as random activities that could not bring about the solution of her problem.
4. She may try to squeeze herself out of the bars, bite them, scratch the floor with her claws or run about. In the course of the new response pattern, her paw may accidentally fall on the button and the door is opened for her.
5. Out of all the series of responses given by the cat a single one proves to be the correct response— e.g. keeping her paw on the button and pressing it.
6. Immediately following this response she comes out and can take food that has a reinforcing effect. Her success during the first trial may be due to sheer chance.
7. But when the animal is put to the same situation next time there is a definite reduction of the random responses and the successful solution of the problem of the random responses and the successful solution of the problem requires less time than before.
8. This way with practice the errors or wrongs responds are gradually eliminated and the correct response is strengthened.
9. When a person learns to swim or to ride on a bicycle the initial pattern of behavior display a large number of random responses. With practice, all the wrong movements are gradually eliminated.

Laws of Learning by Thorndike

Stages of Trial and Error Learning

1. **Drive:** In the present experiment it was hunger which was intensified with the sight of the food.
2. **Goal:** To get the food by getting out of the box.
3. **Block:** The cat was confined in the box with a closed door.
4. **Random movements:** The cat, persistently, tried to get out of the box.
5. **Chance success:** As a result of this striving and random movement the cat, by chance, succeeded in opening the door.
6. **Selection:** Gradually the cat recognized the correct manipulation of the latch. It selected the proper way of manipulating the latch out of its random movements.
7. **Fixation:** At least, the cat learned the proper way of opening the door by eliminating all the incorrect responses and fixing only the right responses. Now it was able to open the door without any error or, in other words, learned the way of opening the door.

Background of the Theorist

1. Edward L Thorndike a famous psychologist (1874-1949) is known as the propagator of the theory of trial and error learning.
2. Thorndike has written—learning is connecting. The mind is man's connection system.
3. Thorndike named the learning of his experimental cat as trial and error learning. He maintained that the learning is nothing but the stamping in of the correct responses and stamping out of the incorrect responses through trial and error.

Implication of Trial and Error Learning

1. Whatever we want to learn or teach, we must first try to identify the things that are to be remembered or forgotten.
2. What is being thought or learnt at one time should be linked with past experiences and learning on the one hand and with the future learning on the other for utilizing the benefits of the mechanism of association, connection or bonds in the process of learning.
3. The learner should try to see similarities and dissimilarities between the different kinds of responses to stimuli and with the help of comparison and contrast should try to apply the learning of something in one situation to other similar situations.
4. The learner should be encouraged to do his task independently. He must try various solutions of the problem before arriving at a correct one.

LEARNING BY INSIGHT

Introduction

The Gestalt psychologist has offered an altogether different explanation of the learning process. They do not believe that learning is a process of blind habit formation. The learning process studied by Thorndike or the behaviorists occurs, according to Kohler, in a very unnatural and restricted situation, where the animal is denied all possibility of a clear perception of the whole situation.

Definition

Insight may be defined as sudden awareness of the relationships among various elements that had previously appeared to be independent of one another.

Background of the Theorist

1. Insight learning introduced by a group of German psychologist called Gestalts; Wolfgan Kohler in particular originated a learning theory known as insight learning.
2. The nearest English translation of gestalt is configuration or more simply an organized whole in contrast to a collection of parts. Gestalt psychologists consider the process of learning as a gestalt—an organized whole.
3. In practical sense, Gestalt psychology is primarily concerned with the nature of perception.
4. Gestalt psychologists tried to interpret learning as a purposive, exploratory and creative enterprise instead of trial and error or simple stimulus-response mechanism.

Concept of Insight Learning

1. It involves mental exploration and understanding of what is being learned. It implies some insight, some awareness of the consequences of performing an act.
2. The Learner perceives the reactions which the problem involves or the significant characteristics of the situation and connects the right response with the solution by using his intelligence.
3. He uses his past learning and his ability to generalize from one situation to another.
4. The principles involved in any learning process depend upon the nature of the learning situation.
5. Kohler in his experiments on learning offered different types of situation and eventually arrived at totally different conclusions regarding the principles involved in the learning process.
6. Insight involves a perceptual reorganization of elements in the environment such that new relationships among objects and events are suddenly seen.

7. It is goal directed and oriented towards the solution of a problem. When the organism is put to a problematic situation, it starts to tackle it. Such tackling involves the perception of the problem.

Kohler's Insight Learning Experimentation

1. Some of the well known experiments of Kohler performed on chimpanzees had the following plan—the hungry chimpanzee was kept in a cage and a bunch of bananas was hung from the ceiling.
2. A number of wooden boxes were lying about. The chimpanzee tries to jump high to reach the bananas. When it was impossible to reach the highest he tries to jump from a celling.
3. When this too was found to be failure he gave up the efforts for some time. All of a sudden the chimpanzee got some new idea and started putting one box upon the other.
4. Finally by getting up on the topmost he could successfully grab the bananas.
5. In the situation described above, there was no evidence of a blind trial and error procedure where the corrected responses occurred gradually.

TRANSFER OF LEARNING

Introduction

Learning one skill sometimes influences the acquisition of other skills. This influence may be positive that can facilitate the new learning. It can also be negative when it interferes with the acquisition of new learning. In the first case we have positive transfer of training, often referred to as merely "Transfer of training" or transfer of learning. In the second case we have what is commonly called habit interference.

Definition

According to Sorenson, transfer refers to the transfer of knowledge training and habits acquired in one situation to another situation.

Meaning of Transfer of Learning

1. Transfer of training or learning influences to carry over the learning from one task to another. The learning or skill acquired in one task is transferred or carried over to other tasks.
2. Transfer of training is the carry—over of habits of thinking, feeling or working of knowledge of skills from one learning area to another usually is referred to as the transfer of training.
3. One of the simplest examples of positive transfer is to be found in experiments showing improvement in performance with the left hand as a result of practice with the right hand. This is called bilateral transfer or cross education.

Characteristics of Transfer Learning

1. **Transfer to a similar activity:** Learning one activity sometimes easier the learning of another activity.
2. **Transfer in verbal learning:** Transfer is also evident for several verbal skills. When comparable lists of nonsense syllabus are learned one after the other, there is a gradual reduction in the trials required to learn successive list.

Types of Transfer

1. **Positive transfer:** Transfer is said to be positive when something previously learned benefits performance or learning in a new situation.

2. **Negative transfer:** When something previously learned hinders performance or learning in a new situation, we call negative transfer.
3. **Zero transfer:** In case the previous learning makes no difference at all to the performance or learning in a new situation, there is said to be zero transfer.

Principles of Transfer

1. **Similarity of contents:** A person familiar with several card games will learn the rules of new card game readily. This is possible as the rules are like those he already knows. Learning to drive one model of car a person any soon master the control of another, since many of the activities involved in driving cars are identical.
2. **Similarity of techniques:** When subjects were given practice to toss a ball in air and then catch it in a cup with their right hand, there was bilateral transfer when they performed the same task with their left hand.
3. **Similarity of principles:** Transfer of principles is not always different from transfer of techniques because the use of techniques may involve the application of principles.
4. **Formal discipline:** Transfer was once sought to be explained on the basis of the doctrine of formal discipline of mental faculties. The mind was supported to be a bundle of independent faculties of reasoning, memory imagination, etc. Transfer of training was thus supposed to be automatically achieved. Through the exercise of mental faculty.

Bagly's Transfer of Training

1. The transfer of training or learning can also be explained on the basis of the theory of ideals put forward by WC Begley.
2. According to this theory, transfer of learning or training takes place in the form of ideals.
3. The experience we have, the generalization or conclusions we arrive at, all do transfer if they are imbibed as ideals of some value or desirable by the individual.
4. Bagley (1922) the ideals of neatness developed on the basis of stress laid on doing things quite neatly in school is likely to transfer in performing all other activities in a quite neat and clean way.
5. If we wish to seek positive transfer from one situation to another we must strive for the formation of general attitude for an ideal.

NURSES ROLE IN LEARNING

1. Learning is fundamental to the development and modification of behavior, thus knowledge of the learning process may be usefully applied to many clinical situations and academic work.
2. Many of our subjective feelings, emotions and attitudes are probably conditioned responses. Through generalization it becomes difficult to identify the origin of our emotional responses. Both our adaptive emotional responses as well as unadaptive responses are learned and can be unlearned through principle of learning.
3. Learning methods have wide applications in educational setting. In programmed learning the material to be learned is broken up into small easy steps, so that the learner can accomplish without frustrations. Also with programmed learning, learner can master the task at his own pace; with versatile and flexible learning, the learner can improve learning style.
4. Applications of reinforcement principles can often increase productivity both in studies as well as in vocation.

5. A nurse should understand the nature of learning and the factors which will affect learning. As learning modifies our behavior, it is necessary for a nurse to learn only the right things so that modification takes place in the right direction.
6. She must have a well-defined purpose and goal in all learning situations.

BIBLIOGRAPHY

1. Arnold MB (Ed). The Nature of Emotion, Baltimore, Penguin, 1968.
2. Bandura A. Principles of Behaviour Modifications, Holt, Rinehart and Winston, New York, 1969.
3. Carison NR. Psychology of Behaviour, Allyn and Bacon, Boston, 1977.
4. Furguson ED. Motivation: An Experimental Approach. bit, Rinehart and Winston, New York, 1976.
5. Goddard FA. The Human Senses (2nd edn), Wiley, New York, 1972.
6. Hochberg JE. Perception (2nd edn), Englewood Cliffs, Prentice Hall, NJ, 1978.
7. Korman AK. The Psychology of Motivation, Englewood Cliffs, Prentice Hall, NJ, 1974.
8. Lindsay H, Nirman DA. Human Information Processing (2nd ed), Academic Press, New York, 1977.
9. Morgan CT. A Brief Introduction to Psychology, Tata McGraw-Hill, New Delhi, 1975.
10. Morgan T, King RA. Introduction to Psychology, 6th edn, Tata McGraw-Hill, New Delhi, 1982.
11. Mueller CG. Sensory Psychology, Englewood Cliffs, Prentice Hall, NJ, 1965.
12. Munn Norman L. Introduction to Psychology, Oxford and IBH, New Delhi, 1973.
13. Robinson DN. An Intellectual History of Psychology, Macmillan, New York, 1976.
14. Strongman KT. The Psychology of Emotion, Wiley, New York, 1973.
15. Thompson RF. Introduction to Psychological Psychology, Harper and Row, New York, 1975.

11 *Motivation*

DEFINITIONS

1. **Motive:** Motive is a state within the individual that under appropriate circumstances initiates or regulates behavior in relation to a goal.
2. **Need:** A need as the lack of something which, if present, would tend to further the welfare of the organism or of the species or to facilitate its usual behavior.
3. **Drive:** A drive is a tendency initiated by shifts in physiological balance, tissue tension, sensitivity to stimuli of a certain class and response in any of a variety of ways that are related to the attainment of a certain goals.
4. **Interest:** It is a tendency to give selective attention to one activity or activities rather than to others in interest.
5. **Instinct:** It is usually defined as a faculty of acting in such a way as to produce certain ends, without foresight of the ends and without previous education in the performance.
6. **Needs:** Needs are general wants or desires and are said to be the very basis of our behavior. Our behavior and feelings about ourselves and others, our values and priorities we set for ourselves all relate to our physiological and psychological needs. Every human being has to strive for the satisfaction of his basic needs if he is to maintain and actualize or enhance himself in this world.
7. **Biological drive:** Biological needs give birth to biological drives such as hunger, thirst, sex and escape from pain. The biological drives are basically unlearned in nature. They arise from our biological needs as a result of a biological mechanism called homeostasis.
8. **Incentives:** Anything that incites rouses or encourages a person is termed as an incentive. Drives are influenced and guided by incentives. Praise, appreciation, regards, bonus, etc. are examples of incentives. Incentive works as a reinforcing agent, as it adds more strength to a drive like adding fuel to the already ignited fire. A piece of candy, chocolate or a toy may work as an incentive for a child to give more strength to his drive and as a result he may be further motivated to act or behave in a desirable way.
9. **Frustration:** Frustration is the feeling of being blocked or thwarted in satisfying a need or attaining a goal, individual perceives as significant.
10. **Conflict:** Conflict means a painful emotional state which results from a tension between opposed and contradictory wishes.

INTRODUCTION

The human behavior is controlled, directed and modified through certain motives, when a person is hungry and is searching for food or constructing a house or mating or learning new skills, we will always be able to trace some such elements which his activities, guide them and his behavior in the lights of his success or failures.

Motivation is that force which impels or incites individual's action, determines the individual's direction of action and his rate of action. When the individual gets any motives, his experiences a tension and disequilibrium and becomes restless. His activities are then initiated. The individual feels a push to behave in a certain direction.

MEANING OF MOTIVATION

1. Motivation is something which prompts, compels and energizes an individual to act or behave in a particular fashion at a particular time for attaining some specific goal or purpose.
2. The term 'Motivation' has been derived from the word 'Motive'. A motive is an inner state that activities, energizes or moves an individual and channelises his behavior towards goals.
3. Motivation is the art of understanding these motives and satisfying them to direct and sustain behavior towards the accomplishment of organizational goal.
4. Motivation is concerned with how behavior gets started, is energized, sustained, directed and stopped. As motivation is the process of inspiring and impelling people to take required actions by providing stimuli that satisfy their needs and motives.
5. Motivation is the complex of forces which propel an individual into action and keep them at work. It reflects the will to work.

DEFINITIONS OF MOTIVATION

1. Motivation means a process of stimulating people to action to accomplish desired goals. It refers to the way in which urges, drives, desires, aspirations, stirrings or needs direct, control or explain the behavior of human being.—*Scott*
2. Motivation is an inspirational process which impels the members of the team to pull their weight effectively, to give their loyalty to the group, to carry out properly the tasks that they have accepted and generally to play an effective part in the job that the group has undertaken.—*Brech*
3. Motivation is the willingness to exert high levels of effort toward organizational goals, conditioned by the effort's ability to satisfy some individual needs.—*Stephen P Robbins*
4. Motivation refers to the degree of readiness of an organism to pursue some designated goal, and implies the determination of the nature and laws of the focus including the degree of readiness.—*Encyclopedia*

NATURE OF MOTIVATION

1. Motivation is a psychological concept. It is concerned with the intrinsic forces operating within an individual which impel him or act or not to act in a particular way.
2. Motivation is a dynamic and continuous process as it deals with human being which is an ever changing entity modifying itself every moment.
3. Motivation is a complex and difficult function. Every person adopts a different approach to satisfy his needs and one particular need may cause different behavior on the part of different people.

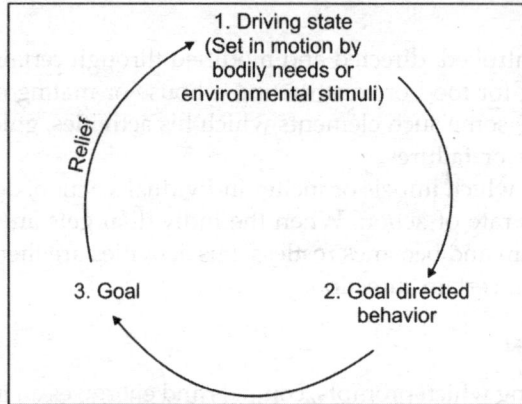

Fig. 11.1: The motivation cycle

4. Motivation is a circular process. Feeling of an unsatisfied need causes tension and an individual takes action (drive) to reduce this tension (Fig. 11.1).
5. Motivation is different from satisfaction. Motivation is the process of stimulating an individual or a group to take desired action.
6. Motivation is the product of anticipated value from a given course of action and the perceived probability that the action will lead to these values.

THE MOTIVATION PROCESS

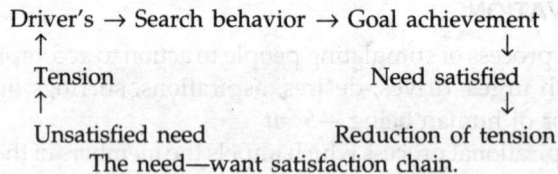

Driver's → Search behavior → Goal achievement

Tension   Need satisfied

Unsatisfied need   Reduction of tension

The need—want satisfaction chain.

1. An unsatisfied tension which stimulates drives, with in the individual. This drives generate search behavior to find particular goals that if attained, will satisfy the need and lead to reduction of tension.
2. In order to relieve this tension, they engage in activity. The greater tension, the more activity will be needed to bring about relief.
3. Therefore, when we see people working hard at some activity, we can conclude that they are driven by a desire to achieve some goal that they perceive as having value to them.

MOTIVE

Meaning of Motive

1. Motive is a force that determines the activity of an individual. It energizes and directs his behavior along this or that channel.
2. When a motive is at work, it creates tension and these tensions arouse the individual towards an activity that will relieve the tension.
3. A motive is the force that initiates, sustains and directs the activity of an organism. A stimulus is an internal or external object which exiles the receptor or activates a sense organ.

Definitions of Motive

1. Caroll, "A need give rise to one or more motives. A motive is a rather specific process which has been learned. It directed towards a goal".
2. Fisher, "A motive is an inclination or impulsion to action plus some degree of orientation or direction".
3. Rosen, Fox and Gregory, "A motive may be defined as a readiness or disposition to respond in some ways and not others to a variety of situations".

Classification of Motive

Physiological Motives

1. **Temperature regulation:** An organism is further active in maintaining a comfortable state of warmth and cold. This motivated activity is the result of the impulses sent to the brain by the skin receptors meant for the sensation of warmth and cold.
2. **Pain:** The sense receptors for pain are distributed in all the bodily organs like skin, internal organs, blood vessels, etc. they are in the form of free nerve ending in theses organs. Whenever, they are stimulated by some sort of injury to the body there is pain sensation. The organism puts in all possible efforts, consciously or at reflex level to avoid such pain.
3. **Sleep:** Need for sleep is one more physiological motive. Though it curtails all activity of the organism unlike other motives and makes him assume an inactive position it can be observed, however, that the inactive position is the goal and the motive of sleep actually drives the individual to more all possible efforts to go to sleep.
4. **Hunger:** When we feel emptiness in our stomach, we are hungry. When we are hungry they occur two kinds of changes. One if the change in our external behavior and other is the change in our internal conditions. The motive of hunger gives rise to the hunger pangs. The actual sensation a person gets in a type of acting sensation.
5. **Thirst:** When deprived of water over some period, the organism becomes excessively restless and needs intake of water. This drive for water comes from dryness of the mouth and thirst. However, the feeling of thirst is basically related to the degree of dehydration of the body tissue. Thirst is also a physiological need which promotes activity. This need is very active when it is not immediately satisfied.
6. **Sex drive:** Sex is a very powerful drive which influences the actions of the individual to a very great extent. According to general convention, this drive remains dormant during childhood. The Freudian theory shows evidence for sexual behavior right from infancy. With the onset of puberty the sex glands known as gonads start functioning and as a result, the sex drive is simulated.
7. **Maternal drive:** What has been said about the sex instinct applies equally well to maternal behavior. Prolactin, a hormone from the anterior pituitary gland plays an important role motivating maternal behavior. Human maternal motivation has several aspects. Child rearing practices and attitudes towards children differ from culture-to-culture and from subculture-to-subculture.

General Motives

1. **Activity:** Men as well as animals are found to be spontaneously active. They enjoy it and spend considerable time in moving about. This innate motive for activity is visible even in a child's

behavior. Activity also accompanies other physiological drives when these drives are stronger activity increases. Activity is closely related to sensors stimulations. More the stimulations in the environment, more active is the organism.

2. **Exploratory drive:** People like to explore new environments. We visit new places; mountaineers even risk their lives in exploratory expeditions. When animals are put in to mazes they are found to explore them without any specific aim to satisfying a physiological drive like hunger. This drives of exploration in stronger when the organism finds itself in a new situation.

3. **Curiosity:** This is a motive which is close to exploration. Exploration is a drive that aids the satisfaction of curiosity. Animals as well as men including children are curious about the several things around them. A small child's curiosity tempts him even a break a new toy given to him.

4. **Manipulation:** This is one more motive which is a related aspect of the two previously discussed. It is not so easy to differentiate clearly among the drive of exploration, curiosity and manipulation. All three seem to be different aspects of a single motivated activity. Curiosity leads to manipulation, in turn, is a counterpart of exploration.

5. **Affectional motive:** Love is an important motive of human life; we love our parents, our brothers and sisters, children, friends, etc. The significant people in the environment become love objects through positive contact with him. There is enough reasons to believe that it is also an unlearned motive that emerges with maturation.

6. **Fear:** Fear is varying powerful motive. The motivates escape from fear—production situation. Fear may also interfere with the satisfaction of other motives. Most of the fears are learned. But there is enough reason to believe that some fears are unlearned.

Social Motives

1. **Affiliation:** Our need for affiliation is well-expressed through our affiliation with clubs and other institutions. Though marriage is partly a means of satisfy many other needs including the need for affiliation. The motive of affiliation is usually seen in all human cultures. This motive perhaps has its roots in our childhood experiences when the helpless infant has to associate himself with others for his basic need satisfaction.

2. **Social approval:** We seek social approval for all the things we do similarly, we try our best to avoid doing anything that may evoke social disapproval. We often show an almost compulsive tendency to confirm to the norms set by our social group. This may be the result of constant parental directions in childhood as to what is right and what is wrong for the child to do.

3. **Status:** All people are common motivated to achieve status among their fellowmen. This motive varies in strength from person-to-person. Some people show the minimum need for status in the form of the desire to the thought well of and heave a respectable position in their professional field or in community.

4. **The need for power and prestige:** The need for prestige is expressed in the form of our striving to feel better than other persons with whom we compare ourselves. In daily life there are many ways in which prestige is sought and achieved, such symbols as dress, money and other belongings are regarded as ways of feeling superior in comparison to others. The need of power is almost similar though, it differs slightly in its expression.

5. **Security:** An urge for feeling of security is also an important motive especially in complex modern societies. This feeling involves the ability to hold on to what one has and continue with the assurance to keep it up on the other hand, insecurity is a haunting feeling that one may lose what he now has.

6. **Achievements:** Achievement is a powerful motive in some societies. This is the motive to accomplish something, to succeed in one's undertaking and to avoid failure. The importance

of this varies from culture-to-culture and from subculture-to-subculture. The strength of achievement motives depends partly on the past success of an individual.

Unconscious Motives

1. Not all our motives are conscious. A number of them are operating without our awareness. In our own behavior we come across instances of acts, the explanation of which cannot be found. All such instances of behavior can be explained with reference to unconscious motives.
2. Origin of unconscious motives can be found in the unconscious. The term unconscious should not be taken to mean that it is a part of mind separated from unconscious mind.
3. The repression itself is a function of the unconscious. Hence, constant repression enlarges the domain of the unconscious. Since the material is related to our motives it is dynamic in nature and does not remain quiet in the unconscious.
4. According to Freud the material of the unconscious is extremely difficult to top because a considerable part of it is originated in infantile preverbal ideas which have never become conscious.

Instinctive and Behavior

1. McDougall defines an instinct, "an inherited or innate psychophysical disposition which determines its possessor to perceive and to pay attention to objects of a certain class, to experience an emotional excitement of a particular quality upon perceiving such an object and to act in regard to it in a particular manner or at least to experience an impulse to such action".
2. According to McDougall instincts are innate tendencies which have a cognitive aspect, emotive aspect to feel certain emotion towards these objects, to act towards them in a particular way.
3. The human instincts sucking, crying, locomotion, curiosity, sociality, shyness, cleanliness, pressing downward on the feet, imitation, pugnacity, fear of dark places, acquisitiveness, love and jealousy.

Hierarchy of Motives

1. Hierarchy of motives helps us to understand the potency of different motives in understanding man's behavior.
2. According to White, motives at the lowest rung are those originating from homeostatic mechanism. Thus, all motives important for survival including the safely motives are included in this class. Affiliation motives are placed still higher. These motives include the need for social acceptance and belongingness.
3. According to Maslow, the highest type of needs which he calls the need for self actualization? The need for self actualization is complicated concept which needs some further explanation.

THEORIES OF MOTIVATION

Drive Reduction Theory

1. One of the earlier theories of motivation was the drive reduction theory. It was proposed by Clark Hull.
2. This theory proposes that organisms' experiences the arousal of a drive when an important need is not satisfied, and they engage in behavior to reduce the arousal and satisfy the need.

3. Primary drives are those that motivate the organism to fulfill some basic need necessary for its survival such as hunger, thirst or sex.
4. An important component of the drive reduction theory is homeostasis. The term homeostasis refers to a state of balance or equilibrium necessary in many physiological systems.
5. Primary drives are biological drives necessary for personal and species survival. Acquired drives develop through learning.
6. The drive is the force that motivates an organism to action. Which action the organism finally performs depends on the strength of the organism's habit.
7. A habit is a response to some stimulus. The strength of the habit depends on the connection between the stimulus and the response that influences what kind of behavior the drive will energize.

Optimum Level of Arousal Theory

1. The optimum level of arousal theory states that drives do not necessarily motivate an organism to seek the lowest level or arousal. Instead they provide motivation to seek an optimum level of arousal.
2. Robert Uerles and JD Dodson (1908) conducted an experiment to examine the effects of different arousal levels on learning. They varied arousal levels in mice by changing the intensity of electric shocks and by observing how well the animals performed in simple and complex mazes.
3. The Yerkes-Dodson law states that performance on a learning task is related to arousal; the best performance results from intermediate levels of arousal. Performance is also related to the difficulty of the task.
4. Yerkes and Dodson found that the mice performed simple tasks better when the stimulation was more intense. For complex tasks, low to intermediate arousal was the best.

Cognitive Theory

1. A cognitive theory (the word comes form the Latin for knowing) emphasizes some sort of understanding or anticipation of events through perception or thought or judgment as in the estimation of probabilities or in making a choice on the basis of relative value.
2. Any organism with memory is capable of recognizing some similarities between the present and the past and hence is able to form some sort of experience with regard to the consequences of its behavior.
3. According to a cognitive theory, motivated goal seeking behavior comes to be regulated by these conditions, which are based on the past, modified by circumstances of the present and includes expectations about the future.
4. Cognitive Dissonance theory: Festinger (1957) proposed a theory in which certain kinds of unbalanced cognitions are described as dissonant and the subject is under stress to remove this dissonance.

Expectancy Theory

1. Expectancy theory emphasizes the importance of rewards and goals as well as how person's expectations of consequences can influence his behavior. This theory stresses 'pull' rather than 'push'.
2. According to expectancy theory, the hunger drive is only part of the reason a hungry rat is motivated to find its way through a maze. It is also motivated because of previous learning experiences in which it has come to expect a bit of food at the end.

3. Motivation is composed of two major features: The valence or attractiveness of the goal and the expectancy or the likelihood that its behavior will lead to the goal.
4. A simple way of explaining the expectancy theory is to say that; motivation = valence × expectancy. The actions that hungry people take to satisfy their hunger depend very much on valence and expectancy.
5. Economic theories assume that the individual can assign value or utility to possible incentives and that he makes his decision according to the risk involved.

Psychoanalytic Theory of Modification

1. Freud believed that all behavior stemmed from two opposing groups of instincts. The life instincts (Eros) that enhance life and growth and the death instincts (Thanatos) that pushes toward destruction.
2. The energy of the life instincts is libido, which involves mainly sex and related activities. The death instinct can be directed inward in the form of aggression towards others. Freud pointed to several forms of behavior:
   a. In dreams, we often express wishes and impulses of which we are unaware.
   b. Unconscious mannerisms and slips of speech may reveal hidden motives.
   c. Symptoms of illness (particularly symptoms of mental illness) often can be shown to serve the unconscious needs of the person.

Maslow's Hierarchy of Needs (Fig. 11.2)

1. The behavior of an individual at a particular moment is usually determined by his strongest need. These needs nave a certain priority.
2. The lower level needs (e.g. physiological needs) have the highest strength until they are reasonably met. When the lower level needs are met, man goes to satisfy the higher needs.
3. The hierarchy needs organized step-by-step to the satisfaction of other needs—physiological needs, safety and security needs, social needs, esteem needs and self-actualization needs. A satisfied need is no longer a motivator of behavior.

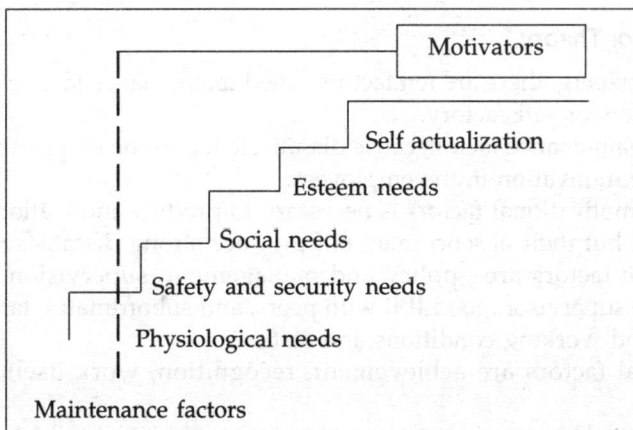

Relationship between Hertzberg and Maslow models

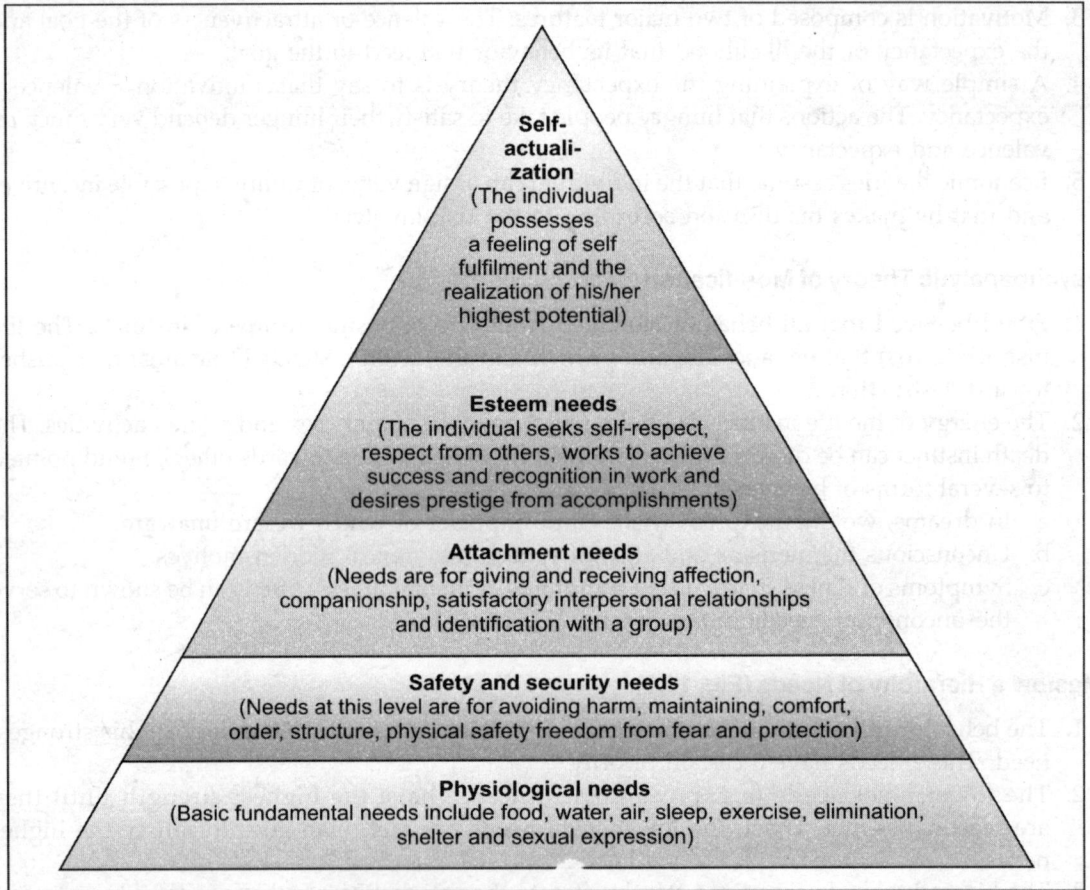

Fig. 11.2: Maslow's Hierarchy of needs

Hertzberg's Two Factor Theory

1. According to Hertzberg, there are ten factors called maintenance factors and six factors called motivational factors or satisfactory.
2. The absence of maintenance factors cause dissatisfaction in the employees, but their presence may not produce motivation in the employees.
3. The presence of motivational factors is necessary to produce motivation and job satisfaction in the individual but their absence may not produce strong dissatisfaction.
4. The maintenance factors are—policy and management, supervision, good interpersonal relationship with supervisor, good IPR with peers, and subordinates, fair salary, Job security, personal life, good working conditions and status.
5. The motivational factors are achievement, recognition, work itself, advancement, and responsibility.
6. The Hertzberg model has given several insights. One of the insights is job enrichment. The idea behind job enrichment is to keep maintenance factors constant or higher while increasing

motivational factors by attaching more responsibility satisfying working conditions and power to the job.

McClelland's Needs Theory

1. McClelland identified three types of basic motivating needs. They are—need for power, need for affiliation and need for achievement.
2. Power motive is the need to manipulate others or the drive for superiority over others. Such individuals are generally seeking positions for leadership.
3. The affiliation motive is concerned with maintaining pleasant social relationships, sense of intimacy and understanding and enjoy in consoling and helping others who are in trouble.
4. Achievement motivated people can be the backbone of most organizations, because they progress faster. They are highly task oriented and work to their optimum capacity.

Carrot and Stick Approach of Motivation

1. Carrot and stick approach of motivation comes from the old story that the best way to make a donkey move is to put a carrot out in front of him or beat him with a stick from behind.
2. The carrot is the reward for moving and the stick is the punishment for not moving.
3. In motivating people for better production in an organization some carrots (rewards) are used such as money, promotion and other incentives.
4. Some sticks (punishments) are used to push the people for desired behavior or to retrain from undesired behavior.

FRUSTRATION

Introduction

When the pursuit of a goal is thwarted or blocked in any situation the result is frustration. That is, frustration is the consequence of the blockage of motives or when competing motives work at the same time and the individual is not in a position to make appropriate choice.

Definition

Frustration is defined as the blocking of a desire or need. It also refers to failure to satisfy a basic need because of conditions, either in the individual or external obstacles.

Meaning of Frustration

1. Frustration is a condition of extreme tension; it is commonly interpreted as a strong emotional tension, caused by the blocking of impulses.
2. The individual is said to be frustrated because he does not to know how to rid himself of his tension. These tensions make the frustrated person highly discomfort able.
3. Frustration involves an insurmountable obstacle and the inability to overcome it and a sense of defeat as well as feeling of stress and strain.

Sources of Frustration

1. **Environmental forces:** The frustration may be caused by environmental situations or conditions which cannot control. Such environmental conditions include a contagious disease, the death of a friend or a beloved relative, us usual rains and storms or floods.

2. **Personal inadequacies:** It may be in the form of poor ability or skill in the individual. On the other hand, the person's level of aspiration may be high which may come in the way of reaching the goals. It may also be due to any physical handicap in the individual.

3. **Conflict of motives:** Sometimes frustration results because of interference of one motive with other motives. For example, in our society sexual motivation is often in conflict with the society's standards of approved sexual behavior.

CONFLICT

Definition

Conflict is a state when two or more incompatible motivations or behavioral impulses compete for expression. In other words, the individual is faced with more than two incompatible demands, opportunities, goals or needs.

Mental conflict is a inner state characterized by tension as a result of the presence, at the same time of mutually exclusive or opposing tendencies, impulses or desires is described as mental conflict.

Types of Conflict

1. **Approach (approach conflict):** In this type of conflict a person is faced with two appealing/ attractive goals or choices and he is forced to choose one of them. For example, a young computer engineer is offered jobs in two popular multinational companies. The young man is in a dilemma choosing between the two.

2. **Avoidance (avoidance conflict):** In this type of conflict an individual has to make a choice between two unattractive goals. Here the individual is repelled by two undesirable alternatives at the same time. For example, a person has a long history of painful backache for which he is advised surgery. Here the person is faced with the prospect of living with painful backache or undergoing dreadful surgery. This conflict is aptly described in the proverb caught between the devil and deep blue sea.

3. **Approach (avoidance conflict):** Here the goal has both attractive and unpleasant aspects. The choice has pleasant and unpleasant consequences. A prospective young professional bride has an offer to marry an non-resident Indian in America. Here going to America is appealing and at the same time leaving the parents in India is distressing.

4. **Resolution of conflicts:** Conflict often produces stress; stress includes a number of unpleasant responses. Every individual is equipped with capacity to overcome obstacles in order to avoid conflict, which is a source of frustration.

CONCLUSION

Motivation is often used to refer an individual's goals, needs, wants, intentions and purpose. For example, when one is hungry, the need is food, and it induces drive. When the food is searched and the drive 'hunger' is reduced and the activity ceases then. All human behavior is motivated by something. Very little human behavior is completely random or instinctive. Most human behavior is goal-directed. People do things for some reason to get certain results. The reasons may not always seem logical or rational, but they do tend to be systematic and hence, behavior is relatively predictable.

BIBLIOGRAPHY

1. Anthikad Jacob. Psychology for Graduate Nurses. 4th edn, Jaypee Brothers Medical Publishers, New Delhi, 2007.
2. Bhatia BD, Craig Margaretta. Elements of Psychology and Mental Hygiene for Nurses in India. Orient Longman: Chennai, 2005.
3. Das G. Educational Psychology, Kind Books, New Delhi.
4. Gross Richard, Kinnison Nancy. Psychology for Nurses and Allied Health Professionals, Hodder Arnold: London, 2007.
5. Hilgard RE, Atkinson CR, Atkinson LR. Introduction to Psychology. 6th edn, Oxford and IBH Publishing Co. Pvt. Ltd, New Delhi, 1975.
6. Hurlock B Elizabeth. Developmental Psychology. A Life Span Approach, 5th edn, Tata McGraw-Hill: New Delhi, 2002.
7. Khan MA. Psychology for Nurses. Academa Publishers, Delhi, 2004.
8. Kupuswamy B. An Introduction to Social Psychology. Media Promoters and Publishers Pvt Ltd, Mumbai, 1994.
9. Mangal SK. Advanced Educational Psychology. 6th edn, Prentice Hall of India Pvt. Ltd., New Delhi, 2007.
10. Mangal SK. General Psychology. Sterling Publishers Pvt. Ltd, New Delhi, 2006.
11. Matlin W Margaret. Psychology. 3rd edn, Harcourt Brace College Publishers: Philadelphia, 1999.
12. Morgan T Cifford, Kind A Richard, Weisz R John, Schopler John. Introduction to Psychology. 7th edn, Tata McGraw-Hill Publishing Company Limited: New Delhi, 2004.
13. Myers G David. Social Psychology. 6th edn, McGraw-Hill College: Boston, 1991.
14. Nagaraja KR, Begum Shamshad B, Sudarshan CY. MCQ5 in Psychology for Nursing and Allied Sciences. Jaypee Brothers Medical Publishers Pvt. Ltd. New Delhi, 2006.
15. Ramnath Sharma. Psychology and Mental Hygiene for Nurses. Kedarnath Ram Nath and Co., Meerut.
16. Robert S Feldman. Understanding Psychology, 6th edn, Tata McGraw-Hill Edition: New Delhi, 2004.
17. Sinclair C Helen, Fawcett N Josephine. Altschul's Psychology for Nurses. 7th edn, Bailliere Tindall: London, 1991.
18. Skinner E Charles. Educational Psychology. 4th edn, Prentice-Hall of India Pvt. Ltd., New Delhi, 1996.
19. Taylor E Shelley. Health Psychology, 6th edn, Tata McGraw-Hill, New York, 2006.
20. Zwemer J Ann. Basic Psychology for Nurses in India. BI Publications Pvt. Ltd., Chennai, 2003.

12

Emotions

DEFINITIONS

1. **Emotion:** Emotion is an affective experience that accompanies generalized linear adjustment and mental and physiological stirred-up states in the individual and that shows itself in his overt behavior.
2. **Negative emotions:** Unpleasant emotions like fear, anger and jealousy which are harmful to the individual's development are termed as negative emotions.
3. **Positive emotions:** The pleasant emotions like affection (love), amusement, curiosity and happiness which are very helpful and essential for normal development, are termed as positive emotions.
4. **Feeling:** Feeling is defined as pleasant or unpleasant experience associated with an idea.
5. **Mood:** Mood is pleasant or unpleasant experience associated with a real or imaginary idea, place or a situation. When an emotion persists for a period, it constitutes mood.
6. **Affect:** Affect is the cross-section of mood.
7. **Primary emotions:** These are those emotions that an individual feels first, as a first response to a situation. These are unthinking and instinctive responses that an individual has for example, if we are threatened, we may feel fear. When we hear of a death, we may feel sadness. Typical primary emotions include fear, anger, sadness and happiness.
8. **Secondary emotions:** These appear after primary emotions, may be caused directly by them, just like primary and secondary colors. They may come from more complex chains of thinking. For example, news of wartime victory may start feelings of joy, but then get tinged with sadness for the loss of life.
9. **Stress** is a physiological or psychological tension that threatens homeostasis or a person's psychological equilibrium. Stress is defined as a broad class of experiences in which tension occurs when demanding situations tax the resources, coping and level of adoption of individual.
10. **Psychosomatic illness:** A psychosomatic or psychophysiologic disorders is an illness whose symptoms are caused by mental processes of the sufferer rather than immediate physiological causes. Psychosomatic symptoms show that a human body can create physical symptoms that compensate for relationship deficiencies. Psychosomatic refers to the relationship between body and mind. Many physical disorders, such as duodenal ulcers or high blood pressure, can be caused due to mental conditions like worry or stress, and are then termed psychosomatic in order to distinguish then from the same conditions having physical or hereditary causes.

INTRODUCTION

Emotions occupy an important place in our life. Life has become enjoyable because of the emotions like love, affection, personal happiness and the like. But all emotions do not have pleasantly toned effect those just mentioned. Emotions like fear, anger and jealousy bring about a good deal of disturbance. Out emotions have a great impact on others when we express them in ways that can be perceived by others. When we perceive the emotional responses of other people, we respond in appropriate ways, perhaps with an emotional expression of our own.

MEANING OF EMOTION

1. An emotion is a strong feeling. It is a conscious stirred up state of our organism.
2. Emotion experienced as certain feelings, pleasant or unpleasant, accompanied by marked physiological changes, involving both visceral and peripheral areas.
3. The subjective experience of an emotion is the cognitive component. Here the conscious experience could be pleasant or unpleasant.
4. The bodily arousal is the physical component; this is reflected by the activation of the autonomic nervous system, which regulates the activity of glands, smooth muscles and blood vessels.
5. Emotion is the mode of experience that accompanies the working of an instinctive impulse.

DEFINITIONS OF EMOTION

1. Emotion is a distinct psychological state, which involves subjective experience, physical arousal and behavioral response. In other words it has a cognitive component, physical component and a behavioral component.
2. Emotion is an affective experience that accompany generalized inner adjustment, mental and physiological stirred-up states in the individual and that shows itself in his overt behavior.
3. Emotion as a complex affective experience that involves diffuses physiological changes and can be expressed overtly in characteristics behavior pattern.

PHYSIOLOGY OF EMOTION

Physiological reactions and changes that are associate with emotions have their roots in our body chemistry. They are controlled by the endocrine glands, the autonomous nervous system and our brain.

Emotion and Autonomic Nervous System

1. Our autonomic nervous system plays a significant role in controlling and regulating our emotional behaviors.
2. The autonomic nervous system consists of sympathetic and parasympathetic system.
3. The sympathetic system activation leads to dilated pupils dryness of mouth, goose pimples of the skin, sweaty palms, dilation of the lung passages, increased heart rate, increased blood supply to the muscles, increased activity of the adrenal glands and inhibited digestion.
4. The parasympathetic system activation leads to constriction of the pupils, salivation, dryness of palm, absence of goose pimples, constriction of lung passages, decreased heart rate, increased blood supply to internal organs, decreased adrenal gland activity and stimulation of digestion.

Emotion and the Brain

1. The brain controls the autonomic responses that accompany emotions. The seat of emotion in the areas of brain is the hypothalamus, amygdale and the adjacent structures in the limbic system.
2. Emotions appear to be triggered by activity in the centers of the brain medicated by neurotransmitters. Dopamine has a major role in pleasant emotions.
3. Reticular formation—this mass of cells discharges impulses diffusely and some of them ascend to the cerebral cortex where they have an alerting function. When the reticular formation is activated, the relaxed or passive organism becomes aroused or alert.
4. Hypothalamus—the limbic system consists of a series of inter-related brain structures which include the hypothalamus and the sepal area both important in emotions. Impulses from the hypothalamus also activate the viscera and muscles, as when the adrenal gland is stimulated to secrete adrenaline.
5. The hypothalamus, in every way, tries to coordinate the activities of the internal organs associated with our emotional behavior. Impulses that come from the hypothalamus increase both smooth muscle (involuntary) and skeletal muscle (voluntary) activities.
6. The connection between the emotional behavior and stimulation of the various parts of the brain has brought the electric stimulation of the brain as a method for treating violent behavior in human being, particularly epileptics whose brain malfunction causes unusual aggressive behavior.

CHANGES IN EMOTION

External Changes

1. Emotions are complex experiences; they are psychical as well as physiological and physical. As psychical experiences the individual feels them as pleasant or unpleasant states of mind.
2. Emotion is a conscious and intellectual perception of a situation, intense and important enough to provoke one emotionally.
3. The body or organism gets stirred up. Changes occur in our breathing, circulation of blood, heart rate and other physiological functions.
4. There are many external changes in the body—changes in our voice, gestures, postures, facial expressions, etc.
5. The changes in facial expressions serve as indices to the nature of emotions. The face of a person experiencing joy is radiated with a smile. The angry man's red face betrays his anger.
6. There is a feeling tone accompanying these physical and physiological changes. All this results in some overt responses or behavior such as laughing, crying, shouting, hitting, crouching and cringing.
7. Bodily postures and gestures too can be used as clues to identify emotions. In sorrow a person tends to slump his face downward and in joy he holds head high and chest out.

Internal Changes

1. There is a greater intensity of heart action results in palpitation.
2. Blood pressure increases during emotional excitement.
3. There is a shift of blood from the viscera to the surface of the body causing flushing of face, for example, in anger.

4. There are many changes in the gastrointestinal tract. For example, churning movements slow down or stop in the stomach and the flow or saliva and other gastric juices necessary for digestion, is reduced by 85 to 90 percent.
5. There is a greater secretion of glycogen into the blood, sweat glands become more active.

CHARACTERISTICS OF EMOTION

1. Emotions are universal-prevalent in every living organism at all stages of development from infancy to old age.
2. Emotions rise abruptly but subside slowly. An emotion once aroused, tends to persists and leave behind emotional hang over.
3. Emotions are personal and thus differ from individual-to-individual.
4. An emotion can give birth to a number of other similar emotions.
5. The emotional experiences are associated with one or the other instincts or biological drives.

KINDS OF EMOTION

Pleasure

1. Pleasure is a reaction to the satisfaction of a motive or the attainment of a goal, i.e. satisfaction of motive states results in the emotion of pleasure.
2. We derive a great deal of pleasure from daydreams in which we think about attaining certain goals.
3. The emotion of pleasure manifest in smiling, laughing, hugging and kissing or in contentment, is evoked by situations which give physical comfort to the infant or a young child.

Fear

1. In general, fear is triggered by situations that are perceived as physically threatening, damaging to one's sense of well-being.
2. Fear is produced in children by sudden happenings, when the child is not prepared for what is coming. In infancy, strange and intense stimuli like noise produce fear.
3. The adolescent boy or girl is afraid of social humiliation and ridicule. In adulthood, we are afraid of situation which threatens our needs to obtain recognitions prestige and economic security.
4. Several factors are important in determining what the specific sources of fear will be for an individual.

Anxiety

1. Anxiety is a vague fear experienced without our knowing just what the matter is. One cause of anxiety can be unconscious memory of a fear stimulus.
2. When we learn a response to a particular situation, we have learned a response to all situations that are similar to the origin born.
3. A child who learns to fear a strict father may later feel uneasy or anxious in the presence of other men.

Anger and Hostility

1. Anger and hostility are reactions to the frustration of motives, insults and threats.
2. Frustrating a motive by imposing restraints an behavior is likely to provoke anger in a person of any age for infants, simple restraints, which frustrates exploratory motive is a common cause of anger.

3. Social frustrations are also common cause of anger adults. We seldom observe outright displays of it. Most frequent are the feelings of anger that we call "annoyance".
4. Ways of expressing anger change with age, among preschool children, anger is likely to take the form of temper tantrums and fighting.
5. An adult feels angry when his prestige is at stake, when his desires are being thwarted, when his plans are being foiled.

Depression and Grief

1. When depressed, people often feel inadequate and worthless, because of their failure to reach important goals. The depressed person losses the joy of living.
2. For most of us, depression does not last long because the situation in the environment changes and we are able to reach at least some of our goals. But for some people, perhaps because of an innate predisposition, depression can be prolonged and serve enough to make suicide.
3. Grief or sorrow and depressions are closely related, but there are differences between them. We usually call the emotion grief, when it is triggered by a specific loss, such as the death of a family member or friend.

EMOTION AND HEALTH

1. Emotions play an important role in human life. We wish to influence another persons actions we can do so by raising the appropriate emotions. They give us energy to carry out the activity.
2. Modern discovers in medicine have shown to us that uncontrolled emotionality plays a vital role in the causation of many physical disorders.
3. Persistent emotional disturbances caused by anger, fear and worries have been found to be one of the causative factors of psychosomatic disorders.
4. The continuous worries, fears and anxieties cause perpetual tensions. As a result, one's mental health is bound to be affected.
5. A relatively new field of investigation known as psychosomatic disease has thrown some light upon it. It has shown how emotional strain can cause bodily harm.
6. Illness like asthma, chronic headache, certain skin diseases, nervous pains, etc. are believed to have a psychosomatic origin. Their symptoms may be physiological but origins are psychological.
7. Other illnesses in which emotions play a vital role are bronchial asthma, high blood pressure, insomnia, chronic constipation and others.
8. Good, pleasant emotions contribute to good health. But intense and unpleasant emotions disturb us sometimes to a great extent if they persist. They may cause certain illnesses or may worsen the conditions of one already ill.
9. The responsibility of a nurse is not only to practice her nursing skills and provide physical comfort; it is also to reduce the intensity of emotional disturbances as much as it is possible for her.

THEORIES OF EMOTION

James-Lange Theory (Fig. 12.1)

1. William James on American psychologist and Lange a Danish physiologist have independently brought forward a theory of emotions that explains the relationship between the components of emotions that explains the relationship between the components of emotions in just the opposite direction of the one given above.

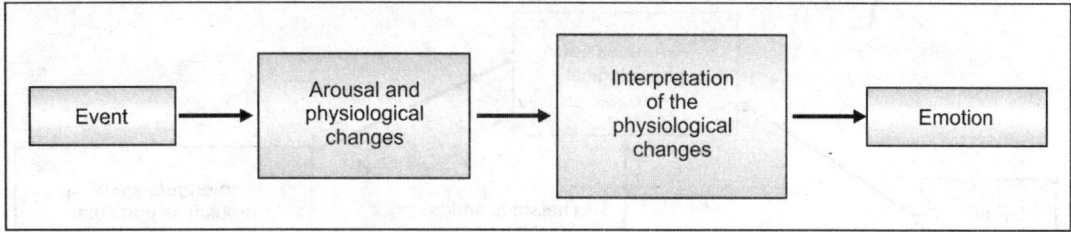

Fig. 12.1: James-Lange theory

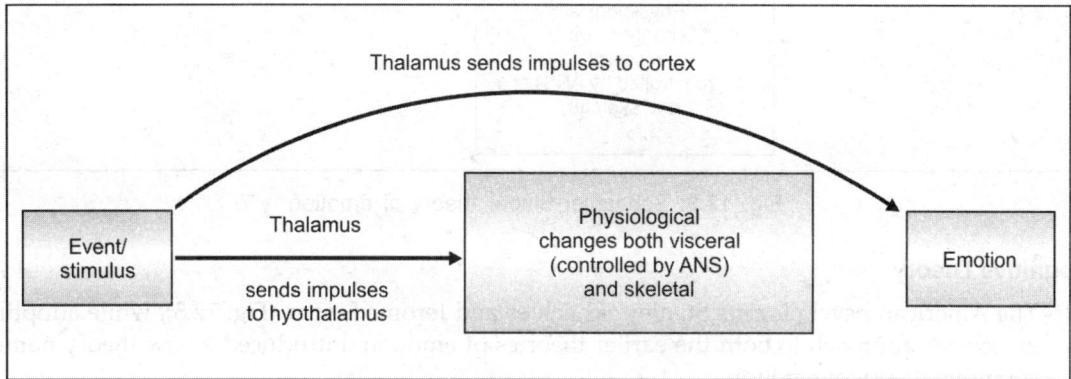

Fig. 12.2: The Cannon-Bard theory of emotion

2. According to this theory, an emotional experience has primarily a physiological basis. The psychical part is the resultant phenomenon.
3. Studies of patients with spinal cord damage have supported the James-Lange theory. These patients have no feedback from their muscles or viscera before the injury and many of them reported that their feelings of emotion changed considerably after the injury.
4. The James-Lange theory of emotions is subject to certain criticisms. The bodily changes in themselves are not seen to be the essential basis of emotions in experimental situations. Such changes brought about by drugs do not cause an experience of emotions.
5. Recently, some scientists have proposed the "facial feedback hypothesis" which suggests that feedback from the facial muscles and the viscera contribute to the experience of emotion.

Cannon-Bard Theory (Fig. 12.2)

1. Walter B Cannon objected to the James-Lange theory for several reasons. Cannon argued that people whose viscera were surgically separated from the central nervous system still reported some kind of emotional experience.
2. This theory emphasizes the role played by hypothalamus in emotional behavior. It says that both the feeling aspect and the bodily changes are set of simultaneously by the hypothalamus.
3. Cannon's theory of emotions suggested that emotions originate in the activity of lower brain areas rather than in the viscera, these circuits then activate both the cortex and viscera. Activity in the brain is critically important for certain emotions.

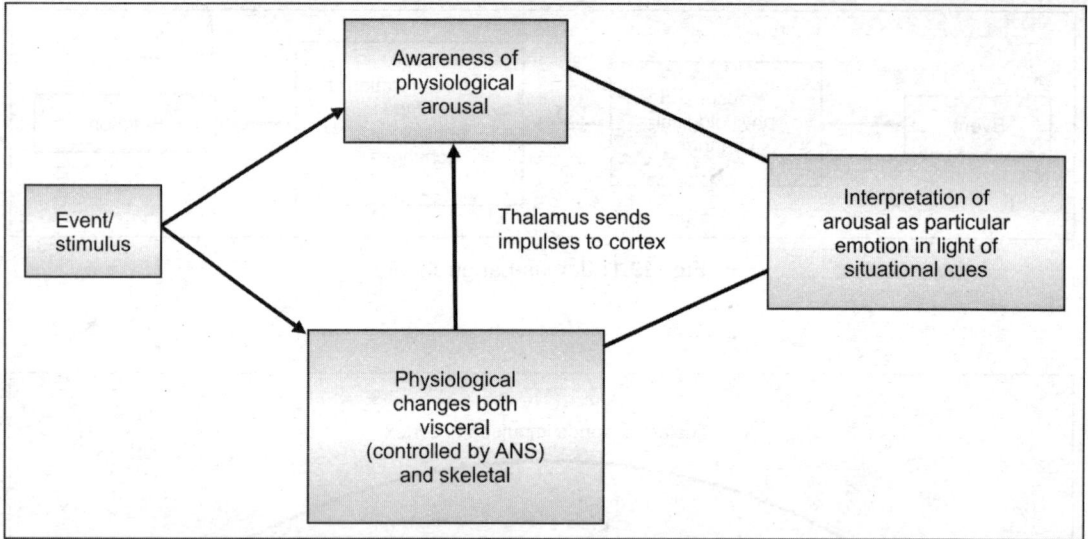

Fig. 12.3: Schachter-Singer theory of emotion

Cognitive Theory

1. The American psychologists Stanley Schachter and Jerome Singer (Fig. 12.3), while adopting an eclectic approach to both the earlier theories of emotion, introduced a new theory named cognitive theory of emotion.
2. This theory suggested that whenever people are emotionally aroused, they decide which emotion they are feeling by cognitively evaluating and appraising situational cues.
3. Network model of emotions is a recent view of the relationship between emotions and cognitions. This theory suggests that manifestations are linked in the brain to memories for the experience in which those emotions were aroused.

Cognitive Physiological Theory of Emotion

1. Schachter (1959) proposed that emotional states are a function of the interaction of cognitive factors and a state of physiological arousal.
2. Feedback to the brain from physiological activity gives rise to an undifferentiated state of affect. But the felt emotion is determined by the "labey" (cognition), the subject assigns to the aroused state. The assignment of a lable is a cognitive process.
3. To interpret his feelings, the subject uses information from past experiences and his perception of what is going on around him.
4. Experienced and inexperienced users of alcohol and other drugs label their bodily sensations differently interms of emotional tone. The initial users have to learn to label the physiological sensations as enjoyable. Hence, emotion is an internal physiological arousal in interaction with cognitive process.

Activation Theory

1. The term activation theory of emotion was actually coined in 1951 by Donald B Linasley. In general activation theory refers to the view that emotion represents a state of lightened arousal rather than a qualitative unique type of psychological, physiological or behavioral process.

2. Arousal is considered to lie on a wide continuum ranging from a very low level such as deep sleep, to such extremely agitated states as rage or extreme anger.
3. According to Lindsley (1951), emotion provoking stimuli activate the reticular activating system in the brainstem, which in turn sends impulses both upward toward the cortex and downward the musculature. For the occurrence of a significant emotional behavior, the reticular formation must be properly activated.

Somatic Theory of Emotions

1. Many psychologists held that consciousness was more directly associated with the muscles than with the brain. Jacobson trained his subjects to relax completely.
2. In this condition, their minds were blank. If the subject thought of moving his arm, electrical potentials showed up in his muscles. Similarly, tension in the region of the eyes accompanied visual images. These experiments clearly show that consciousness is intimately associated with muscular activity.

STRESS AND ADOPTATION

Introduction

Stress is a term that is difficult to define; it is used loosely and means different things to different people. Some use it to describe an upset feeling or response; others use it to describe the source or stimulus for their feeling upset. Study in the field of stress and adaptation has been pursued by researcher in different disciplines, according to their individual conceptual views.

Definition

1. Hans Selye (1976) defined, stress as the state manifested by a specific syndrome which consists of all the nonspecifically-induced changes within a biologic system.
2. George Engel (1960) defines, stress as referring to all processes, whether originating in the external environment or within the person, which impose a demand or requirement up on the organism, the resolution or handling of which necessitates work or activity of the mental apparatus before any other system is involved or activated.
3. Stress is a state produced by a change in the environment that is perceived as challenging, threatening or damaging to the individual's dynamic equilibrium. There is an actual or perceived imbalance in the individual's capability to meet the demands of the new situation.

Nature of Stress

1. Stress is mediated by two factors, the individual's ability to cope and the social support he receives.
2. The change or stimulus that evokes this state is the stressor. The nature of the stressor is variable.
3. Stress is any situation in which a nonspecific demand requires an individual to respond or take action. It involves physiological and psychological responses.
4. Stress can lead to negative or counterproductive feelings or threaten emotional well-being.

Sources of Stress

Physiologic Stressors

1. The primary physiologic stressors are chemical agent, infectious agent, physical agent, faulty immune mechanisms, genetic disorders, nutritional imbalance and hypoxia.
2. All the stressors have both a general effect and a specific effect.
   Stress cycle as shown in Figs 12.4A and B.

STRESSORS

Change stressors
Chemical stressors
Commuting stressors
Decision stressors

Disease stressors
Emotional stressors
Environmental stressors
Family stressors

Phobic stressors
Physical stressors
Social stressors
Work stressors

Distress

Stress overloading

Overstress (hyper)

Behavioral
For example: Excessive eating and drinking alcohol

Physiological
For example: Muscle tension ↑BP AR

Emotional
For example: Heightened anxiety depression, anger

Congnitive
↑Distractibility
↑Concentration

Immediate effects

Behavioral disorders
For example:
Obesity alcoholism

Medical disorders
For example:
Headache, hypertension, heart disease

Emotional disorders
Chronic anxiety and depression, phobias, personality changes and mental illness

Cognitive disorders
For example: Memory problems, obsessive, sleep disorders

Long-term effects

Decreased productivity

Decreased enjoyment

Decreased intimacy

A

Reticular formation

Pituitary gland

Norepinephrine (via bloodstream)

Epinephrine (via bloodstream)

Neural connections

Autonomic nervous system

(ACTH) (via blood-stream)

Neural connections

Adrenal cortex

Adrenal medulla

Steroids (to various sites via blood-stream)

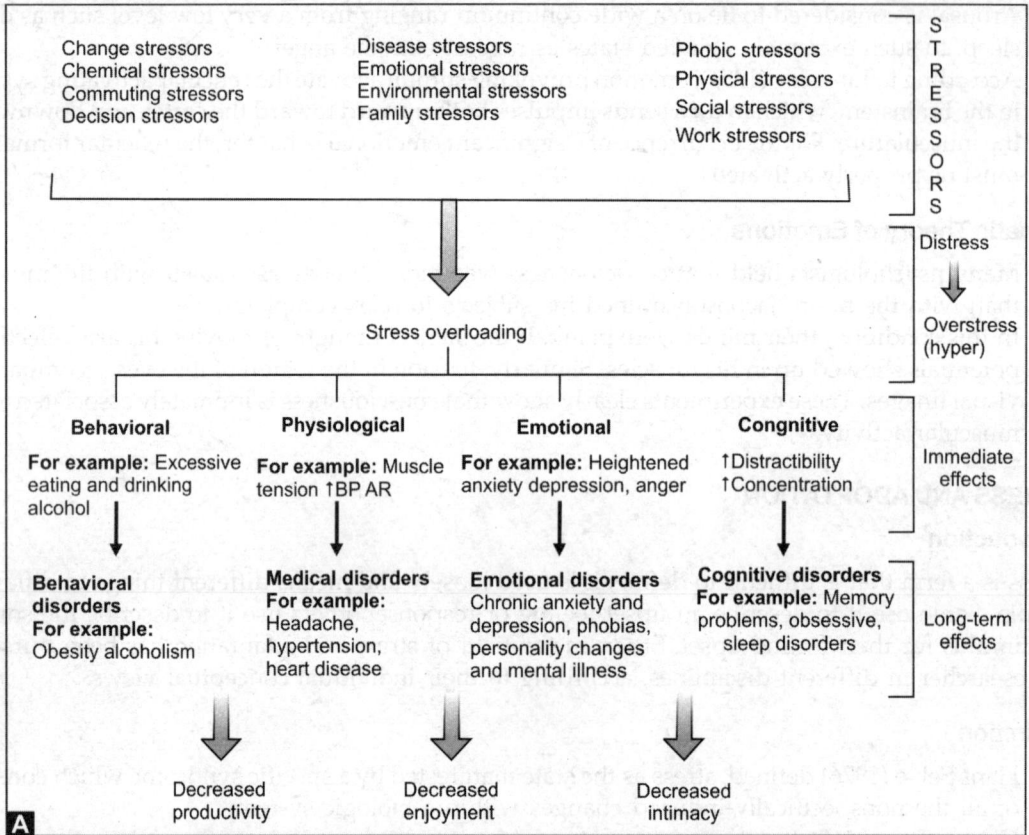

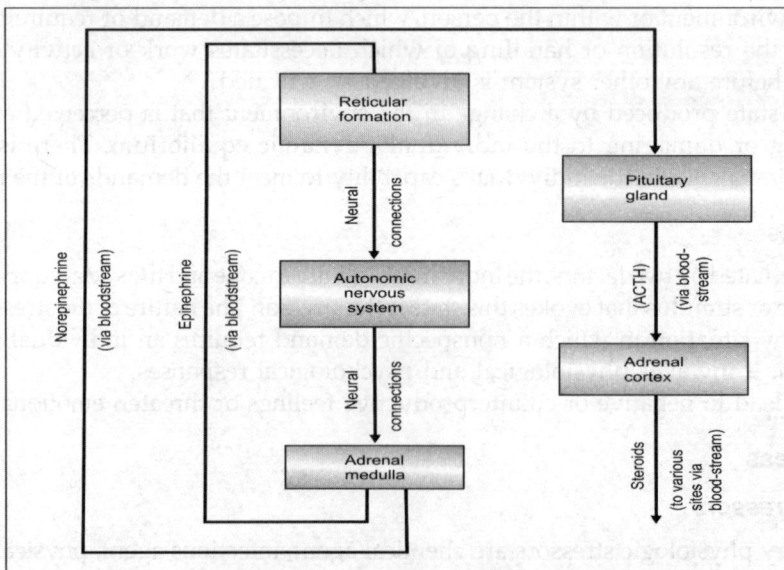

Figs 12.4A and B: Stress cycle

Psychosocial Stressors

1. Accidents and the survivors.
2. The experience of others in our social networks.
3. Horrors of history.
4. Intrapsychic, unconscious conflicts and anxieties.
5. The fear of aggression, mutilation and destruction.
6. The events of history brought into our living room.
7. The changes of the narrower world in which we live.
8. Phase-specific psychosocial crisis.
9. Other normative life crisis-role entries and exits, inadequate socialization, underload and overload.
10. The inherent conflicts in all social relations.
11. The gap between culturally included goals and socially structured means.

Factors Influencing Stressors

The nature of the stressor involves the following factors such as intensity, scope, duration, number and nature of other stressors. Each factor influences the response to a stressor. A person may perceive the intensity or magnitude of a stressor as minimal, moderate or severe. The greater the magnitude of stressor, the greater the stress response. The response to any stressor depends on physiological functioning, personality and behavioral characteristics.

Models of Stress

Response-based Model of Stress

1. The response-based model is concerned with specifying the particular response or pattern of responses that may indicate a stressor.
2. Selye's model or stress is a response-based model that defined stress as a nonspecific response of the body to any demand made on it.
3. Stress is demonstrated by a specific physiological reaction the general adaptation syndrome (GAS). Thus, the response of a person to stress is purely physiological and is never modified to allow cognitive influences.
4. The response-based model does not allow individual differences in response patterns. This lack of flexibility may produce some differences must be identified in the assessment phase.

Adaptation Model

1. The adaptation model proposes that four factors determine whether a situation is stressful. The ability to cope with stress, the first factor, usually depends on the person's experience with similar stressor, support systems and overall perception of the stressor.
2. The second factor deals with the practices and norms of the persons peer group. If the peer group considers it normal to talk about a particular stressor, the client may respond by complaining about it or discussing it.
3. The third factor is the impact of the social environment in assisting an individual to adapt to a stressor.
4. The last factor involves the resources that can be used to deal with the stressor.
5. The adaptation model is based on the understanding that people experience anxiety and increased stress when they are unprepared to cope with stressful situations.

6. Using this model and appropriate interventions, nurses can help clients and families to promote health in all human dimensions.

Stimulus-based Model

The stimulus-based focuses on disturbing disruptive characteristics within the environment. The classic research that identified stress as a stimulus has resulted in the development of the social readjustment scale, which measures the effects of major life events on illness.

Assumptions of the Stimulus-based Model

1. The life change events are normal, and they require the same type and duration of adjustments.
2. People are passive recipients of stress and their perceptions of the event are irrelevant.
3. All people have a common threshold of stimulus and illness results at any point after the threshold.
4. As with the response-based model, the stimulus-based model does not allow for individual differences in perception and response to stressors.

Transaction-based Model

1. The transaction-based model views the person and environment in a dynamic, reciprocal, interactive, relationship.
2. This model, developed by Lazarus and Folkman, views the stressor as an individual perceptual response rooted in psychological and cognitive process.
3. Stress originates from the relationship the person and the environment. This model focuses on stress-related process such as cognitive appraisal and coping.

RESPONSE TO STRESS

The classical research by Selye has identified the two physiological responses to stress; the local adaptation syndrome (LAS) and the general adaptation syndrome (GAS). The LAS is a response of a body tissue, organ or part to the stress of trauma, illness or other physiological change. The GAS is a defense response of the whole body to stress (Fig. 12.5).

Local Adaptation Syndrome

The body produces many localized responses to stress. These include blood clotting wound healing accommodation of the eye to light, and response to pressure.

Characteristics of LAS

1. The body produces many localized responses to stress. These include entire body systems.
2. The response is adaptive, meaning that a stressor is necessary to stimulate it.
3. The response is short-term. It does not persist indefinitely.
4. The response is restorative, meaning that the LAS assists in restoring homeostasis to the body region or part.

Reflex Pain Response

The reflex pain response is a localized response of the central nervous system to pain. It is an adaptive response and protects tissue from further damage.

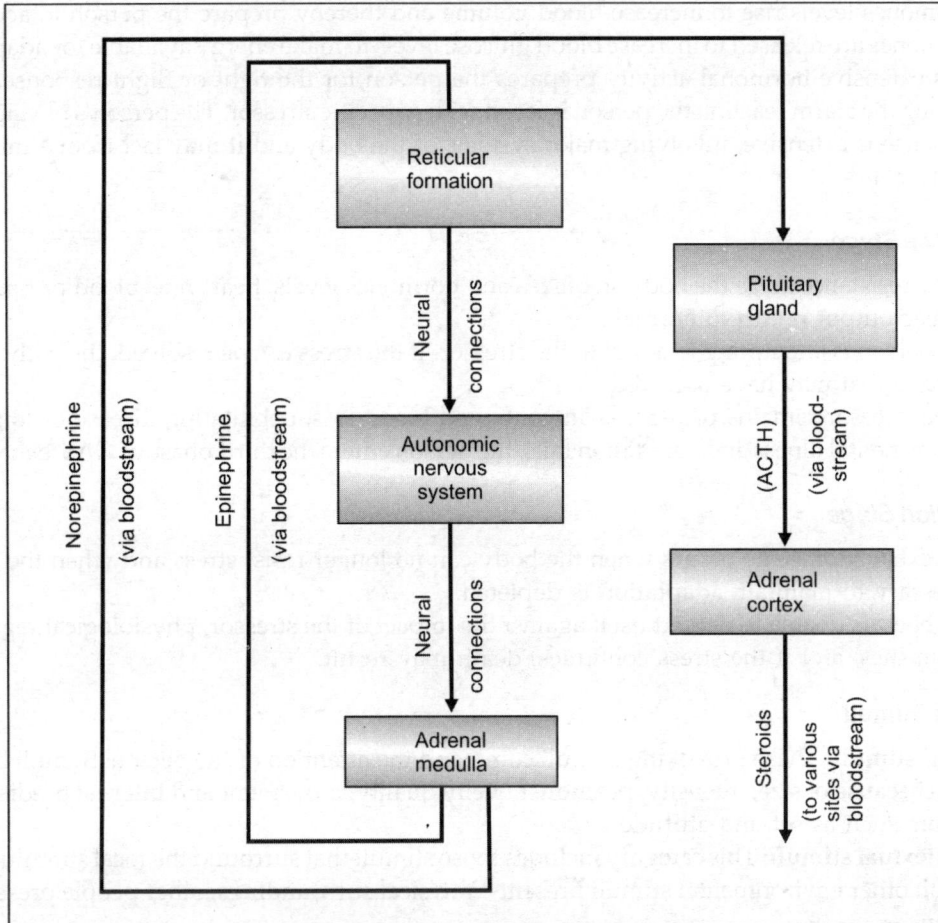

Fig. 12.5: Body's response to stress

Inflammation Response

1. The inflammatory response is stimulated by trauma or infection. This response localizes the inflammation, thus preventing its spread, and promoting healing.
2. The inflammatory response may produce localized pain, swelling, heat, redness and changes in functioning.

General Adaptation Syndrome

The general adaptive syndrome is a physiological response of the whole body to stress. It involves several body systems, primarily the autonomic nervous system and the endocrine system.

Alarm Reaction

1. The alarm reaction involves the mobilization of the defense mechanisms of the body and mind to cope with the stress.

2. Hormones levels rise to increase blood volume and thereby prepare the person to act. Other hormones are released to increase blood glucose levels to make energy available for adaptation.
3. This extensive hormonal activity prepares the person for the fight or flight response.
4. During the alarm reaction the person is faced with a specific stressor. The person's physiological response is extensive, involving major systems of the body and it may last from a minute to many hours.

Resistance Stage

1. In the resistance stage the body stabilizes and hormones levels, heart rate, blood pressure and cardiac output return to normal.
2. The person is attempting to adapt to the stressor. If the stress can be resolved, the body repairs damage that may have occurred.
3. If the stressor remains present, as in continued blood loss, debilitating disease or long-term severe mental illness and adaptation fails, the person enters the third phase of GAS, exhaustion.

Exhaustion Stage

1. The exhaustion stage occurs when the body can no longer resist stress and when the energy necessary to maintain adaptation is depleted.
2. The body is unable to defend itself against the impact of the stressor, physiological regulation diminishes, and if the stress continues, death may result.

Types of Stimuli

1. **Focal stimuli:** These provoking stimuli command the attention of the person. Stimuli become focal because of size, intensity, position, novelty quality, movement and internal predisposing factors such as set and attitude.
2. **Contextual stimuli:** This category includes those stimuli that surround the focal stimulus. They are all other environmental stimuli present—physical surroundings, other people present and so on.
3. **Residual stimuli:** These are recalled remnants of past experiences that influence the meanings attached to other stimuli. Included are attitudes, values, beliefs and other factors that influence an individual's behavior in a given situation.

STRESS ADAPTATION

Introduction

Adaptation is a constant, ongoing process that occurs along the time continuum, beginning with birth and ending with death. Also existing along this lifetime continuum is the dimensions of health and illnesses. Adaptation is a continuous process of seeking harmony in an environment. The desired end goals of adaptation for any system are growth and reproduction. A major nursing objective is to support and promote the efforts of the individual to achieve a healthy adaptation.

Concept of Adaptation

1. Adaptation is a term used to describe the work expended by the body in attempting to maintain homeostasis and toward off the effect of the stressor.

2. The current usage of the term includes the multiplicity of genetic, physiologic, psychic and social phenomena through which adjustment (homeostatic balance) is achieved in response to changes within the environment.
3. According to Helsen's concept of adaptation, constant and varied stimuli impinge on each individual at all times.
4. The basic premise of the adaptation level theory is that an individual's attitudes, values, ways of structuring experiences, judgments of physical, esthetic and symbolic objects, intellectual and emotional behavior, learning and interpersonal relations all represent modes of adaptation to environmental and organism forces.

Modes of Adaptation

In the Roy adaptation theory humans are conceptualized as having four modes of adaptation.

Basic Physiologic Needs

As human respond to environmental changes, they will need to keep balance in exercise, nutrition, elimination, fluid and electrolytes, oxygen, circulation and regulation (temperature, sense, endocrine system).

Self-concept

Self-concept includes all the ideas, feelings, beliefs and attitudes that persons have about them. To maintain psychological adaptation, defense mechanisms may be used to protect the ego when the self concept is threatened.

Role Mastery

In this mode of adaptation humans are viewed as regulating their performance of duties according to their varying positions in society.

Interdependence

Environmental changes may threaten conflict in a person's interactions with other persons.

ADAPTATION CONCEPT IN NURSING

In the conceptual framework of adaptation, nursing intervention becomes the means through which the nurse's knowledge and skill are interposed in supporting and promoting the patient's adaptive potential to the highest level of effectiveness.

Assessment

1. **First level:** Recognizing patient's level of wellness behavior in each adaptive mode.
2. **Second level:** Identifying positive and negative behaviors related to problem areas.

Planning

Selecting appropriate intervention from basic seven.
1. Reducing or limiting stress.
2. Preventing additional stress.

3. Supporting adaptations.
4. Limiting and supporting adaptation.
5. Altering, limiting and supporting adaptations.
6. Interrupting, altering, limiting and supporting adaptations.
7. Supplementing, interrupting, altering, limiting and supporting adaptations.

Intervention

Saxton and Hyland point out seven objectives to nursing intervention related to stress and adaptation.
1. Reduce or limit the extent and intensity of the present stress.
2. Prevent additional stress.
3. Support the individual's adaptations to assist in sustaining and maintaining the defensive responses.
4. Limit and support the individual's adaptations to confine and restrict the compensatory responses.
5. Interrupt, alter, limit and support the individual's adaptations to modify and adjust the symptoms or response.
6. Interrupt, alter, limit and support the individual's adaptations to discontinue or stop the responses that have become stresses.
7. Supplement, interrupt, alter, limit and support the individual's adaptations to complement or replace the responses that are failing to control stress.

Evaluation

Reassessing patient's level of wellness behavior in each adaptive mode to determine satisfactory resolution of problem area or need for reassessment and re-planning.

NURSING IMPLICATIONS ON STRESS REDUCTION
Introduction

Copying behavior should be remembered that the individual is in constant interaction with his environment, both internal and external. This implies that change is constant and that change is necessary for optimal psychosocial and physiological growth. The development of a nursing data base that supplies the essential information for making decisions about patient care is a necessity.

Strategies of Stress Reduction

1. **Modification of the situation:** Techniques to reach these goals may include changing jobs if the work place is the source of excessive stress. Through health appraisals, nurses may identify patient stressors. The stress control requires self-care and motivation and therefore the patient must actively and willingly participate in appraising, identifying and managing his sources of stress.
2. **Modification of the meaning of the problem:** It may require taking a longer range view of situation, or putting it into perspective. Compulsive behavior, deadlines and clock watching may need to be re-evaluated.
3. **Control or management of the symptoms of stress:** The individual needs to be able to anticipate the development of stress and to know how to typically react.

Stress Reduction Methods

1. **Self-regulation of stress:** Sutterley (1982) has described six categories of approaches to self regulation of stress. Proper nutrition, adequate rest and regular exercise improve one's well-

being and help develop resistance to stressors. Regular exercise assists in weight control, decrease a sense of fatigue and monotony and increase the exercise tolerance for patients with angina pector's and peripheral arterial disease.

2. **Biofeedback:** The purpose of biofeedback is to gain some degree of mental control over the autonomic nervous system and possibly decrease blood pressure, control heart rate and prevent migraine headaches, hyperactive stomach, etc. Some form of electronic instrumentation is used to monitor a biological function such as measuring skin conductance with the galvanic skin responder.

3. **Relaxation response:** Benson (1975) has described what he calls the "relaxation response", which is a calming state opposite to the arousal state or stress. Four elements are necessary to produce the relaxation response: A quite environment, a comfortable position, a passive attitude and a mental device or object, such as a word, sound of phrase of occupy the mind and keep out thoughts.

4. **Social supports:** The importance of social support as a mediating resource in stress has already been identified. To reinforce the information, the function of social networks includes the maintenance of positive social identity, the provision of emotional support, the provision of material aid and tangible services, access to information and access to new social contacts and new social roles.

ROLE OF NURSE IN EMOTIONAL CONTROL

A number of patients show emotional reactions like anxiety, worry, fear, irritability, anger and resentment. Such negative feelings need to be replaced by hope, courage, and cooperation. A nurse should listen sympathetically, develop cooperative relationship with the patient, and help him reduce his tensions.

Emotions are controlled as follows:

1. The causes, reactions and consequences of emotions are studied.
2. Emergency situations are avoided because they cause strong emotional reactions. Adequate planning is useful in preventing emergencies.
3. Mental conflicts and emotional tensions are avoided by adopting a sound philosophy of life.
4. Hobbies and sound social relationships are developed so as to direct one's attention away from emotion-provoking situations.
5. Unreasonable and uncontrolled external expression of emotions is avoided, since it increases the intensity of emotions further.
6. Sense of humour is developed. It helps overlook irritations and petty annoyances.

CONCLUSION

An emotion is a conscious, stirred up state of a person. It is a strong feeling. It may be pleasant or unpleasant. It is often accompanied by marked physiological changes. Unpleasant emotions can affect the health adversely. If they are persistent, they can cause an illness or aggravate an existing illness. They can cause conditions like peptic ulcer, epilepsy and ischemic heart disease. They can aggravate diabetes mellitus. If emotions are controlled well, about half of chronic illnesses can be totally prevented.

BIBLIOGRAPHY

1. A Manual of Nursing Education, IGNOU, New Delhi, 2001.
2. Anthikad Jacob. Psychology for Graduate Nurses. 4th edn, Jaypee Brothers Medical Publishers, New Delhi, 2007.
3. Bhatia and Craig. Elements of Psychology and Mental Hygiene for Nurses in India, Orient Longman Ltd, Chennai, 2000.
4. Bhatia BD, Craig Margaretta. Elements of Psychology and Mental Hygiene for Nurses in India. Orient Longman: Chennai, 2005.
5. Das G. Educational Psychology, Kind Books, New Delhi.
6. Denise F Pout, BP Hungler. Nursing Research Principles and Methods, JB. Lippincott Co., 1995.
7. Gdard FA. The Human Senses (2nd edn) John Willey, New York 1972.
8. Gross Richard, Kinnison Nancy. Psychology for Nurses and Allied Health Professionals, Hodder Arnold: London, 2007.
9. Kaplan and Sadock. Synopsis of Psychiatry, Lippincott Williams and Wilkins, 1998.
10. Morgan and King. Introduction to Psychology, Tata McGraw-Hill Publishing Co Ltd, New Delhi 1993.
11. Robert A Bason. Psychology, Prentice Hall of India Pvt Ltd, New Delhi, 2001.
12. Shaw ME. Group Dynamics, McGraw Hill, New York, 1976.
13. Townsend Mary. Psychiatric Nursing, WB Sounders Co, Philadelphia, 2005.
14. Wertheimer M. A Brief History of Psychology, Holt, Rinehart and Winston, New York, 1970.
15. Woodworth RS. Experimental Psychology, Holt, Rinchart and Winston, New York, 1954.

Attention

13

DEFINITIONS

1. **Attention:** Attention is the concentration of consciousness upon one object other than upon another.
2. **Involuntary attention:** It is a type of attention which is given without conscious effort. It is due to the striking qualities of the object of attention, e.g. loud noise. Bright light colorful picture, penetrating odor, etc.
3. **Voluntary attention:** It is given by conscious effort. It is usually against a person's natural inclination, e.g. listening to an uninteresting lecture.
4. **Habitual attention:** It is the attention given with interest because of habit or attitude. For example, attention given by a surgeon to an operation.
5. **Span of attention:** The maximum amount of material that can be attended in one period of attention is called span of attention.
6. **Distraction:** Distraction means any stimulus whose presence interferes with the process of attention or draws away attention from the object which we wish to attend.
7. **Division or divided attention:** Our capacity to attend can be divided among different stimuli so that some receive most of our attention while others less. For example, in any team game, players must divide their attention between many sources of information like the voices of the teammates, crowd, movements of other players, etc. by paying attention to all these aspects can the player pay the attention to one particular stimulus sounds difficult.

INTRODUCTION

We are constantly being exposed to an extensive environment. Stimuli impinging upon us at a given moment are beyond exhaustive enlistment. It is a practical impossibility for a man to take note of all these stimuli collectively. Hence, he selects single stimuli or a few stimuli for observation. This purposive selection of stimuli for observation is called attention. During attention there is a mobilization of various parts of the body muscles and sense organs towards the object of attention. That is why attention is often described as a process of adjustment of the entire body.

MEANING OF ATTENTION

1. Attention is the focusing of consciousness on a particular object or idea at a particular time, to the exclusion of all other objects or ideas.

2. Attention is a selective mental activity; it constantly shifts from one object to another or from one aspect of the situation to another. The process of attention involves motor adjustments on the part of the person who is attending.
3. Out attention is controlled and directed by the intensity of the stimulus as well as a variation in intensity.
4. Attention is the chief characteristic of the conscious mind and is essential to acquiring knowledge.
5. The specific portion which is selected for clear perception is called the focus of attention. Remaining part of the field is called the margin of attention.
6. Attention is not merely a cognitive function but is essentially determined by emotional and conational factors of interest attitude and striving.

DEFINITIONS OF ATTENTION

1. Attention is process of getting an object or thought clearly before the mind—*Ross*.
2. Attention is the concentration of consciousness upon one object rather than upon another—*Dumville*.
3. Attention is being keenly alive to some specific factor in our environment. It is a preparatory adjustment for response—*Morgan and Gilliland*.

IMPORTANCE OF ATTENTION

1. Attention helps in bringing mental alertness and preparedness.
2. Attention helps in our awareness or consciousness of our environment.
3. It makes us better equipped for distinguishing or discriminating the object of attention from others.
4. Attention acts as a reinforcement of sensory process and help in the better organization of the perceptual field for the maximum clarity and understanding of the object or phenomenon.
5. Attention helps in providing proper deep concentration by focusing one's consciousness up on one object at a time rather than two.

TYPES OF ATTENTION

Nonvolitional or Involuntary Attention

1. This type of attention is aroused without the play or will.
2. Nonvolitional attention can be aroused by our instincts as also by our sentiments.
3. Here we attend to an object or an idea without making any conscious efforts on our parts.
4. Example for involuntary attention are mother's attention towards her crying child, attention towards the members of the opposite sex, sudden loud noise, bright colors, etc.
5. Involuntary attention does not require any conscious effort on our part; we cannot ignore the stimulus because of its intensity.

Volitional or Voluntary Attention

1. Voluntary attention demands the conscious efforts on our part. A habit is a learned mode of behaving that is relatively fixed and reliably occurs in certain situations. Frequent repetition or physiological exposure that shows itself in regularity of response acquires a behavior pattern.
2. Volitional attention is further subdivided in to two categories—implicit volitional attention and explicit volitional attention.
   - Implicit volitional attention is single actor volition is sufficient to bring about attention.

- Explicit volitional attention is obtained by repeated acts of will. One as to struggle hard for keeping one self attentive. It requires strong will power, keen attention and strong motives for the accomplishment of the task.
3. Voluntary attention is not given whole-heartedly or spontaneously. It has been give to noninteresting objects, uninteresting tasks and difficult assignments, which have to be done at time when you would like to be doing something else.

Habitual Attention

1. Habitual attend tinting occurs by nature, inclined to take special note of certain things since we have natural interest them.
2. Our physiological make up is such that, we are dragged towards them. Thus, food, drinks, etc. are things in which we have natural interest.
3. **Factors determining attention:** Attention is a selective mental process by which we attend to a particular stimulus is determined by a number of factors. We select one and give up others. It means there is something in these stimuli that makes us attend to them.

FACTORS INFLUENCE ATTENTION

Objective Factors

1. **Intensity:** It is a fact of our everyday experience that a louder sound attracts our attention easily. Similarly, bright color is more effective than a lighter shade.
2. **Size:** Sometimes size also determines the selection of a stimulus. Bigger patch of color would certainly draw our attention more easily than a smaller patch of the same color even of brighter shade.
3. **Repetition:** Certain stimuli are seen to attract our attention only on the strength of their repetition. They may be neither intense nor large size. When we knock at the door, it is habitual to repeat the knocking. For example, we take very little notice of the continuous ticking of the clock in our roomer of the dripping of the tap in our bathroom.
4. **Change:** Although we pay very little attention to the ticking of the clock, we may all of a sudden become aware of it. If it stops, here the factor that operates is change. Many fissions attract attention because of the change involved them.
5. **Movement:** Any thing that moves has an attention value. Electronic signs are always made to move for attraction better attention. We often see infants attending not only to big and bright object but also to tiny insects that move.
6. **Novelty:** Attention is always aroused by some thing new. Some unfamiliar or strange object or a familiar one in some new setting catches attention.
7. **Systematic forms:** Among different things that arouse sensation, we may probably attend to those which have definite systematic pattern or rhythm. A soft melodious tune may be easily heard in the midst of loud noises.

Subjective Factors

1. **Interest:** A person who is interested in a particular field attend to object related to that field. For example, one who is interested in gardening is attracted by a new kind of plant or a girl who is interested in dresses will promptly observe a novel pattern of dress.
2. **Motive:** Our inner motive and desires also determine to a great extent what we things we attend to. A sleeping mother may not be disturbed by the loud noises of traffic outside, but she may

be easily aroused by even a faint cry of her baby. Appeal to certain important motives like self assertion, security or sex are also observed to arouse quick attention.

3. **Organic state:** A person's organic state to determine his attention. Thus, a hungry person is easily attracted by the flavor or sight of eatables.

4. **Moods and attitudes:** If one is in an angry mood, he is proving to notice even the minor mistake of others, but if he is in happy mood he usually overlooks them. Similarly, attitudes towards people and object also determine attention.

5. **Habits:** Habits are enduring types of behavior, which becomes apart of adperson. Habits are acquired over period of time in the course of the development of adperson. For example, a person who has developed the habit of reading sports forest in a paper would look for the sports column in the newspaper.

SPAN OF ATTENTION

1. One more interesting problem of attention is the span of attention, which is also called the span of apprehension. While defining attention, we have emphasized that in strict physiological sense only one object, idea or fact can be the center of consciousness at one particular movement and consequently we can attend to only one thing at time.

2. One of the oldest experiments in the physiological laboratory is concerned with determining how many separate items can thus be apprehended in a single glance. Sir William Hamilton who in the year 1859, first of all tried to perform experiments on the span of attention.

3. Experiments to study the span of visual attention are carried out with the help of an instrument known as tachistoscope. The apparatus tachistoscope that gives a quick exposure of cards containing number of dots or other figures only for a fraction of second. The maximum number of dots or figures that an individual can discarnate correctly gives his span of attention. There are individual differences, but usually four to five letters or numbers can be apprehended by an average individual.

4. The term span of attention may be defined in terms of the quality, size are extent to which the perceptual field of an individual can be effectively organized in order to enable him to attend to a number of things in a given spell of short duration.

SHIFTING OR INFLUCTUATION OF ATTENTION

1. It is a fact of our experiences that we cannot attend to a certain stimulus for a longer time. Our attention oscillates among the stimuli around. Sometimes the center of our consciousness keeps on fluctuating from one stimulus to another or on the different parts of a stimulus; this is known as fluctuation of attention.

2. Fluctuation of attention also involves rapid change in the intensity of the attention. The intensity increases or decreases ranging between the paying of attention and no attention or at least of less attention.

3. While paying attention towards an object, event or phenomenon, it is not possible for us to hold it continuously with the same intensity for a longer duration. In course of time in the center of our consciousness either shifts from one stimulus to another or from one part of the same stimulus to another part, this is called the shifting of our attention.

4. The phenomenon of fluctuation of attention was experimentally recorded the first time by a psychologist named Urbantschitisch (1875). While testing the auditory sensation he observed that the subject was not able to hear the tick continuously of an alarm clock kept at a distance.

THEORIES OF ATTENTION

1. **Broadbent's filter theory:** Broadbent (1958) explains that information from senses passes in parallel' to short-term store, a temporary 'buffer system' which holds information until it can be processed further and effectively extends the duration of a stimulus (Fig. 13.1). Then, the information passes through a selective filter, which operates on the basis of the information's physical characteristics, 'selecting one source' for further analysis and rejecting all others. The information allowed through the filter is analyzed in that it is recognized, possibly rehearsed and then transferred to the motor effectors (muscles), producing an appropriate response.

2. **Treisman's attenuation model:** According to Triesman (1960, 1964), competing information is analyzed for things other than its physical properties, including sounds, syllable patterns, grammatical structure and the information's meaning (Fig. 13.2). He suggested that the non-shadowed message is not filtered out early on, but that the selective filter attenuates it. So, a message that is not selected on the basis of its physical properties and would not be rejected completely, but its 'volume' would be 'turned down'. Both non-attenuated and attenuated information undergo further analyses and response is processed.

3. **Deutsch-Norman theory** of focused attention this theory completely rejected Broadbent's claim that information is filtered out early on. According to the Deutsch-Norman model, filtering or selection only occurs after all inputs have been analyzed at a high level, e.g. after each word has been recognized by the memory system and analyzed for meaning (Fig. 13.3). The filter is placed nearer the response end of the processing system. Hence, it is a late selection filter. Some information will have been established as pertinent (most relevant) and have activated particular memory representations. When one memory is selected for further processing, attention becomes selective.

DISTRACTION

Distraction means any stimulus whose presence interferes with the process of attention or draws away attention from the object which we wish to attend (HR Bhatia-1968)

These alterations in attention reduce the efficiency of work.

Sources of Distraction

The sources of distraction vary very much. They affect the individual according to his own mental set-up and personality characteristics. The conditions which cause distraction to an individual may prove helpful in sustaining attention to others.
• External factors! Environmental factors
• Internal factors

External factors: Noise, music, improper lighting, uncomfortable seats, unfavorable temperature, inadequate ventilation, defective methods of teaching, defective voice of the teacher, etc.

Internal factors: Emotional disturbances, ill-health, boredom, lack of motivation, fatigue, etc.

The nurse should take great care to get away all possible causes of distractions in working area so as to sustain attention.

Types of Distraction

Continuous Distraction

The distraction is continuous in nature. For example, the sound of radio played continuously, the noise at the market place, etc. Experiments have shown that adjustment to continuous distraction takes place quickly.

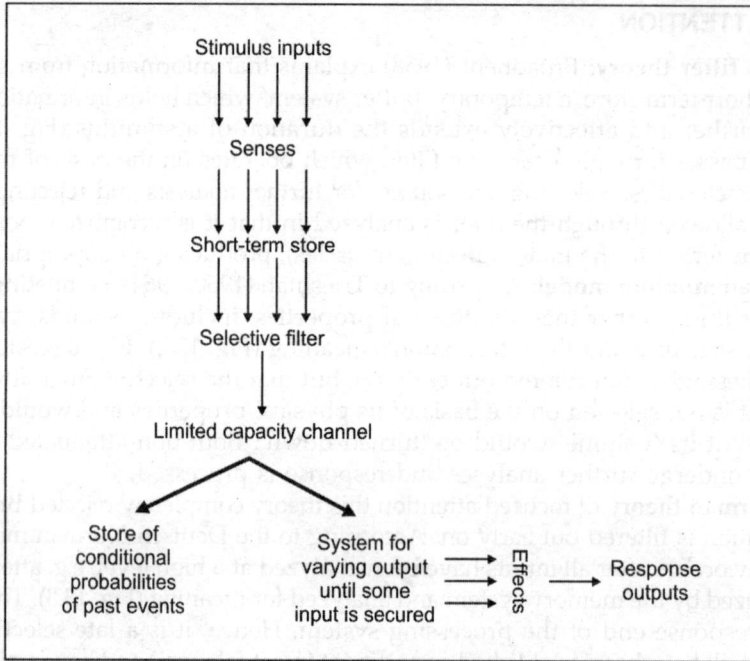

Fig. 13.1: Broadbent's theory of flow of information between stimulus and response

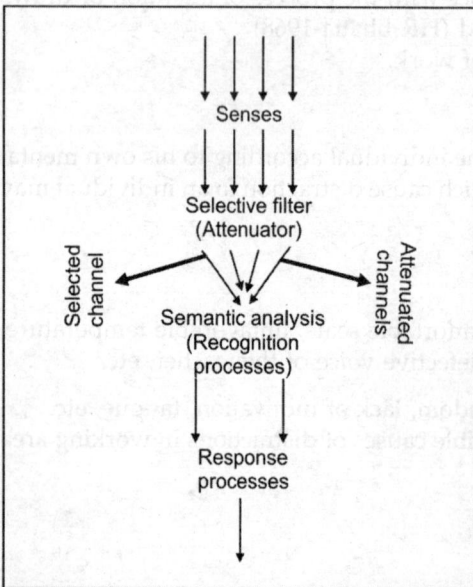

Fig. 13.2: Treisman's attenuation model

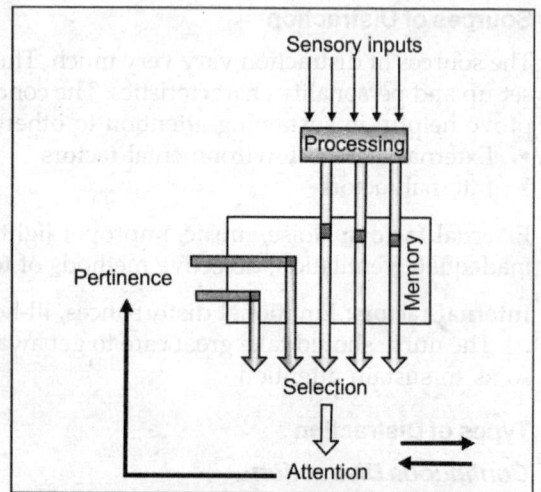

Fig. 13.3: The Deutsch-Norman theory

Discontinuous Distraction

It is irregular. For example, the hearing of somebody's voice every now and then. It interferes with work because of the impossibility of adjustment.

Some major means of removing distractions are:
- Being active in work
- Disregard for distraction
- Making the distraction a part of the work.

DIVISION OF ATTENTION

1. The attention is divided between two tasks, if more than two tasks are attended and performed simultaneously then the attention will have to be divided among those tasks.
2. Many researchers have tried to study the effect of the division of attention on the work product. It has been found that the work products suffer less if both the tasks are simpler but in the case of difficult and similar tasks, the division of attempts proves disadvantages.

Sustained Attention

1. Sustained attention occurs if one desires to be successful in the operation of a task, he has to begin with paying attention or concentrating his energies on the operation of that task. But is the beginning of a process and not the end.
2. After paying initial attention, care is to be taken to hold it for a long enough duration. The individual should be absolutely absorbed in handling the task, unmindful of anything else going on, without getting disturbed in the least.
3. One has to make serious and deliberate efforts for sustaining ones attention by taking care of all the factors responsible for maintaining attention and eliminating or reducing the forces of distraction.

Distraction of Attention

1. Distraction may be defined as any stimulus whose presence interference with the process of attention or draws away attention from the object which we wish to attend.
2. Distraction represents a sort of interference with our attention. The source of distraction may be external (e.g. noise, improper lighting, uncomfortable seats, etc.) and internal (e.g. lack of motivation, emotional disturbances, ill-health, boredom of fatigue, etc.).

ROLE OF NURSE IN ATTENTION

1. Attention helps in bringing mental alertness and preparedness. As a result the nurse becomes mentally alert and tries to exercise one's mental powers as effectively as possible for providing care.
2. Attention helps the nurse to concentrate by focusing consciousness on one object at a time rather than two.
3. Attention helps the nurse for better organization of the perceptual field for maximum clarity and understanding of the patient condition.
4. Attention provides strength and ability to continue the task of cognitive functioning despite the obstacles laid by the distractions.
5. The nurse can use psychology of attention for invoking not only voluntary but also involuntary attention to her job.

It is clear that knowledge of psychology of observation, sense, perception and attention is necessary for every successful nurse.

CONCLUSION

Thus, attention is essentially process and not a product. It helps in our awareness or consciousness of our environment, which is of selective kind, because in a given time, we can only concentrate or focus our consciousness on a particular object only. The concentration provided by the process of attention helps us in the clarity of the perception of the perceived object or phenomenon. Thus, attention is not merely a cognitive factor but is essentially determined by emotional and conventional factors of interest attitude and working memory. Thus, attention therefore is a process of carried out through cognitive abilities and helped by emotional and conational factors to select something out of the various stimuli present in one's environment and bring it in the centre of one's consciousness in order to perceive it clearly for deriving the desired end.

BIBLIOGRAPHY

1. Carison NR. Psychology of Behavior, Allyn and Bacon, Boston, 1977.
2. Goddard FA. The Human Senses (2nd edn), Wiley, New York, 1972.
3. Hochberg JE. Perception (2nd edn), Englewood Cliffs, Prentice Hall, NJ, 1978.
4. Lindsay IH, Nirman DA. Human Information Processing (2nd edn), Academic Press, New York, 1977.
5. Morgan CT. A Brief Introduction to Psychology, Tata McGraw-Hill, New Delhi, 1975.
6. Morgan T, King RA. Introduction to Psychology, 6th edn, Tata McGraw-Hill, New Delhi, 1982.
7. Mueller CG. Sensory Psychology, Englewood Cliffs, Prentice Hall, NJ, 1965.
8. Munn Norman L. Introduction to Psychology, Oxford and IBH, New Delhi, 1973.
9. Robinson DN. An Intellectual History of Psychology, Macmillan, New York, 1976.
10. Thompson RF. Introduction to Psychological Psychology, Harper and Row, New York, 1975.

Perception

14

DEFINITIONS

1. **Perception:** Perception is a process by which we discriminate among stimuli and interpret their meanings and appreciate their significance. For example, when we hear a sound we are able to identify it as being produced by a car or a bus. Perception gives meaning to sensation.

2. **Illusion:** Illusion is a misinterpretation of actual perception. When the interpretation of a particular stimulus goes wrong, it gives rise to a wrong perception or illusion. For example, a rope in the dark is perceived as a snake.

   Illusions are caused by inadequacies of our sense organs, distance of the object from the sense organ which perceives it, misleading stimuli in the environment, our perceived notions and expectancy.

3. **Hallucination:** Hallucination is identified as one of the major errors of perception. These are sensory perceptions in the absence of any corresponding external sensory stimuli. Hallucinations are imaginary perceptions in which one sees or hears something that is not seen or heard by others around him. An alcoholic may see "pink elephants", a paranoid schizophrenic may hear voices, experience foul odors in the absence of any sensory stimulation. Hallucinations are more common in mentally ill people.

4. **Perceptual constancy:** The tendency to perceive objects as unchanging, despite changes in lighting or distance.

5. **Perceptual illusions:** Instances in which perception and reality do not agree.

6. **Exteroceptive sensation (also termed superficial sensation):** Receptors in skin and mucous membranes tactile or touch sensation (thigmesthesia).

7. **Anesthesia:** Implies complete absence of responses to touch sensation. It is the loss or absence of sensitivity. It may be caused by defective sense organs or effect of drugs.

8. **Hyperesthesia:** Exaggeration of touch sensation, which is often unpleasant. Sick and mentally disturbed often show this in their behavior. When we are tired or exhausted we show hyperesthesia.

9. **Paresthesia:** Abnormal sensations perceived without specific stimulation. They may be tactile, thermal or painful; episodic or constant. Paresthesia is often the outcome of poor health or physiological imbalance.

10. **Extra-sensory perception:** Parapsychology is the search for paranormal phenomena, such its ESP and psychokinesis. Most scientists try to explain observable phenomena. Parapsychologists try to observe unexplainable phenomena. All the other sciences have led us away from

superstition and magical thinking while parapsychology has tried to find scientific basis for magical powers and spirits.

11. **Telepathy:** Literally, "distance feeling". The term is a shortened version of mental telepathy and refers to mind reading or mind-to-mind communication through ESP, a person's awareness of another's thoughts without there being any known communication through sensory channels. Commonly known as mind reading.

12. **Clairvoyance:** Clairvoyance is an alleged psychic ability to see things beyond the range of the power of vision. Clairvoyance is usually associated with precognition or retrocognition.

13. **Precognition:** Precognition is psychic knowledge of something in advance of its occurrence. In other words it is the knowledge a person may have of another persons future thoughts (precognitive telepathy) or of future events (precognitive clairvoyance).

14. **Retrocognition:** Retrocognition is a type of clairvoyance involving knowledge of something after its occurrence through psychic means.

INTRODUCTION

Perception is the selection organization and interpretation of sensory input. It involves giving meaning to sensations. Sensation refers to the immediate experiences that are generated by simple and isolated stimuli. Perception involves the organization and interpretation of these stimuli to give them meaning. For instance, in listening to a person who sings, we experience the qualities of loudness and pitch as sensations, while our ability to hear the sequence of sounds as a song is an act of perception. At the next level, if we understand and recognize the words of the song, our perception blends into 'cognition', a more complex interpretive process that involves memory and thought.

MEANING OF PERCEPTION

1. Perception is the selection, organization and interpretation of sensory input. It involves giving meaning to sensations. In other words, it is the activity of selecting, organizing and interpreting sensations with ones past experiences.

2. Perception is very essential to deal with the world around us as it influences our memory, thinking, reasoning emotions, etc. our behavior is very much a reflection of how we react to an interpret stimuli from the world around us. The process of perception helps in becoming aware of objects quality or relations by way of sense organs.

3. Perception is an intellectual and psychological process because a subjective process based on the different people, here they assume according to their environment and interpret accordingly to their own views.

4. Perception is the intellectual process though which a person selects the date from the environment, organize it and obtains meaning from it. Sensations are the first stage of receiving stimuli; it is the experience we get, when the receptors of the sense organs send impulses to specific areas of the brain. The activity of the organism is converting a sense impression into the awareness of some meaningful situation is called perception.

5. Perception is a highly individualized process that helps an organism, in organizing and interpreting one complex pattern of sensory stimulation for giving them, the necessary pattern meaning to initiate his behavioral responses.

6. It is a complex process, determined by both physiological and psychological characteristics of the organism.

DEFINITIONS OF PERCEPTION

1. Perception is a process by which individual organize and interpret their sensory impressions in order to give meaning to their environment.
2. Perception is the appearance of things that is the focus of attention rather than objective reality.
3. Perception is the experience of objects, events or relationships obtained by extracting information from and interpreting sensations.
4. Perception is the organizing process by which interprets our sensory input.
5. Perception defined as all the processes involved in creating meaningful patterns out a jumble of sensory impressions fall under the general category of perception.
6. Perception is an individual's awareness aspects of behavior, for, it are the way each person processes the raw data he or she receives from the environment, into meaningful patterns.
7. Perception is the intellectual process by which an individual screens, selects, organizes and interprets the stimuli in order to five meaning to their environment.

NATURE OF PERCEPTION

1. Perception is a process—perception is essentially a process rather than being a product or outcome of some psychological phenomenon.
2. Perception is the information extractor—out sensory receptors are bombarded continuously by various stimuli present in our environment. Perception performs this duty by extracting relevant information out of a jumble of sensory impressions and converting them into some meaningful pattern.
3. Perception is the first event in the chain which leads from the stimulus to action.
4. Perception is the act of interpreting a stimulus generated in the brain by one or more sense mechanism.
5. Perception is a mental process in which sensory cues and relevant past experiences organize together to give us meaningfulness to the perceived object.

FACTORS INFLUENCING PERCEPTION

1. **Sense organs:** Perception depends upon sense impressions, which is related to the sense organ concerned with the specific stimulus. To perceive different auditory, stimuli auditory, sense organ must be developed and should function properly.
2. **Brain function:** Brain function provides various frames of references in organizing the past experiences and sensory information, which helps in perception.
3. **Motive:** Our perception often depends upon our motives working at the given moment when we are hung, we perceive certain objects as eatables even though they are not eatables in reality.
4. **Familiarity:** Past experiences is required to associate the sensory information, which helps in apprehension.
5. **Set or readiness:** It has been observed that what we see is influenced by what we are set to see. When we are in good mood we do not perceive the mistakes of others very easily.
6. **Values:** When a person places a high premium on a stimulus he tends to perceive it differently. In an experiment children were asked to compare the size of a chip with the adjustable circle of a light. After a few brails the children were told that the chips could be exchanged for a candy. Thus, the children were taught to value the chips higher than before. They then were rewarded with candy for chips. Subsequently, when the children were asked to compare the size of the chip with the circle of the light most of them perceived the chips as longer than size of the circle.

7. **Expectations:** Anticipation influences one's perception. Sometimes one has a tendency to see what we expect to see. Thus, when subjects were shown a red light and asked to report the sign on a cardboard most of them reported as stop sign even though it was spelt as top.

8. **Cognitive style:** As a person matures each one of us develops a way of dealing with the situation/environment, which is known as cognitive style. Cognitive styles could be viewed differently. In one approach field dependent and field independent approach, in the former the person sees the environment as a whole and does not delineate it into its parts. But in the later the person perceives the elements of the environment with its parts.

9. **Personality:** A person's personality influences the way he perceives. In two studies healthy college were compared to depressed patients or students with eating disorder in terms of their ability to identify words related to food. Persons with depression were able to identify adjectives related to depressed traits.

10. **Culture:** The culture background of a person influences the perception of a person. The way in which a person uses the cues depend on one's culture.

Inaccurate Perceptions

Sometimes our perceptions are inaccurate . We cannot make correct interpretations. The following may be the reasons.

Difference between Sensation and Perception

Sl. No.		Sensation	Perception
1.	Organization	Not organized	Organized
2.	Organs involved	Sense organs	The brain
3.	Meaningfulness	Meaningless	Meaningful
4.	Organs stimulated	Sense organs	It is selection, organization and interpretation of the sensory inputs.
5.	Action	Rudimentary action	Perception is a much higher act

PRINCIPLES OF ORGANIZATION OF PERCEPTION (GESTALT PRINCIPLES)

1. **Figure and ground:** Here the person divides the visual displays into figure and ground. In visual perception the person keeps one as the figure while the other forms the background.

2. **Similarity:** Objects of the same color, size and shape are perceived as a pattern. Here the dark colored dots are perceived as number two rather than a random array of dots.

3. **Closure:** The tendency to perceive an incomplete object as a whole complete object is known as the principle of closure. In the illustration though the circle is not complete one tends to perceive it as a circle.

4. **Continuity:** Objects that continue as a pattern or direction tend to be grouped together. In the illustration one tends to perceive the dots as a straight line even though there is a break in the continuity.

5. **Simplicity:** The tendency to organize and perceive elements in the simplest way possible is known as the principle of simplicity. In the illustration one tends to see: (a) As made up of the elements shown in the simplest alternative, (b) Instead of the more complex alternatives shown in (c) and (d).

PERCEPTION AND CONSTANCIES

A tendency to experience a stable perception in spite of changing sensory input or changes in sensory information is known as perceptual constancy. This may apply to shape, size, brightness or color.

1. **Shape constancy:** The tendency to see an object as the same shape irrespective of the angle in which it is viewed is known as shape consistency. For example, familiar objects are seen as having the same shape though the retinal images may change for different angles.
2. **Size constancy:** The tendency to perceive objects of the same size regardless of the distance from which it is viewed. For example, a beautiful lady standing at 20 feet distance looks the same, as she would be at 10 feet distance even though there is change in the retinal image.
3. **Brightness constancy:** The perception of brightness as the same even though the amount of light reaching the retina changes is known as brightness constancy. For example, the brightness of white paper remains same in sunlight or candle light.
4. **Color constancy:** The tendency to perceive objects, as retaining their color despite changes in sensory information is known as brightness constancy. For example, the red colored Maruti car looks red under street light as well as in the dark garage.
5. **Depth perception:** The process by which one interprets visual cues to know how near or far away objects are is known as depth perception. There are two types of cues namely monocular and binocular that helps in depth perception. Monocular cues are the visual cues requiring the use one eye. Binocular cues are visual cues requiring both the eyes.
   a. We cannot perceive and observe correctly sometimes our sense organs may be functioning defectively. For example, we are suffering from myopia or deafness or any other sensory defect.
   b. Our receptors may not be stimulated adequately because the stimuli were not strong enough to stimulate them or the stimuli were rather vague and indefinite.
   c. We may not perceive correctly because, we do not know what to perceive. In order that a student nurse should perceive correctly in the word for proper nursing care, she needs to be guided by her instructor.
   d. Our span of apprehension and attention is limited. If we try to apprehend more things that we can at a time, we are liable to have inaccurate perceptions.
   e. Sometimes objects or figures are perceived with difficulty because they resemble their surroundings. The figure merges in the ground. For example, a white patch is difficult to detect on a white wall.
   f. We are liable to perceive things wrongly if we are not in good health, sick people's perceptions, at times are not correct for this reason. Our sense organs cannot function adequately and correctly as a result of illness.

Common Sensory Abnormalities and Perceptual Disorders

Anesthesia

1. It implies complete absence/ inability to respond to sensory (touch) sensation. It means a loss is absence of sensitivity.
2. Anesthesia may be caused by defective sense organs, effects or drugs or also by some emotional or functional factors.

3. For example, we some time do not notice a pen or a bunch keys lying before us and make a frantic search of it. We are either emotionally disturbed or preoccupied with some other thoughts.

Hyperthesia

1. It means excessive response to stimuli sick people often shows this in their behavior.
2. They react violently to noises or bright lights. When we are fatigued, we become hypersensitive to lights, to sounds or to the weight of clothing and to odors.

Sensory disturbances of perceptions

Pain sensation	
1. Analgesia	Absence of pain appreciation
2. Hypoalgesia	Decrease of pain appreciation
3. Hyperalgesia	Exaggeration of pain appreciation, which is often unpleasant.

Temperature sensation	
1. Thermanalgesia	Absence of temperature appreciation
2. Thermhypoesthesia	Decrease of temperature appreciation
3. Thermhyperesthesia	Exaggeration of temperature sensation Which is often unpleasant?

Sensory abnormalities	
1. Paraesthesia	Abnormal sensation perceived without specific stimulation.
2. Dysesthesia	They may be tactile, thermal or painful, episodic or constant. Painful sensation elicited by and painful cutaneous stimulus such as a light touch or gentle stroking over affected areas of the body.

Proprioceptive sensation	(deep sensation): (arthresthesia): absence of joint position
1. Joint position sense (arthresthesia)	Sense.
2. Vibratory sense (pallesthesia)	Abscense of vibratory sense
3. Kinesthesia	Perception of muscular motion.

Cortical sensory function	
1. Astereognosis	Inability to recognize and identify objects by feeling them.
2. Graph anesthesia	Symbols written on the skin.
3. Topagnosia	Inability to localize stimuli to parts of the body.
4. Sensory extinction	Inability to perceive a sensory stimulus when corresponding areas on the opposite side of the body are stimulated simultaneously.

ERRORS IN PERCEPTION

It has been observed that we get the experience of objective reality through our perception. But perceptions are at times descriptive. They do not always give us the correct experience of facts that exist. Some erroneous illusive experience is the result of such descriptive perceptions. False perceptions occur when perceptual stimulus fails to correspond with the real stimulus in the environment. Two frequently occurring errors in perceptions are discussed under two different phenomena, namely illusion and hallucinations.

ILLUSION

Actually, we always evaluate the world around us with our perceptual habits that help us respond quickly and effectively to our normal environment. Sometimes our perceptual process may distort the images we receive, rather than correcting them with superficial changes in appearance.

An illusion is a mistaken perception of an object. In such cases the stimulus is, no doubt, present giving rise to definite sensory impulses. But while interpreting the sensory impulses in the form of a meaningful experiences, fears or expectations.

Definitions

1. Illusion is one such perceptual distortion. Illusions may create bias in us to distort reality consequently we make faulty interpretation of the environment .
2. An illusion is a wrong or inaccurate or mistaken perception of an existing sensory stimulus.

Nature of Illusion

1. An illusion is a wrong perception , mistaking a rope for a snake, a tree for an animal and mistake it for something that is not really there.
2. Most of our illusions are visual and auditory but others are also possible. Illusions are caused by inadequacies of our sense organs which has to perceive it, misleading stimuli in the environment, our preconceived nations and expectancy.
3. These illusion are usually referred as any interpretation of sense in formations, psychologists usually distinguish illusions in to two groups.

Perceptual Illusion

1. Physical illusions occur because of the distortion of information. For example, when a portion of a sick is dipped in water there appears a bent to the sick. Many physical illusions are created by our natural tendency to view two dimensional scenes as projections of three dimensional realities.
2. Perceptual illusions occur because when the stimulus contains misleading cues that cause perceptions that are inaccurate or impossible.

Classification/Types of Illusions

1. **Moon illusions:** Moon appears large near the horizon that it does later at night, when it is directly overhead. One explanation says that moon illusion depends a visual constancy, i.e. when it is close to the horizon we have cues of distance and while it is overhead we do not get any cues to distance.
2. **Railroad or ponzo illusion:** In simple forms ponzo illusion consists of two gradually converging lines that give the impression of increasing depth in between, two crosswise parallel lines.
3. **Horizontal vertical illusions:** Though both the horizontal and vertical lines are equal in length, the vertical line is perceived as longer than the horizontal.
4. **Poggendorff's illusion:** A straight line appears to become slightly displaced as it passes through two parallel rectangles.
5. **Zollner illusion:** When two parallel lines are interested by numerous short diagonal lines slanting in opposite direction, when the parallel lines are perceived as diverging. All these illusions originate from our perceptual processes, creating an internal representation based on inaccurate and misleading information caused by visual illusions.

6. **Ponzo illusions:** The geometrical illusions that a horizontal in appearing within the smaller end of a pair of divergent vertical lines is lender that an equal length line located at a point at which the vertical lines are farther apart.

7. **Müller-Uger illusion:** It is a geometrical illusion where one line is longer than another equal length when the former has obtuse angles at both ends while the later has acute angles at both ends.

HALLUCINATION

Hallucination is a false perception that is idiosyncratic, not shared by others in the same situation. It is generally seen in some mental disorder like schizophrenia, alcoholic intoxication or drug abuse. Some people claim that their perceptions are quite vivid and life like and they think them real. They may even become confused with reality. They are extreme forms of inaccurate observation. Such observations are usually associated with serve psychological disorders, but they occasionally occur among even nonmentally ill individuals as well.

Definitions

1. Hallucinations are vivid sensory experiences that occur in the absence of external stimulus.
2. Hallucination is the imaginary perceptions, it is a gross error of perception seeing objects that do not exist. They are an extreme form of inaccurate observation in which one sees or hear something that is not seen or heard by others around him.

Nature of Hallucinations

1. Hallucinations appear most frequency in the life of mentally disordered persons. The person hearing sounds that all false, seeing objects moving in a room are called hallucinations.
2. Hallucinations are deceptive perceptions are at times caused purely because of our subjective makeup. The perception has no basis of a real sensory stimulus.
3. Hallucinations are found to be most common with auditory and visual perceptive. Hallucination is also caused due to certain organic condition such as damage of cerebral cortex or sense organs, certain drugs and alcohol can also produce hallucination.
4. Hallucinations are directly related to sensation; they can be classified into visual hallucination, auditory hallucination, taste hallucination, smell hallucination and cutaneous hallucination.

DIFFERENCE BETWEEN ILLUSION AND HALLUCINATION

Though illusions and hallucinations are common experiences the I cadence of hallucination is more serve. It is a serious from of mental illness. Illusion and hallucination shows us that our perception depends to a large extend on subjective factors like set, attitudes and inner needs.

	Illusion		Hallucination
1.	In illusion there will always be one or more stimuli	1.	In hallucination, external stimulus are completely absent
2.	Objective	2.	Subjective
3.	Stimulus is present	3.	Stimulus is not present
4.	Normal or universal	4.	Abnormal
5.	Mistaken perception	5.	False perception

Hallucinations usually occur when individuals lose the capacity to differentiate between inner sensation and the outer environment. Both hallucination and illusion have in pact on behavior and distort our knowledge leading to many personal, social and psychological problems.

EXTRA SENSORY PERCEPTION

If there are so many influences upon perception other than those coming from the presented stimuli, are there perhaps perceptions that require no sense organ stimulation what so ever? The answer to this question is the source of a major controversy within contemporary psychology over the status of extrasensory perception (ESP). Parapsychology is the search for paranormal phenomena, such as ESP and psychokinesis.

Parapsychologists by to observe unexplainable phenomena. All other sciences have led us away from superstition and magical thinking while parapsychology has tried to find a scientific basis for magical power and spirits.

Terminology Used in ESP

1. **Psi (Pronounced sign):** It is a term commonly used by parapsychologist to refer to both ESP and kinesis taken together. The term was coined by BP weisner and recommended by RH Thousless.
2. **Telepathy:** It is the perception of objects or events not influencing the senses.
3. **Clairvoyance:** It is the perception of objects or events not influencing the senses.
4. **Precognition:** It is the perception of a future event. Precognition is psychic knowledge of something in advance of its occurrence. In other words it is the knowledge a person may have of another persons future thoughts.
5. **Retrocognition:** Retrocognition is a type of clairvoyance involving knowledge of something after its occurrence through psychic menaces.
6. **Psychokinesis (PK)** whereby a mental operation affects a material body or an energy system. For example, wishing for a number affects what number comes up in the throw of dice.

Definition

Extrasensory perception is perception occurring independently of sight, hearing or other sensory processes. EPS also refers to telepathy, clairvoyance and precognition. It influencing of physical events by mental operations are the source of controversy in contemporary psychology.

Characteristics of ESP

1. It is a most unstable ability, disappearing suddenly or gradually, often without recognized causes.
2. The extra sensory perception process is diametric in its function, encompassing more than a single object in its scope.
3. The extra sensory perception process is entirely unconscious, i.e. it is not thus far found reliability available to introspection in any way or degree. The extra sensory perception is variable and undependable effect upon performance in the tests.
4. The extra sensory perception does not seem to subject to development through use as other specific capacities.

Nature of ESP

1. The experiments go at work in accordance with the usual Niles of science and generally, Disavow the connection between this work and spiritualism, super naturalism, mediumistic phenomena and other occult effects.
2. Many psychologists who are not convinced would find it congenital to accept evidence that they found satisfactory.
3. The case for ESP is based largely on experiments in card-guessing, in which, under various conditions, the subject attempts to guess the symbols on cards randomly arranged in packs.

PERCEPTION AND NURSE

In caring the sick, nurse needs to remember the words of Plato, the treatments of a part should not be attempted without treatment of the entity. It emphasizes that wholeness of something is more than the sum of its parts because a part is meaningful only in the context of the whole.

1. Our perception of the world outside is greatly affected by current state of mind. For example, we may feel particularly anxious when we tend to perceive our own different disturbed state of mind. A nurse needs to understand the role of sensation and attention in acquiring knowledge of environment, which depends to larger extent on the sensation received by the sense organs.
2. Perception is essential to deal with the world around us as it influences our memory, thing, reasoning and emotions, etc. a nurse should understand and any to interpret the whole environment and apply different types of perceptual skills to understand his patients. In caring the sick, nurse needs to remember the words if Plato, the treatment of a part should not be attempted without treatment of the entity. It emphasizes that wholeness of something is more than the sum of its parts because a part is meaningful only in the context of the whole.
3. The perception of the nurse and that of the patient may be different in the hospital environment. The nurse is familiar with the hospital environment and also well accustomed. The nurse being a healthy and energetic person is working with a positive outlook and enthusiasm to help the patient.
4. The hospital may seem an alien and frightening environment to the patient. Because the new and unfamiliar hospital environment creates a lot of anxieties in the patient. It may influence the thought, behaviors and perceptual set of the patient. Emotional maturity is also another important factor influencing a person's perception of sensory data.
5. A nurse should share the worries, fears and emotions of the sick and help them to solve then. As a nursing student, she must lean to assess all factors with accuracy and efficiency.

CONCLUSION

Perception depends upon sense impressions, which is related to the sense organ concerned with the specific stimulus. To perceive different auditory stimuli auditory sense organ must be developed and should function properly. If any of our sense organ is injured or damaged the concerned stimulus from the environment cannot be perceived. Perception is very essential to deal with the world around us as it influences our memory, thinking, reasoning and emotions, etc. Our behavior is very much a reflection of how we react to and interpret stimuli from the world around us. The process of perception helps in becoming aware of objects qualities or relations by way of sense organs.

BIBLIOGRAPHY

1. Arnold MB (Ed). The Nature of Emotion, Baltimore, Penguin, 1968.
2. Baddeley AP. The Psychology of Memory, Basic Books, New York, 1976.
3. Bandura A. Principles of Behaviour Modifications, Holt, Rinehart and Winston, New York, 1969.
4. Carlson NR. Psychology of Behaviour, Aflyn and Bacon, Boston, 1977.
5. Furguson ED. Motivation An Experimental Approach. Holt, Rinehart and Winston, New York, 1976.
6. Goddard FA. The Human Senses (2nd edn), Wiley, New York, 1972.
7. Hilgard ER, Bower GH. Theories of Learning (4th edn), Englewood Cliff, Prentice Hall, NJ, 1974.
8. Hochberg JE. Perception (2nd edn), Englewood Cliffs, Prentice Hall, NJ, 1978.
9. Hulse SH, Deese J, Egekk H. The Psychology of Learning (4th edn), McGrawHill, New York, 1975.
10. Johnson DM. Systematic Inventory Psychology of Thinking, Harper and Row, New York, 1972.
11. Korman AK. The Psychology of Motivation, Englewood Cliffs, Prentice Hall, NJ, 1974.
12. Lindsay PH, Nirman DA. Human Information Processing (2nd edn), Academic Press, New York, 1977.
13. Morgan CT, King RA. Introduction to Psychology, 6th edn, Tata McGraw-Hill, New Delhi, 1982.
14. Morgan CT. A Brief Introduction to Psychology, Tata McGraw-Hill, New Delhi, 1975.
15. Mueller CG. Sensory Psychology, Englewood Cliffs, Prentice Hall, NJ, 1965.
16. Munn Norman L. Introduction to Psychology, Oxford and IBH, New Delhi, 1973.
17. Robinson DN. An Intellectual History of Psychology, Macmillan, New York, 1976.
18. Strongman KT. The Psychology of Emotion, Wiley, New York, 1973.
19. Thompson RF. Introduction to Psychological Psychology, Harper and Row, New York, 1975.
20. Vinacke WE. The Psychology of thinking (2nd edn), McGraw Hill, New York, 1974.

15 *Memory*

DEFINITIONS

1. **Memory:** The power that we have to 'store' our experiences, and to bring them into the field of consciousness sometime after experiences have occurred, is termed memory.
2. **Registration:** Registration is the short-term storage of the sensory input. Most of the information briefly held in the sensory register is lost. However, we pay special attention to some of the information in the sensory register. When we do this the attended information is passed onto the short-term store. The sensory register holds information for such a brief time that some psychologists prefer to discuss it as related to perception rather than memory.
3. **Retention:** Retention refers to a permanence of what was learnt. When the active process of learning ceases, a comparatively passive process of retaining takes place. The material is retained when we are not thinking about it. People differ in their retentive capacity which is largely due to genetic constitution.
4. **Short-term memory (STM):** STM holds a relatively small amount of information, about seven items, for a short period of (15-30 seconds) time though not nearly as short-lived as the immediate memory.
5. **Long-term memory (LTM):** LTM has the unlimited capacity to store information for days, months, years and even a lifetime. LTM codes information according to meaning, pattern and other characteristics. With the help of LTM we can store, retain and remember most of the things in our life, at record notice, and thus make things quite easy.
6. **Iconic memory:** A form of sensory memory that holds visual information for almost quarter of a second or more. It makes visual world appear smooth and continuous despite frequent blinks and an eye movements.
7. **Echoic memory:** A momentary sensory memory of auditory stimulus, if attention is elsewhere, sounds and words can still be recalled within 3-4 seconds. It would playback auditory information and gives you time to recognize sounds as words.
8. **Semantic memory:** It is the accumulation of facts and experience gained over a lifetime. Semantic memory is used for remembering everyday types of facts and information. It is also called knowledge. Unlike other forms of memory, you usually do not remember where or when you learned the information in semantic memory.
9. **Episodic memory:** It concerns information specific to a particular context, such as a time and place. It is used for more personal memories such as sensations, emotions and personal associations of a particular place.

10. **Visual memory:** It is part of memory preserving some characteristics of our senses pertaining to visual experience. We are able to place in memory information that resembles objects, places, animals or people in sort of a mental image.

INTRODUCTION

The problem of retention is an important problem for a student of learning. He is curious to know as to how much amount of learning is retained by him. He also wants to know why he forgets, at times, certain common things. Remembering and forgetting are the opposite sides of the same coin. What can be directly measured is only the amount that is retained. But this it has a reference to the amount that is forgotten. Our concept of memory is somehow associated with verbal memory. No doubt, we have to memorize a majority of verbal facts; but in actual life-situation, all forms of memory need not involve verbalization. Thus, we remember someone's look, we remember places and we remember the taste of a particular food which requires no verbalization, moreover, our concept of memory indicates that it is single function. Memory denotes the ability or a power of mind to retain and reproduce learning. This ability helps in the process of memorizing. Memory consists of remembering what has previously learned. Thus, the process begins with learning and ends with its retrieval and reproduction.

MEANING OF MEMORY

Memory is a general word which includes several mental activities, like recall, recognition. We see indications of memory all around as, a person or animal experiences ease in relearning any activity which he had learnt previously but had forgotten. This proves very obviously that the previous learning had not been wiped out completely but had left an impression on the mind or a change in the nerves which facilitated relearning. People do not completely forget the story of any motive they have seen but recount it with ease when they are requested to do so by a friend.

Memory can be called the structural mental process, in which the person bring the learned material to his conscious mind and then tries to recall it. To remember or memorize, it is essential to first learned the subject and then retain it. The meaning of memory in Latin and Greek words to be mindful or to remember. Effective memory is not a function of how much time is spend on the material to be remembered, but is directly influenced by the kind of strategy and method of organization imposed on the material to be remembered.

DEFINITIONS OF MEMORY

1. Memory means showing the signs of earlier learned activities in present activities—*Hillguard and Atkinson.*
2. Memory is the capacity of a person to represent the information in response to the collection of previously learned activities and specific stimuli—*HJ Isenk.*
3. Memory defined as the power that we have to store our experiences, and bring them into the field of unconscious sometimes after the experiences have occurred—*Ryburn.*
4. Memory is the ideal revival so far as ideal revival is merely reproductive….. This productive aspect of ideal revival requires the object of past experiences to be reinstated as far as possibility in the order and manner if their original occurrence—*Stout.*
5. Memory consists in remembering what has previously been learned—*Woodworth and Marquis.*

QUALITIES OF GOOD MEMORY

1. Good retention power of the person.
2. Representing the facts quickly.
3. Quick and clear recognition.
4. Learning the subject matter quickly and immediately.
5. Using the facts and thoughts at the suitable time.
6. Using the facts and thoughts at the suitable time.

COMPONENTS OF MEMORY

Memory operates through four important components which are registration, retention, recall and recognition.

1. **Registration:** It is the short-term storage of the sensory input. Most of the information briefly held in the sensory register is lost. However, we pay special attention to some of the information in the sensory register. When we do this the attended information is passed on to the short-term store. The sensory register holds information for such a brief time that some psychologist prepares to discuss it as related to perception rather than memory.
2. **Retention:** It refers a performance of what was learnt. When the active process of learning ceases, a comparatively passive process of retaining takes place. The material is retained when we are not thinking about it. People differ in their retentive capacity which is largely due to genetic constitution.
3. **Recall:** It is the third aspect of memory. Things are learned in order to recall them whatever need arises. Recall is affected by a number of conditions as interference, set; attitude, etc. failure to recall does not necessarily indicate the absence of retention. Without retention there cannot be recall. But there are can be retained without recall.
4. **Recognition:** It is closely related to recall. It is the act of affirming that a particular object or situation has been seen or experienced before. During the process of recalling our co-native effort is more obvious and hence we may think that recall is an active process whereas recognition is a passive state. But in fact recognition also is an active phenomenon.

FACTORS OF MEMORY

We feel that a certain person has good memory whereas some other person has a bad memory. Experiments in memory show that although there is a general factor of memory, the actual functioning of memorizing is seen through specific operation that differ from person-to-person. People may differ in their visual memory, auditory memory or olfactory memory. The following factors are influencing on memory (Fig. 13.1).

1. **Learning:** It will be quite in keeping with the context to give a brief description of each of these activities. As has been mentioned above, the first step or activity is learning. If the learning is good, memory will also be good. Thus, the methods which assist learning do the same for

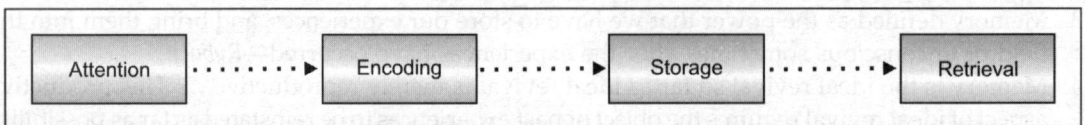

| Attention | ·······▶ | Encoding | ·······▶ | Storage | ·······▶ | Retrieval |

Fig. 13.1: Memory process

memory. Learning creates memory traces on the mind on the basis of which recollection is effected.

2. **Retention:** Retention means making permanent the remains of experience. The remains of experiences are left on the mind in the form of memory traces where they are safe though they are acted upon the interest and other mental states. The proofs of retention are recollection, recognition and relearning.

3. **Observation:** Correct observation gives us correct and accurate information. Observation keeps us alert and informed of latest events happening which helps in remembering.

4. **Attention:** Attention here denotes concentrating our mind on the purpose, which helps in collecting information. Therefore, if we pay attention it will help in retaining.

5. **Sense-perception:** It is the process by means of which we become aware of our environment. Sense perception is necessary for accurate observation of object, event, thing, person, etc.

Favorable Conditions in Retention

1. **Duration:** A sensation which continues for a longer time can be retained for a longer time in mind. A sensation of a shorter duration will be, correspondingly, retained for a shorter duration.

2. **Amount of material:** The subject being pursued is long it will be retained for a longer time while a shorter subject will take less time before it is forgotten. The amount of material to be learnt has favorable effect on its retention.

3. **Nature of material:** Intensity, distinctness, meaning help in its retention to a large extent.

4. **Amount of learning:** The extent of retention is directly proportional to the amount of learning, that is to say that retention will be more if the amount of learning is large. A subject studied more stays longer in the mind while studied less will remain in the mind for a shorter period. Over learning has a favorable effect on the retention.

5. **Methods of learning:** Learning by the whole method instead of the part method, the spaced method and the active method instead of the passive method result in better and longer retention.

6. **Speed of learning:** The faster the learning, the better the retention. This is the principle in accordance with which people learning faster seem to retain the subject learned for longer periods as compared to the slow learners.

7. **Feeling:** Freud and other psychologist assert that we retain pleasant experiences for a longer time whereas we forget painful experiences quickly.

8. **Attention:** While studying a subject if greater attention is paid to the subject the retention will be better. On the contrary, the retention will be weakened by inattention.

9. **Sleep:** Sometimes elapses after study, before the subject is retained in the mind and if this time of strengthening and retention is used for sleep, the memory traces get a good opportunity to be etched upon the memory.

10. **Mental review:** If some experiences is incessantly contemplated upon its retention it is better than one about which the mind does not trouble itself. Really speaking by mental review a repetition of the subject is caused which strengthen retention.

11. **Mental set:** A person retains those things for a longer period which coincide with his mental inclinations. A religious person remembers ideas relating to religion for long-time and a sensuous man remembers things of sexual interest.

12. **Apperception:** Apperception means the assimilating of learned subjects with the knowledge already present. The retention of a newly learned subject is greatly facilitated if it is assimilated with the present store of knowledge to start with. And on the other time is needed for retention if this assimilation is not effected.

13. **Intention:** If the subject is learned with the express intention of being retained, the aim will be fulfilled with extraordinary success. But if there is not such retention, the subject removes itself from the memory of the person after sometimes. Learning gathered with a view to appearing in the examinations is remembered better and things picked up here and there, in the ordinary course, are easily forgotten unless the person has a special inclination towards them.

14. **Massive experience:** The retention will be more if the experience is massive. If a person has ever loved, he never forgets it because it affects his whole personality and it is a fact that we remember that thing longer which affects us more.

Favorable Conditions in Recall

1. **Suitable mental and physical conditions:** Recall is comparatively easy when both the mind and the body are healthy and fresh. And, adverse and indifferent physical and mental conditions hinder recollection.

2. **Perfection of clues:** Recall is done with the help of clues which are stimulators of recall. To take an example if we learn a poem, we cannot recall it without the help of the title, the first line or the clue to some part of it and clue are necessary for the recall of anything in mind.

3. **Mental set:** The mental set of the individual, too, affect recall. A religious minded person remembers religious subjects easily while sensuous person will find it easy to remember things associated with sex.

4. **Motives:** When a person is under the extreme influence of a motive, he has such clear recollection of related incidents that he sometimes has hallucination.

5. **Feelings:** Recollection is not immune to feelings of pleasure and pain. These feelings and experiences of pain and pleasure are recollected easily than indifferent feelings while pleasurable experiences are comparatively easily recollected.

6. **Effort:** This has a very significant effect on recollection. Unless the extreme limit of effect has been passed, recollection generally increases with the effort.

7. **Absence of inhibition:** Recollection is better in the absence of any inhibition, because inhibition obstructs recollection and it may be caused by the conflict of the simultaneous arising of two activities or by repression and again, by fear or other emotions.

Favorable Conditions in Recognition

1. **Mental set:** Recognition is helped by the mental set, in the manner in which other factors assists memory. Recognition is correct when the mental set is favorable and it is incorrect when the mental set is unfavorable.

2. **Confidence:** This, too, is an indispensable element in recognition. In its absence even correct recognition becomes infested with doubt and mistake is the outcome.

TYPES OF MEMORY

Short term memory is the immediate memory which refers to storage of learning for a few seconds. Long-term memory differs from it in that the information is stored for a long duration. The limited storage capacity of short-term memory is seen from the fact that our memory span for a single repetition is not more than seven items long. Whenever it appears that one has a longer span it is because of recording the material in convenient chunks. Most of us learn to break the material and organize it in groups. Thus, even though the material retained is longer the units retained are fewer. The six or seven digit telephone numbers have a reference to span of immediate memory (Figs 13.2 and 13.3). The main differences between short-term and long-term memory are as follows:

1. **Immediate memory:** Immediate memory or sensory memory is that memory which helps an individual to recall something a split second after having perceived it. Immediate memory is needed when we want to remember a thing for a shorter time and then forget it. We enter the cinema hall; see the seat number given on our ticket. After occupying the seat, we forget the seat number. We look up a telephone number from the directory and remember it. But after making the call, we usually forget it. In such type of memory retentive time is extremely brief, generally from a fraction of a second to several seconds.

2. **Short-term memory:** Short-term memory can hold items fairly well for the first few seconds. After 12 seconds however, recall is poor and after 20 seconds the information has disappeared entirely unless we have kept repeating the material to ourselves. A phone number that we look up and dial is often forgotten by the time the call is answered. Short-term memory can also call as working memory.

3. **Long-term memory:** Long-term memory is relatively permanent in which information is stored for us at a longer time. Material enters a storehouse of almost unlimited capacity. Long-term memory seems to be much more complex, for it stores many different aspects of ones experiences. Remembering our identifying data like our name, father's name, date of birth, date of marriage, etc. is the simplest example of our long-term memory.

4. **Permanent memory:** Under permanent memory it is possible to remember a thing permanently. Remembering of our name is the simplest example of our permanent memory. It may or may not involve understanding and insight.

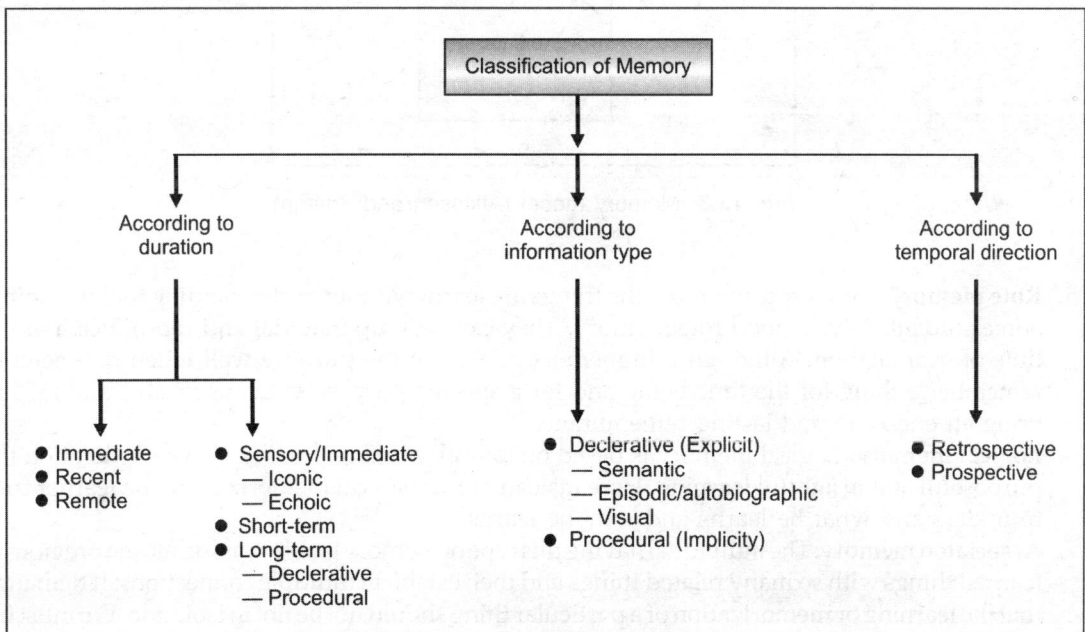

Fig. 13.2: Classification of memory

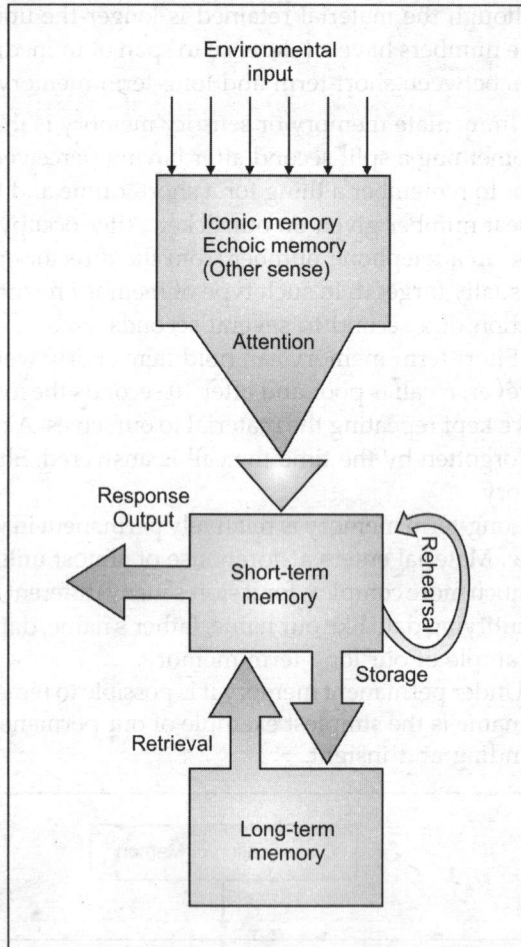

Fig. 13.3: Memory model (Atkinson and Shiffrin)

5. **Rote memory:** Under rote memory, the things are learnt without understanding their meaning. Some students have a good rote memory. They can mug up material and reproduce it at the time of examination. Although rote memory can serve the purpose well when it is need to remember a thing for the time being and for a specific purpose yet is unreliable and fails to bring an enduring and lasting remembrance.
6. **Logical memory:** Logical memory is based on logical thinking. It takes into consideration the purposeful and insightful learning. Here instead of mechanical memorization, the learner tries to understand what he learns and why he learns.
7. **Associated memory:** The individual having this type of memory is able to associate the previously learned things with so many related things and then establish multiple connections. It demands that the learning or memorization of a particular thing should not be not in isolation. We must try to connect or associate it with as many other things as we can. It will help our memory to maintain

multiple relationships. We can be able to have a memory of so many things at a time by adopting the principle of association of ideas and images and make maximum use of our memory.

8. **Active memory:** In active memory, one has to remain active or make deliberate attempts for recollecting past experiences. In answering the question in examination hall we are required to make use of this type of memory.

9. **Passive memory:** In passive memory, the past experiences are recalled spontaneously without any serious attempt or will, for example, when somebody comes form our native village the mere sight of him is enough to remained us about our fields, neighbors and other so many things.

Differences between short- and long-term memory

Sl.No.	Short-term memory	Long-term memory
1.	Short-term memory is carried by active neural process.	Long-term memory on the other hand is carried by permanent structural changes in nervous system.
2.	Short-term memory traces decay spontaneously.	Long-term memory traces show resistance to such spontaneous decay.
3.	The short-term memory storage capacity is limited. It is easily subject to interference.	A single exposure to stimuli is not seen to produce long-term retention in human verbal learning. Many trials are usually for longer-term retention.

MEASUREMENTS OF SHORT- AND LONG-TERM RETENTION

Short-term Retention

The subject is presented a stimulus in the form of nonsense syllable by a three digit numbers. He is given some task like counting the number in reverse or something similar to prevent further rehearsal on his part. He is then asked to reproduce the stimulus when a signal is given. Thus, recall was elicited after every 3 seconds. The recall was seen to drop down considerably till it was almost non-existent after 18 seconds. This effect of reduction becomes more permanent after first few trials. This shows that previous activity interferes with retention. It is known as proactive interference.

Long-term Retention

There are several ways in which long-term retention is measured.

1. **Recall:** The method of recall is used in studying retention of verbal material, e.g. a poem or paragraph from a book. The subject then has to reproduce what has learnt without any cues. It is either estimated in terms of the amount that was initially assimilated or in terms of saving of learning in a relearning situation. This former type of examinations with essay type questions utilizes recall method for measuring retention.

2. **Recognition:** Another method of measuring retention is recognition. Recall and recognition are measured as two independent entities. We may fail to recall the face of the person we met at a certain social function. But if we happen to see him, we may easily recognize him.

Between recognition and recall, the former is considered to be a more reliable criterion of retention. In most of the memory experiments retention is measured by recognition rather than recall. After presenting a list of nonsense syllables, they are intermingled with new and unfamiliar nonsense syllables. The subject has to recognize from among this bigger list, those that were presented to them. Similar experiments are conducted by using photographs of persons or sceneries instead of nonsense syllables. The modern trend of examination with objective questions in place of the essay type questions is mainly based upon the belief that recognition is a better indication of memory than recall. In the essay type questions, where the pupil has to be recalled, it may happens that one with adequate retention may fail to recall due to a number of emotional and situational factors. If he is asked to recognize, as is done by the objective questions there are less chances of the above mentioned factors affecting the expression of the level of retention. Actually, so far as the experience in life is concerned, we are more often required to recognize than recall.

3. **Saving:** This method is frequently used in psychological experiments. The subject is made to learn a certain task. The trials required to master the task are noted. He is again made to relearn the task after a lapse of some time interval. The measure of retention is the difference in number of trails required in the original learning and relearning situations. Such as method is sensitive and reliable. The saving method can show the retention long after other methods have caused to show any degree of it.

THEORIES OF MEMORY

Sl. No.	Theory	Description
1.	Fading of the memory	The theory regards the memory trace as resembling the marks of a pencil on a piece of paper, or a path worn into a plot of grass. It can be kept functioning through use as a pencil mark can be emphasized by tracing and retracing and a pathway can be kept clear by continuing to walk over it. But without use, the memory trace may vanish, as a pencil mark fades with time and pathway becomes over grown when abandoned. Memory theorists continue to believe that memory trace has some physical quality that changes with passage of time, thus reducing, the likelihood that it can be retraced or reactivated. Indeed they think of it as having two qualities. The first is its strength- meaning how likely it is to pop into mind. This quality the strength of the memory trace is at its peak immediately after learning and declines with the passage of time. The second quality is resistance to extinction, meaning how well the trace can manage to survive and become immune to fade.
2.	Failure in retrieval theory	This theory believes that memory trace, once it has been established as part of long-term memory, probably persists for as long as we live. But information held in memory is of no use to us unless it remains not only stored but available. To remember it, we must be able to find it and call upon it when needed, a process called retrieval. If we cannot call upon it we say we have forgotten it. Thus, forgetting may be not a failure in memory, but rather a failure in retrieval. As one psychologist has put it: In this respect memory is like a huge ware house in which all sorts of things are stored but which less than perfectly organized is. So that it is not always easy to find a given item upon demand, there is evidence that forgetting may be a failure in retrieval.

Contd...

Contd...

Sl. No.	Theory	Description
3	Interference theory	This theory holds that our memory for what we learn today is often adversely affected by what we have learned in the past and also by what we will learn in the future. The various pieces of information complete for attention and survival and not all of them can prevail. When old information causes us to forget new information, this process is called proactive interference the phenomenon of proactive interference can be demonstrated very strikingly through simple laboratory procedures. Such as asking subjects to try to learn and remember several lists of words. A steady decline in the ability to remember new material was caused by more and more proactive interference from prior learning. In proactive interference, old information gets in the way of remembering new information. The opposite situation, when new information causes us to forget old information is called retroactive interference.
4.	Motivated forgetting	The fact that we seem to forget something deliberately has already been mentioned in connection with the processes that take place in short-term memory. Motivated forgetting has been widely studied by psychoanalysis, who have found it often plays a part in certain forms of abnormal or neurotic behavior.

FORGETTING

The term forgetting seems to be a part of our day-to-day speech. Forgetting is a spontaneous or gradual process in which old memories are unable to recall from memory storage it is called forgetting. In other words it refers to inability to recall.

Definitions

1. Forgetting is the loss, permanent or temporary of the ability to recall or recognize learned earlier—*Munn*.
2. Forgetting means failure at any time to recall an experience, when attempting to do so or to perform an action previously learned—*Drever*.
3. Forgetting is the failure of the individual to revive in consciousness an idea or group of ideas without the help of the original stimulus—*Bhatia*.

Curve of Forgetting

The studies made by the psychologist Ebbinghaus (1885) present the earliest systematic works in studying the phenomenon of forgetting. He memorized a list of nonsense syllables and then test himself at intervals from 20 minutes to a month to see how much of the list he remembered. The results in terms of the percentage of material forgotten with the lapse of time found in the following order.

Sl. No	Time elapsed	Amount forgotten
1.	20 minutes	47%
2.	One day	66%
3.	Two days	72%
4.	Six days	75%
5.	Thirty-one days	79%

He tried to plot the above data on a piece of graph paper. The curve obtained on the graph paper by plotting the amount forgotten as a function of time was named him as curve of forgetting.

Ebbingghaus concluded the following:

1. Amount of learnt material forgotten depends upon the time lapsed after learning.
2. The rate of forgetting is very rapid at first and then gradually diminishes proportionately as the interval lengthens.

Causes of Forgetting

1. **Interpolated activity:** As far as behaviorists are concerned, it is the interpolated activity after learning which causes forgetting, the extend of forgetting depending upon the divergence of these activities from the material learnt.
2. **Disuse:** The theory of disuse postulates that any learnt activity or accumulated knowledge will be gradually forgotten if it is not regularly practiced.
3. **Retroactive inhibition:** Some learning tends to contradict some previous learning, a tendency entitled retroactive inhibition, meaning the fatal effect of interpolated activity on learning.
4. **Repression:** The psychologists believe that the major cause of forgetting is repression, i.e. the pushing of the experience or thoughts into the unconsciousness.
5. **Deficiency of thinking and repetition:** Mental thinking and repetition assist retention and recollection and in the same manner these factors also affect forgetting, i.e. in absence of these factors forgetting increases.
6. **Deficiency of the mental set:** Mental set is factor assistance in the retention and recollection of a subject so that its greater concurrences will reduce forgetting.
7. **Brain injury:** Often when a person suffers a brain injury he forgets many incidents and experiences and the extent of the forgetting depends upon the seriousness of the injury.
8. **Uses of stimulants:** Wine and other stimulants have a detrimental effect on the brain, because they weaken the memory traces. Thus, forgetting will be increased if such intoxicants are used.
9. **Altered stimulus condition:** If there is an association between the stimulus and the situation of the stimulus, then forgetting is facilitated by any change in the situation or condition of the stimulus. People who stay abroad for long forget their correct dialect.
10. **Ziegornic effect:** According to Ziegornic completed tasks are forgotten more than the uncompleted task. Her theory is based on Levin's field theory. According to this theory when the individual undertakes a task, tension develops within him and it persists until the task is completed that motivates the learner. This enables the learner to remember the task. Incase of completed task the tension disappears and forgetting will be more.
11. **Lack of rest and sleep:** Continuous learning without rest and sleep may lead to greater forgetting due to inefficient consolidation. Experimental studies have shown that sleep following learning favors retention; it also has been found that saving (retention) is definitely greater after sleep especially with 8 hours interval. Forgetting may slow during sleep.
12. **Raise in emotion:** Emotions play an important role in learning and forgetting. Sudden rise of emotions blocks the recall. During the high emotional state blood sugar level is impaired to maintain the balance adrenal gland produces cartisole that disturbs memory cells.

Types of Forgetting

1. **Passive or natural forgetting:** The kind of forgetting in which there is no intention of forgetting on the part of individual is known as passive or natural forgetting. In this kind of forgetting

one has not to make any deliberate efforts. In a quite normal way, with the lapse of time, one gradually forgets so many things experienced and learned earlier.

2. **Active or morbid forgetting:** It is also known as abnormal forgetting. In this forgetting one deliberately tries to forget something. This kind of forgetfulness, as Freud explains, originates from expression. Under this process, the painful experience and bitter memories are deliberately pushed into the unconscious layer of the mind and are left there for forgetting.

THEORIES OF FORGETTING

1. **The Trace Decay Theory:** According to many psychologists, time is the cause of much forgetting, what is learnt or experienced is forgotten with the lapse of time. The cause of such natural forgetting can be explained through a process known as decay of the memory trace. It says that learning results in neurological changes leaving certain types of memory traces or engrams in the brain. With the passage of time through disuse, these memory traces of learning impressions get weaker and weaker and finally fade away. It leads us to conclude that the older an experience, the weaker its memory and as time passes, the amount of forgetting goes on increasing.

   This theory has proved a failure in many instances of forgetting. In long-term memory, such as learning to ride a bicycle forgetting does not occur even after years of neglect. However, this theory has provided good results in explaining forgetfulness in the case of short-term memory. Drill, practice, rehearsal or repetition of learning always results in preventing decay.

2. **The Interference Theory:** Mechanism of interference is responsible for forgetting. Interference is caused on account of the negative inhibiting effects of one learning experience on another. We forget things because of such interference. The interfering effects of things previously learnt and retained in our memory with the things of our recent memory can work both ways, backward and forward. The psychological term used for these types of interference is retroactive inhibition and proactive inhibition.

   In retroactive inhibition the acquisition of new learning works backward to impair the retention of the previously learned material. For example, a second list of words, formulations or equations may impair the retention of a first list.

   Proactive inhibition is just the reverse of retroactive inhibition. Here the old learning or experiences retained in our memory works forward to disrupt the memory of what we acquire or learn afterwards. For example, learning a new formula may be hampered on account of the previously learned formulae in one's memory.

   In both types of the above inhibitions, it can be easily seen that similar experiences when follow each other produce more interference than dissimilar experiences. Because in this case all experiences are so intermingled that a state of utter confusion prevails in the mind of an individual and consequently he faces a difficulty in retention and recall.

   Interference theory as a whole has been proved quite successful in providing adequate explanation for natural and normal forgetting for both the short-term and long-term memory.

3. **The Repression Theory:** The 'Repression Theory' is put forward by Freud's psychoanalytic school of psychology. Repression, according to this school, is a mental function that safeguards the mind from the impact of painful experiences. As a result of this function we actually push the unpleasant and painful memories into the unconscious and thus try to avoid at least consciously the conflicts that bother us. As a result of the repression we forget the things which we do not want to remember.

People under a heavy emotional shock are seen to forget even their names, homes, wives and children. Apart from causing abnormal forgetting, an impaired emotional behavior of an individual does also play its part in disrupting his normal memory process. For example, a sudden rise of emotions in excess may completely block the process of recall. When one is taken over by emotions like fear, anger or love, one may forget all he has experienced, learned or thought before hand. During these emotions one becomes so self-conscious that his thinking is paralyzed. That is why a child fails to recall the answer to a question in the presence of a teacher whom he fears very much.

Abnormal Forgetting

It is seen that forgetting is a function of times as shown in the curve of retention. The other explanation of forgetting is also discussed. But the cause of forgetting frequently has an emotional background. We have already referred to the affective nature of memory. Over-excitement or nervousness is often seen to prevent recall. One facing a big audience for the first time may be well prepared with his speech but also may not be able to utter a word on the stage.

Emotional blocking also results from repression. The defense mechanism or repression has already been discussed by us. It shows how the experiences that bring disgrace or a feeling of guilt to us are pushed to the unconscious. Facts that are in keeping with our attitudes or those that support our view better remembered than those of a contrary nature. Similarly, memories of happy events are seen to be more lasting than those of unhappy events.

When experiences are forgetting as a result of repression, not only that the said experience is forgotten but any associated idea likely to call back the repressed experience to consciousness will be also be clamped down. Sigmund Freud in his book psycholopathology of everyday life has discussed the events of such forgetting at length. He has analyzed a number of memory lapsed of this kind showing how recent events too can be easily forgotten due to emotional blocking.

One interesting thing to know about the process of forgetting is that it is not simply a passive progress involving gradual elimination of the facts retained. It is partly active too, while the originally retained facts are eliminated, the gaps are filled up by entirely new details. So whatever portion that is remembered goes through constant distortion. Our needs, interests, attitudes and prejudices play an active role in filling up the gaps of memory. Sir Frederic C Barlett has shown by has interesting experiments how is reproducing by memory, though the outline is maintained, the details go through a number of changes. In his experiments, on memory for form, the subject were shown some drawing and asked to reproduce them out of memory. A number of details were either seen to be changed or omitted in the reproductions.

It is this quality of memory that really facilitates the spreading of rumors. Since rumors are circulated from person-to-person, at every juncture some of the details are omitted and some new filled in. That is why there is a world of difference between the actual event and the rumor concerning it. The distortion is not intentional. It is the outcome of the nature of the memory process.

ECONOMICAL METHODS OF MEMORIZATION OR REMEMBERING

The problem of having economy in memorizing something has persuaded many psychologists to devise various methods of memorization.

1. **Recitation method:** In this method, the learner first reads the matter once or twice and then tries to recite and recall without looking at that material. In this way, the recitation method provides continuous self-appraisal. Learner evaluates himself from time-to-time and notes the points which he has been unable to recall. To these points due attention can be paid and thus

he is saved of unnecessarily repeating the already memorized material. Moreover, the recitation method is more stimulating than the continued and avoids them by close attention.

2. **Whole and part method**: There are two methods of memorizing a thing, for example, poem. One is to read the poem again and again from the beginning till the end as a whole. This is called whole method of memorization. In other method- part method, the poem is divided into parts and each part is memorized separately.

3. **Spaced or unspaced method:** In the spaced or distributed practice method of memorization, the subject is not required to memorize the assigned material in one continuous sitting. After memorizing for some time some rest is provided and in this way the principle of work and rest is followed in this method. For example, if one has to memorize a piece of poetry by this method, then in beginning he will be advised to go repeating it. After some time he will be given some rest again he will memorize it and take rest. In this way with repeated intervals of work and rest he will be able to have mastery over the assigned piece.

4. **Active and passive methods:** Memorizing by utterance is the active method while mental repetition is the passive method. Many experiments have been carried out to measure the economy which this method may affect.

5. **Rote and intelligent methods:** If a person is learning or memorizing something without understanding it, he is said to be using the rote or unintelligent method. This is no apperception in this. On the other hand, by the use of the intelligent method it involves the understanding of the subject and apperception does come about.

6. **Grouping and rhythm:** Memorization is considerably facilitated by rhythm and grouping. It is easier to memorize poetry than prose but by rhythm and grouping. It is easier to memorize poetry than prose but by the rhythm scheme. One couplet contains enough meaning to be spread over several pages but the rhythm makes their memorization easier.

7. **Association:** Association as a factor which keeps memorization is no less importance than the other, suppose that we have to remember that the first step in the solution of arithmetical problems is the bracket and successive step are of, division, multiplication, subtraction and addition and in order to facilitate it.

IMPROVEMENT OF MEMORY OR MEMORY TRAINING

One is, at time worried that is capacity for memory is being deteriorated. He may be considered with the consideration whether his ability to memorize can be improved. The answer to such question is that memory is not single faculty and moreover, it does not improve nor does it deteriorate. Psychology deals with process of memorizing and not with a composite faculty of memory. Experiments on the process of memorizing show that whatever assimilation is superior, retention is more durable and eventually recall or recognition is prompt. Since assimilation is more closely connected with the process of learning, a thing better learned has more chances of being better memorized.

Hence, to facilitate memory that entire one can do happens to be in the field of learning. All devices that promote learning are seen to help memory. Nothing can be independently done in the field of memory alone since memory is a counterpart of learning. The factors bringing about more permanent learning are obviously contributory for superior memory.

1. **Will to learn:** There must be firm determination or strong will to learn foe achieving desired success in learning. Where there is a will there is a way. Materials read, heard or seen without intention or mood are difficult to be remembered at later times.

2. **Interest and attention:** Interest as well as close attention is essential for effective learning and memorization. One who has no interest in what one learns, cannot give due attention to it and

consequently will not be able to learn it. Therefore, every care should be taken to create the desired interest in the material by making its purpose clear and link it with one's natural instincts and urges.

3. **Adopting proper methods of memorization:** There are so many economical methods of memorization but all are not suitable on all occasions for all individuals. Therefore, a judicious selection should be made in choosing a particular method in a given situation.

4. **To follow principle of association:** It is always good to follow the principle of association in learning. A thing should never be learnt in a complete water tight compartment. Attempts should be made to connect it with one's previous learning on one hand and with so many related things on the other. Sometimes for association of ideas special techniques and devices are used that facilitate learning and recall.

5. **Grouping and rhythm:** Grouping and rhythm also facilitate learning and help in remembering. Rhythms also prove as an aid in learning memorizing. Children learn effectively the multiplication tables in the sing-song fashion.

6. **Utilizing as many senses as possible:** Senses are said to be the gateway of knowledge and it has also been found that the things are better learned and remembered when presented though more than one senses. Therefore, attempts should be made to take the help for audio-visual aid material and receive impressions through as many senses as possible.

7. **Arranging better learning situation:** Environmental factor also affect the learning process. Therefore, due care should be taken to arrange better learning situation and environment. A calm and quite atmosphere and stimulating environment proves an effective aid to learning.

8. **Internal factors within the learner:** Besides the external factors there are things within the learner which affect his learning and reproduction. His physical and mental health and state of the mind at the time of learning as well as reproduction counts a lot to memory.

9. **Provision for change and proper rest:** Adequate provision for change of work, rest and sleep should be made as it help in removing fatigue and monotony. A fresh mind is necessarily able to learn more and retain it for a long time than a tried and dull one.

10. **Repetition and practice:** An intelligent repetition with full understanding, always help in making the learning effective and enduring. The things repeated and practiced frequently learning effective and enduring. The things repeated and practiced frequently and remembered for a long-time. Therefore, due to care should be taken for drill work, practice and review, etc. in the process of memorization and learning.

11. **Pulling it all together:** Organizing and ordering information can significantly improve memory. As learning a large amount of unconnected and unorganized information from various classes can be very challenging. By organizing and adding meaning to the material prior to learning it, you can facilitate both storage and retrieval.

12. **The funnel approach:** This means learning general concepts before moving on to specific details. When you understand the general concepts first, the details make more sense.

13. **Vivid associations:** When you learning something new and unfamiliar, try pairing it with something you know very well. Such images, puns, music, etc.

14. **Active learning:** Active learning facilitates your memory by helping you attend to the process information. All of the memory techniques require active learning.

15. **Talk it out:** Repeat ideas verbatim, repeat the ideas in your own words, repeating information aloud can help you encode the information and identify how well you have learned it.

16. **Mnemonic:** It is a memory aid, and most serve as an learning purpose. It is a powerful technique helps in remembering some specific things. One common mnemonic for remembering lists

consists of an easily remembered word, phrase or rhyme whose first letter are associated with the list items. Mnemonic rely not only or repetition to remember facts, but also an associations between easy to remember constructs and lists of data, based on principle that the human mind much more easily remembers data attached to spatial, personal or otherwise meaningful information that occurring in meaningless sequences. The sequences must make sense.

AMNESIA

Amnesia is a condition in which memory is disturbed. The cause of amnesia is organic or functional. Organic causes include damage to the brain, through trauma or disease or use of certain drugs. Functional causes are psychological factors, such as defense mechanisms. Hysterical post-traumatic amnesia is an example of functional amnesia. Amnesia may also be spontaneous, in the case of transient global amnesia.

Types of Amnesia

Sl. No.	Types	Description
1.	Anterograde amnesia	New events are not transferred to long-term memory, so the sufferer will not be able to remember anything the occur after the onset of this type of amnesia for more than few moments. The complement of this is retrograde amnesia, where someone will be unable to recall events that occurred before the onset of amnesia.
2.	Dissociative amnesia	It is used to refer to inability to recall information, usually about stressful or traumatic events in person's lives. A common form of dissociative amnesia involves amnesia for person identity but intact memory of general information.
3.	Long-term alcoholism	It can cause a type of memory loss known as Korsakoff's syndrome. This is caused by brain damage due to a vitamin B_1 deficiency and will be progressive if alcohol intake and nutrition pattern are not modified.
4.	Lacunar amnesia	It is the loss of memory about one specific event.
5.	Childhood amnesia	It also known as infantile amnesia, is the common inability to remember events from one's own childhood.
6.	Global amnesia	It is total memory loss. This may be a defense mechanism which occurs after a traumatic event. This global type of amnesia is more common in middle-aged to elderly people, particularly males, and usually lasts less than 24 hours. Post-traumatic stress disorder can also involve the spontaneous, vivid retrieval of unwanted traumatic memories.
7.	Posthypnotic amnesia	It is where events during hypnosis are forgotten or where past memories are unable to be recalled.
8.	Psychogenetic amnesia	It results from a psychological cause as opposed to direct damage to the brain caused by head injury, physical trauma or disease, which is known as organic amnesia.
9.	Source amnesia	It is a memory disorder in which someone can recall certain information, but they do not know where or how they obtained it.

CONCLUSION

In psychology, an organism's ability to store, retain, and subsequently retrieve information is known as memory. The process of memory begins with learning or experiencing something and ends with its revival and reproduction. Therefore, memory is said to involve four stages: Learning, or experiencing something, its retention and finally its recognition and recall. Learning occupies a significant place in one's life. Whatever is learned need to be stored in the mind so that it can be utilized whenever required in the future. Memory denotes the ability or a power of mind to retain and produce learning. Thus, this process begins with learning and ends with its retrieval and reproduction. Forgetting has positive and negative values of life. It is a great blessing to mankind. Forgetting is the temporary or long-term loss in our ability to reproduce the thing that has been previously learned.

BIBLIOGRAPHY

1. Arnold MB (Ed). The Nature of Emotion, Penguin, Baltimore, 1968.
2. Baddeley AP. The Psychology of Memory, Basic Books, New York, 1976.
3. Bandura A. Principles of Behaviour Modifications, Holt, Rinehart and Winston, New York, 1969.
4. Furguson ED. Motivation: An Experimental Approach. Rinehart and Winston, Holt, New York, 1976.
5. Hilgard ER, Bower GH. Theories of Learning, 4th edn, Prentice-Hall, Englewood Cliff , NJ, 1974.
6. Hulse SH, Deese J, Egeth H. The Psychology of Learning, 4th edn, McGraw-Hill, New York, 1975.
7. Johnson PM. Systematic Introduction to the Psychology of Thinking, Harper and Row, New York , 1972.
8. Korman AK. The Psychology of Motivation, Prentice Hall, Englewood Cliffs, NJ, 1974.
9. Lindsay IH, Nirman DA. Human Information Processing, 2nd edn, Academic Press, New York, 1977.
10. Morgan CT, King RA. Introduction to Psychology, 6th edn, Tata McGraw-Hill, New Delhi, 1982.
11. Morgan CT. A Brief Introduction to Psychology, Tata McGraw-Hill, New Delhi, 1975.
12. Munn Norman L. Introduction to Psychology, Oxford and IBH, New Delhi, 1973.
13. Robinson DN. An Intellectual History of Psychology, Macmillan, New York, 1976.
14. Strongman KT. The Psychology of Emotion, Wiley, New York, 1973.
15. Vinacke WE. The Psychology of Thinking, 2nd edn, McGraw-Hill, New York, 1974.

16 *Intelligence*

DEFINITIONS

1. **Intelligence:** Intelligence is the aggregate or global capacity of the individual to think rationally, to act purposefully and to deal effectively with the environment.
2. **Analytical intelligence:** It is academic problem solving skills, based on combined operations of execution, performance and knowledge. These three operations will enable us to encode stimuli, hold information in short-term memory, make calculations, perform mental calculations, mentally compare different stimuli, retrieve information from long-term memory.
3. **Creative intelligence:** It involves insights, synthesis and the ability to react to noval situations and stimuli. It consists of ability which allows people to, think creatively and adjust creatively and effectively to new situations. Novel tasks or situations are good measures of intellectual ability because they assess an individual's ability to apply existing knowledge to new problems.
4. **Practical intelligence:** It is the intelligence which operates in the real world. People with this type of intelligence can adapt to, or shape their environment. It is not only influenced by mental skills but also attitudes and emotional factors.
5. **Concrete intelligence:** Concrete intelligence is related to concrete materials. This type of intelligence is applicable when the individual is handling concrete objects or machines. The person uses this intelligence in the operation of tools and instruments. For example, engineers, mechanics generally have this type of intelligence.
6. **Social intelligence:** Social intelligence is the ability of an individual to react to social situations in daily life. It includes the ability to understand people and act wisely in human relationships. Persons having this type of intelligence know the art of winning friends and influence them. For example, Leaders, ministers, salesmen, diplomats are socially intelligent.
7. **Abstract or general intelligence:** It is the ability to respond to words, numbers and letters, etc. This type of intelligence is acquired by study of books and related literature. Mostly good teachers, lawyers, doctors, philosophers have this type of intelligence.
8. **Intelligence quotient (IQ):** It is a measure of intelligence obtained by dividing the individual's mental age as determined by his performance on standardized test items, by his chronological age and multiplied by 100. It can be defined as the ratio between mental age and chronological age multiplied by 100. IQ.
9. **Mental age:** The average age of individual's who achieve a particular level of performance test.
10. **Mental retardation:** Having significantly below-average intellectual functioning and limitations in at least two areas of adoptive functioning.

INTRODUCTION

The term intelligence is derived from Latin word. It is coined by Cicero, and is used to cover all mental process. The individuals differ from one another in their ability to understand complex ideas, to adapt effectively to the environment, to learn from experience, to engage in various forms of reasoning, to overcome obstacles by taking thought. Owning to his intelligence, man is considered be better than other animals. Some people are very intelligent while others do not have that ability. Intelligence is not a single trait or character; rather, it is combination of many triads. Intelligence is a composition of capabilities that makes a person rational, able to think correctly, act purposefully, person can learn through signs and symbols and can adjust effectively with his environment. Most of the people have an intuitive notion of what intelligence is, and many words in English language distinguish between different levels of intellectual skills- bright, dull, smart, stupid, clever, slow and so on. It is necessary for a nurse to learn about intelligence because difference in the amount and quality of intelligence bring and in their ability to make adjustments to situations around them. Intelligent patients want more explanations for their treatment they are getting, whereas less intelligent patients will be satisfied with a little or no explanations.

MEANING OF INTELLIGENCE

Intelligence is one of the most studied and debated personal qualities of the human being. It is invisible, cannot be directly seen, yet it is studied at greater length and is considered to be one of our most important qualities. The study of intelligence has made psychology a more interesting subject but still psychologists are not unanimous about the nature of intelligence. Many aspects of intelligence are included in intelligent behavior because intelligence is a conceptual structure with many characteristics, it is difficult to perceive intelligence in physical form but intelligent behavior can be assessed by the practicality, success in exams and objectives, mental maturity, and ability to adjust, etc. other than these ability to express himself, sharpness of memory, ability to perceive, foresight, ability to forecast results, etc. also help in determining the intelligent behavior of person. Potential to accept challenges and passing the exams with good division, behaving as per one's age, position, prestige, and social status are also the indicators of intelligent behavior.

DEFINITIONS OF INTELLIGENCE

1. Intelligence is the potential or ability of a person to adjust to new conditions—*William Stern.*
2. Intelligence can be defined as the ability of a person to act purposefully, think rationally and deal effectively with his environment—*DL Weschler.*
3. Intelligence can be described as the ability to learn quickly at a given time and to remember the learned material—*Hobour and Freud.*
4. Intelligence is organized around an ideal protype. One's intelligence is defined by the degree of resemblance to this prototype. Since, there exist multiple prototypes; there would be no validated concept of intelligence—*Nesser.*
5. One's adaptation to the environment is called intelligence—*Piaget.*
6. Intelligence defined as a biological mechanism by which the effects of the complexity of stimuli are brought together and given a somewhat unified effect in behavior—*Peterson.*
7. Intelligence is the capacity to learn and adjust to relatively new and changing conditions—*Wagnon.*
8. An individual is intelligent in proportion as he is able to carry on abstract thinking—*Terman.*

9. Intelligence means intellect put to use. It is the use of intellectual abilities for handling a situation or accomplishing any task—*Woodworth and Marquis.*
10. Intelligence defined as a mental activity consisting of grasping the essentials in a situation and responding appropriately to them—*Heim.*
11. Intelligence defined as the effective all-round cognitive abilities to comprehend, to grasp relations and reasons—*Vernon.*
12. Intelligence is the capacity to learn and adjust to relatively new and changing conditions—*Wagnon.*
13. Intelligence is the property of recombining our behavior patterns so as to act better in a novel situation—*Wells.*
14. Intelligence is an ability demand in the solution of problems which require the comprehension and use of symbols—*Garret.*
15. An intelligent person uses past experience effectively, is able to concentrate and keep his attention focused for longer periods of times, adjusts himself to a new and unaccustomed situation rapidly, with less confusion and with fewer false moves, variability of responses, is able to see distinct relationships, can carry on abstract thinking, has a great capacity of inhibition or delay and is capable of exercising self criticism—*Husband.*
16. Intelligence may be defined as the power of good responses from the point of view of truth or facts—*Thorndike.*

NATURE OF INTELLIGENCE

1. It is an innate mental ability which grows and is influenced by the environment.
2. It shows the capacity to adapt to new or changed situations quickly and correctly.
3. It consists in the ability to carry on the higher mental processes each as reasoning, criticism, application and judgment.
4. It implies the capacity to learn difficult tasks and the ability to solve increasing difficult problems.
5. It shows the capacity to observe relationships and detect absurdities.
6. Intelligence may be regarded as a sort of mental energy (in the form of mental or cognitive abilities) available with an individual to enable him to handle his environment in terms of adaptation and facing novel situations as effectively as possible.

TYPES OF INTELLIGENCE

According to Sternberg's Triachic Theory of Human intelligence (1995), it is of three types:

1. **Analytical intelligence:** It is academic problem solving skills, based on combined operations of execution, performance and knowledge. These three operations will enable us to encode stimuli, hold information in short-term memory, make calculations, perform mental calculations, and mentally compare different stimuli, retrieve information from long-term memory.
2. **Creative intelligence:** It involves insights, synthesis and the ability to react to novel situations and stimuli. It consists of ability which allows people to think creatively and adjust creatively and effectively to new situations. Novel task or situations are good measure of intellectual ability because they assess an individual's ability to apply existing knowledge to new problems.
3. **Practical intelligence:** It is the intelligence which operates in the real world. People with this type of intelligence can adapt to, or shape their environment. It is not only influenced by mental skills but also attitudes and emotional factors.

Gardner (1999) Proposes Eight Type of Intelligence

1. **Linguistic intelligence:** Involved in reading, writing, listening, and talking.
2. **Logical:** *Mathematic intelligence:* Involved in solving logical puzzles, deriving proofs, and performing calculations.
3. **Musical intelligence:** Involved in playing, composing, singing, and conducting, furthermore, Gardner believes that auto mechanic and cardiologists may have this kind of intelligence in abundance.
4. **Spatial intelligence:** Involved in moving from one location to another or determine one's orientation in space.
5. **Intrapersonal intelligence:** Involved in understanding oneself and having insight into one's own thoughts, actions and emotions, e.g. self-understanding.
6. **Bodily:** *Kinesthetic intelligence:* Involved in using one's own body (or parts of it) to perform skillful and purposeful movements, e.g. dancer, athletes and surgeons.
7. **Naturalistic intelligence:** It involves the ability to understand and work effectively in the natural world, e.g. biologists and zoologists.
8. **Interpersonal intelligence:** Involved in understanding of others and one's reaction to others. Being high in social skills psychologists, teacher and politicians are supposed to be high in this type of intelligence.

FACTORS INFLUENCING INTELLIGENCE

1. **Biochemical factors:** From the recent studies it is found that the disturbances of biochemical balances of the body may underlie various disorders of learning and intelligence. For optimum functioning of the nervous system sufficient supply of oxygen and various nutrients are necessary. Apart from these, body temperature, pH balance and hormones also influence neural activities and there by affect intellectual performances.
   a. It is found that the defective genes may lead to defective enzyme functioning and this in turn produces a rare condition known as phyenylpyruvic oligophrenia a type of feeble mindedness.
   b. Cretinism is another type of mental deficiency caused by under activity of the thyroid gland in childhood.
   c. Mongolism idiocy is caused by defective cerebral metabolism. If the mother becomes pregnant nearing to menopause, the biochemical imbalances in her during pregnant may cause Mongolian idiocy. Thus various factors affect the growth of intelligence.
2. **Sociocultural factors:** All the intelligence tests, to some extent or the other, are subjected to the influence of sociocultural factors because the test items are drawn from the culture from whom the test is developed. The tests reflect the cultural experiences and reveal how well an individual deals with cultural factors.
   a. **Parent's occupation:** It is found from the studies that there are pronounced difference in the IQ's of children, who parents belong to different occupational groups. The children of professional parents have a mean IQ of about 115; children day laborers have a mean IQ of 94 and of intermediate occupational groups range between these two extremes. The rationale behind this is, that only higher intellectual ability can reach higher occupation.
   b. **Socioeconomic status:** This is more comprehensive factor than occupation. It includes factors like education, source and level of income, ethnic and residential area, etc. the socioeconomic differences in IQ are attributed to the factors which account for occupational differences.

In any society, more intelligent man tend to rise up in the socio-economic scale and remains there, while the less intelligent man comes down and remains in the lower strata.

c. **Regional influences:** Regional location is correlated with performance on intelligence tests. According to McNemar, the mean IQ of urban children was 108; of suburban children 107; and of rural children 96. City offers better schools, better educational facilities, affords wide variety of extracurricular and recreational facilities and thus provide a greater challenge to the growing child.

d. **Environment:** The environment wherein the educational facilities are poor and outside contacts are rare, will reduce the IQ as they grow older. In short the poor environment will have progressively adverse effect as the age increases. On the other hand enriched environment provided to the children. But it will have more beneficial effect it provided very early in life. If it is provided after seven years of life it will have no effect. Thus various biochemical and environmental factors contribute their share to the intellectual growth of the individual.

INTELLIGENCE QUOTIENT (IQ)

The intellectual capacity of the person can be assessed through IQ. This works as a guide in the future but it is essential to know the stability and limits of IQ. IQ of 80% of people is either 100 or around 100. According to modern concept, IQ is a measurement of quality and assessment of intelligence. Stanford-Binet had invented the method of quantifying or measuring intelligence. IQ can be obtained by multiplying the ratio of mental age and chronological age by hundred. This can be explained by following formula:

$$IQ = \text{Mental age} \times \text{Chronological age}/100.$$

Mental age: This represents the development of performance level of a child at certain age. In other words, if 5 years old child is able to do the tests meant foe a 6 years old, his mental age would be counted as 6 years. Failures in the tests meant for a particular age group reduces the mental age.

Chronological age: This is the physical age of the child that is based on his date of birth.

Distribution of IQ: Psychologists have described level of intelligence in many ways. Given below are the normal levels of IQ, which have been explained through a table.

Levels of Intelligence

Sl. No.	IQ	Description
1.	140 and above	Genius
2.	120-139	Very superior
3.	110-119	Superior
4.	90-109	Normal
5.	80-89	Low normal
6.	70-79	Borderline.
7.	50-69	Moron
8.	25-49	Imbecile
9.	0-24	Idiot

Intelligence quotient is determined by both hereditary and the environment. Hence, level of intelligence may change as result of environment. Similarly, repeated tests and using different types of tests may show a change in intelligence level.

INTELLIGENCE TESTS

History of intelligence tests: In the beginning mental tests were devised to study individual differences among college students. These tests were used to measure the speed of reaction, sensory acuity and other simple psychological processes. The primary interest was to study the extent of individual differences and not to assess the level of intelligence of the individual.

In 1896, Binet, a French psychologist who was studding process of school suggested special classes for children showing poor progress in class work. Eight years later the French government requested Binet to discover children in public school who were not having sufficient intelligence to benefit themselves by usual instruction.

Measurement of intelligence tests can be categorized in the following categories:

1. **Individual intelligence tests:** These tests measure the intelligence of one person at a time. These are used to measure the intelligence of retarded children or to provide treatment and guidance. Major limitations of these tests include the skills of examiner and problems of qualification. Financially, these tests are more expensive. These tests can be administered not only individually but not a group at a time. For example: Alexander Battery of performance test, Bhatia tests of intelligence, form board test, Stanford-Binet, Wechsler test, etc.

2. **Group intelligence tests:** This method of measuring intelligence is used to measure the intelligence of more than one person. These tests are very popular. Group intelligence tests were also used in World War I to measure the intelligence of the literature and illiterate soldiers. These tests can be administered to be a large number of individuals at a time, for example, Army alpha, army beta and RPM.

3. **Verbal intelligence test:** In this test, intelligence of a person is measured on the basis of his answer or reactions to the given questions. This is a reliable test and is useful for both the individuals and group, but the examinees should have the knowledge of language or words. Examiner should be highly skilled to get maximum results from these tests.

4. **Nonverbal performance test:** It involves no language but require duplication of block patterns, completion of Jig-Saw, Puzzle, arrangements of pictures, drawing, etc. For example, Goddard's from board, Link's from board, Alexander's Battery of performance tests, Raven's progressive matrices, etc.

5. **Verbal, non-verbal combined tests:** These tests include, both verbal and non-verbal items. For example, Wechsler test for children and adults, Bhatia tests of intelligence, Army alpha and beta test of performance, Army general classifications test (AGCT), Armed Force qualification test (AFQT), etc.

6. **Power tests:** These tests allow sufficient time to the subject to try most or all the items he can do. The score he obtains as an indicator of his achievement, for example, RPM.

Uses of Intelligence Tests

Intelligence tests are used in many walks of life to determine the levels of IQ of an individual which is of utmost importance for success in any walk of life. Hence, innumerable tests have come into existence and this reveals its importance in life. Some of the areas in which intelligence tests are useful are mentioned here under.

1. Intelligence tests have helped use to understand fully the nature of the intelligence.
2. As intelligence plays a very significant role in the determination of personality, intelligence tests are used as a part of personality assessment.
3. Intelligence tests are useful to dispel the wrong notions of racial differences, sex differences, caste differences, etc. these tests have ruled out the superiority of any race, sex or caste in intelligence over others.
4. Intelligence tests are useful in educational guidance of children. By determining the IQ of a child he may be guided to take up a particular course of study for which he is studied.
5. Intelligence tests are used in many educational institutions to select the students for admission. If the student is found below the required level of intelligence for the courses they offer, he may be rejected.
6. Intelligence tests are also used as a part of vocational guidance. The success in any vocation partly depends upon intelligence in addition to aptitude and interest.

Other uses are:
1. Studying the individual differences.
2. Identifying the retarded children and treating them.
3. Help in the field of education.
4. Finding the solution of disciplinary problems.
5. Use in business skills.
6. Use in armed forces.
7. Help in research work.

THEORIES OF INTELLIGENCE

Sl.No	Theory	Description
1.	Monarchic theory or Unitary theory	The theory holds that intelligence is one power or energy which affects all the activities of the individual. According to Victoria Hazlitt, intelligence is a general ability which determines the various specific abilities. The theory has been proved to fallacious. Prominent people show a less than average ability in many activities. The theory has been proved to be fallacious. Prominent people show less than average ability in many activities. For example, Darwin had a very bad handwriting.
2.	Oligarchic theory	This theory postulates that intelligence is an aggregate of mutually independent powers. Binet believed this theory. Experiments disproved this theory by showing the mental powers are interdependent.
3.	Multifactor or Anarchic theory or group factor theory (Thurstone 1933)	Thorndike is the most prominent among those who believed this theory. This theory holds that intelligence is the mean of undetermined independent rudimentary elements. But Spearman has criticized this theory.
4.	Two factor theory (Spearman-1927)	This theory was conceived by Spearman who holds that intelligence has two parts 1. General intelligence or G and 2. Specific intelligence are confined to specific activities. General intelligence is found in lesser or greater degree in every one. Specific intelligence is of various types the several types being independent of each other. They differ from individual to individual. This intelligence of a person depends on his general intelligence.

Contd...

Contd...

Sl.No	Theory	Description
5.	Structure of intellect model (Guilford-1959)	In structure of intellect model, postulated many factors of intelligence. He categorized these factors under three board dimensions: 1. The process or operation performed, 2. The kind of product involved, 3. The kind of material or content involved. He then subclassified under each of these dimensions five operations, six types of products and four types of contents.

Spearman's Two Factors Theory

Charles Spearman has proposed this two factors theory of intelligence, according to Spearman intelligence constitutes two factors, there two factors are:

1. General intelligence factor called G factor
2. Specific or special factor called S factor.

He further said the G factor varies from person to person. Depending upon the amount of G they posses, people are described as generally brought bright or generally dull. Intelligence tests measure the amount of G factor which individual possess. The amount of S factor varies within the same individual. For example, a student may be very good in mathematics but poor in spatial relations.

Louis Thurston, another psychologist objected to Spearman's two factor theory. Thurston said that human intelligence could broken down into a number of primary abilities. His statistical studies lead to the following primary abilities.

Sl.No	Primary abilities	Description
1.	Verbal comprehension	The ability to understand the meaning or words. Vocabulary test intelligence measures this factor.
2.	Word fluency	The ability to think words quickly.
3.	Number	The ability to work with numbers and perform computations.
4.	Space	The ability to visualize space-from relationships, example, recognizing the same figure presentation in different orientation.
5.	Memory	The ability to recall verbal stimulus such as pars of words or sentences.
6.	Perceptual speed	The ability to grasp visual details and to see similarities and differences between picture objects.
7.	Reasoning	The ability to find a general rule on the basis of presented instances.

GROUP FACTOR THEORY

LL Thurstone an American psychologist, while working on a trust of primary mental abilities, he came to the conclusion that certain mental operations have in common a primary factor which gives them psychological and functional unity and which differentiates them from other mental operations. These mental operations constitute a group factor. So there are a number of groups of mental abilities each of which has its own primary factor. Thurstone and his associates have differentiated nine such factors they are:

Sl.No	Factors	Description
1.	Verbal factor (V)	Concerns comprehension of verbal relations, words and ideas.
2.	Spatial factor (S)	Involved in any task in which the subject manipulates an object imaginatively in space.
3.	Numerical factor (N)	Ability to do numerical calculations, rapidly and accurately.
4.	Word fluency factor (W)	Involved whenever the subject is asked to think of the isolated words at rapid rate.
5.	Inductive reasoning factor (RI)	Ability to draw inferences on conclusions on the basis of specific instances.
6.	Memory factor (M)	Involving the ability to memorize quickly.
7.	Deductive reasoning (DR)	Ability to make use of general results.
8.	Perceptual factor (P)	Ability to perceive objects accurately
9.	Problem-solving ability factor (PS)	Ability to solve problems with independent efforts.

The weakest link in the group factor theory was that it discarded the concept of common factor. It did not take Thurston very long to realize his mistake and to reveal a general factor in addition to group factors.

MENTALLY HANDICAPPED PERSONS

Mentally handicapped person is one whose mental ability develops at a very slower rate than normal children of his age. He does not achieve the full intellectual functions of normal adult. He finds difficulty in learning social adjustment and economic productivity. He will have physical and anatomical peculiarities and will be physically interior.

General Characteristics

1. They have difficulty in learning useful information and skills. Poor in adaptation to new problems and conditions of life. Profitless from experience. Abstract and creative thinking is nil. Critical judgment is absolutely poor. Reading, writing and arithmetic are so poor, that are excluded from normal school. They forget soon unless reinforced by reviewing.
2. They are incapable of self-care, self-support or self-management in society. Need a lot of assistance during childhood. They must be fed, dressed, taken care against accidents and need supervision while playing. Incapable of personal and social affairs even during adulthood. If not guided and controlled they may engage in delinquent acts. In short they are incapable of adjusting to social environment by themselves.
3. It is difficult to draw and to hold their attention, interests are few, memory span is limited, and thinking is strenuous and hence avoids it.
4. The development of drives and emotions vary greatly with the degree of feeble mindedness. Laughing and giggling for no reason is common.
5. No two feeble minded are exactly alike in personality but individual differences are less compared to normal. They are rarely dynamic, charming, forceful, etc. they are submissive and easily subjected to influence, usually stable and apathetic.
6. They are very poor in physical resistance to illness and hence mortality is more.

7. They learn to walk and talk very much later than normal children. Their speech is defective, i.e. speech is pedantic and walk with shuffling gait. Their visual and auditory defects are common at all levels. They are seemingly deaf, poor eye contact, unusual body language. These are some of the characteristic features of mentally handicapped.

Causes of Mental Retardation

There are more than two hundred known causes and many more unknown causes. Some of the causes operate before birth, some during birth and some other after birth.

Prenatal Risk Factor

1. If the mother's age is under 15 years or over 40 years at the time of pregnancy, there is an increased risk of chromosomal abnormalities or pre maturity.
2. History of difficult previous pregnancy like miscarriage, still birth, premature birth, etc.
3. Mother with chronic health disease like diabetes mellitus, syphilis and hypertension.
4. Parents with family history of congenital anomalies like PKU muscular dystrophy.
5. Parental risk of biological origin, i.e. infections contacted during first 3 months of pregnancy.- Rubella, toxoplasmosis, CMV, etc.
6. Subjecting pregnant lady (within 3 months) to frequent X-ray treatment.
7. Excessive drugging.
8. Taking certain drugs like carbon monoxide, antititanic serum, typhoid vaccine, etc. affect brain growth and development and cause mental deficiency.

Perinatal Hazards (during birth)

1. Injury to head at the time of birth.
2. Anosmia (no respiration immediately after birth).
3. Deficiency of thiamine and Glutamic acid.
4. Ineffective fevers like encephalitis or meningitis and brain tumor.
5. Prematurely and low birth weight (intrauterine growth retardation) may cause congenital malformation and biological dysfunction.
6. Low blood pressure.
7. Premature separation of placenta.
8. Compression of cord.
9. Postmaturity hypoglycemia and polycythemia.
10. Pre-eclampsia (Toxemia of pregnancy).
11. Rh incompatibility along with kernicterus.

Postnatal Condition

1. Meningitis.
2. Chronic lung diseases.
3. Meconium aspiration.
4. Persistent pulmonary hypertension.
5. Drugs.
6. Poisoning.
7. Poor nutrition or malnutrition.
8. Trauma during first two years of life.

9. Parent child separation.
10. Very poor environment which is not stimulating during babyhood and childhood.
11. Encephalitis, etc. affect the growth of intelligence and cause mental deficiency.

Classification of Mental Retardation

1. **Borderline mental retardation:** Their IQ is 68 to 83. These are slow learner and cannot understand complex ideas. Verbal training is slower than motor learning. They can make adequate adjustment to society and some time the require help of others.
2. **Mild mental retardation:** These people will have an IQ ranging between 52-67. They are equal to 8 to 11 years boys. They lack imagination, inventiveness and judgment. They need some supervision. With parental assistance and special attention, they can adjust socially and master simple skills and can become self-supporting.
3. **Moderate mental retardation:** There IQ is between 36-51 which is equal to 4-7 years old boys. They read and write a little but very slow in learning. They look clumsy and suffer body deformities and motor coordination. With parental help and training, can take care of themselves and economically useful.
4. **Severe mental retardation:** These will have an IQ of 20-35, their motor and speech developments are severely retarded. Sensory defects and motor handicaps are common. They can develop limited personal hygiene and self-help skills. They can perform simple occupational tasks, under supervision.
5. **Profound mental retardation:** These will have an IQ of 2 years child. Absolutely deficient in adoptive behavior. Speech is very rudimentary, they will have severe physical deformities, retarded growth, convulsive seizures, mutism, deafness, etc. They largely depend on others. Resistance to disease is very low and short-lived.

Clinical Types of Mental Retardation

1. **Cretinism:** It is a condition of mental deficiency and lack of physical and mental development caused by thyroid deficiency during prenatal and postnatal growth period.
2. **Down's syndrome (Mongolism):** This term given to certain types of amentia who have monoglian features, eyes are narrow slant and upward, and poor muscular coordination. Mongoloids are particularly susceptible to circulatory, respiratory and gastrointestinal disorders.
3. **Hydrocephalus:** It is a rare condition in which the accumulation of an abnormal amount of cerebrospinal fluid within cranium causes damage to the brain tissues and enlargement of the cranium. So the skull looks very large. The head is either already enlarged at birth or begins to enlarge soon afterwards. This may be due to prenatal disturbances in the formation, absorption or circulation of the cerebrospinal fluid. The clinical picture depends on the extent of neutral damage, this in turn, depends on the age at which the on set and duration and severity of the disorder. The degree of intellectual development varies depending, upon the amount of pressure extorted on the brain tissue and damage caused to it.
4. **Macrocephalus (Sclerotic amentia):** It is a condition of enlarged head due to excessive development of glial cells, or cells which support the active nerves cells. Here both skull and the face are grossly enlarged. On the basis of the shape of the head and skull this can be differentiated from hydrocephalus. The main symptoms are pronounced mental defect, convulsions and fatty tumors of the face. Intelligence is below the level of imbecile. The mental age ranges between 3 to 7 years.

5. **Microcephalus:** The term microcephaly means small headedness. The head is usually small and cone shaped and they are called pin-headed people. The circumference is usually less than 17 inches, as against normal 22 inches. The chin and forehead recede, hair is coarse, thick and wiry. The brain is small in size and less in weight. The convolutions are less and simpler than the normal. They are below average in stature and have a relatively short span of life. Microcephalics are uninhibited in their emotional expressions, and restless and hence quick in movement and repetition is much.

6. **Phenylketnuria (PKU):** This is a rare metabolic disorder. They constitute 1% of the mentally retarded population. The baby appear normal at birth but lacks an enzyme needed to breakdown phenylalanine, which is an amino acid found in protein foods. If this condition is not detected the phenylalanine accumulates in the blood and damages the brain. This appears between 6 to 12 months after birth with symptoms of vomiting, a peculiar odor, infantile eczema and seizures. The extent of retardation depends upon the degree of the disease progressed.

7. **Congenital syphilis:** Children born to syphilitic mothers are sometimes infected with disease through placental circulation while still in uterus. Many of these are terminated in abortion or still birth. Of those born alive many have normal mental development, but others are mentally retarded. These children will have generally physical handicaps-paralysis of the limbs, epilepsy, blindness and deaf-mutism. Some children, who are infected show normal mental growth until puberty and then deteriorate, are diagnosed to have juvenile paresis.

8. **Amaurotic family idiocy:** This is also known as Tay-Sachs disease, which is very rare. This essentially a neurological disorder characterized by diffused degeneration of brain cells, which leads to progressive blindness, wasting the limbs and mental enfeeblement. The mode of transmission is through mating of persons who are free of overt symptoms, or carriers of the defective genes. This is more with the off spring of pedigrees of consanguineous mating.

9. **Traumatic amentia:** Brain injuries account for 5-10% of mental retardation. The cerebral damage may be inflicted before, during or after birth. Many cases are due to intracranial lesions and hemorrhages occurring during birth. In the later cases there is always a history of difficult labor, with or without instrumental delivery. Severe head injuries occurring before or after birth sometimes result in mental deficiency. The degree of mental deficiency present in traumatic amentia ranges from idiocy to high grade morality.

10. **Pseudodementia:** The ability is present but not used. He is an extreme introvert. External response is inadequate because the patient is pre-occupied with subjective problems. The mental ability is present but is undeveloped because of inability to see or hear.

Treatment, Rehabilitation and Prevention

Mental retardation is not an illness and hence the question of treatment and cure do not arise when it sets in it is a lifelong condition. No amount of training or medical care will transform a mentally retarded child into normal child. However, certain condition contributory to mental retardation can be improved or cured. For example deafness, poor vision, emotional disturbances, poor living conditions, deficiency of nutrition, glandular imbalance make child appears retarded. Early detection can help to lessen the degree of handicap. It is mainly a problem of education and rehabilitation. The treatment for mentally retarded lies in the stimulation and education from the earliest possible moment to develop their limited potentialities to the maximum possible extent. Mental ability grows when nourished by love and care.

1. **Parent education:** The parents of the mentally retarded must be educated to accept the child's limitation and the permanency of mental retarded. Generally parents refuse to admit that

something is wrong with their child. Even when they realize that the child is subnormal, they believe that special education and good medical attention can make them normal, and hence spends a lot of money but will be disappointed. So, it is essential to provide intensive parental counseling to enable family to provide love and security to the retarded child.

2. **Home training:** Home is the natural place for the beginning of training. Almost all mentally retarded remain at home during infancy and even during adulthood. Here mother's emotional attitude is of major importance. Some mothers reject and ignore their mentally retarded child and some are over-protective, even at the cost of normal children. In spite of the fact that a mentally retarded child is slow in learning and has poor memory.

   a. The mother should make every effort to teach the child to feed and dress himself, talk, walk and acquire habits of personal cleanliness.
   b. As he grows up, he should be given responsibilities and duties to his mental abilities.
   c. Special attention must be given for moral and personality training.
   d. Misdeeds and temper outbursts should be checked and pleasant disposition must be encouraged
   e. The sibling and other children in the family should be encouraged to accept the sibling as less intelligent but an equal member of the family.
   f. Opportunity to play with other children in the neighborhood should be permitted but care must be taken to see that other children do not ridicule or exploit the defective child.'

3. **School training:** Idiots and imbeciles cannot be sent to school because they cannot be educated. Only morons can be sent to school at the age of eight and not earlier because of slow growth of mental ability. It is better to put them with other feeble minded of the same age to special classes. This has many advantages.

   a. He need not have to compete with bright children and avoid ridicule and humiliation for failure.
   b. In special classes the competition will be with equals and hence can experience some measure of achievement and success.
   c. The curriculum of the special classes can be fitted to the capacity of the defective children.
   d. The class can go slow, with more emphasis on developing motor coordination, speech, and desirable social traits.
   e. The teacher can devote more time and attention to each pupil which is very essential.

4. **Institutionalization:** Generally, these are over-crowded. Children sent to these schools are of two groups. One group is chiefly of idiots and imbeciles, who are generally handicapped. The parents are unwilling or unable to care for them at home. The second group consists of morons. These children (older) due to undesirable or delinquent behavior necessitate segregation from society. A large number of these are discharged after a period of social and occupational training but the former group remains in the institution till their death.

5. **Vocational training and rehabilitation:** Higher grade defectives can be taught a variety of occupations, which will make them work in sheltered workshops or in open employment and can become self supporting. Imbeciles can be trained for simple farming, Landry, dairy and kitchen work. Morons can be trained to assist carpenters, bakers, tailor, shoe maker, electricians, etc. they can also trained to do complex farmwork, poultry and livestock and to operate many kind of machines, etc. thus they can be made self-supporting.

6. **Family care:** This is more economical and desirable way of segregating the mentally retards, by putting them under families in rural homes. This is better and keeping them in institution.

7. Legal facilities, insurance and trust schemes for the retards must be provided, to make them economically independent.

8. Child guidance clinics to help diagnosis the handicap and assess the children must be set up so that necessary action can be taken to improve their lots.
9. Home nursing and parent counseling program must be established to help the parents care for their children and to manage day to day problems.
10. Trained personnel like teachers, psychologists, occupational therapists, specialists in the concerned medical fields and social worker must be provided to cater to their special needs.
11. Specialized diagnostic facilities and special wards must be provided for them in all major hospitals and specialty in children's hospitals.
12. The Government should recognize their functional rights.

Prevention of Mental Retardation

1. **Sterilization:** Sterilization of all the imbeciles and morons on social ground is desirable and especially to girls. Defective boys rarely marry or produce children because they cannot compete with normal boys for female attraction.
2. **Institutionalization:** If not sterilized promiscuous defective girls must be institutionalized for the entire period of reproductive years. However, sterilization as a social measure is found to be useful.
3. **Routine health measures:** For the pregnant mother, precautions against possibility of intrauterine or birth damages and use of various diagnostic measures to detect and correct abnormalities early, can help prevent such births.
4. **After, detecting the defect early:** If normal stimulating environment is provided may kinds of mental retardation, which were once thought to be hereditary and inevitable can be prevented to a great extent.
5. **Genetic counseling:** It is realized now that chromosomal anomalies lead to faulty development. Tests are developed to identify parents who have these anomalies and to provide them genetic counseling which will help prevention of such births.
6. Another way of prevention is alleviation of sociocultural conditions which deprive children the necessary stimulation, motivation and opportunity for normal learning and mental development.

APPLICATIONS OF INTELLIGENCE IN NURSING

1. Hospitalized children who are in the sensor motor stage have not achieved object permanence and therefore suffer from separation anxiety. They are best off if their mothers are allowed to stay with them overnight.
2. Children at the preoperational stage, who are unable to deal with concepts and abstractions, benefit more from role playing for medical procedures and situations than by having them verbally described in detail, e.g. a child who is to receive IV therapy is helped by acting out the procedure with a toy IV set and dolls.
3. As the children could not understand the cause and effect may interpret physical illness as punishment for bad thoughts or deeds.
4. Adolescent's thinking may appear abstract.

   Nurse can explain the procedure to an individual on the basis of his intellectual ability. She knows to what extent, she can explain. Otherwise she educate the parents/relatives about necessary details of the patient.

During any nursing procedure, the nurse must always understand the particular age and his/her cognitive ability.

NURSES ROLE IN INTELLIGENCE

1. Knowledge about the nature of intelligence and its measurement is useful to the nurse in understanding herself, her colleagues as well as her patients.
2. Nurse's explanations or guidance to the patient would be according to the patient's intellectual level.
3. As a student and later as a teacher the knowledge of intellectual function is useful for a nurse. Teaching method, content of the subject matter and expectations from students should be based on student's intellectual functioning.
4. Knowledge regarding intelligence helps the nurse in diagnosing a patient with mental sub-normality or with very superior intelligence.
5. In diseases related to neuropsychiatry disorders, epilepsy, psychiatric disorders and some of the endocrinal disorders, assessment of intelligence is of great assistance in their management.
6. Knowledge about abnormalities in newborns and development of their intelligence helps the nurse in providing suitable care.
7. Aging patients though physically slow, retain their levels of intelligence. Respect and encouragement with the right mix of nursing care has to be ensured.

Every individual is unique, especially when intelligence is the judging factor. A nurse in the course of discharging her duties has to heavily rely on verbal and nonverbal communication patterns. She may have to interact with the patient, his family members, explain and clarify procedures and medications. The intelligence level of the patient and his family members decides how effectively the nurse is able to communicate and discharge her duties. Lower the levels of intelligence, more the time and patience the nurse will have to invest in caring for the patient. The instructions may have to be simple and repeated more often. However, where the patient is more intelligent he can be expected to take an active part in his own health care in the future.

CONCLUSION

The term intelligence is a very popular term used widely to mean many things-quick understanding, fast learning, accuracy in learning, cleaver talking, quick doing, good memory, etc. Intelligence is generally mistaken for intellect. The concept of intelligence is defined by psychologists in different ways. There is little agreement regarding the suitability of the definition of intelligence. The most general definition stresses versatility or flexibility of adjustment. Alfred Binet, the pioneer in this field, defines intelligence as something which sensory acuity tests or reaction time experiments measure. As child grows older his intelligence also grows correspondingly. Under normal conditions, both chronological age and mental age increases proportionately up to 13th years. According to the studies, the growth of intelligence in the early childhood is rapid. It begins to slow down around the age of 12 or 13. The yearly increment becomes smaller and smaller until the growth ceases.

BIBLIOGRAPHY

1. Binet A, Simon T. The Development of Intelligence in Children, Baltimore: Williams & Wilkins, 1916.
2. Brody EB, Brady N. Intelligence: Nature, Determinants and Consequence, Academic Press, New York, 1976.
3. Butcher HJ. Human Intelligence: Nature and Assessment. Methuen, London, 1968.
4. Cronbach LJ. Essentials of Psychology Testing, 3rd edn, Harper and Row, New York, 1970.
5. Drever J, Collins M. The Performance Tests of Intelligence, Oliver and Boyd, Edinburgh, 1948.
6. Griffith JH. The Psychology of Human Beharior, George Allen, London, 1933.
7. Guilford P. The Nature of Intelligence, Mc Graw-Hill, New York, 1967.
8. Morgan CT, King RA. Introduction to Psychology, 6th edn, Tata McGraw-Hill, New Delhi, 1982.
9. Morgan CT. A Brief Introduction to Psychology, Tata McGraw-Hill, New Delhi,1975.
10. Munn, Norman L. Introduction to Psychology, Oxford and IBH, New Delhi, 1973.
11. Pillai NY, Pilllai KS, Nair KS. Psychological Foundations of Education, Kalaniketon, Trivandrum, 1972.
12. Robinson DN. An Intellectual History of Psychology, Macmillan, New York, 1976.
13. Shankar Udai, Exceptional Children, 2nd edn, Sterling, Delhi, 1984.
14. Spearman CE. The Nature of Intelligence and Principles of Cognition. Macmillan, London, 1923.

17 *Thinking*

DEFINITIONS

1. **Thinking:** Thinking is a complex mental activity. It is symbolic in character, initiated by a problem which the individual is facing, involves the response of the individual to this problem. Thinking is a problem solving process in which we use ideas or symbols in places of overt activity.

2. **Images:** Images, as mind pictures, consist of personal experiences of objects, persons or scenes once actually seen, heard or felt. These mind pictures symbolize the actual objects, experiences and activities. In thinking, we usually manipulate the images instead of actual objects, experiences or activities.

3. **Concepts:** A concept is a symbol that stands for common properties of things. Concepts enable us to divide things into classes. Objects with common features are grouped under the same class. For example, we use the concept of flowers to refer to jasmine, lotus, etc. with the concept of 'soft' we sort out objects into soft and hard. The concepts as a tool economize our efforts in thinking. For example, when we listen to the word 'elephant' we are at once reminded not only about the nature and qualities of the elephants as a class but also our particular experiences and understanding about them emerges from our consciousness that stimulate our present thinking.

4. **Languages:** Language is the most efficient and developed vehicle used for carrying out the process of thinking. When one listens or reads or writes words, phrases or sentences or observes gestures in any language, one is stimulated to think. Reading and writing of the written documents and literature also helps in stimulating and promoting our thinking process. The language broadens our thinking.

5. **Perceptual or concrete thinking:** It is the simplest form of thinking. The basis of this type of thinking is perception, i.e. interpretation of sensation according to one's experience. It is also named as concrete thinking as it is carried by the perception of actual or concrete objects and events. It is thinking of a lower order. Such type of thinking is present in animals and children.

6. **Conceptual or abstract thinking:** Like perceptual thinking it does not require the perception of actual objects or events. It is an abstract thinking where one makes use of concepts, the generalized ideas and languages. It is regarded as a superior type of thinking to perceptual thinking as it economizes efforts in understanding and problem solving.

7. **Reflective thinking or logical thinking:** It aims at solving complex problems rather than simple problems. It requires reorganization of all the relevant experiences and finding new ways of

reacting to a situation. Mental activity in reflective thinking does not undergo any mechanical trial and error type of effort. There is an insightful cognitive approach in reflective thinking. It takes logic into account in which all the relevant facts are arranged in a logical order, in order to get to the solution of the problem in hand.

8. **Creative thinking:** This type of thinking is chiefly aimed at creating something new. It is in search of new relationships and associations to describe and interpret the nature of things, events and situations. It is not bound by any pre-established rules. The individual himself usually formulates the problem and is free to collect evidence and invent tools for its solution. The thinking of the scientists or inventors is an example of creative thinking.

9. **Critical thinking:** It is a higher order well-disciplined thought process, which involves the use of cognitive skills like conceptualization, interpretation, analysis, synthesis and evaluation for arriving at an unbiased, valid and reliable judgment of the gathered or communicated information or data as a guide to one's belief and action.

10. **Convergent thinking:** The ability to produce responses that are based primarily on knowledge and logic.

INTRODUCTION

The primary basis of man's progress is thinking. Many problems can be solved with help of thinking. Various processes of teaching are accomplished due to thinking only. It is possible to change the attitudes and thoughts of a person through thinking. Perception, memory, imagination and reason are included in thinking, therefore, thinking is considered to be a complex process. Thinking is an incredibly complex process and a most difficult concept in psychology to define or explain. Thinking, the mental solution of problems, makes use of the symbols of objects instead of the objects. Thinking attempts the solution of problems by employing the trial and error method. There is a kind of flow in the activity of thinking, one problem leading to the thinking of another by reminding the person of that other problem.

NATURE OF THINKING

Thinking is the process of mentally solving the problems. It includes a flow of thoughts. Thoughts continue to come one after the other and this internal process continues till they are expressed. Here attempts are made to solve the problems through trail and error method. If the person arises, its solution is sought through thinking or any new thought is evolved. Along with analysis, thinking also involves synthesis, foresight and hindsight. Here, one thinks about tangible objects through intangible signs and symbols, here thinking is a symbolic behavior. The main form of thinking is reason and this is a process of mental research healthy saves time and behavior.

1. Thinking is essentially a cognitive activity.
2. It is always directed to achieve some end or purpose. In genuine thinking, we cannot let our thoughts wonder on without any definite end in mind as happens in the case of day dreaming and imagination.
3. Thinking is described as a problem-solving behavior. From the beginning to the end, there is some problem around which the whole process of thinking revolves. But every problem- solving behavior is not thinking. It is only related to the inner cognitive behavior.
4. In thinking there is mental exploration instead of motor exploration. One has to suspend immediately one's overt or motor activities while engaging in thinking through some or other types of mental exploration.

5. Thinking is a symbolic activity. In thinking there is a mental solution of the problem which is carried out through some signs, symbols, and mental images.
6. Thinking can shift very rapidly, covering an expanse of time and space almost instantaneously.

DEFINITIONS OF THINKING

1. Thinking is the cognitive process that begins with the problem or work facing the person. It includes trial and error but is affected by the readiness of person and ultimately, it ends at the solution of problem or conclusion—*Warren*.
2. In strict psychological discussion it is well to keep the thinking for an activity which consists essentially of a connected flow of ideas which are directed towards some end or purpose—*Valentine*.
3. Thinking is mental activity in its cognitive aspect or mental activity with regard to psychological objects—*Ross*.
4. Thinking is behavior which is often implicit and hidden and in which symbols (images, ideas, and concepts) are ordinarily employed—*Garrett*.
5. Thinking is an implicit problem-solving behavior—*Mohsin*.
6. Thinking is a problem-solving process in which we use or symbols in place of overt activity—*Gilmer*.
7. Thinking is the organization and reorganization of current learning in the present circumstances with the help of learning and past experiences—*Vinake*.
8. Thinking is a perceptual relationship which provides for the solution of the problem—*Maier*.
9. Thinking is a complex cognitive form of behavior which occurs only at a relatively advanced stage of development, when simpler and more direct methods of dealing with environment have proved ineffective and simple memory is adequate to solve a problem thinking occurs—*Whittaker*.

TYPES OF THINKING

1. **Imaginative thinking:** Here, thinking takes place without any basic sensory stimulus. Daydreaming and only being aware of future plans are major examples of imaginative thinking.
2. **Creative thinking:** This thinking is related to creative activities; it is the basis of adopting new thoughts and attitudes in life, inventions, research and other creative activities. Creative thinking is chiefly aimed at creating something new. It is in search of new relationship and associations to describe and interpret the nature of things, events and situations. It is not bounded by any pre-established rules. Creative thinkers are great boons to the society as they enrich the knowledge of mankind.
3. **Positive thinking:** Here, the thoughts of person are of optimistic and positive point of view. This thinking identifies the good mental health.
4. **Negative thinking:** Here, person gives more important to negative thoughts. This type of thinking is not good for health.
5. **Perceptual or concrete thinking:** It is the simple form of thinking. The basis of this type of thinking is perception, i.e. interpretation of sensation according to one's experience. It is also named as concrete thinking as it is carried over the perception of actual or concrete objects and events.
6. **Conceptual or abstract thinking:** It does not require the perception of actual objects or events. It is also called abstract thinking as it makes the use of concepts or abstract ideas. It is superior

to perceptual thinking as it economizes efforts in understanding and helps in discovery and invention. It is an abstract thinking where one makes use of concepts; the generalized ideas and language. It is economizes effects in understanding and problem-solving.

7. **Nondirected or associative thinking:** In strict psychological sense, what we have discussed above in terms of the types of categories of thinking constitutes real or genuine thinking. It is essentially a directed thinking which pertains to reasoning and problem-solving procedure aimed at meeting specific goals.

8. **Reflective thinking:** It is somewhat of a higher form of thinking. It can be distinguish from simple thinking in the following ways:
   a. It aims at solving complex problems rather than simple problems.
   b. It requires reorganization of all the relevant experiences and finding new ways of reacting to a situation or of removing an obstacle instead of simple association of experiences or ideas.
   c. Mental activity in reflective thinking does not undergo any mechanical trial and error type of effort. There is an insightful cognitive approach in reflective thinking.
   d. It takes logic into account in which all the relevant facts are arranged in a logical order, in order to get to the solution of the problem in hand.

CHARACTERISTICS OF THINKING

1. A number of mental processes are included in thinking.
2. Thinking is affected by motives.
3. Thinking begins from general to specialty.
4. Analysis and synthesis have an important role in thinking.
5. Thought and language are very important in thinking.
6. Thinking begins with the beginning of problem.
7. Thinking can solve problem.
8. Brain remains active during thinking process.
9. Thinking enjoys challenges.
10. Thinking able to suspend judgments.
11. Thinking challenges assumptions.
12. Thinking seeks problems as opportunities.

ELEMENTS OF THINKING (TOOLS OF THINKING)

1. **Images:** Images, as mind pictures, constant of personal experiences of objects, persons or scenes once actually seen, heard or felt. These mind pictures symbolize the actual objects, experiences and activities. In thinking, we usually manipulate the images instead of actual objects, experiences and activities. The uses of images in thinking depend in no small measure upon the method of thinking which the individual employs. Some people use other symbols in their thinking instead of images.

2. **Concepts:** Concepts are the abstract forms of past experiences. Humanity is the quality of the human species, found equally in all human beings. A concept is a general idea that stands for a general class and represents the common property of all the objects, or events of this general class. The concepts as a tool economies our efforts in thinking. Concept formed with the help of abstraction is mental. Concepts extend the limits of thinking to include both the past and the future. Reasoning cannot be done without concepts which are both the past and the future.

3. **Symbols and signs:** Symbols and signs represent and stand as substitutes for actual objects, experiences and activities. In this sense they cannot be confined to words and mathematical numerals and terms. Traffic lights, railway signals, school bells, badges, songs, flags, and slogans all stand for the symbolic expression. These symbols and signs stimulate and economies thinking.

4. **Language:** Language is the most efficient and developed vehicle used for carrying out the process of thinking. When one listens or reads or writes words, phrases or sentences or observes gesture in any language, one is stimulated to think. Reading and writing of the written documents and literature also help in stimulating and promoting our thinking process.

5. **Muscle activities:** Thinking in one way or the other shows evidence of the involvement of a slight incipient movement of groups of our muscles. It can be easily noticed that there are slight muscular responses when we think of a word, resembling the movements used when we utter the word aloud. A high positive correlation has been found to exist between the thinking and muscular activities of an individual. The more we engage ourselves in thought, the greater is the general muscular tension and conversely as we proceed toward muscular relaxation, our thought processes gradually diminish.

6. **Brain function:** Whatever may be the role of muscles, thinking is primarily a function of our brain. Our mind or brain is said to be the chief instrument or reservoir for carrying out the process of thinking. The mental picture of images can be stored, formed, reconstructed or put to some use only through the functioning of the brain.

STAGES OF THINKING

John Dewey says that there are distinct stages in thinking:

1. **Awareness of the problem:** According to John Dewey reason for thinking is confusion or doubt and hence whenever we are aware or confronted with a problem we start thinking. Therefore being aware of the existing problem is essential if we have to think. For instance the student who is not aware that his behavior would lead to problem may not think before showing the behavior.

2. **Defining the difficulty:** Following the awareness of the problem one should be able to understand the kind of problem he/ she has this is important to find out the root cause of the problem.

3. Discovering the relationships and formulating the possible solutions to the problems is the third step. This helps in manipulating the information or as we have discussed in insight learning, this is helps in perceptual reorganization assisting in problem-solving.

4. **Evaluation:** Testing the solution. This helps in taking the effective steps to solve a problem.

5. Applying the solution is the last stage where we show the problem solving behavior that is the result of thinking.

ELEMENTS IN THINKING

Favorable Elements in Thinking

1. **Interest and attention:** Both interest and attention favor thinking. Conclusive or authoritative thinking is extremely difficult if not impossible when the subject is such as does not interest us. Attention, too, is difficult in the absence of any interest. On the contrary, both attention and thinking are natural in a subject which does interest us.

2. **Strong motivation:** Strong motivation is needed in valid thinking, the latter being impossible in the absence of motivation. Organized and controlled thinking needs strong motivation. Thinking involves the solution of problems. The effort of the mind in thinking corresponds to the strength of motivation for the solution of problems. Motivation maintains enthusiasm and postpones fatigue.

3. **Alertness and flexibility:** Alertness and flexibility also favor valid thinking, because they serve to keep external faults, from containing thinking. Alertness checks mistakes and fallacies from creeping into thinking. Flexibility keeps thinking freeform conservation and blind beliefs. An alert person has new methods, ways and views and makes use of them in thinking whenever necessary.

4. **Time limit should not be rigid:** When a solution to some problem is being sought, the time limit provided should not be too rigid because id it so, then, normal thinking is hampered and our mental facilities become invalid. Very inflexible and short-time limit cannot admit of valid thinking. Time limit for any interesting problem is superfluous because as it is every person exerts himself to the maximum.

5. **Wide range of wisdom:** The wide range of wisdom is also a favorable factor in thinking. Thinking needs insight, which is constituted of hindsight and foresight. A proper development of the faculties of the mind is essential for these activities.

6. **Incubation:** Another factor which favors thinking is incubation. If the solution of some problem proves elusive despite strenuous and persistent effort it is advisable to lay aside the problem and to involve oneself in some other activity. While one is engaged in this work, the mind ponders over the earlier problem and just as eggs are hatched by incubation, a solution is evolved through pondering in this manner.

Unfavorable Elements in Thinking

1. **Emotion:** Emotion hinders thinking because strong emotion disturbs the mental equilibrium and thereby obstructs thinking. Even if thinking is pursued in an emotional state it will be extremely one-sided and biased. If the emotion is very faint, the speed of thinking will be augmented instead of being hindered. But, for correct thinking it is better to have control over the emotions.

2. **Suggestion:** Suggestion also obstructs thinking, because it makes it one-sided. Thinking moves along the path suggested. If for example, someone is told the he will not live for any length of time; his thinking will be very badly affected, making him a pessimist. But is not essential that suggestions be invariably harmful to thinking because healthy suggestions assist thinking.

3. **Superstition:** Superstition is just as harmful as a prejudice. It contradicts reasoning; superstition is belief in something without any thinking or reasoning. Superstition is unreasoned belief. If for example, we superstitious believe some theory, opinion or person, we will always think in favor of him and never see his faults. The people who believe superstitious in a certain religion believe mutually contradictory things but never mentally reason them out.

4. **Prejudice:** Prejudice, like the two a foreside factor, has a detrimental effect on thinking, the only point of distinction being the extent of damage, which is more in this case than in the two cases discussed earlier. The word prejudice suggests the meaning namely some preconceived idea. If we are going to start thinking on some problems with an inclination in a particular direction all our thinking will be colored by our bias and will not be impartial.

ASSESSMENT OF REASONING AND PROBLEM-SOLVING

Wisconsin Card Sorting Test (WCST)

1. This test assesses abstract reasoning and flexibility in problem-solving stimulus cards of different color, form and number are presented to patients to sort into groups according to the principle established by the examiner but unknown to the patient (e.g. to sort by color, ignoring form and number).
2. As the patient sots the cards, he/she is told whether the responses are correct or incorrect, and the number of trials required to achieve 10 consecutive correct responses is recorded. When the patient has mastered the task, the examiner changes the principle of sorting, and the number of trials required to achieve correct sorting is recorded.
3. The procedure, repeated several times, measures the capacity for abstract thinking (i.e. the number of trials required to achieve a solution) and flexibility (perseverated error on successive sorting trials).
4. Persons with damage to the frontal lobes or to the caudate and some person with schizophrenia give abnormal response.
5. Patients with cerebral disease are likely to loose the capacity to reason abstractly and to lack flexibility in problem-solving or adopting to change situations.

REASONING

Reasoning plays a significant role in adjusting to one's environment. It is not only controls one's abilities, but also the total behavior and personality is affected by the proper or improper development of one's reasoning ability. Reasoning depicts a higher type of thinking which is quite careful, systematic and organized in its functioning. Reasoning is solving a problem by putting two or more elements of past experience together in a logical sequence to arrive at something new. Most human reasoning makes use of symbols- especially the verbal symbols. The process of reasoning follows some standard rules are rigid in nature and can be used as standards for reasoning. The rules are called logic. They prescribe what kind of implication statements can have and what kinds of conclusions it is permissible to draw from them.

Meaning of Reasoning

Reasoning is a form of thinking itself. When thinking process is guided by some logical principles, it is called reasoning. Good thinking and reasoning are clearly related. One facilitates the other. Reasoning is goal directed as is thinking in general. But in reasoning, the goal is imposed upon the process at every step. Every step weighs the advancement of the process in terms of the accuracy in inaccuracy of the condition. When facts of data are put together according to the logical principles, reasoning is correct. Reasoning is mostly directed towards getting at certain definite conclusions and inferences. In this process the facts relevant to the particular problem.

Definitions of Reasoning

1. Reasoning is step-wise thinking with a purpose or goal in mind—*Garrett*.
2. Reasoning is the term applied to highly purposeful controlled selective thinking—*Gates*.

3. In reasoning, items (facts or principles) furnished by recall, present, observation or both; are combined and examined to see what conclusion can be drawn from the combination—*Woodworth*.
4. Reasoning is the word used to describe the mental recognition of cause and effect relationships. It may be the prediction of an event from an observed cause or the inference of a cause from an observed event—*Skinner*.
5. Reasoning is combining past experiences in order to solve a problem, which cannot be solved by mere reproduction of earlier solutions—*Munn*.

Characteristics of Reasoning

1. It is genuine thinking; it involves a definite purpose or goal.
2. It is also an implicit act and involves problem-solving behavior.
3. Like thinking here one makes use of one's previous knowledge and experiences.
4. Like thinking there is mental exploration instead of motor exploration in reasoning as we try to explore mentally the reason or cause of the event or happening.
5. Like thinking, reasoning is a highly symbolic function. The ability to interpret various symbols, development of concepts and linguistic ability helps much in reasoning.

Steps of Reasoning

1. Identification of the goal or purpose for which reasoning is to be directed.
2. The mental exploration or search for the various possibilities, cause and effect relationships or solutions for releasing the set goal or purposes based on previous learning or experiences and present observation or attempts.
3. Selection of the most appropriate possibility or solution by careful mental analysis of all the available alternatives.
4. Testing the validity of the selected possibility or solution, purely through mental exercise and thus finally accepted or reject it for actual solution of the problem.

Types of Reasoning

1. **Inductive reasoning:** In this type of reasoning we usually follow the process of induction. Induction is a way of proving a statement or generalizing a rule or principle by proving or showing that if a statement or a rule is true in one particular case, it will be true in cases which appear in some serial order and thus it may be applied generally to all such type of cases.
2. **Deductive reasoning:** Deductive reasoning is just opposite to inductive reasoning. Here one starts completely agreeing with some already discovered or pre-established generalized fact or principle and tries to apply it to particular cases.

CREATIVE THINKING

At times, thinking leads to fertile results. Such thinking that brings about novel results is known as creative thinking. The creative thinkers like artists, writers, or scientific try to create something new and nonexistent in the world. In contrast with ordinary problems-solving creating solutions are new ones that other people have not thought of before. Creative thinking results in offering new and unique ways of conceptualizing the world around us. The word new is of importance in creative thinking. Usually it appears that a creative thinker becomes aware of a new idea suddenly. The sudden appearance of new ideas is called insight. In fact, instead of being sudden such an insight is based on unconscious deliberations. All the discoveries or inventions of the scientists are instances of creative thinking.

Steps Involved in Creative Thinking

1. **Preparation:** In a way, all education is a preparation for creating thinking in general. But specific problems require special training and preparation in that particular field. The creative results in such thinking are mostly the results of insightful inspiration. But this inspiration is possible within the relevant field of training and experience. It cannot take place in a vacuum. Much emphasis is, therefore, placed on training for creative thinking in the field of modern day educational psychology.
2. **Incubation:** The new ideas take some time to ripen or to get mature. They are to be hatched. The productive solution does not occur the movement it is started upon. Often the thinker has to struggle hard for the solution. Sometimes he may even given up thinking about it in despair.
3. **Illumination:** When the solution occurs after the period of incubation, it occurs all of a sudden in the form of illuminating insight. Naturally, the thinker feels that something like inspiration is at work. He cannot explain it in terms of his own attempts. He feels that the solution occurs by a sudden flash. But illumination can be well explained, taking the incubation period into account.
4. **Verification:** The solution of idea that results from illumination cannot be the final stage of creative thinking. The idea should well fit in the system of existing knowledge. Hence, evaluation of the solution is the essential stage following the solution. Especially, for the scientific invention it is necessary to get idea verified and see whatever, it is correct and workable.
5. **Revision:** The final stage is that of revision where the new solutions are further tested by applying them to other situations. Many thinkers find it necessary to get their ideas revised and modified before the results of their thinking are satisfactory.

PROBLEM-SOLVING

Problem-solving in an important characteristic of thinking is that it is a problem-solving behavior. It is always directed towards the solution of a problem. Whenever a need arises, man tries to satisfy it by some already established pattern of behavior. A problematic situation arises when this fixed pattern fails to satisfy the need. Man is constantly faced by some problems or the other, as his needs are numerous. Even when the needs necessary for his physical and social well-being are satisfied, he may still have a number of intellectual or spiritual needs which has to get satisfied. Being thus constantly confronted with problems, man has to keep on thinking all the time. If he stops thinking, the problems due to the unsatisfied needs may affect his adjustment to life. He has to think in the most diverse possible manner.

Definitions of Problem-Solving

1. Problem-solving behavior occurs in novel or difficult situations in which a solution is not obtainable by the habitual methods of applying concepts and principles derived from past experience in very familiar situations—*Woodworth and Marquis.*
2. Problem-solving is a process of overcoming difficulties that appear to interfere with the attainment of a goal. It is a procedure of making adjustment in spite of interferences—*Skinner.*

Scientific Methods of Problem-Solving

1. **Problem-awareness:** The first step in the problem-solving behavior of an individual concerns his awareness of the difficulty or problem that needs a solution. He must be confronted with some obstacle or interference in the path of the realization of his needs or motives and consequently the must be conscious of the felt difficulty or problem.

2. **Problem-understanding:** The difficulty or problem felt by the individual should be properly identified by a careful analysis. He should be clear about what exactly is his problem. The problem then should be pinpointed in terms of the specific goals and objectives.

3. **Collection of the relevant information:** In this step, the individual is required to collect all the relevant information about the problem through all possible sources. He may consult experienced persons, read the available literature, revive his old experiences, think of possible solutions, and put in all relevant efforts for widening the scope of his knowledge concerning the problem in hand.

4. **Formulation of hypothesis or hunch for possible solutions:** In the light of the collected relevant information and nature of his problem, one may then engage in some serious cognitive activities to think of the various possibilities for the solution of one's problem.

5. **Selection of a proper solution:** In this important step, all the possible solutions, thought of in the pervious step, are closely analyzed and evaluated. Gates and others (1946) have suggested the following activities in the evaluation of the assumed hypotheses or solution:

   a. One should determine the conclusion that completely satisfies the demand of the problem.

   b. One should find out whether the solution is consistent with other facts and principles which have been well established.

   d. One should make a deliberate search for negative instances which might cast doubts on the conclusion.

6. **Verification of the concluded solutions or hypothesis:** The solution arrived at or conclusion drawn must be further verified by utilizing it in the solution of the various likewise problem. In case, the derived solution helps in solving these likewise problems, then and then only, one is free to agree with his findings regarding the solution of his problem.

An important step in problem-solving is the direction or set. A wrong direction may interfere with the correct solution of the problem. A flexibility of mental set is often helpful in giving the proper direction to problem-solving. The thinking which is done in problem-solving is goal directed and is motivated by the need to reduce discrepancy between one state of affairs and another. The direction required for problem-solving is given by the rules associated with the solutions of most of the problem. In everyday problems these rules are supplied by our social experience. In some formal problems they are the part of the problem itself.

Some of these rules when followed correctly guarantee a solution to a problem. In most problems where such rules are not supplied we fall back on our past experiences with problems which are likely to lead to a solution. The problem at hand is broken down in smaller such problems each of which is a little closer to the end goal. However, there is no guarantee of correct solutions. Hence, thinking may be described as an implicit problem-solving behavior.

ATTRIBUTION

Social perception is the process through which one seeks to know and understand others. It the most basic aspect of social life. We always try to understand others current or present feelings, moods, emotions, etc. the process through which we seek to determine the causes behind others behavior is known as attribution. In other words, attribute refers to our effects to understand the causes behind behavior and on some occasions, the causes behind our behavior. Attribute are influences that people draw about causes of events, others behavior and their own behavior. Attribution is necessary to understand our experiences. If we can attribute others behavior it will help in making adjustments with others and to maintain self-image.

Theories of Attribution

1. **Kelly's co-variation model:** It is based on assumption that people attribute behavior to factors that are present when the behavior takes place and absent when it dies not. According to Kelly, when people attempt to infer the cause of an actor's behavior. They usually consider three types of behavior:
   a. **Consensus:** At first, we consider to the extent to which an individual responds in the same manner to different stimuli or different situation.
   b. **Consistency:** We consider constancy the extent to which this reacts to this stimulus or event in the same way on other occasions.
   c. **Distinctiveness:** The extent to which the person reacts in the same manner other different stimuli and events.
   According to Kelly, low consistency favors an external attribution, but high consistency is compatible with either an internal or external attribution.

2. **James Davis-correspondent inference theory:** This theory describes how with information about others behavior is used as a basis for inferring their stable traits and hence, when we are making attributions about the people, we compare their action with alternative actions, evaluating the choices they have made. Information's about five factors is sought to make there inferences:
   a. Whether the behavior being considered is voluntary and freely chosen.
   b. What is unexpected about the behavior (rare effects)?
   c. Whether the behavior is socially desirable.
   d. Whether the behavior impacts the person doing the inferring.
   e. Whether the behavior is of personal interest the person doing the inferring.

WAYS TO IMPROVE THINKING

1. Keep yourself only with current project, clutters create confusion. Get organized and work with fresh canvas. On an average, we spend about 45 minutes a day looking for things.
2. Dedicate an hour of focus time to your most important task: multi-tasking is highly over-rated and cause a loss of up to 40% efficiency. Get yourself one hour of focused seclusion to work on your most important task.
3. Stir up your visual sense and creative talents with exposure to the arts: Go to a gallery. Pick up an art book or spend time with nature.
4. Learn how to mind map: this is a best practice that allows you to visualize and map your projects, and strategies. It is also a life-saving memory device that will help you remember more and organize your thinking.

5. Give rest for thinking: when you have been working on something for more than an hour, you start losing concentration and focus. So stop, get up and walk around and go back to your work.

ALTERATIONS IN THINKING

Psychosis

Psychosis is a major psychiatric disorder in which reality testing is not intact; behavior may violate gross social norm. It is just opposite to nervous in which reality testing is intact and behavior may not violate social norms. Many psychiatric disorders such as schizophrenia, mania, depression, etc. come under psychosis. It includes various disturbances in thinking.

DELUSION

Delusion is a false, persistent, irrational belief not shared by persons of some age, race, education, standard which cannot be altered by logical arguments.

Types of Delusions

Sl. No	Type	Description
1.	Persecutory delusions	The individuals feel interfered, discriminates against, threatened or mistreated, e.g. the patient says, my family members wants to kill me.
2.	Delusion of reference	The individual feels that others are talking about him, other's remarks/actions have special significance for him.
3.	Delusions of influence/ passivity	The individual believes the he is influenced by and controlled by others. For example, the cardiologist puts transmitter near heart that controls my feelings and thoughts.
4.	Delusion of sin and guilt	The individual has a belief that he has committed unforgivable sin/ some wickedness in past leads to calamity to others. So he is evil and worthless.
5.	Hypochondrical delusions	These are delusions of some bodily diseases.
6.	Delusion of grandeur	The individual has an exaggerated feeling of importance, power, knowledge or identity.

CONCLUSION

Thinking starts with a problem and concludes with its solution. This activity of thinking continuous till either the solution is found or till the person becomes fatigued by the effort. There cannot be any thinking in the absence of some problem. Problems in human life come in an incessant stream and they have to be solved by thinking. Thinking, the mental solution of problem, makes use of the symbols of objects instead of the objects. Thinking attempts the solution of problems by employing the trial and error method. There is a kind of flow in the activity of thinking, one problem leading to the thinking of another by reminding the person of that other problem. The instruments of thinking-images, imagination, signs, indications and such are also called internal. Thinking continues to be an internal activity unless and until it takes form of verbal thinking.

BIBLIOGRAPHY

1. Bartlett F. Thinking, Basic Books, New York, 1958.
2. Borirg EC, Langfield HS, Weld HP (Ed). Foundation of Psychology, (Indian Edi), John Wiley, New York, 1961.
3. Davis G. Psychology of Problem Solving. Basic Books, New York, 1973.
4. Fentino E, Reynold G. Introduction to Contemporary' Psychology, W.H. Freeman & Co, San Francisco, 1975.
5. Garrett HE. General Psychology (Indian Edi), Eurasia Publishing House, New Delhi, 1968.
6. Gates AG. Elementary Psychology (Reprint), Macmillan, New York, 1947.
7. Gates Al, et. al. Educational Psychology, Macmillan, New York, 1947.
8. Gilmer B, Vonhaller. Psychology (International Edi), Harper, New York, 1970.
9. Mohsin SM. Elementary Psychology, Asia Publishing House, Kolkata, 1967.
10. Morgan CT, King RA. Introduction to Psychology, 6th edn, Tata McGraw-Hill, New Delhi, 1982.
11. Morgan CT. A Brief Introduction to Psychology. Tata McGraw-Hill, New Delhi, 1975.
12. Munn NL. An Introduction to Psychology (Indian Edi.) Oxford & IBH, New Delhi, 1967.
13. Munn Norman L. Introduction to Psychology, Oxford and IBH, New Delhi, 1973.
14. Robinson DN. An Intellectual History of Psychology, Macmillan, New York, 1976.
15. Ross JS. Ground of Educational Psychology, George O. Harrap & Co, London, 1951.
16. Skinner CE (Ed). Essentials of Educational Psychology, Prentice-Hall, Englewood, Cliffs, New Jersey, 1968.
17. Valentine CW. Psychology and its Bearing on Education, The English Language Book Society & Methuen, London, 1965.
18. Vinacke WE. The Psychology of Thinking (2nd edn), McGraw-Hill, New York, 1974.
19. Wertheimer M. Productive Thinking. Harper, New York, 1945.
20. Woodworth RS, Marquis DG. Psychology 5th edn, Henry Holt & Co, New York, 1948.
21. Woodworth RS. Psychology, Methuen, London, 1945.

18 *Aptitude*

DEFINITIONS

1. **Aptitude:** Aptitude is a combination of characteristics indicative of an individual's capacity to acquire (with training) some specific knowledge, skill or set of organized responses, such as the ability to speak a language, to become a musicians, to do mechanical work.

2. Mechanical aptitude is not a single unitary function, it is a combination of sensory and motor capacities plus perception of spatial relations, the capacity to acquires information about the mechanical matters and the capacity to comprehend mechanical relationships.

3. **Clerical aptitude test:** Clerical aptitude is also a composite function it involves several specific abilities like, perceptual ability, intellectual and motor ability.

4. **Professional aptitude:** The aptitude related to the activities of various professions and occupations are included in this category. These aptitudes are able to predict the future success of an individual in the field or profession related to these aptitudes.

5. **General aptitude test:** Battery developed by the employment service bureau of USA has 12 tests, eight of which are paper pencil tests as for name comparison, computation, vocabulary, arithmetic, reasoning from matching, test matching, three dimensional spaces, etc. The other four require the use of simple equipment in the shape of moving pegs on boards, assembling and dissembling rivets and washers.

6. **Differential aptitude test (DAT):** Differential aptitude test developed by USA psychological corporation. It has proved more successful in predicting academic success and found especially useful for providing educational and vocational guidance to secondary school children.

7. **Abstract reasoning test:** This test is intended as a verbal measure of the student's reasoning yielding ability. It has many picture test yielding ambiguous scores because they require the student to discriminate between lines and areas which differ slightly in size and shape. This test supplements the general intelligence aspects of the verbal and numerical tests.

8. **Graphic art test:** It requires the subject to produce sketches from given patterns of lines and figures. The created sketches of the subject are then evaluated according the standard given by the author of this test.

9. **Verbal reasoning:** It is a measure of ability to understand concepts framed in words. It is aimed at evaluation of the student's ability to abstract or generalize and to think constructively, rather than simple fluency or vocabulary recognition. The words used in these items may come from history, geography, literature, science, or any other content area.

10. **Space relations:** It is the ability to visualize a constructed object from a picture of a pattern and an ability to imagine how an object would appear if rotated in various ways for

measurement of space perception. It means that these tests require mental manipulation of objects in three dimensional spaces.

INTRODUCTION

It is an observable fact the people differ from one another and within themselves in their performance in one or the other field of human activity such as leadership, music, art, mechanical work, teaching, etc. We usually come across the individuals who under similar circumstances excel the other persons in acquiring certain specific jobs. Such persons are said to possess certain specific abilities or aptitudes, besides general intellectual abilities or intelligence, which help them in achieving success in some specific occupations or activities. Therefore, in a simple way, aptitude may be considered a special ability or specific capacity besides the general ability which helps an individual to acquire a required degree of proficiency or achievement in a specific field.

MEANING AND CONCEPTS OF APTITUDE

An aptitude is the capacity of a person to achieve along special lines. It is a special tendency, bent, fitness or aptness due to a special neural or muscular organization possessed by the individual. Aptitudes make for special abilities and our achievements in special areas. Some of the well-known aptitudes are the mechanical, artistic, musical, numerical or nursing aptitudes. Aptitude is to be distinguished from present ability. It shows that although a certain individual does not possess certain ability, he can acquire it or have it, provide the opportunities are available. Specific aptitudes can be assessed by means of specific aptitude tests. They can help us in knowing people who will be able to acquire a high degree of proficiency in fairly specific skills within minimum of training. The results of aptitude teats can be used for vocational guidance and adjustment.

1. An aptitude may be considered a special ability or specific capacity besides the general intellectual ability which helps an individual to acquired degree of proficiency or achievement in a specific field.
2. An aptitude is the interaction of heredity and environment. An individual is born with certain potentialities and begins to learn immediately. Therefore, everything he learns enables him to learn still more.
3. It embraces any characteristics which predisposes to learning including intelligence, achievements, personality, interests and special skills.
4. Intelligence is concerned with the general mental ability of an individual, but aptitude is related to specific abilities. Thus, the knowledge of intelligence of an individual predicts his success in a number of situations involving mental function or activity.
5. Usually, interest and aptitude go hand in hand. A person must have aptitude for activity and an interest in a given activity to desirable success. But interest and aptitude both are not one and same way.
6. Aptitude is measured by tests of general mental activity which are used to facilitate prediction of scholastic success.

DEFINITIONS OF APTITUDE

1. Aptitude refers to those qualities characterizing a person's ways of behavior which serves to indicate how well he can learn to meet and solve certain specified kinds of problems—*Bingham*.
2. Aptitude is a condition a quality or a set of qualities in an individual which is indicative of the probable extent to which he will be able to acquire under suitable training, some knowledge, skill or composite

of knowledge, understanding and skill, such as ability to contribute to art or music, mechanical ability, mathematical ability to read and speak a foreign language—*Traxler*.

3. An aptitude is a combination of characteristics indicative of an individual's capacity to acquire (with training) some specific knowledge, skill or set of organized responses, such as the ability to speak a language, to become a musicians, to do mechanical work—*Freeman*.

DIFFERENCE BETWEEN INTELLIGENCE AND APTITUDE

Area	Intelligence	Aptitude
Ability	They exist usually test the general mental ability of an individual.	Aptitudes are concerned with specific abilities.
Knowledge	The knowledge of intelligence of an individual we can predict his success in a number of situation involving mental function or activity.	The knowledge of aptitudes acquaints us with those specific abilities and capacities of an individual which give an indication of his ability or capacity to succeed in a special field or activity.
Prediction	Predicting achievements of intelligence for general ability.	Predicting achievement in some particular job, training, courses or specialized instruction we need to know more about one's aptitudes (specific abilities).

MEASUREMENT OF APTITUDE

The term intelligence, ability, and aptitude are often used interchangeably to refer to behavior that is used to predict future learning or performance. However, subtle differences exit between the terms. Like intelligence tests, aptitude tests measure a student's overall performance across a broad range of mental capabilities. But aptitude tests also include items which measure more specialized abilities-such as verbal and numerical skills that predict scholastic performance in educational programs.

Specific nature of aptitudes tests:
1. Mechanical aptitude tests.
2. Musical aptitude tests.
3. Art judgment tests.
4. Professional aptitude tests, i.e. tests to measure the aptitudes for professionals like teaching, salesmanship, research work, etc.
5. Scholastic aptitude tests, i.e. tests to measure the aptitude for different course of institution.

Mechanical Aptitude Test

Some persons have a specific bent of mind for the tasks related to the use of mechanical abilities and thus demonstrate their aptitude for all tasks and job that require the use of mechanical abilities. The term mechanical aptitude is not a single unitary function. It is a combination of sensory and motor capacities plus perception of spatial relations, the capacity to acquire information about mechanical matters and the capacity to comprehend mechanical relationships. Some of the well known mechanical aptitude tests are:
1. Minnesota mechanical assembly test.
2. Minnesota spatial relation test.
3. The revised Minnesota power form board (1948).

4. Stenquist mechanical aptitude tests (part-I and III).
5. LJO Rourke's mechanical aptitude tests (part-I and III).
6. SRA mechanical aptitude test.
7. Bennet tests of mechanical aptitude tests (Hindi) prepared by mano-vigyanshala, Allahabad.
   Usually these tests contain the items of the following nature.
   a. Asking the subject to put together the parts of mechanical devices.
   b. Asking to replace cut-outs of various shapes in their correct holes in the board.
   c. Requiring the ability to solve problems in geometric terms.
   d. Asking questions concerning the basic information about tools and their uses.
   e. Questions relating to comprehension of physical and mechanical principles.

Clerical Aptitude Tests

Clerical aptitude is also a composite function. According to Bingham, it involves several specific abilities like:
1. **Perceptual ability:** Ability to perceive words and numbers with speed and accuracy.
2. **Intellectual ability:** Ability to grasp the meaning of words and symbols.
3. **Motor ability:** Ability to use various types of machines and tools like typewriter, duplicator, cyclostyle machine, punching machine, etc.

Some of the popular clerical aptitude tests are:
1. Detroit clerical aptitude examination.
2. Minnesota vocational test for clerical works.
3. The clerical ability test prepared by the Department of Psychology University of Mysore, Mysore, Karnataka, India.
4. Clerical aptitude test Battery (English and Hindi), Bureau of Education and Vocational Guidance, Patna, Bihar, India.
5. Test of clerical aptitude prepared by the Parsee Panchayat Guidance Bureau 209, Hornby road, Mumbai, Maharashtra, India.

Sensory Aptitude Test

In this category, we can include all those aptitude which are related to the sensory capacities and abilities of the children. One may have aptitude in the task related to the use of his sense of hearing; other may have aptitude in the task related to the use of the sense of sight, sense of smell, sense of taste or sense of touch. Here depending upon their present ability concerning the particular sensory capacity, we can have an idea of their future success in the area or professions where the use of such sensory ability or capacity is most demanded.

Musical Aptitude Tests

These tests have been devised for discovering musical talent. One of these important musical aptitude tests is discovered below;
   Seashore measure of musical talent: it gives consideration to the following musical components:
1. Discrimination of pitch.
2. Discrimination of intensity of loudness.
3. Determination of time interval.
4. Discrimination of timbre.
5. Judgment of rhythm.
6. Tonal memory.
The instruction in these tests is of following nature:

You will hear two tones which differ in pitch. You are to judge whether the second is higher or lower than the first. If the second is higher, record H; if lower, record L.

Aptitude for Graphic Art

These tests are devised to discover the talent for graphic art. The two important tests of this nature are:

1. The meier art judgment test.
2. Horne art aptitude inventory.

   In meier art judgment test there are 100 pairs of representational pictures in black and white. One member of each pair is an acknowledged art masterpiece while the other is a slight distortion of the masterpiece. It is usually altered from the original so as to violate some important principle of art. Tests are informed regarding which aspect has been altered and are asked to choose from each pairs the one that is better- more pleasing, more artistic, more satisfying. Another important test of measuring aptitude for graphic art is the horn art aptitude inventory. It requires the subject to produce sketches from given patterns to lines and figures. The created sketches of the subject are then evaluated according to the standard given by the author of this test.

Professional Aptitude

The aptitude related to the activities of various professions and occupations are included in this category. These aptitudes are able to predict the future success of an individual in the field or profession related to these aptitudes.

Tests for Scholastic and Professional Aptitudes

For helping in the proper selection of students for the studies of specific courses of professions like engineering, medicine, law, business, management, teaching, etc. the various specific aptitude tests have been designed. Some of these aptitude tests are:

1. Stanford scientific aptitude test by DL Zyve.
2. Science aptitude test (after higher sec. stage) NIE, Delhi.
3. Moss scholastic aptitude test for medical students.
4. Ferguson and Stoddard's law aptitude examination.
5. Tale legal aptitude test.
6. Pre-engineering ability test (education testing services, UAS).
7. Minnesota engineering analogical test.
8. Coxeorleans prognosis test of teaching ability.
9. Teaching aptitude test by Jai Prakash and RP Shrivastav, University of Saugar (MP).
10. Shah's teaching aptitude test.
11. Teaching aptitude test by moss, FA and others, George Washington University Press.

Contemporary Trend in Aptitude Testing

Instead of utilizing specific aptitude tests for measuring specific aptitude in very specific field or area, the trend at present, has now been changed towards multiple aptitude tests battery to find the suitability of people for different professions requiring different abilities on the basis of scores in the relevant aptitude tests in the battery. The examples of such tests are general aptitude test battery (GATB) and differential aptitude test (DAT).

General Aptitude Test (GATB)

Battery developed by the employment service bureau of UAS has 12 tests, eight of which are paper-pencil tests as for name comparison, computation, vocabulary, arithmetic, reasoning form matching, test matching, three dimensional spaces, etc. the other four require the use of simple equipment in the shape of moving pegs on boards, assembling and dissembling rivets and washers. From the scores obtained by the subject, the experimenter is able to draw inferences about the nine aptitude factors intelligence, verbal aptitude, and numerical aptitude, spatial aptitude from perception, clerical perception, motor coordination, finger dexterity, and manual dexterity. The GABA has proven to be one of the most successful multiple aptitude batteries particularly for the purposes of job classification.

Differential Aptitude Test (DAT)

Developed by UAS psychological corporation. It has proved more successful in predicting academic success and found especially useful for providing educational and vocational guidance to secondary school children. The test induced in the battery of DAT is the following:

1. **Verbal reasoning:** It is a measure of ability to understand concepts framed in words. It is aimed at evaluation of the student's ability to abstract or generalize and to think constructively, rather than simple fluency or vocabulary recognition. The word used in these items may come from history, geography, literature, science or any other content area.

2. **Numerical ability:** These items are designed to test understanding of numerical relationships and facility in handling numerical concepts. This test is a measure of the student's ability to reason with numbers, to manipulate numerical relationships to deal intelligently with quantitative materials, educationally, it is important for prediction in such fields as mathematics, physics, chemistry, engineering and other curricula in which quantitative thinking is essential. Various amounts of numerical ability are required in occupations such as laboratory assistant, book-keeper, statistical and shipping clerks as well as in professions related to the physical sciences.

3. **Abstract reasoning:** This test is intended as a verbal measure of the student's reasoning ability. It has many picture test yielding ambiguous scores because they require the student to discriminate between lines are areas which differ but slightly in size and shape. This test supplements the general intelligence aspects of the verbal and numerical tests.

4. **Clerical speed and accuracy:** This test is intended to measure speed of response in a simple perceptual task.
   a. **Perceptual ability:** Ability to perceive words and numbers with speed and accuracy.
   b. **Intellectual ability:** Ability to grasp the meaning of words and symbols.
   c. **Motor ability:** Ability to use various types machines and tools like writer, duplicator, cyclostyle machine, punching machine, etc.

5. **Mechanical reasoning:** This tries to test mechanical aptitude which is a combination of sensory and motor capacities plus perception of spatial relations, the capacity to acquire information about mechanical matters and the capacity to comprehend mechanical relationships.

6. **Space relations:** It is the ability to visualize a constructed object from a picture of a pattern and an ability to imagine how an object would appear if rotated in various ways for measurement of space perception. It means that these tests require mental manipulation of objects in three dimensional spaces.

7. **Language usage:** This test has two sections:
Language usage-1: Spelling
Language usage-2: Grammar.

VALUES OF APTITUDE TESTING

1. They are excellent predictors of future scholastic achievements.
2. They provide ways of comparing a child's performance with that of others children in the same situation.
3. They provide a profile of strength and weaknesses.
4. They assess differences among individuals.
5. They have uncovered hidden talents in some children, thus improving their educational opportunities.
6. They are valuable tools for working with handicapped children.

USES OF APTITUDE TESTS

1. **Instructional:** Teacher can use aptitude test results to adopt their curricula to match the level of their students, or to design assignments for students who differ orderly. Aptitude tests score can also help teachers from realistic expectations of students. Knowing something about the aptitude level of students in a given class can help a teacher identify which students are not learning as much as could be predicted on the basis of aptitude scores. For instance, if a whole class were performing less will than would be predicted form aptitude test results, then curriculum, objectives, teaching methods or student characteristics might be investigated.
2. **Administrative:** Aptitude test scores can identify the general aptitude level of a high school. This can be helpful in determining how much emphasis should be given to college preparatory programs. Aptitude tests can be used to help identify students to be accelerated or given extra attention, foe grouping, and in predicting job training performance.
3. **Guidance:** Guidance counselors use aptitude tests to help parents develop realistic expectations for their child's school performance and to help students understand their own strengths and weakness. These tests are found to be very useful in helping the youngsters as well as youth in the selection of special courses of instruction, fields of activities and vocations.
4. **Educational and vocational:** Aptitude tests can be safely used for the purpose of education and vocational selection. They help us in making scientific selection of the candidates for various educational and professional courses as well as specialized jobs as Munn puts it. The chief values of aptitude testing is, in fact, that it enables us to pick out from those who do not yet have the ability to perform certain skills, those who, with a reasonable amount of training, will be most likely to acquire the skills in question and acquire them to a desirable level of proficiency.

APTITUDE AND NURSING

Aptitude is to be distinguished from present ability. A certain nurse may not at present have the ability to act as a operation theater nurse working with the surgeon, but she is clever and quick, able to think ahead and foresee what will be needed. She possesses a high degree of aptitude for theater work and has good chances with proper training of becoming a very successful operation theater nurse. Nursing is an arts and science, which requires high degree of aptitude for being a good bedside nurse. The nurse needs to foresee the need and progress of the patient. The aptitude differs from one area to another based on their application of nursing.

CONCLUSION

Aptitude tests properly anticipate the future potentialities or capacities of an individual and thereby, help us in making selection of those individuals who are best fitted for a particular profession and course of instruction or those who are likely to be more benefited by the pre-professional training or experiences. Aptitude testing when combined with the other information received through interest inventory, personality tests, intelligence tests and cumulative record, etc. can help, to a greater extent, in avoiding the huge wastage of human as well as material resources by placing the individuals to their proper places and lines of work.

BIBLIOGRAPHY

1. Bhatia HR. Element of Educational Psychological, Orient Longman (3rd edn reprint), Kolkata, 1968.
2. Bigge Moris L. Learning Theories of Teachers (First Indian reprint), Universal Book Stall, Delhi, 1967.
3. Biggie ML, Hunt MP. 'Psychological Foundations of Education, Harper and Row, New York, 1968.
4. Bingham WV. Aptitude and Aptitude Testing, Haper & Brothers, New York, 1937.
5. Binnet A, Simon T. The Development of Intelligence in Children, Williams and Wilkins, Baltimore, 1916.
6. Blair GH, Jones RS, Sirnpsonn RH. Educational Psychology, Macmillan, New York, 1954.
7. Boring EC, Lang Field HS, Weld HP (Eds). Foundations of Psychology, New York.
8. Brown JF. Educational Sociology (5th edn), Prentice Hall, New York, 1960.
9. Brown JF. The Psychodynamics of Abnormal Behaviour (Indian Reprint), Asia Publishing House, New Delhi, 1969.
10. Hull CL. Aptitude Testing, World Book Co, Youkers, New York, 1928.
11. Korman AK. The Psychology of Motivation, Prentice Hall, Englewood Cliffs, NJ, 1974.
12. Seashore CE. Seashore, Measures of Musical Talents, Psychological Cooperation, New York, 1960.

Attitude

19

DEFINITIONS

1. **Attitude:** Attitude is evaluation expressed by terms such as liking-disliking, pro-anti, favoring-not favoring and positive-negative. They are the feeling tone aroused by any attitude object. Attitude is thought to guide behavior. e.g. if you are unfavorable toward smoking, you will show negative attitude towards smokers.

2. **Cognitive dissonance:** When two contradictory feelings, beliefs or behaviors exist, it creates a state of tension and the person tries to reduce tension by changing their feelings, beliefs or behaviors. For example, if a student nurse studies hard for a test, she expects to do well. But if she studies hard and fails, dissonance is aroused.

3. **Unconscious motivation:** Some attitudes are held because they serve some unconscious function for an individual. For example, a person who is threatened by his homosexual feelings may employ the defense mechanism of reaction formation and become a crusader against homosexuals.

4. **Rational analysis:** Involves the careful weighing of evidence for and against a particular attitude. The nurses giving health education to slums will influence their attitude for personal hygiene when informing about rationale of unhygienic conditions.

5. **Commitment:** It is the extent to which he feels reluctant to give up his initial position (attitude). Greater the strength of commitment to his own attitude, it is harder for the individual to change his attitude.

6. **Resistance to change/persuasion:** Attitudes socialized early in life and to which the person is highly committeed, do not change very much in adulthood. They are largely unaffected by mass communications or life changes like aging, geographical mobility, social mobility.

7. **Attitude relevance:** Because our world abounds with attitude issues, each of us can be concerned only with a limited number of issues, those which are of special importance to us. It has been suggested recently that relevant attitudes are a better guide to subsequent behavior than are irrelevant attitudes. That is, for any given attitude issue, the link or correlation between attitudes and behavior should be much stronger for those individuals for whom the attitude is relevant than for those for whom it is not. This effect has been demonstrated for experimentally induced relevance.

8. **Selective attention and interpretation:** Whether a message will influence a recipient depends upon how it is perceived and interpreted. Most important, it depends upon whether the message is attended to in the first place.

9. **Influenceability:** Most personality traits are not related to the ease with which someone is persuaded. A person's general personality profile will be of little use in predicting whether

a given message will be persuasive. It is known, however, that some people are more easily influenced than others and that some people are downright gullible. The latter, bombarded with conflicting viewpoints, will believe the one they heard most recently. As might be expected, there are group differences in this trait. Obviously, children are more easily influenced than are adults, and poorly educated people are more easily influenced than are the well-educated.

10. **Suggestion:** Advertisers and propagandists often rely on suggestion, the uncritical acceptance of a statement. They design their messages in hopes that people will accept a belief, form an attitude, or be incited to action by someone else's say-so, without requiring facts.

INTRODUCTION

Attitudes are not innate or unlearned like our physiological motives or some emotional reactions. They are acquired by us. Some of them are built by us by our effort. Others are absorbed by us passively and spontaneously from the social environment into which we are born and in which we grow. Many of our attitudes are the result of reflection and purposeful thinking or the outcome of training and suggestion from others, especially our parents and teachers. Attitude is the evaluation of an object, person, behavior or event based on beliefs guiding behavior of an individual. Psychologists have defined an attitude in any diverse ways. Kimball Young defines an attitude as a predisposition to respond, in a persistent and characteristic manner……. In references to some situation, idea, value, material objects or class of objects or person or group of persons. This can be positive, negative or neutral views of an attitude object, example, person, behavior or an event.

DEFINITIONS OF ATTITUDE

1. An attitude denotes an adjustment of the individual towards some selected person, group or organization—*Kuppusamy*.
2. An attitude is the entire package of particular beliefs, feelings, and response tendencies of the individual towards the appropriate object—*Kerch and others*.
3. Attitude is a mental structure of framework that includes motivational, perceptual, emotional and cognitive reactions. The positive or negative reaction of a person to his environment, other persons and objects is based on his attitude.
4. Attitude is a permanent disposition of a person towards an object, subject or thought that tends him to react in accordance with his interests.
5. Attitudes are the manifestation of a person's concepts, thoughts or imaginations, which direct his behavior towards a specific direction.

COMPONENTS OF ATTITUDE

1. **Cognitive component:** The opinion or belief segment of an attitude. It is made up of thoughts and beliefs the people hold about the object of the attitude. It is therefore, what we have learned about something. It is what we believe to be true about it. For example, vegetarian food is healthy.
2. **Affective component:** It is the emotion or feeling segment of an attitude. The affective component is the matter of liking or disliking something. This consists of the emotional feelings stimulated by the object of the attitude. For example, I like vegetarian food.
3. **Behavioral component:** An intention to behave in a certain way towards someone or something. The action component of attitudes refers to a readiness to respond. Thus expressed attitudes usually have a consistent relationship to behavior. For example, I always eat vegetarian food.

NATURE OF ATTITUDE

Attitudes are universal; they are either positive or negative and are found towards social as well as nonsocial aspects of the environment. These attitude are not innate, they are acquired. It implies subject-object relationship. Attitude of respect towards our elders is a positive attitude, whereas, an attitude of hatred towards a certain community is a negative attitude. It is a way we perceive, think and feel more or less permanently in relation to something. It is a sort of mental readiness or a tendency to react to certain situations, in a more or less consistent manner. We have acquired certain set ways of reacting to religious rituals to political democracy, to social equality, to our parents and teachers, to various racial, communal and religious groups, to people exercising authority over us, to our colleagues who work us, to our own profession and its prestige, and to other professions.

1. Attitude is evaluation expressed by terms such as liking-disliking, pro-anti, favoring-not favoring and positive-negative. They are the feeling tone aroused by any attitude object.
2. Attitudes are thought to guide behavior. Example: if you are unfavorable toward smoking, you show negative attitudes towards smokers.
3. The expressions that one makes publicly to others are not always the same as the expressions one makes privately to one self.
4. They are feeling tones aroused by any attitude object. Attitudes can be formed about many things. The object of attitudes can be entities (a lecture, a restaurant), people (my parents, siblings, prime minister, myself) or abstract concepts (abortion, civil rights, foreign aid).
5. The attitude varies. The attitude may be similar towards some of the objects and different towards others.
6. Individuals are not fully aware of their attitudes, and this accounts in part for possible inconsistency of attitudes with one another.
7. The attitude attempts to understand the motives they serve for the individual.
8. It provides a ready basis for interpreting the world and processing new information.
9. It is a way of gaining and maintaining social interaction.
10. Attitude is a hypothetical construct that represents an individual's likes or dislikes for an item.
11. Attitudes that are accompanied by strong feeling tones are called sentiments. These can be positive or negative. We may have sentiments of love for our country, a sentiment of respect for our elders or a sentiment of hatred for dishonesty and lying.

MOTIVATIONAL FUNCTIONS OF ATTITUDE

Katz (1960) has suggested four motivational functions of attitudes; they are knowledge, social adjustment, value expression and ego defenses.

1. **Knowledge function:** People seek a degree of practicability, consistency and stability in their perception of the world.
2. **Social adjustment function:** It refers to the favorable responses the individual achieves from others by displaying socially acceptable attitudes.
3. **Value expression function:** The value expressive function of attitudes, the individual achieves self-expression with regard of cherished values.
4. **Ego-defensive function:** The ego-defensive function allows the individual to be protected from acknowledging personal deficiencies.

DEVELOPMENT OF ATTITUDES

Attitudes of person are the permanent ways of one's behaving. These are the acquired characteristics of a person, which are reflected in his work and behavior. Many of our attitudes are the result of reflection and purposeful thinking or the outcome of training and suggestion from others, especially our parents and teachers. Children whose parents show respect and courtesy to others acquire attitudes of respect and courtesy to most human being without being especially told about it. The simply take suggestions from their parents unconsciously. Our motives, our emotional conditions, our schooling, cultural norms, the type of parent-child relationships that obtains in childhood, the way we have been taught to perceive thing, propaganda-all these factors affect the growth of our attitudes.

Our attitude also influenced by the type and quantity of the factual knowledge that we acquire about situation, things and person. Many a time we may develop hostile attitudes towards a person because what we have been told about him does evoke hostility or aggression. Many of our attitudes are the result of wrong or false knowledge that is available to us. The best expample is our prejudices and biases. We may have acquired this knowledge from newspaper, journals, books, the movie, or the political speeches. The cognitive components of attitudes are assumed to be learned in the same ways as are any facts, knowledge of beliefs. The basic processes of association, reinforcement and imitation determine this acquisition.

1. **Association and reinforcement:** Child exposed to certain things about the world. He is reinforced for expressing some cognitions or attitudes or for actual acting on the basis of them, thus he learns them.
2. **Imitation/Identification:** It is important in the learning process. A child spends a great deal of time with his parents and after a while begins to believe as they do simply by copying them, even when they do not deliberately try to influence him.
3. **Classical conditioning:** It involves involuntary responds and is acquired through the pairing of two stimuli. Two events that repeatedly occur close together in time become fused and before long the person responds in the same way to both events. Example pleasant and unpleasant experiences with members of a particular group could lead to positive or negative attitudes towards the group.
4. **Social (Observational):** Learning is based on modeling. We observe others. If they are getting reinforced for certain behaviors or expression of certain attitudes, makes it more likely that we, too will behaves in this manner or express this attitude.
5. **Cognitive dissonance:** When two contradictory feelings, beliefs or behaviors exist it creates a state of tension and the person tries to reduce tension by changing their feelings, beliefs, or behaviors.
6. **Unconscious motivation:** Some attitudes are held because they serve some unconscious function for an individual. For example, a person who is threatened by his homosexual feelings may employ the defense mechanism of reaction formation and become a crusader against homosexuals.
7. **Rational analysis:** Involves the careful weighing of evidence for against a particular attitude. The nurse giving health education to slums will influence their attitude for personal hygiene when informing about rationale of unhygienic conditions.
8. **Other factors:** Even after a child develops attitudes, he continues to be exposed primarily to information that supports it. At this stage, various socio-economic factors determine what he hears. His neighborhood, newspaper, school, church, friend's, etc. tend to be more homogeneous than the rest of the world.

CHANGING ATTITUDES

An individual attitude are formed during the childhood stages as a result of socialization and later on when he meets and interacts with the peer group in later childhood, adolescence and early childhood. When an individual says a smoker is confronted with communication from the communicator that cigarette smoking causes lung cancer. Now, the stress is produced by the discrepancy between the individual's attitude and the attitude expressed in the communication. This stress has been called conflict, incongruity, imbalance, or just inconsistency. Therefore, there is pressure on the individual to resolve the discrepancy. If the individual changes his attitude in the direction advocated by the communication, the discrepancy is reduced. Hence, the stress is resolved.

Attitude change can be either:
1. **Congruent change:** Example, already negative attitude will increase too negatively or positive attitude will increase too positively, i.e. change in the same direction.
2. **Incongruent change:** Example, the attitude change from positive to negative or from negative to positive. In other words, the change will be in the same direction.

Change of Attitude

Once the attitudes and beliefs have been formed they have a tendency to persist or continue. It is therefore, difficult to change the attitudes that have been established. There are many reasons for our inability to change them easily. One of the reasons is that we don't want to change on account of the social support we have acquired for them in order to change attitudes and beliefs we should a. change perceptions by new experiences and factual knowledge, b. control emotions and motivational factors in early childhood when most of our daily attitudes are formed, and c. tap the various formative agencies.

CHARACTERISTICS OF ATTITUDES

1. Attitudes are related to the needs and problems of the person.
2. Unconscious mind plays an important role in the formation of attitudes.
3. A series of emotional experiences is attached to attitudes.
4. Attitudes direct the activities or actions of person.
5. The reaction of a person towards an object, issue or environment can be predicted by knowing his attitudes.
6. Attitudes are related to some thoughts, images and external objects.

EFFECTS OF ATTITUDES ON BEHAVIOR

Attitudes manifest the nature of person, and they direct the behavior of person. Hence, favorable or positive attitudes (kindness, service, and assistance) are the indicators of good behavior, while unfavorable or negative attitudes (hate, non-cooperation, selfishness, etc.) express the bad behavior of person. It is easy to provide nursing to the patients having favorable attitude towards hospital, while the behavior of patients with negative attitudes towards hospital, may create obstacles in their nursing treatment. Similarly, nurses and doctors should adopt a professional attitude towards the patients.

THEORIES OF ATTITUDE CHANGE

Balance Theory

1. This theory given by Heider (1946, 1958) emphasized the positive and negative valences of attitudes towards or persons which might not agree with one another.

2. There is always movement toward a balance state, a situation in which the relations fit together harmoniously, and then there is no stress.
3. The basic concept of the balance is that a tendency exists for individuals to restore balance to attitude which are not of the same sign.
4. Heider's P-O-X Model explains situations in which there are two person, a perceiver P and an other O, each of whom might have an attitude toward a given object, X.
5. If P likes O, the assumption is that O's attitude toward X should be the same as P's for example, two staff nurses might share a common positive attitude toward ward sister. If they differed on that issue, than an imbalance state would exist. In that case, they might try to persuade each other or also avoid the topic until the duty was over in order to retain at least apparent balance.
6. These theory statements are shown by plus or minus signs. It predicts that when all signs are positive, a state of balance exists. If there is one negative sign or three negative signs, the outcome is negative leading to an imbalance state (just like multiplication of two minuses yields a plus). Therefore, balance occurs when there are either in negative sign or two negative signs.

Congruity Theory

1. Osgood and Tannenbanum (1955) postulates that imbalance between attitudes is resolved by summing the amount of their positive or negative quality. There is a pair of attitudes on which one has a positive sign and one has a negative sign.
2. The greater the amount of the positive or negative quality of an attitude, the less likely it is to change when paired with something of an opposite sign. The valence goes from +3 to -3 on the usual attitude scale.
3. Suppose you dislike a public figure at the highest scale value of +3 and then learn that he favors a policy which you dislike at the relatively moderate level of -1.
4. The prediction is that you are more likely to alter the attitude toward the policy, in a more favorable, a positive direction rather than the attitude toward the political figure in an unfavorable direction.
5. However, the actual results may be a less negative or neutral attitude, rather than a positive one. Abelson's and Rosenberg (1958) gave three rules of cognitive interaction, are:
   a. A likes B and B likes C that A likes C ALSO.
   b. A likes B and B dislikes C implies that A dislikes C.
   c. A dislikes B and B dislikes C implies that A likes C.

Cognitive Dissonance Theory (Festinger, 1957)

1. When related cognitions, feelings or behaviors are inconsistent or contradictory, it creates an unpleasant state of tension that motivates people to reduce their dissonance by changing their cognitions, feeling or behavior.
2. For instance a person who starts out with a negative attitude toward marijuana and finds themselves enjoys the experience.
3. The dissonance they experience is thus likely to motivate to change their attitude toward marijuana, or to stop using marijuana.

MEASUREMENT OF ATTITUDES

Self Report Methods

It includes attitude scales, questionnaires, interviews and projective tests. When you are asked to express your preferences, likes and dislikes to an interviewer or to write your evolution of something on a questionnaire.

1. Attitudes are measured by attitude scales which deal with an issue or set of related issues. These depict the direction of an attitude, the degree or extent in that direction and the intensity of feeling that goes with the attitude.
2. Sometimes these components may be a part of questionnaire studies and interviews in which people are asked, first, how (pro or con) they feel about something and then how strongly they feel. Finally these rates are highly related.
3. Attitudes scales typically consist of a number of statements with which a person may agree or disagree with several scale points, usually ranging from highly agree or highly disagree. In this way, both the direction and the degree are indicated by the response to each statement or item.
4. Typically, these items relate to some common social thing, person, issue, person's overall attitude.
5. Attitude scales commonly used are Thurstone's scale, Likert's scale, paried comparison method and rank order method.

Thurstone's Scale (Methods of Equal-appearing Intervals)

1. Louis L Thurstone and EJ Chave (1929) in their classic study of attitudes towards the church developed an interval scale by using the method of equal-appearing intervals.
2. Since, the scale represents an evenly graduated series of attitudes as in the foot rule the method is named so.
3. Every statement in Thurstone's scale has a numerical value already determined.
4. The subject has to place a tick mark against each item with which he/she agrees. The attitude score is the mean of the scale value.

Likert's Scale (Summated Rating)

1. For the Likert's scale, various opinion statements are collected, edited and then given to a group of subjects to rate the statements on a five-point scale: strongly disagree, agree undecided, disagree and strongly disagree.
2. The subject expresses the degree (1-5) of their personal agreement or disagreement with each of the statements.
3. The respondent's attitude score in the sum of her/his rating of all the statements. For this reason, the Likert's scale is also known as the scale of summated ratings.

Bogardus Social-Distance Scale

1. ES Bogardus developed an attitude scale in 1933, called the social-distance scale, which become a classic instrument to measure attitudes towards ethnic group.
2. He was the first one to design a technique for the specific purposes of measuring and comparing attitudes toward different nationalities, particularly measuring tolerance of out-group.
3. The subject is asked to indicate the extent of his willingness to accept members of different social groups into various social institutions.

Observations of Behavior

1. It is a method of studying the behavior, consists of the perception of an individual's attitude under conditions by the other individuals and analysis of his perceived attitude by them.
2. By this method, we can infer the mental processes of other persons through the observation of their.
3. For example, observing the actual overt behavior of students in natural situation.

ATTITUDE AND NURSE

While giving nursing services in the hospital, the nurse has to deal with patients having all kinds of attitudes, simultaneously: she also has to adjust with her personal and professional attitudes. A nurse should try to understand her patient's attitudes. Some of them enter hospital ready and willing to cooperate, others enter hospital afraid or resentful or event definitely antagonistic to the ideas of receiving treatment and to the rigidity of ward routine.

Kempf and Averill list the following attitudes for a successful and efficient nurse:
1. Ambition to do her task.
2. Conformity with the rules and regulations of the profession for which she is preparing.
3. Willingness to work and to work with effectiveness.
4. Cheerfulness and optimism.
5. Interest in the problems and difficulties of other people.
6. Co-cooperativeness, industriousness, respect for the opinion and judgment of others.
7. Interest in increasing the fund of knowledge underlying effective nursing care.
8. Determination to grow professionally.
9. Maintenance of poise and self-control in all professional situations.
10. Maintaining a consistent pride in their profession.
11. Arising to the unexpected without undue panic.
12. Determination to make the patient comfortable by giving attention to small details that mean so much to the patient's well-being.

CONCLUSION

Attitudes are not inborn but acquired. A person develops his behavior pattern in accordance with knowledge, experiences and emotions. Such behavior becomes a relatively permanent basis of his actions. Parents, teachers, religious leaders, literature and media, etc. have an extensive impact on the development of attitudes. Healthy attitudes like kindness, generosity; self-less service, etc. must be encouraged. The nurse needs to develop and cultivate professional attitude which will contribute to her being successful in her work. The nurse should try to find out the cause of the unfavorable attitudes and should change them to favorable ones, because favorable attitudes help in treatment and recovery.

BIBLIOGRAPHY

1. Aggarwal JC. Education Vocational Guidance and Counseling revised and enlarged 8th edn, Doaba House; New Delhi; 1998, Chapter 23, 257-71.
2. Basvanthappa BT. Nursing Education. 2nd edn, Jaypee Brothers Medical Publications, New Delhi.
3. Best W John, Kahn V James. Research in Education. 7th Edn; Asoke K Ghosh; Prentice Hall of India Pvt Ltd, New Delhi, 2002, 25, 26, 106-07.
4. Flippo Edwin B. Principles of Personnel Management, McGraw Hill, New York, 1975.
5. George K Aleyamma. Principles of Curriculum Development and Evaluation; Vivekananda Press, Nammakkal, Tamil Nadu 2002, Chapter 5, evaluation, 120-90.
6. Gupta CB. Principles and Practice of Management, 4th edn, National Publishing House, New Delhi 316-30.
7. Hall CS, Lindzey G. Theories of personality (2nd edn). Wiley, New York 1970.
8. Hall E. A conversation with Jean Piaget and Barbel Inhelder. Psychology Today, 1970; 3, 25-32, 54-56.
9. Heidgerhen H Loretta. Teaching and Learning in School of Nursing. Principles, 3rd edn, Konark Publishing Pvt Ltd, Delhi, 1994; 629-68.
10. Maslow A. Motivation and Personality, Haper & Row, New York, 1954.
11. White Alan R. Attention, Oxford: Blackwell, 1964.

20 *Mental Health and Mental Hygiene*

DEFINITIONS

1. **Mental health:** Mental health is a sound, efficient mind and controlled emotions. It is the total and harmonious functioning of the whole personality of an individual for optimum functioning with maximum realization. A positive mental health shows an individual's ability to cope with the present and to adjust satisfactorily in future. A state of compromise and adaptation to a situation in his life leads to better adjustment. He fulfils his responsibilities, function effectively and is satisfied with his interpersonal relationships arid himself.

2. **Mental hygiene:** Mental hygiene is an art and science which includes application of scientific principles and practices for the promotion, preservation and maintenance of mental health and prevention of mental disorders, enjoys healthy practices to lead productive, happy and contended life.

3. **Defense mechanism:** Defense mechanism is a pattern of adjustment through which an individual relieves or decreases anxieties caused by an uncomfortable situation that threatens self-esteem. Ego defense mechanism is consciously or unconsciously operating device to keep confliction issues out of consciousness of the individual to bring some protective measures.

4. **Denial:** It is protecting self from unpleasant reality by refusal to perceive it or face it. It is a defense mechanism in which a person is faced with a fact that is too painful to accept and reject it. The individual may deny the reality of the unpleasant fact altogether, admit the fact but deny its seriousness or admit both the fact and seriousness but denies responsibility. The concept of denial is particularly important to the study of addiction.

5. **Distortion:** A gross reshaping of external reality to meet internal needs.
   For example, mentally ill patients have no intact contact with reality. These patients are suffering with psychosis.

6. **Delusional projection:** Grossly frank delusions about external reality, usually of a persecutory nature. This defense mechanism is common feature of psychotic mental illnesses like schizophrenia, delusional disorder, etc.
   These delusions are the false beliefs of the person which are not shared by race, age, educational background, etc. Like, the person says that his family members are planning to kill him very soon.

7. **Hypochondriasis:** The transformation of negative feelings towards others into negative feelings toward self, pain, illness and anxiety. Hypochondrias (or hypochondria), sometimes referred to as health phobia, refers to an excessive preoccupation or worry about having a serious illness.

Often, hypochondria persist even after a physician has evaluated a person and reassured him/ her that his/her concerns about symptoms do not have an underlying medical basis.

8. Adjustment is defined as an interaction between a person and his environment by which he adapts depends upon his personal characteristics and circumstances of a situation producing a more harmonious relationship between himself and his environment.

9. **Stress:** Stress may be defined as "an adjustive demand placed on the organism. The condition or force or object giving rise to this demand may be internal or external and is designated as the stressor".

10. **Super ego:** According to Freud, the part of the personality that acquires the values and ideals of the parents and society and imposes constraints on the id and ego, the conscience.

INTRODUCTION

Mentally healthy person is the one who is able to make adjustments, fully mature, able to evaluate him, leading a regular life, having balanced behavior and satisfied with his job, etc. Mental health is the ability of a person to make personal and social adjustments. Actually, it is essential to be mentally healthy for optimum health and well-being. Mental health is an important constituent of optimum health. Mental health is essential for a healthy and successful life. Mental health and physical health are inter-related, and that is the reason behind the popularity of saying healthy mind lives in healthy body. Ancient saints of India have stressed the importance of emotional balance. It means, mental health is the balanced department of a person's personality and emotional attitudes because of which, he becomes capable of living happily with his friends, relatives and environment.

NATURE AND MEANING OF MENTAL HEALTH

1. Mental health is influenced by both biological and social factor.
2. Major importance of mental health is related to the ability of a person to develop pleasant relations with other. Also, it stresses the constructive and positive contribution or participation in the changes of physical and social environment.
3. Mental health is the ability of a person to establish personal and social balance.
4. Mental health is the balanced development of a person's personality and attitudes, which makes him capable of living in harmony with himself and his relatives.
5. Mental health is that ability of a person through which he builds harmonious relations with others and participates or creatively contributes in the changes of his social, physical, or spiritual environment.
6. Mental health is a state of the individual's mind, where he can adjust and adapt to the situations in a harmonious manner, body and mind work together in same direction in order to lead a happy and protective life.
7. A good mental health is the ability to respond to many varied experiences of life with flexibility and a sense of purposes.

DEFINITIONS OF MENTAL HEALTH

1. A mentally healthy person is the one who is comfortable with himself, lives peacefully with his neighbors, brings up his children to be healthy civilians and after completing his basic duties he has the energy and strength to do something for the welfare of society—*PV Luken.*
2. Mental health is a process of adjustment which involves compromise, adaptation, growth, and continuity—*Bhatia and Craig.*

3. Mental health defined as the capacity in an individual to form harmonious relations with others and to participate in, or contribute constructively to the changes in his social and physical environment—*WHO*.
4. Mental heath concerns with the development of wholesome balanced personality, one who does not comfort himself like a series of compartmentalized selves, honest on Sunday, dishonest on Monday, generous today, crabbed tomorrow, reasonable and logical at times, at other times confused and inconsistent—*Waltin, JEW*.
5. Mental health is the full and harmonious functioning of the whole personality—*JA Hadfield*.
6. Mental health is defined as the adjustment of human being to the world and to each other with a maximum of effectiveness and happiness. It is the ability to maintain even temper an alert intelligence, socially considerate behavior and a happy disposition—*KA Menninger*.
7. Mental health is the ability which helps us to seek adjustment in the different situations of our life—*Cutts and Moslay*.
8. Mental health defined as simultaneous success at working, living and creating the capacity for mature and flexible resolution of conflicts between instincts, conscience—*American Psychiatric Association*.
9. Mentally health is defended as a positive but relative quality of life. It is a condition which is characteristic of the average person who meets the demands of life on the basis of his own capacities and limitations—*John, Sutton, and Webster*.

CHARACTERISTICS OF MENTALLY HEALTHY PERSON

Mental health also a state like physical health, this condition can be recognized by its characteristics.

1. **Self evaluation:** A mentally healthy person is aware of his limits, accepts his shortcoming and tries to overcome these. He also introspects to reduce his problem and is able accurately estimate his potential.
2. **Adjusting capacity:** A mentally health person lives in present not in the past dreams of future. He adjusts with the new condition with minimum of pain and sorrow. He is well acquainted with the fact change is the rule of life. Therefore, he is ready for every change.
3. **Maturity:** A mentally healthy person exhibits emotional maturity. He behaves in a responsible manner and expresses his feelings and thoughts clearly. His sexual behavior is also mature.
4. **Non-extremist:** Excess of everything is bad is the right principle for mental health. Excess of any behavior or desire has an adverse effect on health. Being excessively courageous, excessive speaking, lewd or ambitious does not let the person relax, which has an ill effect on health. Therefore, excessive (extremism) should be avoided for the development of mental health.
5. **Regular life:** Healthy habits are the basis of mental health. Regularity of habits, as those of living, eating, sleeping and walking, etc. are essential. Regular habits save time and energy. Mentally healthy people are able to accomplish all works of life in a natural and mature manner, without any problem.
6. **Good social relationship:** A mentally healthy person maintains good social relations with the people of society, colleagues and family members. Mutual cooperation helps in the building and development of personality. Goodwill and good behavior is more important for such people. Balanced relations in society help in the development of mental health.
7. **Job satisfaction:** Being satisfied with one's job or occupation is essential for mental health. Dissatisfaction with work gives birth to frustrations. Hence, one should increase interest in his job by making adjustments to achieve satisfaction and thus the standard of mental health can be increased.

8. **Other characteristics:** Mentally healthy person do not daydream, they expert in social etiquettes. They exhibit the capacity to tolerate stress and exhibit the ability to take decisions as per the situation. Mentally healthy person pay attention to make balance in every aspect of life, work and behavior. They take responsibility of their actions.

9. **Personal worth:** He has a sense of personal worth, feels worth while and important. He has self-respect and feels secure in a group.

10. **Sense of personal security:** He has sense of personal worth, feels worthwhile and important. He has self-respect and feels secure in a group.

11. **Well-balanced life:** He has a variety of interests and generally lives a well-balanced life of work, rest and recreation. He has the ability to get enjoyment and satisfaction our of his daily routine job. According to Fromm, a mentally healthy person has developed a zest of living that includes a desire for activity which is reflected in an attitude of utilizing wherever possibilities he possesses in productive forms of behavior.

12. **Rational attitude:** He has a rational attitude towards problems of his physical health. He maintains a daily routine of health practices which promote healthful living. He practices good health habits with regard to nutrition, sleep, rest, relaxation, physical activity, personal cleanliness and protection from disease.

13. **Philosophical life:** He has developed a philosophy of life that gives meaning and purpose to his daily activities. This philosophy belongs to this world and discourages the tendency to withdraw or escape from the world. It makes him to something concrete about his problems as they rise. He does not evade responsibility or duty.

14. **Faith in his ability:** He has faith in his ability to succeed; he believes that he will do reasonably well whatever he undertakes. He solves his problem largely by his own initiative and effort. He feels confident of everyday life, more or less effectively.

15. **Mental health is a dynamic concept:** Mental health denotes a state od balance or equilibrium of our mind. This balance is not static, it is quite dynamic. The circumstances in our life are never static, they are changeable and so is our adjustment.

FACTORS INFLUENCE MENTAL HEALTH

1. **Heredity:** It provides raw material, or the potentialities of the individual. It sets the limits for his mental health. What individual inherits is the potentialities in relation to growth, appearance, intelligence and the life. The development and utilization of these potentialities is determined to a large extent by environmental opportunities. Investigations shown that hereditary may predispose a person to the development of a particular type of mental illness which he is placed under extensive stress. In the words of Wallin, defective heredity may furnish a fertile soil for the development of mental and nervous diseases but so far as minor personality maladjustments are concerned, heredity supplies only a predisposing condition.

2. **Physical factor:** Physical health factors make a significant contribution to mental health. You will agree that an erect posture, a winning smile, color in the cheeks, a feeling of exhilaration promote a sense of personal security and have a marked influence on other people. People with greater strengths, better looks and robust health enjoy a social advantage in the development of personality characteristics. An individual with a feeling of physical well-being ordinarily a good disposition and is enthusiastic and intellectually alert. Sick people find it more difficult to make adjustments to new situations than healthy people. Vitamin deficiencies have been found to be the causative factors in many personality difficulties.

3. **Social factor:** Social factor pertains to the individual's society in which he lives, the interactional process and his social functioning with other persons. It is the social environment which shapes the knowledge, the skills, interests, attitudes, habits, values and goals that he acquires. Every individual is born into a society which influences the content of his behavior. Of our social factors, the most important are the home, the school, and the community.

4. **Satisfaction of fundamental or basic needs:** From the discussion of the physical and social factor it will be clear that mental health in childhood and later depends very much on the adequate satisfaction of our fundamental or basic needs. Our basic needs are physical, organic as well as emotional or psychological. The organic needs are to be satisfied for marinating physical well-being. Hunger, thirst, fatigue, lack of sleep, physical pain, exercise, heat or cold and the like set up certain tension in the individuals which must be relived.

5. **Environmental factor:** It has now been established account of various researches in the field of mental hygiene that environmental forces—family, school, and society are more responsible for bringing mental illness than the hereditary or constitutional forces.

PRINCIPLES CONTRIBUTING TO MENTAL HEALTH

1. One should respect his own and other's personality.
2. One should be aware of the limitations of the self and others and should also have the knowledge of others abilities.
3. This fact should be understood that every behavior has some reason.
4. Person should be evaluated according to his total behavior.
5. Important needs or drive should be recognized and efforts should be made to fulfill these.

NEEDS OF MENTAL HEALTH

To develop ideal mental health, one should pay attention to the important needs, which are given below:

1. Need for love and attachment.
2. Desire for being independent and self-sufficient.
3. Desire for achievements.
4. Need for recognition and respect.
5. Need for self-actualization.
6. Need for the identification of personality.

Major Foundations of Mental Health

1. Sound physical health.
2. Fulfillment of the basic needs of person like physical, psychological, and social.
3. Development of healthy habits, education, philosophy of life, etc.
4. Various components related to hereditary and environment.

Skills Needed for Positive Mental Health

World Health Organization has recommended some life skills, which may be used for promotion of mental health. These skills should taught every person to maintain the positive mental health.

1. **Problem solving:** Learning steps of problem solving and generating solutions to difficult problems.
2. **Decision making:** Learning basic steps for decision making.
3. **Creative thinking:** Developing creativity in thinking and developing adaptation behavior.
4. **Critical thinking:** Through making objective judgment about risks and choices.
5. **Effective communication:** Developing positive communication skills during the stress period.
6. **Interpersonal relationship:** Learning importance of interpersonal relations, making support groups for the need of time.
7. **Self-awareness:** Identifying one's own qualities, strengths and weaknesses.
8. **Coping mechanisms:** Understanding the emotions, their affects and coping with emotional distress and stressful situations.
9. **Empathy:** Through caring of people and avoiding prejudices and discriminations.

NURSES RESPONSIBILITIES IN PROMOTION OF POSITIVE MENTAL HEALTH

Nurses are responsible to provide mental health care to all sections of the people community and hospitals. In this regard some important activities of community health nurse are given:
1. Educating the community about mental health, its importance and needs.
2. Educating the parents and other specific sections of society, this may be responsible for psychological development of children. It is necessary to caution against over protection.
3. Preventing infection, trauma, and poisoning before, during and after birth which may lead to various mental health problems in the life span of a person.
4. Providing anticipatory guidance and counseling to prevent psychological problems.
5. Providing school mental health care services.
6. Avoiding misconceptions, superstitions about mental illness.
7. Educating the individuals about coping mechanisms.
8. Providing counseling services to parents of mentally and physically handicapped children.
9. Identifying the high-risk groups in the community and preventing them from forthcoming mental problems.
10. Providing mental health care services to sufferer of mental diseases.
11. Implementing the National Mental Health Program.

IMPORTANCE OF MENTAL HEALTH

Health is rightly said wealth. It involves one's physical as well as mental health. As said earlier, mental health has much wider scope than physical health as it aims for the development of wholesome balanced and integrated personality.
1. **Mental health helps in the development of desirable personality:** Mental health helps in the development of a wholesome, well-balanced and integrated personality.
2. **Mental health helps in proper emotional development:** There is a close relationship between one's mental health and emotional behavior. The individual who enjoy good mental health are supposed to demonstrate proper emotional maturity in their behavior.
3. **Mental health helps in proper social development:** One's mental health helps one is becoming quite sociable and establishing proper social relationships in the society.

4. **Mental health help in proper moral development:** The individuals who enjoy sound health are usually found to behave as a man of integrity and character by following the ethical standards of the society.
5. **Mental health helps in proper esthetic development:** Proper mental health helps the individual in the development of appropriate esthetic sense, artistic tastes and refined temperament.
6. **Mental health help in actualizing one's potentialities:** Everyone of us has a fund of natural abilities and potentialities that can be actualizing through proper efforts. Exercising such effort and striving towards the actualization of one's mental health.
7. **Mental health helps in seeking proper adjustment:** A mentally healthy individual is an adjusted person. He is able to seek adequate adjustment with his self and his environment. He is able to adjust his needs to the demands of the situations and well-being of the society.
8. **Mental health helps in seeking goals of life:** Mental health helps the individual to strive properly for the realization of the goals of his life. These goals may differ from person-to-person depending upon their life styles and philosophy of life.
9. **Mental health helps in the progress of the society:** Mental health helps the individuals to develop as well balance useful citizens who are conscious not only for their rights but for their responsibilities also. They take essential from the society for their proper development and living but also ready to give something to the society for its progress and development.
10. **Mental health helps in the prevention of mental illness:** Mental health helps the individual in protecting him against abnormalities of behavior, maladjustment, illness and mental diseases in the same ways as physical health is helpful in saving him from the physical illness, ailments and diseases. A sound mind and balanced personality has enough resistance for fighting with the odds of life and bearing the accidental stresses and strains of life in comparison to the people having impaired mental health.

SYMPTOMS OF POOR MENTAL HEALTH

1. Emotionally unstable and easily upset.
2. Apprehensive, suspicious and insecure.
3. Lack of self-confidence and willpower.
4. No adequate adjustment with the self and environment—physical, social, and professional.
5. Failure in setting a proper level of aspiration.
6. Suffering from frustrations, unresolved conflicts, strains and stresses.
7. Always remains in the state of over-anxiousness and tension.
8. Lack of enduring power and tolerance.
9. Lack of decision making ability.
10. Poor self-concept and achievement motivation.
11. Unrealistic attitude towards life and people.
12. Suffering from mental disturbances, disorder, ailments and diseases.
13. Always dissatisfied with his achievements and tries to seek over perfection in his or other's work.
14. Lives in the world of his own imagination and fantasy.

MENTAL HYGIENE

Mental hygiene is concerned with realization and maintenance of mind's health and efficiency or in other words it deals with healthfulness of mind. Mental hygiene is concerned with the study of factors which go against mental health and efficiency. Mental hygiene means the balanced and integrated development of personality. It is a science that deals with human welfare and pervades all fields of human relationships. The aim of mental hygiene is to aid people to achieve more satisfying and more productive lives, through the preventive and anxieties and maladjustments. According to dictionary, mental hygiene is the science or arts of maintaining mental health and preventing the development of maladjustment and neurosis.

Prof W Beers is called the father of mental hygiene. Once, when he was suffering from some ailments, he realized that various ailments are caused due to failure of the individual to adjust him with situation and requirement of environment. This maladjustment also leads to the development of various mental ailments. It is necessary to do away with them. With this aim in view an International Mental Health Society was established in 1908. The society believed in the slogan sound mind resides in sound body.

Definitions

1. It is concerned with the principle and practice in promotion, maintenance of the mental health and prevention of mental disorders—*JA Hadfield*.
2. The means by the process of mental health is related it is a way of life and involves that influences what one feels, says, and does—*HW Bernard*.
3. Mental health defined as the realization and maintenance of the mind's health and efficiency—*DB Klein*.
4. Mental hygiene is defined as the science and art of preserving and maximizing the mental health—*English and English*.
5. It is organized attempts to effort human adjustment through the application of principles and practices of living—*Bhatia BD and M Craig*.
6. Mental hygiene means establishment of environmental conditions, emotional attitudes and habits of thinking that will resist an onset of personality maladjustments. It is the study of principles and practices in the promotion of mental health and prevention of mental disorder—*Dictionary of Education*.
7. Mental hygiene defined as the application of a body of hygienic information and technique called from sciences of psychology, child study, education, sociology, psychiatric, medicine and biology for the purpose of observation and improvement of mental health of the individuals and the community; for the prevention and care of minor and major mental diseases and defects and mental, educational, and social maladjustments—*Wallace-Wallin*.

Spheres of Mental Hygiene

There are two spheres of mental hygiene, prophylactic hygiene and meliorative hygiene.
1. **The prophylactic mental hygiene:** It is oriented towards the prevention of diseases, breakdown, weakness, disaster and death.
2. **The meliorative mental hygiene:** It is oriented towards the acquisition of better health, more energy and abundant life. It stresses the normal and the ideal as opposed to the abnormal and pathological.

Mental Health in Different Age-groups

Sl.No.	Age-group	Description
1.	Prenatal and postnatal period	Emotional level of pregnant mother affects the mental behavior of child. Some women are much tensed during pregnancy or pregnancy can be an existing and frightening experience for them. Therefore, along with the physical care of mother, she should also be given due emotional support. Maintaining a healthy and creative mental level by mother during pregnancy is very important for the mental hygiene of child. The psychiatric nurse should give health education to mother during antenatal and postnatal period about the importance of healthy living for healthy baby. After birth the baby needs mother protection, food, love for normal growth.
2.	Infancy (1 month to 1 year) and childhood (toddler to 12 years)	In the womb, the fetus feels more comfortable and enjoys warmth. But the newborn is full of fear when he comes to this open world. Primary childhood is the foundation of mental health. It is essential that during this period, parents should have loving and close relations with other children. Any incident that occurs in the school is imprinted in his mind. Therefore, behavior of other children in the school, student-teacher relations and environment of school should be friendly and assisting in providing the emotional satisfaction to the child. Parent responsibility is to provide happy and conductive environment for the child to grow. Understanding and sympathetic approach in meeting child's need is essential as adequate satisfaction of physical needs which forms a basis for adequate mental health.
3.	Adolescence (13-18 years)	Adolescence is the most sensitive period from the point of normal health. Mental illnesses arising in adolescences, can be prevented by recognizing the needs of adolescence, proper adjustment with opposite sex, giving due importance to the freedom of teenagers and the balanced and understanding behavior of parents.
4.	Adulthood (20-40 years)	Adulthood is a period, person should be complete mentally healthy, but the tensions of the responsibility of family, social beliefs, financial limitations and other environment-generated stresses affect the mental health of the person.
5.	Old age (60 and above)	Mental problems of elderly have increased significantly owing to various factors. These include reduction in the important of joint family system, changing moral and life values, industrialization and urbanization, financial dependence, physical disabilities and diseases, etc.

DEFENSE MECHANISM

The human individual is as much equipped with mental capacities to protect himself against conflicts and frustrations as with physical energy and powers to safeguard against physical dangers or distress. These mental capacities give rise to protective devices known as mental mechanisms or adjustment mechanisms or defense mechanisms. This adjustment mechanism helps the individual in overcoming threats to his ego and thus in maintaining inner balance or harmony. Mental mechanisms interact and overlap in our behavior. They are not mutually exclusive, nor do they generally operate as separate entities. Both well-adjusted and maladjusted individuals make use of these mechanisms in their daily behavior.

Definitions

1. Defense mechanism is a pattern of adjustment through which an individual relieves or decrease anxieties caused by an uncomfortable situation that threatens self-esteems.
2. Ego defense mechanism is consciously or unconsciously operating devices to keep conflictual issues out of consciousness of the individual to bring some protective measures.
3. Ego defense mechanisms are learned, usually during early childhood and are considered to be maladaptive when they become the predominant means of coping with stressors.
4. When psychological equilibrium is threatened by severe emotional trauma, frustrations, or conflicts, the mind resorts to a variety to protective subterfuges and detours called mental mechanisms or dynamisms—*Page.*
5. An adjustment mechanism is a device resorted to in order to achieve an indirect satisfaction of a need so that tension will be reduced and self-respect maintained—*Carroll.*
6. Certain patterns of behavior that are employed for protection against threat or anxiety are called defense mechanisms or adjustments mechanisms. Sometimes, they are referred to as ego defense mechanisms since they are serve to defend the ego or the self from threat—*Arkoff.*
7. A defense mechanism is a strategy, unconsciously utilized, that serves to protect the ego from anxiety—*Davison and Neale.*

Functions of Defense Mechanism

1. Protecting individuals from dangerous situations.
2. To deal with minor, hurt, pain, anger, anxiety, sadness, and self-devaluation.
3. Removing anxiety and hurt.
4. Plays an important role in normal adjustment mechanism.

Characteristics of Defense Mechanism

1. The purpose of defense mechanism is to reduce anxiety.
2. Defense mechanism is compromise solutions.
3. The pattern of defense mechanism depends on one's stability.
4. The same individual may use varied mechanisms are his need.
5. Defense mechanisms may be used consciously but usually act at unconscious or subconscious level.
6. Defense mechanisms are devised in the forms of a certain pattern of behavior.
7. These mechanisms provide protection against whatever threatens our ego or self-esteem.
8. There are many situations in our environment and also within us which threaten our psychological equilibrium.
9. Defense mechanism may be evolved by anything in conflict with minimum ideal of what the self must be.
10. Defense mechanisms are quite temporary defense against anxiety and inadequacies. By resorting to them one tries to deceive himself more than somebody else.

11. Defense mechanisms are largely unconscious. They do tend to operate in a machine-like or automatic way. In fact, they are always, in corresponding degree, self-deceptive and thus aim at softening or disguising what is unaccepted to us in terms of our failure or inadequacies.

12. Defense mechanisms should not be confused with symptoms of neuroses or other abnormal conditions. These mechanisms are purely psychic or mental devices or ways of perceiving and desiring.

Types of Defense Mechanism

Level I: Psychotic

Sl. No.	Classification	Description
1.	Denial	It is protecting self from unpleasant reality by refusal to perceive it or face it. It is a defense mechanism in which a person is faced with a fact that is too painful to accept and reject it. The individual may deny the reality of the unpleasant fact altogether, admit the fact but deny its seriousness or admit both the fact and seriousness but denies responsibility.
2.	Distortion	A gross reshaping of external reality to meet internal needs. For example, mentally ill patients have no intact contact with reality. These patients suffering with psychosis.
3.	Delusional projections	Gross frank delusions about external reality, usually of persecutory nature. The delusions are the false beliefs of the person which are not shared by race, age, educational background, etc.

Level II: Immature

Sl. No.	Classification	Description
1.	Fantasy	It is gratifying frustrated desired by imaginary achievements. It is the defense mechanism involving tendency to retreat into fantasy in order to resolve inner and outer conflicts.
2.	Projection	It is unconscious denial of unacceptable feelings and emotions in one while attributing to others. It is primitive form of paranoia.
3.	Hypochondrias	The transformation of negative feeling towards others into negative feelings towards self, pain, illness, and anxiety. Hypochondrias sometimes referred to as health phobia, refers to an excessive preoccupation or worry about having a serious illness.
4.	Passive aggression	Aggression towards others expressed indirectly or passively. Passive aggressive defense create or disorder known as passive aggressive personality disorder is said to be marked by a pervasive pattern of negative attitudes and passive, usually resistance in interpersonal or occupational areas.

Contd...

Contd...

Sl. No	Classification	Description
5.	Acting out	Direct expression of unconscious wish or impulse without conscious awareness of the emotion that derives that expressive behavior. This behavior is very common in children with temper tantrum, oppositional defiant disorder, truancy etc.
6.	Regression	It is returning to an earlier stage of behavior when stress creates, problem at the present stage, involving less mature responds and usually lower level of aspiration. Regression mechanism of going from the present pattern to the past level of behavior. The individual returns to patterns of behavior that were successful in earlier stages of development.
7.	Idealization	Subconsciously choosing to perceive another individual as having positive qualities he/she may actually have.

Level III: Neurotic

Sl.No	Classification	Description
1.	Displacement	Defense mechanism that shifts sexual or aggressive impulses to a more acceptable or less threatening target; redirecting emotion to a safer outlet; separation of emotion from its real object.
2.	Dissociation	It is temporary drastic modification of one's personal identity or character to avoid emotional distress; separation or postponement of a feeling that normally would accompany a situation or thought.
3.	Isolation	It is separation of feelings from ideas and events. For example, describing a murder with graphic details with no emotional response.
4.	Intellectualization	It is avoiding unavoidable emotions by focusing on the intellectual aspects. It is separating from emotional contents of an event, focusing instead on the facts.
5.	Reaction formation	Converting unconscious whishes or impulses that are perceived to be dangerous into their opposites; behavior that is completely the opposite of what one really wants or feels; taking the opposite beliefs because of true causes anxiety.
6.	Repression	Repression acts to keep information out of conscious awareness. Repression is more complicated mechanism in which unpleasant or unacceptable experiences, emotions or motivations are actively forced into the unconscious and kept there. Repression operates wholly on an unconscious level. Unacceptable feeling are unconsciously kept out of awareness. A man is jealous of his good friend's success but is unaware of his feelings or jealously.

Level IV : Mature

Sl.No.	Classification	Description
1.	Altruism	This is constructive service to others that brings pleasure and personal satisfaction. Altruism loves others as oneself, behavior that promotes the survival chances of others at a cost to one's own. In other words, it is self-sacrifices for the benefit of others.
2.	Sublimation	The transformation of negative emotions or instincts into positive actions, behavior or emotion is sublimation. Sublimation is a defense mechanism that allows us to act out unacceptable impulses by converting these behaviors into a more acceptable form.
3.	Suppression	Suppression is a device where a conscious effort is made by the individual to dismiss the impulses, feelings and thoughts that are unpleasant to the preconscious mind. So unacceptable feelings and thoughts are consciously kept out of awareness.
4.	Humor	Overt expression of ideas and feelings (especially those that are unpleasant to focus or too terrible to talk about) that gives pleasure to others.
5.	Identification	The unconscious modeling of one's self upon another person's character and behavior. Some individuals try to resemble with another person's character. A lonely teenager being copying the clothes and action of a popular peer.
6.	Introjections	It is identifying with some ideas or objects so deeply that it becomes a part of that person. It is complete acceptance of another's opinion and values as one's own.

ADJUSTMENT

The word adjustment means to fit, make suitable, adapt, arrange, harmonize, correspondence with. Adjustment is defined as the series of techniques, methods or processes by which an individual tries to meet the environmental, spatial or psychological changes and maintains a satisfactory equilibrium (balance) with his world. This also called adaptation. There are different types of changes to which a person has to adjust himself. These changes can be environmental example change in temperature, humanity, oxygen level. Spatial example change of a place and psychological example, the husband leaves the job; family members face a problem of change of job of the head of the family.

Definitions

1. Adjustment can be defined in that form of social process in which two or more people or groups interact to end or reduce conflict—*Fitcher*.
2. Adjustment is that special process through which a person is able to develop the tendency of cooperation in his environment—*MacIver and Page*.
3. Any operation whereby an organism becomes more favorably related to the environmental and internal—*Warren*.
4. It is the establishment of satisfactory relationship, as representing, harmony, conformance, adoption etc—*Webster*.
5. A continual process in which a person varies his behavior to produce a more harmonious relationship between himself and his environment—*Gates and Jersild*.

6. The process of finding and adopting modes of behavior suitable to the environment or the change in the environment—*Cater V Good*.
7. An individual's adjustment is said to be adequate, wholesome or healthful to the extent that he has established harmonious relationship between himself and the conditions, situations and persons who compromise his physical or social environment—*Crow and Crow*.
8. Adjustment is psychological survival—*Vonhaller*.

Nature of Adjustment

1. **Continuity:** The process of adjustment is continued throughout life long. Individual from birth to death has to adjust one-way or the other. The individuals who are able to adjust themselves to changing situations in their environment can live a harmonious, happy and continued life.
2. **Mental peace:** Conflict upsets a person, whereas adjustment provides peaceful.
3. Universality: adjustment is prevalent in all the aspects of life example, social, economic, political, religious, etc.
4. **Social necessity:** Adjustment is necessary to prevent society.
5. **Harmonious relationship:** Harmonious relationship between individual, their needs and environment is essential. The individual meets demands either by adopting, modifying previous ways of doing or facing the challenges.
6. **Day-to-day demand:** Adjustment will help the individual to change his way of life according to the demand of the situation and gives strength and ability to bring about the necessary changes in the environment conditions.
7. **Two-way process:** Adjustment is a process of fitting oneself into available circumstances, but also the process of changing the circumstances to fit one's own needs. In majority of cases, adjustment is compromise between two extremes.
8. **Conscious/unconscious activity:** To adjust in a society, the individual learns morals, traditions, etc. from birth to death in conscious and unconscious manner to adjust and accommodate to the needs and demands of self and society.

Aims of Adjustment

1. To maintain harmonious and active relationship between structural components of society.
2. For social reform and social construction.
3. To lead a harmonious social life.
4. To perform functions effectively in relation to their culture customs, values and beliefs.
5. To provide good interpersonal relationship.
6. To promote character building.
7. To develop orderly social unity.
8. To manifest collective behavior in terms of state, religion, economic agencies, organization and social group.

Measurement of Adjustment

1. **Testing techniques:** To assess the individual characteristic at the unconscious level.
2. **Projective techniques:** To assess the individual's characteristics at the unconscious level.
3. **Sociometric techniques:** To measure social relationships and provide clues to the level of social adjustment.

4. **Scaling techniques:** Opinions, views are collected from other person about the adjustment pattern of a particular interval known to the respondents.
5. **Inventory techniques:** They may have many advantages to the techniques.

Methods of Adjustment

Direct Method

1. **Improving efforts:** To improve the behavioral process and to solve difficult situations in the environment, he will increase his efforts to improve his efficiency.
2. **Compromising methods:** Individual changes his efforts in a different direction to fulfill his aspiration.
3. **Withdrawal and submissiveness:** Accepts his own defeat and surrounding himself to the powerful environmental forces.
4. **Making proper choices and decisions:** A person adapts himself and to serves harmony with his environment by making use of his intelligence for the proper choices and wise decision particularly when faced with conflicting situations and stressful moments/situations.

Indirect Method

By using defense mechanism/coping strategies, the individual will try to adopt himself to the changing situation and accommodating new life styles.

Improvement of Adjustment

It is very important to establish positive adjustment by finding out reasons of stress, hopelessness, frustration and maladjustments.

1. Find patterns of behavior that satisfy basic needs and solve problems effectively.
2. Assume conscious control of your behavior.
3. Use problem solving to find the best possible solution for a problem situation instead of acting impulsively.
4. Use emotion constructively when appropriate; express feelings at the time they are experienced.
5. Self evaluate in a constructive sense. Look for ways to improve but avoid feelings of guilt or inadequacy.
6. **Avoid burnout:** Perform effective stress management techniques such as yoga, meditation, exercises, etc.
7. **Adapting to new situation:** When a change occur in your life situation of your patterns of behavior in order to achieve a state of good adjustment in new situations.

MENTAL ILLNESS

Definition

Mental and behavioral disorders are understood as clinically significant conditions characterized by alterations in thinking, mood (emotions) or behavior associated with personal distress and/ or impaired functioning (WHO, 2001).

Characteristics of Mental Illness

1. Changes in one's thinking, memory, perception, feeling and judgment resulting in changes in talk and behavior which appear to be deviant from previous personality or from the norms of community.

2. These changes in behavior cause distress and suffering to the individual or others or both
3. Changes and the consequent distress cause disturbance in day-to-day activities, work and relationship with important others (social and vocational dysfunction).

Features of Mental Illness

The features of mental illness are classified under four headings:
1. Disturbances in bodily functions
2. Disturbances in mental functions
3. Changes in individual and social activities
4. Somatic complaints

Disturbances in Bodily Functions

1. **Sleep:** Disturbed sleep throughout the night, or no sleep at all, or difficulty in falling asleep, or waking up in the middle of night and failing to fall asleep again. In addition, the individual may experience lethargy and lack of freshness in the morning.
2. **Appetite and food intake:** Increased appetite or decreased appetite, weight loss or weight gain, nausea, vomiting.
3. **Bowel and bladder movement:** Diarrhea or constipation, increased micturition, bed-wetting.
4. **Sexual desire and activity:** Decreased interest in sex, premature ejaculation, impotence or lack of sexual satisfaction. In some conditions, there can be excessive sexual desire or lack of social inhibitions.

Disturbances in Mental Functions

1. **Behavior:** The patient may exhibit over activity, restlessness, irritability, may be abusive to others for trivial or no reasons at all, or the patient may become dull, withdrawn and not respond to external or internal cues. At times the patient may behave in a bizarre way which the family members may find irritating. Sometimes the patient's behavior can be dangerous to self or others.
2. **Speech:** Patient talks excessively and unnecessarily or talks very little or stays mute. The talk becomes irrelevant and un-understandable (incoherent).
3. **Thought:** Patient expresses peculiar and wrong beliefs which others do not share.
4. **Emotions:** Patient may exhibit excessive emotions like excessive happiness, anger, fear or sadness. Sometimes emotions can be inappropriate to situations. He may laugh to self or weep without any reason.
5. **Perception:** The patient may perceive without any stimulus. There can be misinterpretation of perception. For example, a mentally ill person can see things or hear sounds or feel objects which do not exist or which others do not see. This is known as hallucinations. A patient who is hallucinating is seen talking to self, laughing or weeping to self, wandering in the streets and behaving in a manner which others may find abnormal.
6. **Attention and concentration:** Patient may have decreased attention and concentration; he may get distracted easily, or have selective inattention.
7. **Memory:** Patient may lose his memory and start forgetting important matters.
8. **Intelligence and judgment:** In some mental illnesses, intelligence and the ability to take decisions deteriorate. Patient loses reasoning skills and abilities, may not be able to perform simple arithmetic, or commits mistakes in routine work.

9. **Level of consciousness:** In some mental illnesses due to possible brain damage, there may be changes in the level of consciousness. Patient fails to identify his relatives. He can be disoriented to time and place. He may remain confused or become unconscious.

Changes in Individual and Social Activities

Patients may neglect their bodily needs and personal hygiene. The patient may also lose social sense. They behave in an inappropriate manner in social situations and embarrass others. They behave strangely with their family members, friends, colleagues and others. They may insult, abuse/assault them.

Somatic Complaints

Patient may complain of aches and pains in different parts of the body, fatigue, weakness, involuntary movements, etc.

Common Signs and Symptoms of Mental Illness

Disturbances in Motor Behavior:
Motor retardation, stupor, stereotypes, negativism, ambitendence, waxy flexibility, echopraxia, restlessness, agitation and excitement.

Disorders of thought, language and communication:
Pressure of speech, poverty of speech, dysarthria, flight of ideas, circumstantialities, loosening of association, tangentiality, incoherence, perseveration, neologism, clang association, thought block, thought insertion, thought broadcasting, echolalia, delusions, obsessions and phobias.

Disorders of perception illusions, hallucinations, depersonalization, derealization

Disorders of emotion: Blunt affect, labile affect, elated mood, euphoria, ecstasy, dysphoric mood, depression, anhedonia.

Disturbances of consciousness: Clouding of consciousness, delirium and coma.

Disturbances in attention: Distractibility, selective inattention.

Disturbances in orientation: Disorientation of time, place or person.

Disturbances of memory: Amnesia, confabulation.

Impaired judgment

Disturbances in biological function: Persistent deviations in temperature, pulse and respiration, nausea, vomiting, headache, loss of appetite, increased appetite, loss of weight, pain, fatigue, weight gain, insomnia, hypersonmia and sexual dysfunction.

Concepts of Normal and Abnormal Behavior

Psychiatry as evident from the above is concerned with abnormal behavior in its broadest sense, but defining the concepts of normal and abnormal behavior as such has been found to be difficult. These concepts are much under the influence of sociocultural factors.

Several models have been put forward in order to explain the concept of normal and abnormal behavior.

Medical Model

Medical model considers organic pathology as the definite cause for mental disorder. According to this model, abnormal people are the ones who have disturbances in thought, perception and psychomotor activities. The normal are the ones who are free from these disturbances.

Statistical Model

It involves the analysis of responses on a test or a questionnaire or observations of some particular behavioral variables. The degree of deviation from the standard norms arrived at statistically, characterizes the degree of abnormality.

Statistically normal mental health falls within two standard deviations (SDs) of the normal distribution curve.

Sociocultural Model

The beliefs, norms, taboos and values of a society have to be accepted and adopted by individuals. Breaking any of these would be considered as abnormal. Normalcy is defined in context with social norms prescribed by the culture. Thus cultural background has to be taken into account when distinguishing between normal and abnormal behavior.

Behavior Model

Behavior that is adaptive, is normal, maladaptive is abnormal. Abnormal behavior is a set of faulty behaviors acquired through learning.

Problems of Mental Disorders

1. Self-care limitations or impaired functioning related to mental illness.
2. Significant deficits in biological, emotional and cognitive functioning.
3. Disability, life-process changes.
4. Emotional problems such as anxiety, anger, sadness, loneliness and grief.
5. Physical symptoms that occur along with altered psychological functioning.
6. Alteration in thinking, perceiving, communicating and decision making.
7. Difficulties in relating to others.
8. Patient's behavior may be dangerous to self or others.
9. Adverse effects on the well-being of the individual, family and community.
10. Financial, marital, family, academic and occupational problems.

Burdens of Mental Disorders

Mental disorders are common, affecting more than 25 percent of all people at some time during their lives. They are also universal, affecting people in all countries and societies, individuals of all ages, women and men, the rich and the poor, from urban and rural environments. They have an economic impact on societies and on the quality of life of individuals and families.

1. Mental disorders at any point of time are present in about 10 percent of the adult population. Around 20 percent of all patients seen by primary health care professionals have one or more mental disorders.
2. During the last two decades many epidemiological studies have been conducted in India, which show that mental disorders prevail in 18 to 207 per 1000, with median 65.4 per 1000 at any given time. About 2.3% of the population suffers from seriously incapacitating mental disorders or epilepsy. A large number of adult patients (10.4 to 53.0%) coming to the general outpatient department are diagnosed as mentally ill.
3. It is estimated that in 2000, mental disorders accounted for 12% of the total disability adjusted life years (DALYs) lost due to all diseases and injuries. Common disorders, which usually cause

severe disability, include depressive disorder, substance use disorders, schizophrenia, epilepsy, Alzheimer's disease, mental retardation and disorders of childhood and adolescence.

4. More than 450 million people today suffer from mental and behavioral disorders. Within the next 20 years depression will have the dubious distinction of becoming the second biggest cause for global burden of disease.

5. Worldwide 70 million people suffer from alcohol dependence, 50 million from epilepsy, 24 million from schizophrenia and another 20 million people attempt suicide every year.

6. Global Burden of Disease (GBD) 2000 estimates show that mental and neurological conditions account for 30.8% of all years lived with disability (YLD). Depression causes the largest amount of disability, accounting for almost 12% of all disabilities. Six neuropsychiatry conditions figured in the top twenty causes of disability worldwide which include:
   • Unipolar depressive disorders
   • Alcohol use disorders
   • Schizophrenia
   • Bipolar affective disorders
   • Alzheimer's and other dementias
   • Migraine

7. Mental illnesses cause massive disruption in the lives of individuals, families and communities. Individuals suffer the distressing symptoms of disorders. They also suffer because they are unable to participate in work and leisure activities often as a result of discrimination. They worry about not being able to shoulder their responsibilities towards their family and friends and are fearful of being a burden to others. Mental illnesses are common to all countries and cause immense suffering. People with these disorders are often subjected to social isolation, poor quality of life and increased mortality. These disorders are thus the cause of staggering economic and social costs.

8. It is estimated that one in four families has at least one member currently suffering from a mental illness. These families are required not only to provide physical and emotional support, but also to bear the negative impact of stigma and discrimination present in all parts of the world.

9. Families in which one member is suffering from a mental disorder make a number of adjustments and compromises that prevent other members of the family from achieving their full potential in work, social relationships and leisure. These are the human aspects of the burden of mental disorders that are difficult to assess and quantify.

10. The impact of mental disorders in communities is large and manifold. There is the cost of providing care, the loss of productivity and certain legal problems associated with some mental disorders.

Misconception about Mental Illness

Beliefs about mental illness have been characterized by superstition, ignorance and fear. Although time and advances in scientific understanding of mental illness have dispelled many false ideas, there remain a number of popular misconceptions. Some of them are:

1. Mental illness is caused by supernatural power and is the result of a curse or possession by evil spirit: Many people do not consider mental illness as an illness, but possession by spirits or curse that has befallen on the patient or family because of past sins or misdeeds in previous life.

2. **Mentally ill people show bizarre behavior:** Patients in mental hospitals and clinics are often pictures as a weird lot, who spend their time exhibiting useless bizarre behavior like twisting of hands, etc.

3. **Mentally ill people are dangerous:** People who have or had a mental illness are viewed with suspicion and as dangerous persons.
4. **Mental illness is something to be ashamed of:** This idea arouses an unsympathetic, cruel attitude towards a mentally ill person. This is the reason why many people hide mental illness in the family.
5. **Mental illness is not curable:** People object to have normal relationship with mentally ill people, or to give them employment even after being cured, or even to accept them as neighbors.
6. **Mental illness is contagious:** The fear that it is contagious is the main false notion which leads people to view suspiciously, or object to marital relations with a person belonging to the household of the mentally ill.
7. **Mental illness is hereditary:** It is not a rule that children of mentally ill patients should become mentally ill.
8. **Marriage can cure mental illness:** A mentally ill person can get worse if he gets married when he is ill, as marriage can become an additional stress. A patient who has recovered can get married and live a normal life like any other person.
9. Mental hospitals are places where only dangerous mentally ill individuals are treated and restraint is a major form of treatment: People hesitate to take their relatives to mental hospitals for treatment because of fear. Further, as expatient of a mental hospital, he, as well as his family members is often isolated. Therefore, people seek help from mental hospitals only as a last resort.

General Attitude toward the Mentally Ill

1. In general, the community responds to the mentally ill through denial, isolation and rejection. There is also a lack of understanding of mental illness as any other illness, and a lack of tendency to reject both the patients' and those who treat them.
2. Mentally ill are viewed as people with no capacity for understanding.
3. People feel mental illness cannot be cured, and even if the patient gets better, complete physical rest is considered essential.
4. The mentally ill are by and large perceived as aggressive, violent and dangerous.

An individual's values and personal beliefs affect his attitude about mental illness, the mentally ill and treatment of mental illness. There still exists a stigma surrounding individuals who need or use Psychiatric Mental Health Services. The need continues for public education to modify or alter misconceptions about mental illness and people with mental disorders.

Mental Health Team or Multidisciplinary Team

Multidisciplinary approach refers to collaboration between members of different disciplines who provide specific services to the patient.

The multidisciplinary team includes:

- A psychiatrist
- A psychiatric nurse
- A clinical psychologist
- A psychiatric social worker
- An occupational therapist or an activity therapist
- A pharmacist and a dietitian
- A counselor

A psychiatrist is a medical doctor with special training in psychiatry. He is accountable for the medical diagnosis and treatment of patient. Other important functions are:
1. Admitting patient into acute care setting
2. Prescribing and monitoring psychopharmacologic agents
3. Administering electroconvulsive therapy
4. Conducting individual and family therapy
5. Participating in interdisciplinary team meetings
6. Owing to their legal power to prescribe and to write orders, psychiatrists often function as leaders of the team.

A psychiatric nurse is a registered nurse with specialized training in the care and treatment of psychiatric patients; she may have a Diploma, MSc, MPhil or PhD in psychiatric nursing. She is accountable for the bio-psychosocial nursing care of patients and their milieu. Other functions include:
1. Administering and monitoring medications.
2. Assisting in numerous psychiatric and physical treatments.
3. Participate in interdisciplinary team meetings.
4. Teach patients and families.
5. Take responsibility for patient's records.
6. Act as patient's advocate.
7. Interact with patients' significant others.

A clinical psychologist should have a Master's Degree in Psychology or PhD in Clinical Psychology with specialized training in mental health settings. He is accountable for psychological assessments, testing, and treatments. He offers direct services such as individual, family or marital therapies.

A psychiatric social worker should have a Master's Degree in Social Work or PhD degree with specialized training in mental health settings. He is accountable for family care work and community placement of patients. He conducts group therapy sessions. He emphasizes intervention with the patient in social environment in which he will live.

An occupational therapist or an activity therapist is accountable for recreational, occupational and activity programs. He assists the patients to gain skills that help them cope more effectively to gain or retain employment, to use leisure time.

A counselor provides basic supportive counseling and assists in psychoeducational and recreational activities.

CONCLUSION

Mental health is an important aspect of one's total health status. It is another word for adjustment or properly integrated living. A mentally healthy person feels, thinks, and acts harmoniously. He is self-confident, adequate and free-from continuous internal conflicts, he is able to make adaptations to a social set-up. Waltin and Hadfield consider mental health as a means and measures for the development as well as functioning of a wholesome well balanced and integrated personality. Considering this way, mental health has wider scope than physical health. It concerns with an all round development of the personality of the child and not merely with the development of one's physical or bodily aspects. Moreover, it aims at the balanced personality, a personality like the balanced physical system who is able to stand firmly in the mildest of stress and strain and who can exhibit adequate emotional maturity and balance between his needs and circumstances.

BIBLIOGRAPHY

1. Ahuja N. A Short Textbook of Psychiatry, 3rd edn. Jaypee Brothers Medical Publishers, New Delhi, 1999.
2. Anthikad Jacob. Psychology for Graduate Nurses. 4th edn, Jaypee Brothers Medical Publishers, New Delhi, 2007.
3. Bhatia BD, Craig Margaretta. Elements of Psychology and Mental Hygiene for Nurses in India. Orient Longman, Chennai, 2005.
4. Bhatia MS. A Concised Textbook on Psychiatric Nursing, 1st edn. CBS Publishers, New Delhi, 1997.
5. Bimla Kapoor. Textbook of Psychiatry Nursing, 1st edn, Kumar Publishing House, New Delhi,1998.
6. Boyd AM. Psychiatric Nursing Contemporary Practice. Lippincott-Raven Publishers, New York, 1998.
7. Das G. Educational Psychology. Kind Books, New Delhi.
8. Gabor D. First contact body language. In: How to start a conversation and make friends. Revised Edn. Rockefeller center, Fireside Publications, New York, 2001:21.
9. Gelder M, Gath D, Mayou R, Cowen P. Oxford Textbook of Psychiatry, 3rd edn. Oxford University Press, New York, 1996.
10. Grant. Child development in India, 3rd edn, Ashish Publishing House, New Delhi, 1992.
11. Gross Richard, Kinnison Nancy. Psychology for Nurses and Allied Health Professionals, Hodder Arnold, London, 2007.
12. Kaplan IH, Sadock JB. Synopsis of Psychiatry: Behavioral Sciences/Clinical Psychiatry, 8th edn Waverly Pvt Ltd, New Delhi, 1998.
13. Lalitha K. Mental Health and Psychiatric Nursing, 1st edn. Gajanana Publishers, Bengaluru, 1995.
14. Morgan CT, King RA. Introduction to Psychology, 6th edn, Tata McGraw-Hill, New Delhi, 1982.
15. Morgan CT. A Brief Introduction to Psychology, Tata McGraw-Hill, New Delhi, 1975.
16. Morrison M. Foundation of Mental Health Nursing. Mosby, Philadelphia, 1997.
17. Munn Norman L. Introduction to Psychology, Oxford and IBH, New Delhi, 1973.
18. Nambi S. Psychiatry for Nurses. Jaypee Brothers Medical Publishers, New Delhi, 1998.
19. Namboodiri VMD, John CJ, Subhalakshmi TP. Clinical Methods in Psychiatry, 2nd edn. Churchill Livingstone, New Delhi, 1999.
20. Rawlins RP, Williams SR. Mental Health Psychiatric Nursing:A Holistic Life cycle Approach, 3rd edn. CV Mosby, Toronto, 1993.
21. Robinson DN. An Intellectual History of Psychology, Macmillan, New York, 1976.
22. Santrock JW. Child Development, 7th edn, Brown and Bench Mark Publishers, Sydney, 1996.
23. Schultz MJ, Videbeck LS. Lippincott's Manual of Psychiatric Nursing Care Plans, 6th edn. Lippincott Williams and Wilkins, Philadelphia, 2002.
24. Stuart WG, Laraia TM. Principles Practice of Psychiatric Nursing, 7th edn. Harcourt Private Limited, New Delhi, 2001.
25. Stuart WG, Sundeen JS. Principles Practice of Psychiatric Nursing, 5th edn. CV Mosby Company, 1995.
26. Taylor CM. Comprehensive Textbook of Psychiatry, 14th edn. CV Mosby, London, 1982.
27. Tendon BN, et al. Management of severely malnourished children by village workers through ICDS in India. Journal of tropical pediatrics, 1984;30:274.

21 *Personality*

DEFINITIONS

1. **Personality:** The distinctive patterns of behavior, thought, and emotions that characterize an individual's adaptation to the situations of his or her life. Personality is the individual's characteristic (and relatively enduring) organization (or integration) of ways of behaving (or traits, interests, abilities, attitudes), and modes of adjustment to others and to his total environment.
2. **Psychoanalysis:** The method of psychotherapy based on Freud's psychoanalytic theory of personality; its basic premise is that the unconscious mind contains buried impulses and desires that must be brought to the surface if anxiety is to disappear.
3. **Psychoanalytic theory:** Freud's theory that all human behavior is dominated by instinctual biological urges that must be Controlled; it is the conflict between the urges and the efforts to control them that leads to emotional problems.
4. **Psychodrama:** A method of therapy in which one acts out scenes in order to bring out their emotional significance of behavior
5. **Intelligence:** It is capacity of an individual to learn and to solve problems and adjust to relatively new and changing conditions. There are individual differences but it is desired from well-balanced personality ir which intelligence is supplemented by healthy social being.
6. **Emotionality:** Emotionality has a powerful role to play is personality. The emotional stability and maturity is required for health) personality.
7. **Personality disorders:** Personality disorders are psychological disorders characterized by lifelong maladaptive behavior patterns See antisocial personality disorder, schizotypal personality disorder, compulsive personality disorder, histrionic personality.
8. **Personality dynamics:** Personality dynamics (1) The interactions among perroeatuy characteristics, especially motives (2) The behavioral expression of personality characteristics in the process of adjusting to the environment. (3) In psychoanalysis, the management of the personality's energy system through the interactions of the Ed, ego, and superego.
9. **Personality structure:** In general, the unique organization of traits, motives, and ways of behaving that characterizes a particular person; in psychoanalytic theory, the conception of the personality in terms of Ed, ego, and superego. See personality.
10. **Personality tests:** Tests to measure the characteristic ways a person behaves, thinks, and feels. Compare ability tests, achievement tests. Personalized system of instruction (PSI) An educational application of instrumental conditioning/operant conditioning in which the material in a course

is divided into small units, each of which must be mastered at a high level of proficiency before the next unit is attempted.

INTRODUCTION

Etymologically, the word personality has been derived from the Latin word persona. Persona means mask used by actors on the stage. Personality in the modern usage of the term means the real individual. Personality in the modern usage of the terms means the real individual. Personality covers the whole nature if an individual and hence it is very difficult to define it. The personality system is a complex product of biological endowment, cultural shaping, cognitive style and spiritual groups. When psychologist talk of personality they mean a dynamic concept describing the growth and development of person, as a whole, which is composed of habits, interests, attitudes, will, character, etc. Watson (1930), the father of behaviorism, taking clues from his behavioral studies, tried to conclude that personality is the sum of activities that can be discovered by actual observations over a long enough period of time to give reliable information.

CONCEPTS OF PERSONALITY

1. Personality is a combination of all the behavioral, emotional, temperamental and mental attributes that shape the unique character of a person.
2. Personality includes both physical-mental characteristics of the person, which determine his general and specific qualities. The distinct identity of the person is only determined by his personality.
3. The impact of personality can always be seen on the behavior, thoughts, conducts, actions and activities of the person.
4. Personality is also described as the unique pattern of traits which characteristics the individual. Traits are characteristics of an individual like good natured, calm, anxious, shy, and irritable.
5. Personality includes the behavior patterns, a person shows across situation or the psychological characteristics of the person that lead to those behavior patterns.
6. Personality includes the cognitive, affective and psychomotor behavior and covers all the conscious, subconscious and unconscious also.
7. Personality is not static but dynamic in nature. Personality of an individual keeps adjusting itself to the environment on a continuous basis. A fine balance is maintained between the environmental and the inner forces.
8. Personality is the individual characteristic (and relatively during) organization (or integration) of ways of behaving (or trait, motives, interests, abilities, attitudes), and modes of adjustment to others and to his total environment.

DEFINITIONS OF PERSONALITY

1. Personality is the dynamic organization within the individual of those psychophysical systems that determine his unique adjustments to his environment—*Gordon Allport.*
2. Personality may be defined as the most characteristic integration of an individual's structure, modes of behavior, interests, attitudes, capacities, abilities and aptitudes—*M N Munn.*
3. The more or less stable and enduring organization of a person's character, temperament, intellect and physique that determines his unique adjustment to his environment is called personality—*Eysenck.*

4. Personality is that which permits a prediction of what a person will do in a given situation—*Cattell.*
5. Personality is a person's unique pattern of traits—*Guilford.*
6. Personality is the most adequate conceptualization of a person's behavior in all its detail—*McClelland.*
7. Personality is a study concerned with the interaction of the biological organism with the social interaction—*Gardener Murphy.*
8. Personality is the sum total of all the biological innate dispositions, impulses, tendencies acquired by experience—*Morton Prince.*
9. Each individual's characteristically recurring patterns of behavior are known as personality—*Kolb.*
10. Personality refers to the aggregate of the physical and mental qualities of the individual's as these interact and function in characteristic fashion with his environment—*Taylor.*
11. Personality consists of the distinctive patterns of behavior including thoughts and emotions that characterize each individual's adaptation to the situations of his or her life—*Walter Mischel.*
12. Personality is the sum of activities that can be discovered by actual observations over a long enough period of time to give reliable information—*Watson.*
13. Personality refers to deeply ingrained patterns of behavior, which include the way one relates to, perceives and thinks about the environment and oneself—*American Psychiatric association.*
14. Personality is defined as enduring patterns of perceiving, relating to, and thinking about environment and oneself—*DSM-IV (APA).*
15. Personality refers to the organized consistent and general pattern of behavior of a person which helps use to understand his or her behavior as individual—*IGNOU.*
16. Personality is an united multiplex, which means a unity composed of elements. He further stated that personality is continuous in an individual's life, a perpetual and a consistent whole which represent his entire life pattern—*Sterm.*

COMPONENTS OF PERSONALITY

1. **Physical appearance:** It refers the physique of an individual. Some people place much emphasis on looks and judge mental alertness from personal appearances, it cannot be denied that to some extent success and failure is determined by personal appearance which includes not only weight, height, complexion but also voice, dress, other characteristics of personal nature.
2. **Character:** It refers to the ethical or moral aspect of a personality which one possesses. The character of an individual is judged by the level of consistency exhibited in his behavior.
3. **Temperament:** It refers to the deep rooted emotional trends present in an individual. It is a result of secretion of endocrine glands as well as habit formation. Temperament plays an important role in one's ability to adjust to his environment.
4. **Interest:** It refers to a felt need. It is connected to three aspects, the need to know, feel, and perform.
5. **Ability:** It refers to a special natural power to do something well, physical or mental.
6. **Sociability:** It refers to an ability of the individual to socialize himself in a social environment and how others perceive his presence in the group. This trait is present in varying degree in different people. The young child is inclined to be extremely selfish and self-centered, but gradually he learns to share his things and experiences with others. He plays other children and shares his toys with them. this give and take co-operation in childhood lays the foundation of social solidarity at the adult level.

7. **Emotionality:** It refers to the ability of an individual to show mature emotional behavior in suitable situations. Emotionality has a powerful role to play in personality. The emotional stability and maturity is required for health personality.
8. **Moral character:** This trait refers to social approval as to whether we have a balanced personality pursuing well- defined goals that benefit to the individual society.
9. **Intelligence:** It is capacity of an individual to learn and solve problems and adjust to relatively new and changing conditions. These are individual differences but it is desired from well-balanced personality in which intelligence is supplemented by healthy social being.

VARIABLES OF PERSONALITY

There are three basic factors or variable which have to be considered in describing the analyzing the personality.
1. The internal aspects of the individual or organism: The basic drives, covert feelings, the physiological systems, glands and his inherently determined physical features.
2. The social and material stimuli or situations exterior to the individual. These modify and direct his impulses and needs. They include the influence of family and other groups to which one belongs, the influence of customs, traditions and culture.
3. The reaction of behavior or conduct which results from the interaction of the individual and the stimuli.

From these three basic variables, it will be clear that personality is a dynamic thing. It grows in a social set-up, through social experiences. These variables do not stand apart from each other; they are related to each other, they are interconnected and as well as a result of this integration give raise to a characteristic behavior pattern or quality called personality.

FACTORS INFLUENCING PERSONALITY

Physiological Factor

Physiological factors include the physique of the individual size, strength, looks, and constitution. They also include the physical deficiencies and nature of glandular functioning. The physiological conditions of the body, influenced by drugs, disease, diet, toxins and bacterial infections, may also shape our behavior and personality. The changes:
1. Physical appearance is the first thing that attracts our attention when we meet a person and our judgment of him is inevitably colored by it. An attractive physical appearance helps to create self-confidence, poise, self-reliance and other similar personality traits in the individual. A well-built person generally enjoys a forceful and impressive personality. He may develop a tendency to bully or to dominate or to protect. The smaller person may feel be titled in the presence of large and tall people. He may try to compensate for this by being hard-working.
2. Physical attractiveness, strength and general health may determine certain reactions and traits. But it must it must be remembered that these things, in themselves, are not the major factors that determine one's personality.
3. Physical handicaps such as orthopedic defects, a bad squint in the eye, snub nose or deafness may cause shyness, reserve and unsociableness in persons.
4. The endocrine glands produce hormones which have the power to raise or depress the activity of the various organs. They influence emotional behavior and hence color our personality. They bring about changes in physical appearance, motor functioning, intelligence and emotional

stability. The parathyroid gland regulates calcium metabolism. Excitability of nervous system is directly dependent on the amount of calcium in the blood. Deficient working of this gland leads to the development of an irritable, quick-reactive, distracted, nervous and a tense person. Similarly, other glands namely pituitary, the adrenal and the gonads have their tremendous impact on various personality traits.

5. Syphilis infections of the brain or general paralysis may change a truthful, meticulous person into one who is dishonest and unreliable. Encephalitis lethargic or sleeping sickness may cause serious behavior problems in a child who has been a joy to parents and teachers.

6. **Nervous system:** Entire behavior is effectively managed and controlled by the coordination and functioning of the nervous system. The sense impressions, which are received through sense organs, do not bear any significance unless they are given meaning by the nervous system.

7. **Hereditary:** At conception when the egg cell of the female is fertilized by the sperm cells of the male, each new human being receives a genetic inheritance that provides potentialities for development and behavioral traits throughout a lifetime. The principle raw materials of personality- physique, intelligence and temperament are the result of heredity.

Environmental or Social Factor

The social aspects of an individual's environment affect personality significantly. Cruze says, an individual's personality is influenced more by the reactions of other people to him and his reactions to other people than by any other factor in the environment. Of these social factors, the most important are the relationship in the home and the family, the influence of the school and the playground, the social codes and social roles which the individual has to play in the family environment and in the community.

1. **Family:** The reaction of the family environment towards an individual, and the role of parents are very important in the molding of personality. Parents serve as a model that the child imitates, and their influence is considerable on the child. Parents influence the development of a child's personality in a wide variety of ways. Children learn the moral values, code of contact, social norms and methods of interacting with others from parents.

2. **School:** The children spend much of their time in the schools and hence it can play a very significant part in the formation of the personality of the child. A nurturing school atmosphere provides for all round development of the child.

3. **Teacher:** A teacher is the most important person in the school who can help in modifying the children's personalities. He is the most powerful source of stimulation for the child.

4. **Peer group:** Peer group refers to other children of the same age who study with or play with the child. Peer group is much more influential than sibling or parents. The peer group serves as an important reference group in shaping personality traits and characteristics of the growing child. As peer group grows up peers become progressively more influential in molding the child's self-concept.

5. **Culture:** Culture influences personality because every culture has a set of ethical and moral values, beliefs and norms which considerably shapes behavior. Cross-cultural studies have pointed out the importance of cultural environment in shaping our personality.

Psychological Factor

Psychological factors include our motives, acquired interests, our attitudes, our will and character, our intellectual capacities such as intelligence, reasoning, attention and perception and imagination.

These factors determine our reaction in various situations and thus, affect our personality growth and direction.

DEVELOPMENT OF PERSONALITY

"Personality consists of distinctive patterns of behavior (including thoughts and emotions) that characterize each individual's adaptation to the situations of his or her life"—*Walter Mischel, 1976*

Babyhood (Birth-2 years)

1. This period is the true foundation period of life because many behavioral patterns, attitudes and patterns of emotional expressions are being established. These have a lifelong influence on the child's personal and social adjustments.
2. The term 'infant' suggests extreme helplessness. The infant is truly a dependent individual, and his total existence depends on resources outside himself. It is a time of rapid growth and development, and a time of radical adjustments.
3. An average infant weighs 7 lbs and measures 18-19 inches in length. Common responses like spontaneous eye movements, yawning, turning and lifting the head, etc. are present. Gradually dentition, bowel and bladder control develop. The baby grows rapidly and masters some common skills such as self- feeding, self-dressing, walking alone, climbing stairs, etc.
4. The baby's vocalization includes crying, cooing, gurgling, which gradually develop into babbling, and later, speech.
5. Emotional reactions are intense and sudden, whatever the stimulus, These reactions may be described as states of pleasantness (characterized by relaxing of the body) and unpleasantness (characterized by tensing of the body). Later on, emotions such as anger, fear, curiosity, joy, affection are exhibited. Babies who experience more of pleasant emotions are laying the foundation for good personal and social adjustments later on in life.
6. **Personality traits:** Children are born with characteristic temperamental differences, and it is these differences from which the individual personality patterns develop. The infant develops self-trust by trusting in what he sees and hears. The beginning feelings of confidence and faith develop if he receives what is needed. Feelings of distrust develop if the baby's needs are not met. This leads to personality problems such as clinging and demanding behavior, greed, giving up easily, taking rather than giving, etc.

Early Childhood (2-6 years)

Growth during early childhood proceeds at a slow rate as compared with the rapid rate of growth in infancy. Body proportions change markedly. The muscles become longer, stronger and heavier. The average annual increase in height is 3 inches and the average annual increase in weight is 3-5 lbs.

Emotions are especially intense, and they are easily aroused to emotional outbursts such as temper tantrums, fears, and unreasonable outbursts of jealousy. Other emotions of curiosity, joy, and affection also develop.

Personality Traits

1. The most important psychosocial achievement at this time is the development of autonomy or independence. If trust and security do not develop at an early age, autonomy will fail to develop.

There is heightened awareness and curiosity of the self, termed as narcissism. The issue of sexuality also overtly develops.
2. The child also begins to know the difference between right and wrong, and laid down standards of behavior and rules of conscience which will thereafter guide much of his behavior.
3. In this phase specific crisis is between initiative and guilt. If the child successfully passes through this stage, it leads to internalization of values and social sanctions, and from this time onwards, he is able to differentiate between right and wrong and to lay down standards of behavior and rules of conscience that will thereafter guide much of his behavior.
4. The child with faulty autonomy traits will be clinging and dependent. Phase related adult characteristics include stubbornness, over compensatory control, compulsive cleanliness and extreme self control. He may also develop intense anxiety or guilt or an antisocial personality.

Late Childhood (6-11 years)

1. Late childhood is a period of slow and uniform growth. The average annual increase in height is 2-3 inches and the average annual weight increase is 3-5 lbs.
2. Emotional expressions are usually pleasant ones, although outbursts of anger, anxiety and frustration may continue to occur.
Psychosocial Development
3. It is during this stage there is increased ego control over basic drives. Behavioral characteristics like sympathy and concern for others, cleanliness, modesty, co-operation and willingness to share develop. The child now looks beyond the family and begins to interact with the social system.
4. Developmental tasks during this period are the acquisition of social skills, incorporating social values and patterns, and competition and interaction with peers and authority figures. Failure in mastery of the tasks results in emotional instability, low self-esteem, social inferiority and inability to assume expected responsibilities.

Adolescence (12-19 years)

1. The period of adolescence is a period of "storm and stress," an action-oriented phase of life in which feelings and thoughts are primarily expressed through behavior.
2. The important physical changes which occur during this period include changes in body size and proportion, and the development of primary and secondary sex characteristics.
Psychosocial Development
3. A major change from the childhood to the adolescent is the development of self-consciousness. Adolescents become very aware of how others see them and react to them, and this awareness makes teenagers feel apprehensive and extremely self-conscious.
4. This is the period when there is a consolidation of personality and a beginning sense of identity as a mature person. Phase specific tasks for the adolescent may be identified as gaining independence from the family, integrating new found sexual maturity, establishing meaningful relationships with peers of both sexes, and making decisions about life work and goals.
5. Parent-adolescent conflict is very common, as adolescents seek independence from their parents. The approval of their own age group is much more important to them than the approval of adults. Intense conflicts can occur if the values of the group conflict with those of the parents. Being a member of the peer group has a strong influence on the self-identity and self-esteem of the adolescent.
6. The issues of the period of later adolescence (15-19 years) are related to career, marriage and parenthood. This is the period when there is a consolidation of the personality and a beginning sense of identity as a mature person.

7. Characteristic troubles of the adolescent identity crisis may include psychosis, neurosis, delinquency (breaking rules of society), etc.

Early Adulthood (20-40 years)

1. The term 'adult' is derived from the Latin word 'adultus', which means 'grown to full size and strength'. Adults are therefore individuals who have completed their growth and are ready to assume their status in society along with other adults.
2. During this stage, the physical and psychological changes which accompany the beginning of reproductive capacity appear. The Basal Metabolic Rate (BMR) slowly begins to come down, when compared to adolescence, so excess body weight is easily gained.

Psychosocial Development

3. The four major social expectations or tasks for the adult include choice of career, sexual mutuality (marriage/choosing a life partner), generativity and child-rearing, participation in social processes and work.
4. If the young adult has been over-protected by parents, difficulties arise in forming intimate relationships with another person and coping with responsibilities in the working world.

Middle Adulthood (41-60 years)

Physical changes related to ageing become more prominent, such as wrinkled skin, muscular pains and impaired sensory capacities. Faulty lifestyles may bring on diseases such as hypertension, heart disease, cancer, etc. A very major physical change is menopause or the male climacteric. Many physical discomforts and mood changes may accompany menopause, and they may become depressed, hostile and self-critical and have wide mood swings. All these usually disappear once endocrine balance is restored. How successfully women make the adjustment to the physical and psychological changes that accompany menopause is greatly influenced by their past experiences, and especially the social support available to them.

Psychosocial Issues

1. During this age, people become more and more occupied with their work and family. The major adjustments to be made during this period include adjusting to physical and mental changes, occupational responsibilities, approaching retirement and old age.
2. Failure to master these developmental tasks may lead to marital, social or occupational conflicts and failures.

Late Adulthood (Old age 60 years and above)

1. Physical changes include wrinkling of skin, stooped posture, flabbiness of muscles, decreased vision and hearing, a decreased efficiency of cardiovascular system.
2. Psychosocial issues.
3. The theme of this age period is loss, which may be:
   • Loss of physical abilities
   • Loss of intellectual processes
   • Loss of work role and occupational identification (retirement)
   • Loss of intimate ties, such as death of spouse, friends and other acquaintances
4. The major adjustments to be made include adjustment to physical changes, retirement, loss of spouse, post-child rearing period (empty nest syndrome), grandparenthood.

5. If favorable factors such as satisfaction of needs, retention of old friendships, positive social attitudes, etc. are present, they foster ego integrity of the person. However without adequate support to sustain and bear the losses the older adult is vulnerable to a profound sense of insecurity. Despair and disgust can take over the person, including the feeling, time is running out and there are no alternatives possible at this late date.

6. Serious personality breakdown in old age may lead to criminal behavior or suicidal tendencies, as in dementia.

TYPES OF PERSONALITY

Hypocrates Classification (400 BC)

A great physician known as father of medicine based on the individuals temperaments, human being are classified into four characteristic groups according to their temperaments.

Type of fluids in the body	Personality type	Temperamental characteristics
Blood	Sanguine	Optimistic, happy, hopeful, accommodating and lighthearted.
Phlegm	Philegatic	Cold, calm, slow, and indifferent.
Black bile	Melancholic	Sad, depressed, pessimistic, dejected, deplorable, and self-involved.
Yellow bile	Choleric	Irritable, passionate, strong, active, imaginative.

Kretschmer's Classification

Kretschmer classificated all human being into certain biological types according to their physical structure:

Physical structure	Personality type	Characteristics
Fatty body	Pyknic	Sociable, jolly, easy going and good natured.
Balanced body	Athletic	Energetic, optimistic and adjustable.
Lean and thin	Leptosomatic	Unsociable, reserved, shy, sensitive and pessimistic.

Sheldon's Classification

Human being was classified by their physical body structures and attached certain temperamental characteristics to them:

Name	Description	Characteristics
Endomorphic	Person having highly developed viscera but weak somatic structure (fat, soft, round-like pyknic type)	Easy going, sociable, affectionate and fond of eating.
Mesomorphic	Balanced development of viscera and somatic structure—muscular, strong (like athletic type)	Craving for muscular activity, self-assertive, loves risk and adventure, energetic, assertive and bold tempered.
Ectomorphic	Weak somatic structure as well as undeveloped viscera-thin, long fragile (like Kertschmer's leptosomatic)	Pessimistic, unsociable, reserved, brainy, artistic and introvert.

Jung's Classification

Dr Karl G Jung proposes to classify the personality based on complex network of ideas bound together by a common emotion or a set of feeling.

	Extrovert	*Introvert*
Interest	The extrovert are interested in the world around them	The introverts are interested in themselves, their own feeling, emotions and are unable to adjust easily to social situation.
Social interaction	Involves in social participation, they are sociable, not easily upset by difficulties.	Socially they are aloof and withdrawn.
Adjustment	They are successful in adjusting to the realities of their environment, are socially active and more interested in leaving a good impression on others.	They prefer to work alone and avoid social contacts. They are inclined to worry and get easily embarrassed.
Influencing factor	Their behavior is influenced more by physical stimulation than by their inner thought and ideas.	Introverts are the persons who seek the manifestation of their life through inner activities by going inward or dragging up things from within themselves.
Area of occupation	Politicians, social workers, lawyers, insurance agents, salesmen, etc. fall in this category.	Philosophers, scientists, writers, etc.

Hans-Eyseneh's Classification (1967)

Distinct types in his theory of personality are introversion, extroversion, neuroticism, and psychoticism.

Sl.No	*Type of personality*	*Characteristics*
1.	Type A Personality	The characteristics of type A personality are competitive drive, restlessness, hostility, sense of urgency, impatience, hard driving, live under constant pressure. Seeks recognition and advancement, multiple activities with deadliness to meet and cope up more constructively with stressors might be useful.
2.	Type B Personality	Calmer, more philosophical, easy going, non-competitive, little dull, longer life, struggle to control situation, but when they fail to do so, they stop coping.

Gordon Allport's Classification (1937)

Gordon Allport counted 18000 traits terms designated as distinctive and personal forms of behavior and divided into three parts.

Sl. No.	Traits	Characteristics
1.	Cardinal traits	Are traits which are so dominant that nearly all of the individual's actions can be traced back to them? Each term describes a trait so broad and so deep in its impact that it overshadows the influence of other traits in the same individual. He believed that most people have no true cardial traits.
2.	Central traits	Are traits which are major characteristics of a person such as trust, worthiness, honesty or conscientiousness?
3.	Secondary traits	Are less important characteristics that are not central to our understanding of an individual's personality such as particular attitudes, performance and style of behavior.

THEORIES OF PERSONALITY

There are five paradigms that have been chosen to represent personality theories (Herhenhahn, 1944). Each paradigm is named after its central them. All paradigms provide useful information about personality and contribute to understanding personality.

1. **Psychonalytical paradigm:** For example, personality theories of Sigmund Freud and Carl Jung. This paradigm focuses on the analysis of the psyche.
2. **Sociocultural paradigm:** For example, personality theories of Alfred Adler, Karen Horney and Erik Erikson. This paradigm emphasizes the importance of sociocultural factors influencing personality.
3. **Trait paradigm:** For example, personality theories of Gorton Allport and Raymond B Cattell. This paradigm emphasizes the importance of various traits that a person possesses.
4. **Learning paradigm:** For example, personality theories of BF Skinner, John Dollard and Neal Miller, Albert Bandura and Walter Barash. This paradigm emphasizes the importance of learning in personality development.
5. **Sociobiological.**

PSYCHOANALYTICAL THEORY— FREUD'S

Freud (1939), father of psychoanalytical theory, is created as the first to identify development by stages. He believed that the first 5 years of a child's life to be the most important, as he believed that an individual's basic character had been formed by the age of 5.

Freud's personality theory conceptualization:

Sl.No	Theories	Description
1.	Structure of personality	Id, Ego, Superego
2.	Dynamics of personality	Conscious, preconscious, semiconscious, unconscious.
3.	Topography	Cathexis, anti cathexis.
4.	Stages of personality development	Oral stage, anal stage, phallic stage, latency stage and genital stage.

The Structure of Personality

Sl.No	Types	Description
1.	Id	The Id contains all our biological based drives—the urge to eat, drink, and eliminate especially to be sexually stimulated. The Id operates according to the pleasure principle. It aims to achieve immediate gratification. It driven behaviors are impulsive and may be irrational.
2.	Ego	It is based on rational self or reality principle, it develop between ages of 4 and 6 months. It acts as a mediator to maintain harmony among the external world. It experiences the reality of the external world, adapts to it and responds to it.
3.	Superego	It is based on perfection principle. It develops between 3 and 6 years, internalizes the values and morals set fourth by primary caregivers. The superego is important in the socialization of the individual as it assist the ego in the control of Id impulses. When the superego becomes rigid and punitive, problems with low self-confidence and low-self esteem arise.

Dynamics of Personality

Sl.No	Theories	Description
1.	Conscious	Consciousness refers to the perception, thoughts and feelings existing in a person's immediate awareness. The conscious includes all memories that remain within an individual's awareness. It is thought to be under the control of the ego, the rational and logical structure of the personality.
2.	Preconscious	Preconscious includes all memories that may have been forgotten or not in present awareness but that with attention can be recalled into consciousness. Preconscious content on the other hand, is not immediately accessible to awareness.
3.	Unconscious	The unconscious includes all memories that one is unable to bring to conscious awareness. Unconscious material consists of unpleasant or nonessential memories that have been repressed and can retrieved only through therapy, hypnosis and with certain substances that alter the awareness and have the capacity to restructure repressed memories.

Stages of Personality Development/Psychosexual Development

Sigmund Freud (1856-1939), described formation of personality through five stages of psychosexual development:

Sl.No.	Theories	Description
1.	Oral stage (infancy) 1-18 months	During this stage baby's mouth is the focal point of pleasure, children suck, bite and chew anything that fits into their mouth. Infant obtains gratification by taking in, begins to develop self-concepts from the

Contd...

Contd...

Sl.No.	Theories	Description
		response of others. Interest in oral gratification from sucking, eating, mouthing, biting.
2.	Anal stage (early childhood) 18 months to 3 years	Gratification from expelling and withholding feces; coming to terms with society's controls relating to toilet training. In early part of his period, the child freely gratifies his love of self with the pleasurable sensation involved in evacuating the bladder and bowels naturally and without restriction. Freud believed that if great success is placed on the child in relation to remaining clean during this period, he may grow up compulsively clean. Other adult attitudes thought to be rigid toilet training include stubbornness hoarding, collecting excessive concern with bowel function and sadistic or masochistic tendencies.
3.	Phallic stage (later childhood) 3-6 years	Interest in the genitals; coming to terms with edipal conflict, leading to identification with same-sex parent. The focus of pleasurable sensation has shifted from the mouth and the excretory organs to the genitalia. Freud proposed that the development of the Oedipus complex occurred.
4.	Latency stage (6-12 years)	Sexual concerns largely unimportant. During the elementary school years, the focus changes from egocentrism to one of more interest in group activities, learning and socialization with peers. Sexuality is not absent during this period but remains obscure and imperceptible to others. The preference is homosexual; children of this age show a distinct preference for same-sex relationships, even rejecting members of opposite sex.
5.	Genital stage (12-18 years)	Re-emergence of sexual interests and establishment of mature sexual relationships. During puberty and adolescence final stage of personality development is characterized by a reactivation of libidinal energy and focusing of this energy on the genital area. The adolescent is simultaneously drawn towards his parents and driven away from them. This ambivalence is manifested by much conflict between behaving in a dependent, immature, child like way and in an independent, mature adult manner.

Topography of the Mind

Sl.No.	Theories	Description
1.	Psychic energy	It is the force or impetus required for mental functioning. The psychic energy originates in the Id and instinctually fulfills basic physiological needs is called libido. As the child matures, it is diverted from the Id to from the ego and then from the ego to form the super ego.
2.	Cathexis	It is the process by which the Id invests energy into an object in an attempt to achieve gratification.
3.	Anticathexis	It is the use of psychic energy by the ego and the superego to control Id impulses.

PSYCHOSOCIAL THEORY—ERIKSON'S

Erik H Eriksson, born in 1902, build on Freud's theories by identifying eight development stages that encompasses the entire life span, referred as eight ages of man.

Sl.No.	Stages	Description
1.	Trust vs Mistrust (birth to 18 months)	The major development task during this stage is to develop a basic trust with the mothering figure and be able to generalize it to others. The trust depends not on absolute quantities of food or demonstrations of love, but rather on the quality of maternal relationship, when needs, met, trust develops. Distrust can develop if the infant's world is filled with insecurity due to unmet needs, caused by lack of caring on the part of parents and significant others.
2.	Autonomy vs Shame (18 months to 3 years) Early childhood	The major developmental task during this stage is to gain some self-control and independence within the environment. Achievement of the task results in a sense of self-control and ability to delay gratification. Autonomy is achieved when parents encourage and provide opportunities for independent activities. Nonachievement results in a lack of self-confidence, lack of pride in the ability to perform, a sense of being controlled by others and a range against the self.
3.	Initiative vs Guilt (4 - 5 years) Middle childhood	The major development task during this stage is developing a sense of purpose and ability to initiate and direct own activities. Achievement of the task results in ability to exercise restraint and self control of inappropriate social behavior, enjoys learning and personal achievement, achieve, initiative when creativity is encouraged and performance is recognized and positively reinforced. If this initiative and curiosity are discouraged, the child may be prevented from setting future goals by a sense of guilt and shame for holding such ambitions.
4.	Industry vs Inferiority (6 - 11 years) Late childhood	The major developmental task during this stage is to achieve a sense of self-confidence by learning, competing, performing successfully and receiving recognition from significant others, peers and acquaintances. Achievement of the task results in a sense of satisfaction and pleasure in the interaction and involvement with others; master's reliable work habits and develops attitudes of trust worthiness; feels pride in achievement. This industry is achieved when encouraged for activities and responsibilities given in home, school and community. Non achievement results in difficulty in interpersonal relationships owing to feeling of personal inadequacy; neither cooperate and compromise with others in group's activities nor problem solver or complete task successfully.
5.	Identity vs Role confusion (12-20 years) Adolescence	The major developmental task during this stage is to integrate the tasks mastered in the previous stages into a secure sense of self. Childhood comes to an end during this stage and youth begins. Puberty brings on a physiological revolution with each adolescents must learn to cope. Achievement of this task results in a sense of confidence, emotional stability and a view of self as unique individual. Identity is achieved when adolescent are allowed to experience independence by making decisions that influence their values. Nonachievement

Contd...

Contd...

Sl.No.	Stages	Description
		results in sense of self-consciousness, doubt and confusion about one's role in life.
6.	Intimacy vs Isolation (20-30 years) Young adolescence	The major development task during this stage is to form as intense, lasting, relationship or a commitment to another person. Intimacy is achieved by the task results in the capacity for mutual love and respect between two people and the ability of an individual to pledge a total commitment to another, personal sacrifices are made for another; capacity for giving of oneself to another. This is learned when one has been the recipient of this type of giving within the family unit. Nonachievements results in withdrawal, social isolation, aloneness unable to form lasting intimate relationships, often seeking intimacy through numerous superficial sexual contacts.
7.	Generativity vs Stagnation (30 to 65 years) Adulthood	The major development task during this stage is to achieve the life goals established for oneself, while also considering the welfare of future generations. Achievement of the task results in a sense of gratification from personal and professional achievements and form meaningful contributions. Nonachievement results in lack of concern for the welfare of others and total preoccupation with the self becomes withdrawn, isolated and highly selfindulgent with no capacity for giving of self to others.
8.	Ego integrity vs Despair (65 years to death) Old age	The major developmental task during this stage is to review one's life and derive meaning from both positive and negative events while achieving a positive sense if self worth. Achievement of the task results in a sense of selfworth and selfacceptance as one reviews life goals; derives a sense of dignity from his or her life experiences and does not fear death. Nonachievement results in a sense of selfcontempt and disgust with how life has progressed; feels worthless and hopeless to change; feels anger, depression and loneliness; fears death.

LEARNING THEORIES OF PERSONALITY

Social Learning Theory—Bandura and Walter's

1. Albert Bandura and Richard Walter in 1963—gave altogether a new approach to personality in the shape of a social learning theory.
2. The theory emphasizes that what one represents through his personality is very much acquired through a process of continuous structuring and restructuring of his experience through social learning.
3. Observational learning from social situations may involve both real and symbolic models. Children, for example, may learn social etiquette by watching their parents and elders as well as by direct instructions.

Learning Theory of Personality—Dollard and Miller's

1. John Dollard and Neal Miller (1950), in the institute of Human relations at Yale University provided their own theory of personality. In this theory they tried to substitute Freud's concept of a pleasure principle with the principle of reinforcement, concept of ego with the concept of learned drive and learned skills, concept of conflict with competing reinforces, etc.
2. It emphasizes that what we consider as a personality is learned. The child at birth is equipped with two types of basic factors; reflexes and innate hierarchies of response and a set of primary drives, which are internal stimuli of great strength and are linked with known psychological processes.
3. Dollard and Miller's theory of personality stressed the acquisition of personality in the same way as learning of most of the responses and behavior through the process of motivation and reward.

Self Theory—Carl Roger's

1. Carl Ransom Roger, an American psychologist in 1947, brought out a new theory of personality named self-theory quiet distinct from the earlier theories of personality.
2. He stressed the importance of an individual's self for determining the process of his growth and development, and unique adjustment to his environment. There are two basic systems underlying his personality theory- the organism and the self.
3. Roger considers them as system operating in one's phenomenological field (a world of subjective experience, the personal and separate reality of each individual). The organism is an individual's entire frame of reference. The represents the totality of experience—both conscious and unconscious available with him.
4. The second system the self is the accepted, awareness part of experience. The self as a system of one's phenomenal field can perhaps best be understood in terms of our concepts of I, me or myself. Human being have inherited a tendency to develop their self in the process of inter-personal and social experiences which they have in the environment.
5. Roger does not propose a set of specific stages in the development of personality as proposed by Freud in his history, rather his advocate's continuity of growth in terms of the continuous evolution of the concept of self.
6. Once a concept of self is formed, the individual strives to maintain it. In order to do this, he regulates his behavior. What is consistent at conscious level while what threatens the image of self may be totally ignored or buried deep in his conscious?
7. The most unfortunate results in the environment of one's personality lie in the cases where an individual develops some false self-images. This false image is often so strong that obvious reality can be stoutly denied.

TRAIT APPROACH THEORY

Trait Approach GB Allport

GB Allport (1897-1967)—was the first personality theorist who adopted trait approach in providing a theory of personality. According to him, an individual develops a unique set of organized tendencies or traits, generally, these traits are organized around a few cardinal (primary) trait. Allport's theory asserts that no two individuals are alike. Allport regarded traits as responsible for these individual differences according to Allport; triad is a predisposition to act in the same way in a wide range of situations. Allport deeply committed to study of individual traits. He started calling them as personal dispositions. Common traits were simply called as traits. Allport proposed that are three types of personal dispositions.

Sl.No.	Types	Description
1.	Cardinal disposition	A cardinal disposition is so dominant that all actions of the person are guided by it. Very few people possess cardinal dispositions.
2.	Central disposition	These are not a dominant as cardinal dispositions, but they influence the person's behavior in a very prominent way. Therefore, they are called the building blocks of personality.
3.	Secondary disposition	These are not very consistent and are thus less relevant in reflecting the personality of the individual.

Trait Theory—Raymond Cattell's

The most recent advanced theory of personality based on trait approach has been developed by Raymond B Cattell, a British born American researcher. He defined trait as a structure of the personality inferred from behavior in different situation and describes four types of traits.

Sl.No.	Types	Description
1.	Common traits	The traits found widely distributed in general population like honesty, aggression and cooperation.
2.	Unique traits	Unique to a person as temperamental traits, emotional reaction.
3.	Surface traits	Able to recognize by our manifestations of behavior like curiosity, dependability, tactfulness.
4.	Source traits	Underlying structures of source that determine one's behavior such as dominance, submission, emotionality, etc.

According to cattell, personality is that which permits us to predict what a person will do in a given situation. In line with his mathematical analysis of personality, prediction of behavior can be made by means of a specification equation:

$$R = f (S, P)$$

According to this formula the response (R) of the person is a function (f) of the stimulus (S) at a given moment of time, and of the existing personality structure (P). This equation conveys Cattell's strong belief that human behavior is determined and can be predicted.

Trait-Type Theory of Personality-Hans Eysenck's

This approach tries to synthesis the type and trait approaches. Eysenck gave it more specification by grouping traits into definite types. The essence of personality can be arranged hierarchilly. In this scheme certain super traits and types such as extroversion exert a powerful influence over behavior. According to Eysenck's focus has been on a small member of personality types, defined by two major dimensions: Introversion-extroversion, stability-instability (neuroticism).

Sl.No.	Types	Stable	Unstable
1.	Introvert	Calm	Moody
		Reliable	Anxious
		Controlled	Rigid
		Peaceful	Pessimistic
		Careful	Reserved
2.	Extrovert	Leader	Restless
		Easygoing	Aggressive
		Talkative	Impulsive
		Outgoing	Optimistic
		Sociable	Active

Basing on his categorization of personality types, Eysenck constructed an inventory called Eysenck Personality Questionnaire (EPQ). It covers item from each of the personality types identified by them throughout his writing, Eysenck consistently emphasized the role of genetic factors and neurophysiologic factors, role of the cerebral cortex, autonomous nervous system, limbic system, reticular activating system in explaining individual differences in behavior.

PSYCHOMETRIC ASSESSMENT OF PERSONALITY

Personality testing is done for various reasons. A personnel psychologist may want to identify people for a salesman's job. A clinical psychologist often uses personality tests to evaluate psychological disorders. We want to describe it and know what type of personality or the personality traits possessed by us or others. It needs the knowledge and skill for the assessment or measurement of personality.

Subjective Methods of Personality Assessment

It is that approach where methods employed provide an opportunity to the individuals to speak about themselves. The methods followed under this approach are called subjective methods.

Sr.No	Type	Description
1.	Autobiography	The subject (individual) is asked to write his autobiography either on a structured pattern or an unstructured pattern. Generally, only those subjects should be asked of guidance. Such autobiographical material

Contd...

Contd...

Sl. No.	Type	Description
		provides data on the personal qualities of an individual, for instance, goals, aspirations, hopes, wishes, disappointments, frustrations, etc.
2.	Case history method	The case history method takes into consideration the time factor and the changes in the personality of an individual during this time. Following steps should be followed in the case history method. • Identification data. • Family background. • Health history. • Educational achievement. • Emotional and social behavior. • Interpretation of the data. • Evaluation treatment. The above information helps in making predictions about the personality of an individual. This method has a limited application for educational institutions but it is more useful in clinics for the treatment of patients.
3.	Case study method	This method is concerned with the intensive study of an individual with the aim of having an holistic view of that individual. The cases of the problems of an individual are found on the basis of the collected information and remedial treatment is suggested for better adjustment in the society, school or home environment. Following steps should be taken into consideration while following the case study method. • Selection of the subject or the case. • Reason for the selection of the case/subject. • Tools for recording data like cumulative records, tests, medical reports, etc. • General information about the subject. • Health records. • Family background. • Educational data. • Social relations. • Hobbies, interests, attitudes, etc. • Interpretation of data. • Remedial treatment to the case/subject under study. The following points should to take into consideration for selecting a case for case study. • Preferably, problem children, that are those who are truants, delinquents, low-achievers, shy, quite and retiring etc. should be selected for the case study. The teacher is free to select any student for case study depending upon the situation. • Selection of the case by the teacher should be made from his class. • Time and facilities should be taken into consideration for the case study in question.

Contd...

Sl.No.	Type	Description
4.	Questionnaires	A questionnaire is a valuable tool for collecting information directly given by a person. Such an information may consists of personal knowledge, like and dislikes (values and preferences), attitudes and beliefs, experiences (biography) and present status of things or event. This information can be both qualitative (verbal, description, comments or views) and quantitative (numbers, or scores as in the case of rating scale or opinion scores elicited by attitude scales). Any assembly of questions cannot be called a questionnaire. It must reflect an objective, a design and a framework. It is a way of obtaining data about persons by asking them rather than watching them behave or by sampling a portion of their behavior. A good questionnaire embodies a beginning, middle and an end. There is an introductory section comparing a note on the purpose of the questionnaire, an appeal and a direction for responding to the various questions and a basic data part of which is to filled in accurately by the respondents.
5.	Interviews	An interview is face to face talking with a purpose. It is a systematic method by which one person enters more or less imaginatively into the inner life of another who is generally a comparative stranger to him. An interview can be formal or informal. For good interview, there is a need for establishing a rapport between the interviewee and the interviewer.

Objective Methods of Personality Assessment

Objective data are collected by experts using specific tools or devices based upon certain methodologies. These methods which are used to collect objective data regarding varied personality aspects of an individual are called objective methods of assessing the personality of an individual. These methods are also known as observational methods as these are based upon the observation of experts rather than the answers given by individuals an in the case of the subjective methods. The observation methods are rating scales, verbal behavior, situation tests and sociometiric method.

OBSERVATION METHOD

The observation method can be used to observe intellectual functioning, emotional development, interests, and hobbies and to study habits, etc.

Psychological Process

Four psychological processes are involved in collecting data in the observation method: Attention, sensation, perception and conception.

1. **Attention:** It implies a mental set or a state of alertness which an individual assumes in order to perceive selected events and conditions of things.
2. **Sensation:** It means the awareness of the internal and external environment through one's senses. It is the immediate results of a stimulus to the sense organs.
3. **Perception** is the art of liking what is sensed with some past experience to give meaning to sensation.

4. **Conception** is that quality of the mental activity associated with observing by which one removes blocks to perception through the creation of imaginative concepts. It is an intellectual representation of some aspects of reality which is derived from the perception of a phenomenon.

Steps of Observation Method

Following are the four elements of the observational method.
1. Deciding major phenomenon to be observed.
   - Defining the phenomenon to be observed.
   - Modalities for the observation of the phenomenon: Structured, semistructured, or unstructured.
   - Person conducting the observation.
   - System involved in recording various features of the phenomenon: Videotape, tape recorder or any other devices.
2. Recording.
3. Organizing.
4. Interpreting the observations.

Precautions

1. Training of the observer is a must.
2. Subjective of the observer should be involved to be minimum possible extent.
3. The observer should have knowledge of personality aspects.
4. A member of observations should be taken for the purpose of making the observation more reliable.

Phenomena Amenable to Observations

Phenomena amenable to observations include:
1. **Characteristics and conditions of individuals:** Like people's attributes and states such as physical appearance, physiological symptoms that can be observed directly through the senses or with the aid of observational apparatus such as radiography.
2. **Verbal communication behaviors:** Like observing the content and structure of people's conversations .e.g., nurses giving information to parents, nurses conversation with grieving relatives.
3. **Nonverbal communication behaviors:** Include facial expressions, touch, posture, gestures, and other body movements.
4. **Activities:** Like patient's eating habits and trends and aggressive actions among children in the hospital playroom.
5. **Skill attainment and performance:** Like behavior assessment through skill development by patients and nurses.
6. **Environmental characteristics:** Noise levels in different areas of a hospital, cleanliness in homes in a community, safety, hazards of children's classroom, shelters of homeless, etc.

SITUATIONAL TESTS METHOD

In situation tests, certain artificial situations resembling real life situations are created before the students. The reaction of the students are recorded and interpreted. The interpretations on the recorded responses under certain situations reveal the personality of the individual. These tests provide opportunities to observe the behavior in life situations. Traits like leadership, initiative, cooperation, persistence, risk-taking capacity, honesty, flexibility, imagination, etc. can be assessed. Reliability and validity of these tests have not been ascertained.

Group Discussion

It is a general part of the selection procedure for admission. Group discussion is a situational test. A group is given a problem on a certain theme. No one is assigned the duty of a group leader. Every one in the group is free to express ideas on the problem. In this situation, qualities like initiative, imagination, accommodation, suggestibility, flexibility etc can be assessed.

Created Situations to Assess Honesty

A teacher may create the following situations in the class to assess the honesty traits of his students;
1. The teacher holds a class test.
2. He evaluates the written performance but does not show marks on the answer-books.
3. He distributes the answer-book to the student expressing his inability to mark the answer-books due to certain reasons. He asks his students to handover the answer-books the next day.
4. The answer-book is collected again.
5. Those students are located whose awards are found higher due to additions. Thus, some students may reveal their dishonesty trait or honesty trait.

Imaginary Situations

Imaginary situations can be created and responses of students to these imaginary situations may reveal personality aspects of the individuals. For example, suppose one of us comes across an individual who inquire about a certain place and the approach road to reach that place.

Situational Test by May and Hartshorne

May and Hartshorne mention a number of situational tests in their book studies in deceit. One example related to honesty from this book is mentioned. The teacher had a box containing coins. Coins from the box were distributed to some of the students in a class. The coin left in the box was counted and then the box was placed in a corner. Students were asked to place back the coins given to them. The coins were again counted. Some students kept the coins with themselves.

SOCIOMETRIC METHOD

The sociometric method involves studying relationship among the members a group which helps in assessing the personality traits of the members of the group. Mereno devised this method. Social preferences with specific references to a specific criterion are recorded. For example, social preferences of students are recorded on the following questions:
1. With whom would you like to sit in the class?
2. With whom would you like to go on the educational tour?

The sociometric data so obtained can be expressed graphically. Such graphical expression is called a sociogram. A sociogram revels information regarding sub-groups, cliques, stars, isolated, neglected, rejected. Appropriate steps can be taken on the basis of the sociometric data to improve the personality of the individuals.

RATING SCALE

A rating scale is an instrument designed to facilitate appraisals of a number of traits or characteristics by references to a common quantitative scale of values. The rating scale is used to know from others where an individual stands in terms of some personality traits.

Three points are taken into consideration in this method:
1. The specific traits or traits to be rated are specified.
2. The scale range is also decided, i.e. 3 point scale, 5 point scale, 7 point scale or 11 point scale.
3. Those persons are decided who are require to use the scale to quantify the trait regarding a specific person whose personality is to be measured, e.g. we may decide that these specific persons will submit their observations on the scale for a particular trait (s) regarding a person.

Precautions while using a Rating Scale

The rating scale method can be made more effective if the following precautions are taken.
1. The raters should be impartial.
2. A number of rater should give their rating and these should be taken into consideration for framing the final assessment on the traits.
3. Generally, the halo effect is the there in the rating of the raters for different traits. It should be checked. It is a tendency for transfer to occur so that a rater many rate the same individual high or low for many different traits. One impression may color the rest.
4. Avoid being too lenient or too strict in standard.
5. Avoid the tendency to either remain at the neutral points or the extreme points in the rating scale.

Purposes of Rating Scale

According to Freemen (1965), the purposes of rating scales are as follows.
1. Rating scales are chiefly useful for finding out what impression an individual has made of persons with whom he has come in contact with respect to some specified traits or attitudes.
2. It is a device that rates social values, occupational efficienency, group status and the like in certain specified areas.
3. It reflects the impression the subject has made upon the persons who do the rating.
4. For the evaluation of an individual, rating scales are submitted to teachers, counselors, employers, colleagues, parents and others who have had sufficient contact with the person in question.
5. Rating scales may be devised for a variety of traits such as tact, generosity, leadership, co-cooperativeness, resourcefulness, punctuality, industriousness, honesty, personal attractiveness, etc.

Points for the Construction and use of Rating Scale

1. Each trait should be clearly defined.
2. The degree of the trait should be defined. Each trait should be rated on a scale, most frequently of five or seven intervals.
3. The mean or the median of the rating by different judges should be taken for having a reliable rating.
4. Guidance counselors, employers and personnel officers find them helpful if the judges are carefully selected and if the rating are properly made.

5. Overt traits are more reliably rated than convert traits. For example, overt traits like emotional expression, social acceptability, manifest fear and anxiety, aggressive or impulsive acts are related with greater reliability than the covert traits like a person's inner life and feeling about one's self.
6. Degree of certainty of rating should be stated, e.g. very strong, strong, and moderate.
7. Extroverted persons are more reliably judged than introverted ones.

Types of Rating Scales

1. Scoring rating scale.
2. Ranking rating scale.

PROJECTIVE TESTS

Introduction

This technique has been developed by Swiss psychologist, son of an art teacher Mr. Harmans Rorschach. Projective methods involve an unstructured stimulus or situation. In this process, the individual projects his unconscious desires, fears, motives, drives, needs, etc. subjective and objective methods do not clear study the unconscious mind of an individual. Projective methods deal with the conscious as well as the unconscious mind. The unconscious mind is 9/10th of the mind and inner urges, wishes, emotions, etc. are not visible to the outsiders and the individual himself.

Definition

Projective test is an instrument that is considered sensitive to covert or unconscious aspect of behavior. It permits or encourages a wide variety of subject's responses. It is highly multidimensional it invokes rich and profuse response data with a minimum of subject's awareness, concerning the purpose of the test—Lindsey.

Characteristics of Projective Test

According to Rastogi (1983), following are the characteristic features of a projective test:
1. Brief instructions are given to the subjects which are necessary for him/her to respond.
2. The test material is kept ambiguous projects his characteristic ideas, attitudes, strivings, fears, conflicts, aggressiveness, hostility, etc.
3. The purpose of the test is hidden from the subject.
4. The projective tests reflect the influence of psychoanalytical school.
5. The test reveals emotional and social characteristics, maladjustments, attitudes and motives. Certain intellectual aspects of individual behavior are also revealed.

RORSCHACH INKBLOT TEST

Description

This test that was developed by H Rorschach has ten cards with vague inkblot on them. Five of the cards are chromatic stimuli while rest of the five is achromatic stimuli, subjects are asked to tell what they see on these cards. Each response has elaborate scoring system and well developed interpretation. Rorschach Inkblot test reveals structural aspects of personality such as individual stability, value system ego strength, etc.

Procedure

1. The card is presented one at a time in a specific order. When the subject takes his seat, the examiner gives him the first card with necessary instruction. He is asked to say what he sees in it, what it looks like, etc.
2. The subject is allowed as much time as he wants of a given card and it is permitted to give as many responses to it as he wishes. He is also allowed to turn the card around and look at it from any angle to find things in it.
3. Besides keeping a record of the response of the subject concerning these inkblots on different pieces of paper, the examiner notes the time taken for each response, position in which cards are being held, emotional expression and other incidental behavior of the subject during the test period, etc.
4. After all the cards have been presented; the second phase of inquiry follows. It is intended to seek clarification or addition to original responses.

Verbal Projective Test

Present subjects with an ambiguous verbal stimuli rather than a pictorial one. There are two types of verbal methods.

1. **Association technique:** An example of an association technique is word-association method, which represents subjects with a series of words, to which the individual respond with the first thing comes to mind. The word list often combines both neutral and emotionally tinged words, which are included for the purpose of detecting impaired thoughts processes or internal conflicts, anxiety or any problems in relationships.
2. **Sentence completion test:** This test includes a list of incomplete sentences generally open at the end and is asked to complete them in any desired manner. This approach is frequently used as a method of measuring attitudes or some aspect of personality.

Expressive Method

These techniques encourage self-expression, through the construction of some product out of raw materials. The major expressive methods are play techniques, drawing and painting and role playing. It is believed that people express their feelings, needs, motives and emotions by working with or manipulating various materials.

Scoring of Responses

Responses to the test are scored in terms of location, determinants, content and popularity or originality taken for responses.

1. **Location:** The response of the subject in the context of the whole inkblot or a part of it is recorded. The subject may observe the whole ink for giving a response or a part of it. The subject may give large details or small details.
2. **Determining quality:** Scoring is done with specific responses of the subject on the form or shape, shades, movements (human movement, inanimate movement or animal movement) perceived by the subject.
3. **Contents:** The subject may respond on the inkbolt on the basis human figures, human details, parts of human figure, animal figure, details of animal figure, inanimate objects, plants, maps,

clouds, blood, nature (light), sexual objects and other symbols. The responses are recorded keeping in view the above contents of the inkblot.

4. **Popularity or originality:** Some responses are given frequently by normal subjects. These are called popular responses. Some responses may be extremely different which can be considered original responses.

Analysis

The recorded responses are analyzed in the light of location, determining quality, contents and popularity or originality.

Interpretation

Interpretation is done on the basis of the analyzed data. Interpretation of the responses is a different job. Generally, subjectivity comes in the way and reduces the validity of the test as such. There is need for further experimentation on the test to make valid.

A few examples of responses of the subject to Rorschach Inkblot test and the corresponding interpretation.

Sl.No.	Response	Interpretation
1.	The response is associated with the whole inkblot (location).	The subject has the ability to solve his problems in a comprehensive manner. He/she possess high mental ability.
2.	The response is linked with large details (location)	The subject has a practical approach towards problems of life.
3.	The response is linked with small details (location)	The subject expresses emotional conflicts.
4.	The response involved too many colors (determining quality)	The subjects are impulsive.
5.	Predominance of human figure movement (determining quality)	The subject has vivid imagination.
6.	The response frequently involved animal figures (determining quality)	The subject has stereotyped thinking and perhaped he/she is of low intelligence.

THERMATIC APPRECIATION TEST (TAT)

The test consisting of perception of a certain picture in a thermatic manner (revealing imaginative thermes) is called TAT or Thermatic appreciation test. This test was developed by Murray and Morgan in 1935.

Description

The standard test contains 30 pictures for men alone, 10 for women alone and, 10 mixed ones for both men and women. All the pictures are more or less vague. Each picture shows a dramatic or emotional scene that might have a number of explanations.

Administration of the Test

1. The picture is shown to the subject one by one and he asked to develop a story about each picture. The subject is asked to explain the picture and to give an imaginary reconstruction of what went before and what followed. Although a good deal of emotion is portrayed in each picture, yet it is not clear just what the excitement is all about.
2. Thus, a man may be shown pointing excitedly towards something but there is no clue as to what he is pointing at. The subject therefore, reads into the pictures some fantasies or interpretations of his own.
3. In giving meaning to the pictures, a person is certain to reveal something about him.
4. The raw material for a pupil's story comes from his own experiences and is colored by his own personality needs. His stories are scored for evidence of basic, unsatisfied urges and for environmental pressures.
5. The nature of the outcome is also examined, since it is the product of the needs and the pressures. Environmental and psychological aspects can be analyzed.

TAT Type Picture

TAT type pictures are:
1. Achievement motivation.
2. Need for affiliation.
3. Parent-child relationships.
4. Inner fantasies.
5. Level of aspiration.
6. Social and family relationships.
7. Functioning of sex urge.
8. Emotional conflicts.
9. Attitudes to work, minority groups or authority.
10. Outlook towards future.
11. Frustration.
12. Creativity.
13. Fear of success.

Modification of TAT

1. The number of pictures can be reduced depending upon the nature of the subjects and the experience of the expert.
2. Some other pictures can be combined with the original ones.
3. The test can be determined to act as a group test. Pictures can be projected and the group of individuals can be required to write stories after necessary instructions. Stories are evaluated individually to assess the personality of concerned students.
4. Bellaks modified TAT for using it for children of 3 to 11 years. This test is known as children's apperception test (CAT). The test consists of 10 pictures depicting situations of family relationships, toilet training, feeding habits, etc.

CHILDREN APPERCEPTION TEST (CAT)

Children apperception test (CAT) developed by D Leopold Bellak. TAT test is used among adults and adolescents but not suitable for children between 3 and 10 years.

Description

It consists of 10 cards. The cards have pictures of animals instead of human character since it was thought that children could identify themselves with animal figures more readily than with persons. These animals are shown in various life situations. For both sexes, all the 10 cards are needed. Whatever story the child makes, he projected himself. The pictures are designed to produce fantasies relating to the child's own experience, reactions.

Administering the Test

All the 10 cards are presented one-by-one and the subjected is asked to make up stories on them. The child should have confidence and he should take story making a pleasant game to play with.

Interpretation

Interpretation of the stories is centered round the following variables.

1. **Hero:** The personality traits of the hero as revealed by the story.
2. **Theme of the story:** What particular theme has he selected for the story building?
3. **The end of the story:** Happy ending or unhappy, wishful, realistic or unrealistic.
4. **Attitude towards parental figures:** Hatred, respectful, devoted, grateful, dependent, aggressive and fearful, etc.
5. **Family role:** With whom in the family the child identifies himself.
6. **Other outside figures introduced:** Objects of the elements introduced in the story but not shown in the picture.
7. **Omitted or ignored figures:** Which figures are omitted or ignored should be not as they may depict the wish of the subject that the figures were not there.
8. **Nature of the anxieties:** Harassment, lose of love, afraid of being left alone, etc, should also be noted.
9. **Punishment for crime:** The relationship between a crime committed in the story and severity of punishment given for it.
10. **Defense and confidence:** The types of defenses, flight, aggression, passivity, regression etc., the child takes nature of compliance or dependence, involvement in pleasure and achievement sex desire, etc.

WORD ASSOCIATION TEST

A word is presented to a subject and he/she is asked to answer as quickly as possible with the first word that comes in his/her mind. The interpretation depends upon two factors, responses and the reaction time. In this technique there are a number of selected words. The subject is told that:

1. The examiner will utter a series of words, one at a time.
2. After each word the subject is to reply as quickly as possible with the first word that comes to his mind.
3. There is no right or wrong responses.

The examiner than records the reply to each word spoken by him, the reaction time and any unusual speech or behavior manifestations accompanying a given response. The contents of the response along with other recoded things give clues for evaluating the human personality and thus help a psychologist in his work.

SENTENCE-COMPLETION TEST

These tests include a list of incomplete sentences, generally open at the end, which require completion by the subject in one or more words. The subject is asked to go through the list and answer as quickly as possible (without giving a second thought to his answer). For example, we can have the following sentences:

1. I am worried over.............
2. My hope is ....
3. I feel proud when.............
4. My hero is ....

The sentence competition tests are regarded as superior to word association because the subject may respond with more than one word. Also there it is possible to have a greater flexibility and variety of responses and more area of personality and experiences may be tapped.

In addition to the projective techniques mentioned above there are some others which may prove useful in many situation. These are play technique; drawing and painting tests etc. both of these techniques are very useful in the case of small children. In the former, the examiner observes the spontaneous behavior of the children while playing or constructing something with the help of given material and in the later, the natural free hand drawing and painting of the children are the matter of the study. Both of these techniques provide a good opportunity for the careful analysis of a child's personality.

MINNESOTA MULTIPHASIC PERSONALITY INVENTORY (MMPI)

One of the most commonly used personality test in the MMPI. It was developed during 1930's. This test asks for answers of True or False or Cannot say to 567 statements (one for men and another for women) about different personality traits such as attitudes, emotional reactions, physical and psychological symptoms and past experiences. The answers are quantitatively measured and personality assessment is done based on the norm scores. Dr NH Murthy of NIMHANS, Bangalore has reduced it to 100 items called multiphasic questionnaire.

MILLION CLINICAL MULTIAXIAL INVENTORY (MCMAI)

Items on this test correspond more closely than those on the MMPI to the categories of psychological disorders currently used by psychologists. This makes the test especially useful to clinical psychologist, who must find identity individuals problems before recommending specific forms of therapy for them.

NURSE AND PERSONALITY

1. The nurse needs know the basic structure of personality for providing effective care in the community and hospital set-up.
2. The nurse interacts different individual everyday so evaluation of character and personality is essential in planning the care.
3. The nurse should be basic understanding about the uses of defense mechanisms, it is important in making determinations about maladaptive behaviors, in planning care clients to assist in creative change, if desired or in helping clients accept themselves as unique individuals.
4. The nurse is not only to acquire skills and correct knowledge, she should have and develop a pleasing and string personality if she wants to be a successful nurse.

5. Possessing professional qualities are the essential characteristics of a nurse such as integrity, dignity, mental alertness, poise, self confidence and dependency. She ought to have such personal qualities as sympathetic, understanding, friendliness of spirit, gracious manners, kindness and adaptability.

6. The nurse interacts with patients, doctors, co-workers and other important members of society want certain behavior patterns, so the nurse should develop and practice well adjustable personality.

7. The patient appreciate a nurse who brings physical comfort to them with her skills, and is prepared to understand their emotional reaction and difficulties which have been caused by illness.

8. Personality is the total quality of an individual's behavior as it is shown in his habits of thinking in his attitudes, interests, his mammers of acting and personal philosophy, which facilitates quality patient care.

9. Personality is dynamic, growing thing, different in each person. Individuals are different from each other even at birth in physical appearance, motility or temperament, the needs to understand the individual differences while planning the care or education.

10. Many individuals with mental health problems are still struggling to achieve tasks from a number of developmental stages. Nurses can plan care to assist these individual in fulfilling these tasks and moving to a higher developmental level.

11. Assisting teaching and advising the parents, teachers and family's responsibility in developing and achieving developmental task in personality.

12. It incorporates sociocultural concepts into the development of personality.

CONCLUSION

Personality is something that enables a person to stand out has distinct from others. It is the total quality of an individual's behavior. It includes his physical, mental, emotional and temperamental make-up and how it shows itself in behavior. Personality is a dynamic thing it grows in a social setup. It is different in each person. The growth is affected by one's physique, glandular functioning, and physical appearance and physiological conditions of the body brought about by drugs, disease and toxins, the growth is also influenced by one's environmental and social factors as the relationships in the home and the school, social codes and roles which one has to play, the cinema, the agencies of social communication and the radio. Maternal factors influence the growth of our motives, acquired interests, our attitudes, will or character and our intellectual capacities. Personality can assessed or evaluated by means of interview, observation of behavior, rating scales, questionnaire and case study method. A successful nurse needs to develop a pleasing and strong personality such qualities as dignity, mental alertness, self-confidence, dependability, sympathetic understanding, a strong desire to help, a high standard of values and the ability to develop healthy interpersonal relationships, are generally associated with the personality of a successful nurse.

BIBLIOGRAPHY

1. Adler A. Przctiee and Theory of Individual Psychology, Harcourt Brace & World, New York, 1927
2. Allport GW, Personality—A Psychological Interpretation, Moft, New York, 1948.
3. Anastasi A. Psychological testing (2nd edn) Macmillan, New York, 1961.
4. Bandura A, Walters RH. Social Learning and Personality Development, Holt, New York, 1963.
5. Bhatia HR. Elernents of Educational Psychology (3rd edn reprint), Orient Longinan, Kolkata 1996s.
6. Butcher James N. Objective Personality Assessment, Academic Press, New York, 1972.

7. Cattell RB. Quoted by Hall, CS, Lindzey G. (2nd edn) Theories of Personality, John Wiley, 1970.

8. Cohen R, Dirk L Schaeffer. Patterns of Personality Judgment, Academic Press, New York, 1973.

9. Cronbach LJ. Essentials of Psychological Testing (3rd edn) Harper & Row, New York, 1970.

10. Dollard J, Miller NE. Personality and Psychotherapy, McGraw-Hill, New York, 1950.

11. Eysenck H J. Dimensions of Personality, Kegan Paul, London, 1994.

12. Eysenck HJ. the Structure of Human Personality (3rd Ed.), Methuen, New York, 1971.

13. Fordham F. An Introduction to Jung's Psychology, Penguin Books, London, 1953.

14. Freud S. An outline of psychoanalysis, Hogart, London, 1953.

16. Good and Hatt, Methods of SocialResearch, McGraw Hill, New York, 1952.

17. Freud S. An outline of Psychoanalysis, Norton, New York, 1939.

16. Hogan R. Personality Theory-Englewood Cliffs, Prentice Hall, New Jersey, 1976.

17. Janis IL, Mahi OF Kagan J, Holt RR. Personality Dynamics, Development and Assessment, Harcourt Brace, New York, 1969.

18. Jones E. The Life and Work of Sigmund Freud. Lionel Trilling and Steven Marcus (Eds). Garden City, Anchor, New York, 1963.

19. Klopfer B, Kelley D. The Rorschach Technique, World Book Co., Yonkers 1946.

20. Mischel, 'Walter, Personality and Assessment, John Wiley, New York, 1976.

Psychological Assessment, Testing and Evaluation

22

DEFINITIONS

1. **Reliability:** Reliability is concerned with the consistency, stability, and dependability of the results. In other words, a reliable result is one that shows similar performance at different times or under different conditions. If a student takes a test several times and has not grown in the area the test measures, he or she should earn a similar score each time.

2. **Reliability coefficient:** A reliability coefficient is determined by calculating the correlation between obtained and estimated true scores on a given test. If the reliability coefficient equals 0.00, the test reflects total unreliability. If the coefficient equals 1.00, there is no error in measurement whatsoever that is, every individual in the class would have obtained the same ranking on both administrations of the test.

3. **Measurement:** Measurement is a system for observing a phenomenon, attribute, or characteristic and translating those observations into numbers according a rule. We most often think of measurement in terms of equal-sized units that can be counted, such as centimeters on a ruler. Similarly, a child takes a spelling test and the teacher counts the number of correct answers, or a student takes a typing test and the instructor counts the number of words typed per minute. These do not have equal-sized units, but clearly 42 correct items on a test represents higher achievement than does 36. Numbers are assigned according to a procedure that applies equally to everyone, and the rule says that larger numbers represent greater skill than smaller ones.

4. **Testing:** A test is a set of specified, uniform tasks to be performed by students. These tasks are an appropriate sample from the knowledge or skills in a broader field of content. From the number of tasks performed correctly in the sample, the teacher makes an assumption of how the student is likely to perform in the total field.

5. **Evaluation:** Evaluation is the determination of the worth or the value of an event, object, or individual in terms of a specified criterion. Educators evaluate student progress by comparing student performance to the criteria of success based on instructional objectives. They evaluate a program in terms of how well children progress compared to how they might do in an alternative program.

6. **Achievement testing:** An achievement test is a systematic procedure for measuring a representative sample of learning tasks. Although the emphasis is usually on measuring a set of intended learning outcomes, as defined by the instructional objectives, it should not be implied that testing be limited to.

7. **Paper-and-pencil performance:** A paper-and-pencil performance test differs from the more traditional paper-and-pencil test by placing greater emphasis on the application of the

knowledge and skill in a simulated setting. These paper-and-pencil applications might result in desired terminal learning outcomes, or they might serve as an intermediate step to performance that involves a higher degree of realism (for example, the actual use of equipment).

8. **Identification test:** The identification test includes a wide variety of test situations representing various degree of realism. In some cases, a student may simply be asked to identify a tool or piece of equipment and to indicate its function. A more complex test situation might present the students with a particular performance task (for example, locating a short in an electrical circuit) and ask them to identify the tools, equipment, and procedures needed in performing the task.

9. **Student performance:** Student performance emphasizes proper procedure. The student is typically expected to perform the same motions as those required in the actual performance of the task, but the conditions are simulated. In physical education, for example, swinging a bat at an imaginary ball, shadow boxing, and demonstrating various swimming strokes out of water are simulated performances.

10. **Formative evaluation:** Formative evaluation can be defined as the designing and using of tests for only one specific purpose—to promote learning. Formative evaluation enables teachers to monitor their instruction so they can keep it on course. Also, if any student cannot learn excellently from the original instruction, the student can learn excellently from one or more correctives. While most teachers agree that going over test answers in class can help some students learn more about the material, it is essential that there be a much more systematic use of evaluation, separate from grading and aimed only at promoting learning.

11. **Summative evaluation:** Teachers have been using tests almost exclusively for determining grades, it may be assumed that with all that practice teachers are systematic in the way they convert raw scores into letter grades. But this is not so. Each teacher seems to have an individual system, and many teachers use a different system in each grading period. It is so because most teachers never find a system, with which they are satisfied. There is no single system that is right for all classes. Once the strengths and weaknesses of various grading systems are known, the choice can be exercised with greater wisdom.

12. **Competitive evaluation:** All evaluation systems can be grouped into two categories: Those that force a student to compete with other students (no referenced) and those that do not require interstudent competition but instead are based on a set of standards of mastery (criterion reference Traditionally, our schools have required competition among students and many teachers believe that competition among students is necessary for motivating. Many also believe that competition is needed to prepare students for adulthood in a competitive world, especially for getting ahead in their future employment.

13. **Standardized tests:** An example of tests that force students to compete among themselves is the standardized test, which is very popular today. Standardized tests have several features in common. First, they are based on norms derived from the average scores of thousands of students who have taken the test. Usually, these scores come from students throughout the nation, so each student's performance is compared with that of thousands of other students. Standardized tests are usually used to measure or grade a school's curriculum. They are also used to measure teacher success and student success. These tests make the students, teachers and schools accountable.

14. **Validity:** Validity is a characteristic that refers to the appropriateness of the inferences, uses, and consequences that result from the test or other method of gathering information. In other words, is the interpretation made from test results reasonable? How sound is the interpretation of the information? Validity is concerned with the inferences, not the test itself. Thus, it is an

inference or use that is valid or invalid, not the test, instrument, or procedure that is used togather information. Validity means a lot more than simply "the extent to which a test measures what it is supposed to measure".

INTRODUCTION

Evaluation includes a variety of procedures. A vast variety of evaluation procedures are available for measuring the results of teaching and learning. Evaluation procedures can be classified as qualitative and quantitative techniques. It can also be classified in terms of aspects of behavior to be evaluated and in term of evaluative method used.

DEFINITIONS OF EVALUATION

1. Evaluation is a relatively new technical term introduced to designate a more comprehensive concept of measurement than is implied in conventional tests and examination—*Wringhtone.*
2. Evaluation is essential in the never ending cycle of formulating goals, measuring progress towards then and determining the new goals which emerge as a result of new warnings — *Clara M Brown.*
3. Evaluation in education is a process of judging the effectiveness of educational experiences through careful appraisal—*LE Hidgerken.*
4. Evaluation is a process used to determine what has happened during a given activity or in an institution—*John W Best.*

Evaluation requires many skills—skills that are of equal importance with the other elements of the instructional process. A complete evaluation program for a teacher of nursing would encompass evaluation of:

1. Educational objectives
2. Teaching and learning procedures.
3. Student's progress.
4. Outcomes.

NURSING AND EVALUATION

The very essence of nursing requires, the nurses to evaluate constantly the patient's nursing needs as well as her own activities in meeting these needs guiding the patient in his own evaluating of his own health needs, determining how well he is meeting them and planning with him to maintain an optimal level of health.

All of this requires continuous evaluation. The nurses must evaluate the results of the interventions they perform for the patients. By evaluating the condition of patients they can provide better care to their patients.

General Evaluation Plan

1. Evaluation in education is a systematic process which enables to measure the extent to which the student has achieved the educational objectives.
2. This plan should include a list of learning outcomes and the techniques to be used in evaluating the outcomes.
3. It must be planned jointly by teachers and others including students involved in teaching learning process.
4. It should be a group activity.

Steps in Construction of a Test

Groulund summarized the preliminary steps in construction of test as follows:
1. Objectives and specific learning outcomes must be identified and defined in terms of desired changes in pupil behavior.
2. Subject matter contents must be outlined.
3. A table of specification, which relate to the subject matter content should be developed.
4. Specific test questions are constructed in accordance with the table of specification.

Steps in Evaluation

According to L Heidgerken:
1. Starting objectives.
2. Defining changing in behavior expected as outcomes.
3. Listing and briefing describing situations that give opportunity for the expression of the behaviors described.
4. Developing appropriate and systematic means of electing kinds of behavior implied in the objectives to be evaluated.
5. Recording on ways of recording and summarizing (scores, rating, or describing) behavior as the basic of evidence collected.
6. Checking validity, reliability and difficulty of the measures used.
7. Establishing conditions that permit the students to give her best performance.
8. Assigning scores on the basis of the above step.
9. Developing methods of interpretation.

Criteria for Selecting Evaluation Tools or Devices

Major criteria used in selecting and developing evaluation tools are:
1. Sample of objectives.
2. Sampling of the content.
3. Checking validity, reliability, practicability and usefulness.

Evaluation Methodology

There is certain methodology for evaluation. The educational spinal illustrated by Gilberto is given below. It has four steps:
1. Defining objectives.
2. Planning evaluation system.
3. Preparing.
4. Implementing evaluation.

The processes are repeated giving feedback and re-examining the objectives, and making necessary changes in the education system (program). Evaluation is continuous process and the results are used for the educational spiral by Guilbert.

PRINCIPLES OF EVALUATION

1. The objectives of evaluation must be started clearly before evaluation is made.
2. Evaluation techniques should be selected in terms of the purposes to be served.

3. Comprehensive evaluation requires a variety of evaluation techniques.
4. Proper use of evaluation techniques requires an awareness of their limitation as well as on their strength.
5. Evaluation is a means to an end and not an end itself. Evaluation procedures would be related in terms of the decisions to be made.
6. Evaluation procedures must contribute to improved decisions of instruction, guidance and administrative nature.
7. Since evaluation involves getting evidence about the behaviors that are desired as educational objectives an appropriate method of evaluation.
8. Evaluation assures that it is possible to estimate the typical reaction of the students by getting evidence about a sample of his reaction (behavior).

PURPOSES OF EVALUATION

1. Evaluation procedures help the students to know the desired behaviors to be achieved and what the desired behaviors to be achieved and what they should learn.
2. It helps the students to identify their difficulties and problems in learning and know the progress they make.
3. To guide the teacher and students in selecting of future learning.
4. To provide guidance and counseling to the students related to learning.
5. To provide judgment as to the appropriateness and feasibility of determined objectives.
6. To provide the teacher with clues to the effectiveness of the course plan, teaching method and effectiveness of learning experience provided.
7. To decide promotion and placement etc.
8. To report to the parents the achievement of students.
9. To diagnose each student's strengths and weakness and suggest remedial measures.
10. To motivate and encourage students to learn.
11. To determine the level of knowledge and understanding of students at various levels.
12. To gather information needed for administrative purpose such as selecting student's for honors course. Placement of students for advanced standing and meeting graduation requirements evaluation help the administration to determine effectiveness of curriculum, its strengths and weakness, to interpret to the public the goals and accomplishments of the school.

CHARACTERISTICS OF EVALUATION PROCEDURE

Essential Characteristics

1. **Validity:** It is the extent to which the test used really measures what it is intended to measure.
2. **Reliability:** It is the term used to indicate the consistency with which a test measures, what it is designed to measure.
3. **Objectivity:** This is the extent to which independent and competent examiners agree on what constitutes a good answer for each of the item of measuring instruments.
4. **Usability:** This implies such factors as the time taken to conduct the test, the cost of using it and practicability for everyday use.

Other Characteristics

1. **Relevance:** It is the degree to which the centers established for selecting questions so that they confirm to the aims of the measuring instrument.

2. **Equilibrium:** Achievement of correct proportion or balance among questions allotted to each of the objectives of a course and representatives of the sample of the tasks included in the test.
3. **Discrimination:** This refers to the quality of each element of measuring instruments which makes it possible to distinguish between good and poor student in relation to a given variable.

Evaluation Tools

It is divided into three domains:
1. Intellectual skills.
2. Communication skills.
3. Practical skills.

INTELLECTUAL SKILLS

The test and scales that have met the criteria of testing are known as standardized tests.

Characteristics of Standardized Tests

According to Thorndike
1. A fixed set of test items, designed to measure clearly designed sample of behaviors.
2. Specific direction for admistering and scoring the test.
3. Standard content and procedures.

Types of standardized test

They are of five types:
1. Achievement tests.
2. Aptitude tests.
3. Personality tests.
4. Intelligence test.
5. Prognostic test.

Meaning of Intelligence
The meaning of intelligence, Binet describes intelligence as:
1. The tendency of thought to take and maintain a definite direction.
2. The capacity to make adaptation for the purpose of attaining a desired end.
3. The power of self-criticism.

Measurement of intelligence
Intelligence is measured through a complicated process. It involves a comparison and establishment of a relationship between CA (chronological age) and MA (mental age). This relationship is expressed by the term IQ (intelligence quotient). When the mental age is divided by the chronological age and the quotient is multiplied by 100, the result is IQ.

$$IQ = MA \times CA \times 100$$

Classification of intelligence tests
These may be classified under three categories:
1. **Individual tests:** These tests are administered to one individual at a time.
   These cover age group from 2 to 18 years. These are:

   a. The Binet-Simon tests
   b. Revised tests by Terman.
   c. Mental and scholastic tests of Burt.
2. **Group tests:** Group tests are administered to a group of people. Group tests had birth in America, when the intelligence of the recruits who joined the army in the First World War was to be calculated. These are:
   a. The army alpha and beta test.
   b. Terman's group tests.
   c. Otis self-administrative tests.
3. **Performance tests:** These tests are administered to the illiterate person. These tests generally involve the construction of certain patterns or solving problems in terms of concrete material. Some of the famous tests are:
   a. Koch's block design test.
   b. The cube construction tests
   c. The pass along tests.

APTITUDE TEST

Meaning of Aptitude

According to Traxler, Aptitude is a present condition which is indicative of an individual's potentials for the future.

   Hahn and Macheam, aptitude are correctly referred to as latent potentialities, undeveloped capacities to acquire abilities and skills and to demonstrate achievements.

How to measure scholastic aptitude
1. School marks and scholastic aptitude. This is the traditional method of measuring aptitude.
2. Occupation of parents and scholastic aptitude. Mc Nemur tested the IQ's of children following different occupations. He found that children of professional peoples, engineers, doctors, lawyers, etc. got higher IQ at all age levels than children of clinical, skilled trade and retail business people. The lowest IQ was of the children of day laborers. This study indicated a positive relationship between the intelligence of the child and the occupational status of the father.
3. Teacher's observation and scholastic aptitude. The following points may be observed.
   a. Rapidity in comprehending material of study.
   b. Rapidity and accuracy in reading.
   c. Ability in attaching new problems.
   d. Large vocabulary.
   e. Eagerness to answer questions.
   f. Deficiency in one or more skills (a negative criterion).
4. Scholastic aptitude test. The Yale educational aptitude test. The battery contains test designed to measure a person's relative aptitude or ability in the areas.

Measurement of Aptitude

The term intelligence, ability, and aptitude are often used interchangeably to refer to behavior that is used to predict future learning or performance. However, subtle differences exit between the terms. Like intelligence tests, aptitude tests measure a student's overall performance across a broad range of mental capabilities. But aptitude tests also include items which measure more specialized abilities such as verbal and numerical skills that predict scholastic performance in educational programs.

Specific nature of aptitudes tests

1. Mechanical aptitude tests.
2. Musical aptitude tests.
3. Art judgment tests.
4. Professional aptitude tests, i.e. tests to measure the aptitudes for professionals like teaching, salesmanship, research work, etc.
5. Scholastic aptitude tests, i.e. tests to measure the aptitude for different course of institution.

Mechanical Aptitude Test

Some persons have a specific bent of mind for the tasks related to the use of mechanical abilities and thus demonstrate their aptitude for all tasks and job that require the use of mechanical abilities. The term mechanical aptitude is not a single unitary function. It is a combination of sensory and motor capacities plus perception of spatial relations, the capacity to acquire information about mechanical matters and the capacity to comprehend mechanical relationships. Some of the well-known mechanical aptitude tests are:

1. Minnesota mechanical assembly test.
2. Minnesota spatial relation test.
3. The revised Minnesota power form board (1948).
4. Stenquist mechanical aptitude tests (part-I and III).
5. LJO Rourke's mechanical aptitude tests (part-I and III).
6. SRA Mechanical aptitude test.
7. Bennet tests of mechanical aptitude tests (Hindi) prepared by Manovigyanshala, Allahabad. Usually, these tests contain the items of the following nature.
   - Asking the subject to put together the parts of mechanical devices.
   - Asking to replace cut-outs of various shapes in their correct holes in the board.
   - Requiring the ability to solve problems in geometric terms.
   - Asking questions concerning the basic information about tools and their uses.
   - Questions relating to comprehension of physical and mechanical principles.

Clerical Aptitude Tests

Clerical aptitude is also a composite function. According to Bingham, it involves several specific abilities like:

1. **Perceptual ability:** Ability to perceive words and numbers with speed and accuracy.
2. **Intellectual ability:** Ability to grasp the meaning of words and symbols.
3. **Motor ability:** Ability to use various types of machines and tools like typewriter, duplicator, cyclostyle machine, punching machine, etc.

Some of the popular clerical aptitude tests are:

1. Detroit clerical aptitude examination.
2. Minnesota vocational test for clerical works.
3. The clerical ability test prepared by the Department of Psychology, university of Mysore, Mysore.
4. Clerical aptitude test battery (English and Hindi), Bureau of Education and Vocational Guidance, Patna (Bihar).
5. Test of clerical aptitude prepared by the Parsee Panchayat Guidance, Bureau, 209 hornby road, Mumbai-1.

Sensory Aptitude

In this category, we can include all those aptitude which are related to the sensory capacities and abilities of the children. One may have aptitude in the task related to the use of his sense of hearing; other may have aptitude in the task related to the use of the sense of sight, sense of smell, sense of taste or sense of touch. Here depending upon their present ability concerning the particular sensory capacity, we can have an idea of their future success in the area or professions where the use of such sensory ability or capacity is most demanded.

Musical Aptitude Tests

These tests have been devised for discovering musical talent. One of these important musical aptitude tests is discovered below:

Seashore measure of musical talent: It gives consideration to the following musical components,
1. Discrimination of pitch.
2. Discrimination of intensity of loudness.
3. Determination of time interval.
4. Discrimination of timbre.
5. Judgment of rhythm.
6. Tonal memory.

The instruction in these tests is of following nature:
You will hear two tones which differ in pitch. You are to judge whether the second is higher or lower than the first. If the second is higher, record H; if lower, record L.

Aptitude for Graphic Art

These tests are devised to discover the talent for graphic art. The two important tests of this nature are:
1. The Meier art judgment test.
2. Horne art aptitude inventory.

In Meier art judgment test there are 100 pairs of representational pictures in black and white. One member of each pair is an acknowledged art masterpiece while the other is a slight distortion of the masterpiece. It is usually altered from the original so as to violate some important principle of art. Tests are informed regarding which aspect has been altered and are asked to choose from each pairs the one that is better—more pleasing, more artistic, more satisfying. Another important test of measuring aptitude for graphic art is the horn art aptitude inventory. It requires the subject to produce sketches from given patterns to lines and figures. The created sketches of the subject are then evaluated according to the standard given by the author of this test.

Professional Aptitude

The aptitude related to the activities of various professions and occupations are included in this category. These aptitudes are able to predict the future success of an individual in the field or profession related to these aptitudes.

Tests for Scholastic and Professional Aptitudes

For helping in the proper selection of students for the studies of specific courses of professions like engineering, medicine, law, business, management, teaching, etc. the various specific aptitude tests have been designed. Some of these aptitude tests are:

1. Stanford scientific aptitude test by DL Zyve.
2. Science aptitude test (after higher sec. stage) NIE, Delhi.
3. Moss scholastic aptitude test for medical students.
4. Ferguson and Stoddard's law aptitude examination.
5. Tale legal aptitude test.
6. Pre-engineering ability test (education testing services, UAS).
7. Minnesota engineering analogical test.
8. Coxe-orleans prognosis test of teaching ability.
9. Teaching aptitude test by Jai Prakash and RP Shrivastav University of Saugar (MP).
10. Shah's teaching aptitude test.
11. Teaching aptitude test by Moss, FA and others, George Washington University Press.

Contemporary Trend in Aptitude Testing

Instead of utilizing specific aptitude tests for measuring specific aptitude in very specific field or area, the trend at present, has now been changed towards multiple aptitude tests battery to find the suitability of people for different professions requiring different abilities on the basis of scores in the relevant aptitude tests in the battery. The examples of such tests are general aptitude test battery (GATB) and differential aptitude test (DAT).

General Aptitude Test Battery (GATB)

Battery developed by the Employment Service Bureau of UAS has 12 tests, Eight of which are paper-pencil tests as for name comparison, computation, vocabulary, arithmetic, reasoning, form matching, test matching, three-dimensional spaces, etc. The other four require the use of simple equipment in the shape of moving pegs on boards, assembling and dissembling rivets and washers. From the scores obtained by the subject, the experimenter is able to draw inferences about the nine aptitude factors intelligence, verbal aptitude, and numerical aptitude, spatial aptitude from perception, clerical perception, motor coordination, finger dexterity, and manual dexterity. The GABA has proven to be one of the most successful multiple aptitude batteries particularly for the purposes of job classification.

Differential Aptitude Test (DAT)

Developed by UAS psychological corporation. It has proved more successful in predicting academic success and found especially useful for providing educational and vocational guidance to secondary school children. The test induced in the battery of DAT is the following.

1. **Verbal reasoning:** It is a measure of ability to understand concepts framed in words. It is aimed at evaluation of the student's ability to abstract or generalize and to think constructively, rather than simple fluency or vocabulary recognition. The word used in these items may come from history, geography, literature, science or any other content area.

2. **Numerical ability:** These items are designed to test understanding of numerical relationships and facility in handling numerical concepts. This test is a measure of the student's ability to reason with numbers, to manipulate numerical relationships to deal intelligently with quantitative materials, educationally, it is important for prediction in such fields as mathematics, physics, chemistry, engineering and other curricula in which quantitative thinking is essential. Various amounts of numerical ability are required in occupations such as laboratory assistant, book-keeper, statistical and shipping clerks as well as in professions related to the physical sciences.

3. **Abstract reasoning:** This test is intended as a verbal measure of the student's reasoning ability. It has many picture test yielding ambiguous scores because they require the student to discriminate between lines are areas which differ but slightly in size and shape. This test supplements the general intelligence aspects of the verbal and numerical tests.

4. **Clerical speed and accuracy:** This test is intended to measure speed of response in a simple perceptual task.
   a. *Perceptual ability:* Ability to perceive words and numbers with speed and accuracy.
   b. *Intellectual ability:* Ability to grasp the meaning of words and symbols.
   c. *Motor ability:* Ability to use various types machines and tools like writer, duplicator, cyclostyle machine, punching machine, etc.

5. **Mechanical reasoning:** This tries to test mechanical aptitude which is a combination of sensory and motor capacities plus perception of spatial relations, the capacity to acquire information about mechanical matters and the capacity to comprehend mechanical relationships.

6. **Space relations:** It is the ability to visualize a constructed object from a picture of a pattern and an ability to imagine how an object would appear if rotated in various ways for measurement of space perception. It means that these tests require mental manipulation of objects in three dimensional spaces.

7. **Language usage:** This test has two sections.
   Language usage-1: Spelling.
   Language usage-2: Grammar.

INTELLIGENCE TESTS

History of Intelligence Tests

In the beginning mental tests were devised to study individual differences among college students. These tests were used to measure the speed of reaction, sensory acuity and other simple psychological processes. The primary interest was to study the extent of individual differences and not to assess the level of intelligence of the individual.

In 1896, Binet, a French psychologist, who was studying process of school suggested special classes for children showing poor progress in class work. Eight year later the French government requested Binet to discover children in public school who were not having sufficient intelligence to benefit themselves by usual instruction.

Measurement of intelligence tests can be categorized in the following categories:

1. **Individual intelligence tests:** These tests measure the intelligence of one person at a time. These are used to measure the intelligence of retarded children or to provide treatment and guidance. Major limitations of these tests include the skills of examiner and problems of qualification. Financially, these tests are more expensive. These tests can be administered not only individually

but not a group at a time. For example, Alexander Battery of performance test, Bhatia tests of intelligence, form board test, Stanford-binet, Wechsler test, etc.

2. **Group intelligence tests:** This method of measuring intelligence is used to measure the intelligence of more than one person. These tests are very popular. Group intelligence tests were also used in World War I to measure the intelligence of the literature and illiterate soldiers. These tests can be administered to be a large number of individuals at a time, for example: Army alpha, army beta and RPM.

3. **Verbal intelligence tests:** In this test, intelligence of a person is measured on the basis of his answer or reactions to the given questions. This is a reliable test and is useful for both the individuals and group, but the examinees should have the knowledge of language or words. Examiner should be highly skilled to get maximum results from these tests.

4. **Nonverbal performance tests:** It involves no language but require duplication of block patterns, completion of Jig-Saw, Puzzle, arrangements of pictures, drawing, etc. For example: Goddard's from board, Link's from board, Alexander's battery of performance tests, Raven's progressive matrices, etc.

5. **Verbal, non-verbal combined tests:** Include both verbal and nonverbal items. For example: Wechsler test for children and adults, Bhatia tests of intelligence, Army alpha and beta test of performance, Army general classifications test (AGCT), Armed force qualification test (AFQT), etc.

6. **Power tests:** These tests allow sufficient time to the subject to try most or all the items he can do. The score he obtains as an indicator of his achievement, for example: RPM.

Uses of Intelligence Tests

Intelligence tests are used in many walks of life to determine the levels of IQ of an individual which is of utmost importance for success in any walk of life. Hence, innumerable tests have come into existence and this reveals its importance in life. Some of the areas in which intelligence tests are useful are mentioned here under.

1. Intelligence tests have helped use to understand fully the nature of the intelligence.

2. As intelligence plays a very significant role in the determination of personality, intelligence tests are used as a part of personality assessment.

3. Intelligence tests are useful to dispel the wrong notions of racial differences, sex differences, caste differences, etc. these tests have ruled out the superiority of any race, sex or caste in intelligence over others.

4. Intelligence tests are useful in educational guidance of children. By determining the IQ of a child he may be guided to take up a particular course of study for which he is studied.

5. Intelligence tests are used in many educational institutions to select the students for admission. If the student is found below the required level of intelligence for the courses they offer, he may be rejected.

6. Intelligence tests are also used as a part of vocational guidance. The success in any vocation partly depends upon intelligence in addition to aptitude and interest.

Other uses are:

1. Studying the individual differences.
2. Identifying the retarded children and treating them.
3. Help in the field of education.

4. Finding the solution of disciplinary problems.
5. Use in business skills.
6. Use in armed forces.
7. Help in research work.

ASSESSMENT OF REASONING AND PROBLEM SOLVING

Wisconsin Card Sorting Test (WCST)

1. This test assesses abstract reasoning and flexibility in problem solving stimulus cards of different color, form and number are presented to patients to sort into groups according to the principle established by the examiner but unknown to the patient (e.g. To sort by color, ignoring form and number).
2. As the patient sots the cards, he/she is told whether the responses are correct or incorrect, and the number of trials required to achieve 10 consecutive correct responses is recorded. When the patient has mastered the task, the examiner changes the principle of sorting, and the number of trials required to achieve correct sorting is recorded.
3. The procedure, repeated several times, measures the capacity for abstract thinking (i.e. the number of trials required to achieve a solution) and flexibility (perseverated error on successive sorting trials).
4. Persons with damage to the frontal lobes or to the caudate and some person with schizophrenia give abnormal response.
5. Patients with cerebral disease are likely to loose the capacity to reason abstractly and to lack flexibility in problem solving or adopting to change situations.

MEASUREMENT OF ATTITUDES

Self Report Methods

It includes attitude scales, questionnaires, interviews and projective tests. When you are asked to express your preferences, likes and dislikes to an interviewer or to write your evolution of something on a questionnaire.

1. Attitudes are measured by attitude scales which deal with an issue or set of related issues. These depict the direction of an attitude, the degree or extent in that direction and the intensity of feeling that goes with the attitude.
2. Sometimes, these components may be a part of questionnaire studies and interviews in which people are asked, first, how (pro or con) they feel about something and then how strongly they feel. Finally, these rates are highly related.
3. Attitudes scales typically consist of a number of statements with which a person may agree or disagree with several scale points, usually ranging from highly agree or highly disagree. In this way, both the direction and the degree are indicated by the response to each statement or item.
4. Typically, these items relate to some common social thing, person, issue, person's overall attitude.
5. Attitude scales commonly used are Thurstone's scale, Likert's scale, paried comparison method and rank order method.

Thurstone's Scale (Methods of Equal-appearing Intervals)

1. Louis L Thurstone and EJ Chave (1929), in their classic study of attitudes towards the church developed an interval scale by using the method of equal-appearing intervals.

2. Since the scale represents an evenly graduated series of attitudes as in the foot rule the method is named so.
3. Every statement in Thurstone scale has a numerical value already determined.
4. The subject has to place a tick mark against each item with which he/she agrees. The attitude score is the mean of the scale value.

Likert's Scale (Summated Rating)

1. For the Likert scale, various opinion statements are collected, edited and then given to a group of subjects to rate the statements on a five-point scale: Strongly disagree, agree undecided, disagree and strongly disagree.
2. The subject expresses the degree (1-5) of their personal agreement or disagreement with each of the statements.
3. The respondent's attitude score in the sum of her/his rating of all the statements. For this reason, the Likert scale is also known as the scale of summated ratings.

Bogardus Social-Distance Scale

1. ES Bogardus developed an attitude scale in 1933, called the social-distance scale, which become a classic instrument to measure attitudes towards ethnic group.
2. He was the first one to design a technique for the specific purposes of measuring and comparing attitudes toward different nationalities, particularly measuring tolerance of out-group.
3. The subject is asked to indicate the extent of his willingness to accept members of different social groups into various social institutions.

Observations of Behavior

1. It is a method of studying the behavior, consists of the perception of an individual's attitude under conditions by the other individuals and analysis of his perceived attitude by them.
2. By this method, we can infer the mental processes of other persons through the observation of their.
3. For example, observing the actual overt behavior of students in natural situation.

PSYCHOMETRIC ASSESSMENT OF PERSONALITY

Personality testing is done for various reasons. A personnel psychologist may want to identify people for a salesman's job. A clinical psychologist often uses personality tests to evaluate psychological disorders. We want to describe it and know what type of personality or the personality traits possessed by us or others. It needs the knowledge and skill for the assessment or measurement of personality.

Subjective Methods of Personality Assessment

It is that approach where methods employed provide an opportunity to the individuals to speak about themselves. The methods followed under this approach are called subjective methods.

Sl.No.	Type	Description
1.	Autobiography	The subject (individual) is asked to write his autobiography either on a structured pattern or an unstructured pattern. Generally, only those subjects should be asked of guidance. Such autobiographical material provides data on the personal qualities of an individual, for instance, goals, aspirations, hopes, wishes, disappointments, frustrations, etc.
2.	Case history method	The case history method takes into consideration the time factor and the changes in the personality of an individual during this time. Following steps should be followed in the case history method. • Identification data. • Family background. • Health history. • Educational achievement. • Emotional and social behavior. • Interpretation of the data. • Evaluation treatment. The above information helps in making predictions about the personality of an individual. This method has a limited application for educational institutions but it is more useful in clinics for the treatment of patients.
3.	Case study method	This method is concerned with the intensive study of an individual with the aim of having an holistic view of that individual. The cases of the problems of an individual are found on the basis of the collected information and remedial treatment is suggested for better adjustment in the society, school or home environment. Following steps should be taken into consideration while following the case study method. • Selection of the subject or the case. • Reason for the selection of the case/subject. • Tools for recording data like cumulative records, tests, medical reports, etc. • General information about the subject. • Health records. • Family background. • Educational data. • Social relations. • Hobbies, interests, attitudes, etc. • Interpretation of data. • Remedial treatment to the case/subject under study. The following points should to take into consideration for selecting a case for case study. • Preferably, problem children, that are those who are truants, delinquents, low-achievers, shy, quite and retiring, etc. should be selected for the case study. The teacher is free to select any student for case study depending upon the situation. • Selection of the case by the teacher should be made from his class. • Time and facilities should be taken into consideration for the case study in question.
4.	Questionnaires	A questionnaire is a valuable tool for collecting information directly given by a person. Such an information may consists of personal

Contd...

Contd...

Sl.No.	Type	Description
		knowledge, like and dislikes (values and preferences), attitudes and beliefs, experiences (biography) and present status of things or event. This information can be both qualitative (verbal, description, comments or views) and quantitative (numbers, or scores as in the case of rating scale or opinion scores elicited by attitude scales). Any assembly of questions cannot be called a questionnaire. It must reflect an objective, a design and a framework. It is a way of obtaining data about persons by asking them rather than watching them behave or by sampling a portion of their behavior. A good questionnaire embodies a beginning, middle and an end. There is an introductory section comparing a note on the purpose of the questionnaire, an appeal and a direction for responding to the various questions and a basic data part of which is to filled in accurately by the respondents.
5	Interviews	An interview is face-to-face talking with a purpose. It is a systematic method by which one person enters more or less imaginatively into the inner life of another who is generally a comparative stranger to him. An interview can be formal or informal. For good interview, there is a need for establishing a rapport between the interviewee and the interviewer.

Objective Methods Personality Assessment

Objective data are collected by experts using specific tools or devices based upon certain methodologies. These methods which are used to collect objective data regarding varied personality aspects of an individual are called objective methods of assessing the personality of an individual. These methods are also known as observational methods as these are based upon the observation of experts rather than the answers given by individuals an in the case of the subjective methods. The observation methods are rating scales, verbal behavior, situation tests and sociometiric method.

OBSERVATION METHOD

The observation method can be used to observe intellectual functioning, emotional development, interests, and hobbies and to study habits, etc.

Psychological Process

Psychological process involved:

Four psychological processes are involved in collecting data in the observation method: Attention, sensation, perception and conception.

1. **Attention:** It implies a mental set or a state of alertness which an individual assumes in order to perceive selected events and conditions of things.
2. **Sensation:** It means the awareness of the internal and external environment through one's senses. It is the immediate results of a stimulus to the sense organs.
3. **Perception** is the art of liking what is sensed with some past experience to give meaning to sensation.
4. **Conception** is that quality of the mental activity associated with observing by which one removes blocks to perception through the creation of imaginative concepts. It is an intellectual representation of some aspects of reality which is derived from the perception of a phenomenon.

Steps of Observation Method

Following are the four elements of the observational method.
1. Deciding major phenomenon to be observed.
    - Defining the phenomenon to be observed.
    - Modalities for the observation of the phenomenon: Structured, semistructured, or unstructured.
    - Person conducting the observation.
    - System involved in recording various features of the phenomenon: Videotape, tape recorder or any other devices.
2. Recording.
3. Organizing.
4. Interpreting the observations.

Precautions

1. Training of the observer is a must.
2. Subjective of the observer should be involved to be minimum possible extent.
3. The observer should have knowledge of personality aspects.
4. A member of observations should be taken for the purpose of making the observation more reliable.

Phenomena Amenable to Observations

Phenomena amenable to observations include:
1. **Characteristics and conditions of individuals:** Like people's attributes and states such as physical appearance, physiological symptoms that can be observed directly through the senses or with the aid of observational apparatus such as radiography.
2. **Verbal communication behaviors:** Like observing the content and structure of people's conversations, e.g. nurses giving information to parents, nurses conversation with grieving relatives.
3. **Nonverbal communication behaviors:** Include facial expressions, touch, posture, gestures, and other body movements.
4. **Activities:** Like patient's eating habits and trends and aggressive actions among children in the hospital playroom.
5. **Skill attainment and performance:** Like behavior assessment through skill development by patients and nurses.
6. **Environmental characteristics:** Noise levels in different areas of a hospital, cleanliness in homes in a community, safety, hazards of children's classroom, shelters of homeless, etc.

SITUATIONAL TESTS METHOD

In situation tests, certain artificial situations resembling real life situations are created before the students. The reaction of the students are recorded and interpreted. The interpretations on the recorded responses under certain situations reveal the personality of the individual. These tests provide opportunities to observe the behavior in life situations. Traits like leadership, initiative, cooperation, persistence, risk-taking capacity, honesty, flexibility, imagination, etc. can be assessed. Reliability and validity of these tests have not been ascertained.

Group Discussion

It is a general part of the selection procedure for admission. Group discussion is a situational test. A group is given a problem on a certain theme. No one is assigned the duty of a group leader. Everyone in the group is free to express ideas on the problem. In this situation, qualities like initiative, imagination, accommodation, suggestibility, flexibility, etc. can be assessed.

Created Situations to Assess Honesty

A teacher may create the following situations in the class to assess the honesty traits of his students:
1. The teacher holds a class test.
2. He evaluates the written performance but does not show marks on the answer-books.
3. He distributes the answer-book to the student expressing his inability to mark the answer-books due to certain reasons. He asks his students to handover the answer-books the next day.
4. The answer-book is collected again.
5. Those students are located whose awards are found higher due to additions. Thus, some students may reveal their dishonesty traits or honesty trait.

Imaginary Situations

Imaginary situations can be created and responses of students to these imaginary situations may reveal personality aspects of the individuals. For example, suppose one of us comes across an individual who inquire about a certain place and the approach road to reach that place.

Situational Test by May and Hartshorne

May and Hartshorne mention a number of situational tests in their book studies in deceit. One example related to honesty from this book is mentioned. The teacher had a box containing coins. Coins from the box were distributed to some of the students in a class. The coin left in the box was counted and then the box was placed in a corner. Students were asked to place back the coins given to them. The coins were again counted. Some students kept the coins with themselves.

SOCIOMETRIC METHOD

The sociometric method involves studying relationship among the members a group which helps in assessing the personality traits of the members of the group. Mereno devised this method. Social preferences with specific references to a specific criterion are recorded. For example, social preferences of students are recorded on the following questions:
1. With whom would you like to sit in the class?
2. With whom would you like to go on the educational tour?

The sociometric data so obtained can be expressed graphically. Such graphical expression is called a sociogram. A sociogram revels information regarding sub-groups, cliques, stars, isolated, neglected, rejected. Appropriate steps can be taken on the basis of the sociometric data to improve the personality of the individuals.

RATING SCALE

A rating scale is an instrument designed to facilitate appraisals of a number of traits or characteristics by references to a common quantitative scale of values. The rating scale is used to know from others where an individual stands in terms of some personality traits.

Three points are taken into consideration in this method:
1. The specific traits or traits to be rated are specified.
2. The scale range is also decided, i.e. 3 point scale, 5 point scale, 7 point scale or 11 point scale.
3. Those persons are decided who are require to use the scale to quantify the trait regarding a specific person whose personality is to be measured, e.g. we may decide that these specific persons will submit their observations on the scale for a particular trait(s) regarding a person.

Precautions While Using a Rating Scale

The rating scale method can be made more effective if the following precautions are taken.
1. The raters should be impartial.
2. A number of rater should give their rating and these should be taken into consideration for framing the final assessment on the traits.
3. Generally, the halo effect is there in the rating of the raters for different traits. It should be checked. It is a tendency for transfer to occur so that a rater many rate the same individual high or low for many different traits. One impression may color the rest.
4. Avoid being too lenient or too strict in standard.
5. Avoid the tendency to either remain at the neutral points or the extreme points in the rating scale.

Purposes of Rating Scale

According to Freemen (1965), the purposes of rating scales are as follows.
1. Rating scales are chiefly useful for finding out what impression an individual has made of persons with whom he has come in contact with respect to some specified traits or attitudes.
2. It is a device that rates social values, occupational efficiency, group status and the like in certain specified areas.
3. It reflects the impression the subject has made upon the persons who do the rating.
4. For the evaluation of an individual, rating scales are submitted to teachers, counselors, employers, colleagues, parents and others who have had sufficient contact with the person in question.
5. Rating scales may be devised for a variety of traits such as tact, generosity, leadership, co-cooperativeness, resourcefulness, punctuality, industriousness, honesty, personal attractiveness, etc.

Points for the Construction and Use of Rating Scale

1. Each trait should be clearly defined.
2. The degree of the trait should be defined. Each trait should be rated on a scale, most frequently of five or seven intervals.
3. The mean or the median of the rating by different judges should be taken for having a reliable rating.
4. Guidance counselors, employers and personnel officers find them helpful if the judges are carefully selected and if the rating are properly made.
5. Overt traits are more reliably rated than convert traits. For example, overt traits like emotional expression, social acceptability, manifest fear and anxiety, aggressive or impulsive acts are related with greater reliability than the covert traits like a person's inner life and feeling about one's self.

6. Degree of certainty of rating should be stated, e.g. very strong, strong, and moderate.
7. Extroverted persons are more reliably judged than introverted ones.

Types of Rating Scales

1. Scoring rating scale.
2. Ranking rating scale.

PROJECTIVE TESTS

Introduction

This technique has been developed by Swiss psychologist, son of an art teacher Mr Harmans Rorschach. Projective methods involve an unstructured stimulus or situation. In this process, the individual projects his unconscious desires, fears, motives, drives, needs, etc. subjective and objective methods do not clear study the unconscious mind of an individual. Projective methods deal with the conscious as well as the unconscious mind. The unconscious mind is 9/10th of the mind and inner urges, wishes, emotions, etc. are not visible to the outsiders and the individual himself.

Definition

Projective test is an instrument that is considered sensitive to covert or unconscious aspect of behavior. It permits or encourages a wide variety of subject's responses. It is highly multidimensional it invokes rich and profuse response data with a minimum of subject's awareness, concerning the purpose of the test—*Lindsey*.

Characteristics of Projective Test

According to Rastogi (1983), following are the characteristic features of a projective test:
1. Brief instructions are given to the subjects which are necessary for him/her to respond.
2. The test material is kept ambiguous projects his characteristic ideas, attitudes, strivings, fears, conflicts, aggressiveness, hostility, etc.
3. The purpose of the test is hidden from the subject.
4. The projective tests reflect the influence of psychoanalytical school.
5. The test reveals emotional and social characteristics, maladjustments, attitudes and motives. Certain intellectual aspects of individual behavior are also revealed.

RORSCHACH INKBLOT TEST

Description

This test that was developed by H Rorschach has ten cards with vague inkblot on them. Five of the cards are chromatic stimuli while rest of the five is achromatic stimuli, subjects are asked to tell what they see on these cards. Each response has elaborate scoring system and well-developed interpretation. Rorschach inkblot test reveals structural aspects of personality such as individual stability, value system egostrength, etc.

Procedure

1. The card is presented one at a time in a specific order. When the subject takes his seat, the examiner gives him the first card with necessary instruction. He is asked to say what he sees in it, what it looks like, etc.

2. The subject is allowed as much time as he wants of a given card and it is permitted to give as many responses to it as he wishes. He is also allowed to turn the card around and look at it from any angle to find things in it.

3. Besides keeping a record of the response of the subject concerning these inkblots on different pieces of paper, the examiner notes the time taken for each response, position in which cards are being held, emotional expression and other incidental behavior of the subject during the test period, etc.

4. After all the cards have been presented; the second phase of inquiry follows. It is intended to seek clarification or addition to original responses.

Verbal Projective Test

Present subjects with an ambiguous verbal stimuli rather than a pictorial one. There are two types of verbal methods:

1. **Association technique:** An example of an association technique is word-association method, which represents subjects with a series of words, to which the individual respond with the first thing comes to mind. The word list often combines both neutral and emotionally tinged words, which are included for the purpose of detecting impaired thoughts processes or internal conflicts, anxiety or any problems in relationships.

2. **Sentence completion test:** This test includes a list of incomplete sentences generally open at the end and is asked to complete them in any desired manner. This approach is frequently used as a method of measuring attitudes or some aspect of personality.

Expressive Method

These techniques encourage self-expression, through the construction of some product out of raw materials. The major expressive methods are play techniques, drawing and painting and role playing. It is believed that people express their feelings, needs, motives and emotions by working with or manipulating various materials.

Scoring of Responses

Responses to the test are scored in terms of location, determinants, content and popularity or originality taken for responses.

1. **Location:** The response of the subject in the context of the whole inkblot or a part of it is recorded. The subject may observe the whole ink for giving a response or a part of it. The subject may give large details or small details.

2. **Determining quality:** Scoring is done with specific responses of the subject on the form or shape, shades, movements (human movement, inanimate movement or animal movement) perceived by the subject.

3. **Contents:** The subject may respond on the inkblot on the basis human figures, human details, parts of human figure, animal figure, details of animal figure, inanimate objects, plants, maps, clouds, blood, nature (light), sexual objects and other symbols. The responses are recorded keeping in view the above contents of the inkblot.

4. **Popularity or originality:** Some responses are given frequently by normal subjects. These are called popular responses. Some responses may be extremely different which can be considered original responses.

Analysis

The recorded responses are analyzed in the light of location, determining quality, contents and popularity or originality.

Interpretation

Interpretation is done on the basis of the analyzed data. Interpretation of the responses is a different job. Generally, subjectivity comes in the way and reduces the validity of the test as such. There is need for further experimentation on the test to make valid.

A few examples of responses of the subject to Rorschach Inkblot test and the corresponding interpretation.

Sl. No	Response	Interpretation
1.	The response is associated with the whole inkblot (location)	The subject has the ability to solve his problems in a comprehensive manner. He/she possess high mental ability.
2.	The response is linked with large details (location)	The subject has a practical approach towards problems of life.
3.	The response is linked with small details (location)	The subject expresses emotional conflicts.
4.	The response involved too many colors (determining quality)	The subjects are impulsive.
5.	Predominance of human figure movement (determining quality)	The subject has vivid imagination.
6.	The response frequently involved animal figures (determining quality).	The subject has stereotyped thinking and perhaped he/she is of low intelligence.

THERMATIC APPRECIATION TEST (TAT)

The test consisting of perception of a certain picture in a thermatic manner (revealing imaginative thermes) is called TAT or Thermatic appreciation test. This test was developed by Murray and Morgan in 1935.

Description

The standard test contains 30 pictures for men alone, 10 for women alone and 10 mixed ones for both men and women. All the pictures are more or less vague. Each picture shows a dramatic or emotional scene that might have a number of explanations.

Administration of the Test

1. The picture is shown to the subject one-by-one and he asked to develop a story about each picture. The subject is asked to explain the picture and to give an imaginary reconstruction of what went before and what followed. Although a good deal of emotion is portrayed in each picture, yet it is not clear just what the excitement is all about.
2. Thus, a man may be shown pointing excitedly towards something but there is no clue as to what he is pointing at. The subject, therefore, reads into the pictures some fantasies or interpretations of his own.

3. In giving meaning to the pictures, a person is certain to reveal something about him.
4. The raw material for a pupil's story comes from his own experiences and is colored by his own personality needs. His stories are scored for evidence of basic, unsatisfied urges and for environmental pressures.
5. The nature of the outcome is also examined, since it is the product of the needs and the pressures. Environmental and psychological aspects can be analyzed.

TAT Type Pictures

TAT type pictures are:
1. Achievement motivation.
2. Need for affiliation.
3. Parent-child relationships.
4. Inner fantasies.
5. Level of aspiration.
6. Social and family relationships.
7. Functioning of sex urge.
8. Emotional conflicts.
9. Attitudes to work, minority groups or authority.
10. Outlook towards future.
11. Frustration.
12. Creativity.
13. Fear of success.

Modification of TAT

1. The number of pictures can be reduced depending upon the nature of the subjects and the experience of the expert.
2. Some other pictures can be combined with the original ones.
3. The test can be determined to act as a group test. Pictures can be projected and the group of individuals can be required to write stories after necessary instructions. Stories are evaluated individually to assess the personality of concerned students.
4. Bellaks modified TAT for using it for children of 3 to 11 years. This test is known as children's apperception test (CAT). The test consists of 10 pictures depicting situations of family relationships, toilet training, feeding habits, etc.

CHILDREN APPERCEPTION TEST (CAT)

Children apperception test (CAT) developed by D Leopold Bellak. TAT test is used among adults and adolescents but not suitable for children between 3 and 10 years.

Description

It consists of 10 cards. The cards have picture of animals instead of human character since it was thought that children could identify themselves with animal figures more readily than with persons. These animals are shown in various life situations. For both sexes, all the 10 cards are needed. Whatever story the child makes, he projected himself. The pictures are designed to produce fantasies relating to the child's own experience, reactions.

Administering the Test

All the 10 cards are presented one-by-one and the subjected is asked to make up stories on them. The child should have confidence and he should take story making a pleasant game to play with.

Interpretation

Interpretation of the stories is centered round the following variables.
1. **Hero:** The personality traits of the hero as revealed by the story.
2. **Theme of the story:** What particular theme has he selected for the story building?
3. **The end of the story:** Happy ending or unhappy, wishful, realistic or unrealistic.
4. **Attitude towards parental figures:** Hatred, respectful, devoted, grateful, dependent, aggressive and fearful, etc.
5. **Family role:** With whom in the family the child identifies himself.
6. **Other outside figures introduced:** Objects of the elements introduced in the story but not shown in the picture.
7. **Omitted or ignored figures:** Which figures are omitted or ignored should be not as they may depict the wish of the subject that the figures were not there.
8. **Nature of the anxieties:** Harassment, lose of love, afraid of being left alone, etc. should also be noted.
9. **Punishment for crime:** The relationship between a crime committed in the story and severity of punishment given for it.
10. **Defense and confidence:** The types of defenses, flight, aggression, passivity, regression, etc. the child takes nature of compliance or dependence, involvement in pleasure and achievement sex desire, etc.

WORD ASSOCIATION TEST

A word is presented to a subject and he/she is asked to answer as quickly as possible with the first word that comes in his/her mind. The interpretation depends upon two factors, responses and the reaction time. In this technique there are a number of selected words. The subject is told that:
1. The examiner will utter a series of words, one at a time.
2. After each word the subject is to reply as quickly as possible with the first word that comes to his mind.
3. There is no right or wrong responses.

The examiner than records the reply to each word spoken by him, the reaction time and any unusual speech or behavior manifestations accompanying a given response. The contents of the response along with other recoded things give clues for evaluating the human personality and thus help a psychologist in his work.

SENTENCE-COMPLETION TEST

These tests include a list of incomplete sentences, generally open at the end, which require completion by the subject in one or more words. The subject is asked to go through the list and answer as quickly as possible (without giving a second thought to his answer). For example, we can have the following sentences:
1. I am worried over............
2. My hope is ....
3. I feel proud when............
4. My hero is ....

The sentence competition tests are regarded as superior to word association because the subject may respond with more than one word. Also there it is possible to have a greater flexibility and variety of responses and more area of personality and experiences may be tapped.

In addition to the projective techniques mentioned above there are some others which may prove useful in many situation. These are play technique; drawing and painting tests, etc. both of these techniques are very useful in the case of small children. In the former, the examiner observes the spontaneous behavior of the children while playing or constructing something with the help of given material and in the later, the natural free-hand drawing and painting of the children are the matter of the study. Both of these techniques provide a good opportunity for the careful analysis of a child's personality.

Minnesota Multiphasic Personality Inventory (MMPI)

One of the most commonly used personality test in the MMPI. It was developed during 1930's. This test asks for answers of True or False or Cannot say to 567 statements (one for men and another for women) about different personality traits such as attitudes, emotional reactions, physical and psychological symptoms and past experiences. The answers are quantitatively measured and personality assessment is done based on the norm scores. Dr NH Murthy of NIMHANS, Bangalore has reduced it to 100 items called multiphasic questionnaire.

Million Clinical Multiaxial Inventory (MCMAI)

Items on this test correspond more closely than those on the MMPI to the categories of psychological disorders currently used by psychologists. This makes the test especially useful to clinical psychologist, who must find identity individuals problems before recommending specific forms of therapy for them.

BIBLIOGRAPHY

1. Bhatia HR. Element of Educational Psychological, Orient Longman. 3rd edn, Kolkata, 1968.
2. Bigge Moris L. Learning Theories of Teachers, Universal Book Stall (First Indian reprint), Delhi, 1967
3. Biggie ML, Hunt MP. 'Psychological Foundations of Education: Harper and Row, New York, 1968.
4. Bingham WV, Aptitude and Aptitude Testing, Haper and Brothers, New York, 1937.
5. Binnet A, Simon T. The Development of Intelligence in Children, Williams and Wilkins, Baltimore 1916.
6. Blair GH, Jones RS, Simpson RH Educational Psychology, Macmillan, New York 1954.
7. Boring EC, Lang Field HS, Weld HP (Eds); Foundations of Psychology, New York.
8. Brown JF. Educational Sociology, Prentice Hall, New York 1960 (5th Printing).
9. Brown JF. The Psychodynamics of Abnormal Behaviour, Asia Publishing House (Indian Reprint), New Delhi, 1969.
10. Brown, JF. Educational Psychology, Prentice Hall, New York, 1960 (5th Printing).
11. Hull CL, Aptitude Testing, Youkers, World Book Co, New York, 1928.
12. Korman AK. The Psychology of Motivation, Englewood Cliffs, Prentice Hall, NJ, 1974.
13. Seashore CE. Seashore, Measures of Musical Talents, Psychological Cooperation, New York, 1960.

Introduction to Sociology

23

DEFINITIONS

1. **Sociology:** Sociology is the science that deals with social groups, their internal forms or modes of organization, the processes that tend to maintain or change these forms of organization, and the relations between groups.

2. **Social survey:** Social survey is intended to be the study of the social aspect of a community's composition and activities. It aims at the collection of quantitative facts. It makes a concrete study of society, especially the social problems inherent in the society. It presents programs for improvement and development. It is conducted within fixed geographical limit; it is related to problems of social importance and assists in formulating constructive programs.

3. **Social research:** Social research is the discovery of new truths about society. It is a systematic method of discovering new facts or verifying old facts, their sequences, inter-relationships, causal explanations and natural laws. In this way, social researcher discovers new facts about social activities, social circumstances, social assumptions, social groups, social values or social institutions, etc. and investigates the old facts on these subjects. It locates inter-relationship or causal relations among social incidents. It verifies those natural laws which stimulate different phenomena in social life.

4. **Society:** A society is a collection of individuals united by certain relations or modes of behavior which mark them off from others who do not enter into these relations or who differ from them in behavior. In this way, Ginsberg, like Giddings, has accepted society as an organized group, and has professed to a unity in the relations between its members and their modes of behavior. It is this unity which serves to distinguish members of society from people, who do not belong to society, since these latter people do not enter into the organization of that society, differing as they do in their behavior and other aspects from those in the society. Ginsberg's definition is the definition of a society not of the 'society'.

5. **Community:** "By community is to be understood a group of—beings living a common life including all the infinite variety and comple: of relations which result from that common life or constitute it."

6. **Social interaction:** Social interaction is the general process whereby two or more persons are in meaningful contact as a result of which their behavior is modified however slightly.

7. **Social processes:** Social process mean the various modes of interaction between individuals or groups including cooperation and conflict, social differentiation and integration, development, arrest and decay.

8. **Social structure:** Social structure is the basic concept for the proper understanding of society. The term structure is the arrangement, organization or inter-relation of the parts as a whole. Take the example of the human body. It is not a mere assemblage of different organs of the body. But, these organs are to be properly or orderly arranged in relation to one another, then only the structure of human body will come up.

9. **Social pathology:** By social pathology, we mean such serious maladjustment between the various elements in the cultural configurations as to endanger the survival of the group or as seriously to interfere into the satisfactions of the fundamental desires of its members, with the result that social cohesion is destroyed.

10. **Political sociology:** Political sociology studies the relationship between state, society and party system. Politics pervades the entire present society. The scope of Political Sociology includes the effect, social attitudes on political participation, social class and political attitudes, voting and its political and social implications. Political Sociology studies the characteristics of a multigroup society, the political and social implications and nature of modern bureaucracy and its form in different political-social context.

INTRODUCTION

The word sociology is derived from Latin word "Societus" meaning society and the Greek word "Logos" meaning the study of science. Thus sociology means science of society. Sociology essentially and fundamentally deals with the network of social relationship we call "Society". Sociology is one of the youngest of social sciences disciplines.

The term sociology was coined by Auguste Comte, a French philosopher lived between 1978 and 1857, often referred to as the *Father of Sociology*. He introduced the word sociology for the first time in his famous work "Course de Phiolosophe Positif" at about 1839. With the increase in scientific knowledge during the early 19th century, there was a challenge to the religious faith of the people. Thus social thinkers thought that development was scientific in nature. Plato, and Aristotle, the Greek philosophers, were the first to work out a model society, later on social thinker started thinking about the emergence, growth and developments of the society.

Teaching of sociology as a separate discipline:

Sociology is one of the youngest sciences of the social sciences discipline. Sociology was earlier studied as a part of philosophy. The development of science during the last century is closely connected with its separation from philosophy.

Year	Country
1876	United States
1889	France
1907	Great Britain
1925	Egypt and Mexico
1947	Sweden
After World War-I	Poland and India

General concepts of sociology are:
1. Sociology is a science of society.
2. Sociology is a science of social relationships.

3. Sociology is the study of social life.
4. Sociology is the study of human behavior in groups.
5. Sociology is the study of social action.
6. Sociology is the study of forms of social relationships.
7. Sociology is the study of social groups or social systems.

DEFINITIONS OF SOCIOLOGY

1. LF Ward, Sociology is the science of society of social phenomena.
2. M Ginsberg, Sociology is the study of human interaction and inter-relations, their conditions and consequences.
3. Von Wiese, Sociology is a special social science concentrating on inter-human behaviors on processes of sociation, on association and dissociation as such.
4. JE Cuber, Sociology may be defined as a body of scientific knowledge about human relationships.
5. Simmel, Sociology asks what happens to men and by what rules they behave, not in so far as they unfold their understandable individual existences in their totalities, but in so far as they form groups and are determined by their group existence because of interaction.
6. ME Jones, the chief interest of sociology is the people, the ideas, the customs, the other distinctively human phenomena, which surround man and influence him, and which are, therefore, part of his environment. Sociology also devotes some attention to certain aspects of the geographical environment and to some natural as contrasted with human phenomena, but this interest is secondary to its preoccupation with human being and the products of human life in association. Our general field of study is man as he is related to other men and to the creation of other men which surround him.
7. Max Weber, Sociology is the science which attempts the interpretive understanding of social action.
8. Reuter, The purpose of sociology is to establish a body of valid principles a fund of objective knowledge that will make possible the direction and control of social and human reality.
9. Giddings, sociology is an attempt to account for the origin, growth, structure and activities of sociology by the operation of physical causes working together in the process of evolution.
10. PA Sorokin, Sociology is a generalizing science of socio-cultural phenomena viewed in their generic form, types and manifold interconnections.
11. Young and Mack, Sociology is the scientific study of the structure of social life.
12. Authur Fairbanks, Sociology is the name applied to somewhat inchoate mass of materials which embodies our knowledge of society.
13. Arnold Green, Sociology is the synthesizing and generalizing science of man in all his social relationships.
14. MacIver, Sociology is about social relationships, the network of relationships we call society.
15. Samuel Koening, Sociology is the study of man's behavior in groups or of interaction among human beings.
16. August Comte, Sociology is the science of social phenomena.
17. Ely Chinoy, Sociology is the study of human groups, or of human interaction, of social institutions.
18. Alex Inkeles, Sociology concern three major subject areas: Society as a whole, social institutions and social organizations and social interaction and relationships.
19. George Ritzier, et. al. Sociology is the study of the inter-relationships of five basic units: Individuals, groups, organizations, culture and societies.

20. Betty Yorburg, Sociology is the study of the typical ways of thinking, feeling and acting of people who are similarly located in time and physical and social space.

ORIGIN OF SOCIOLOGY

Sociology is a science of recent origin. Sociology as a science and particularly as a separate field of study is of recent origin. The earliest attempts at systematic thought regarding social life in the west may be said to have begun with the ancient Greek philosopher Plato (427-347 BC). Plato's republic is an analysis of the city community in all its aspects, and in Aristotle's ethics and politics we find the first major attempts to deal systematically with the law, the society, and the state.

Romans were mainly occupied with giving Europe the law and hence they did not think in terms of non-legalistic aspects of society. They have produced few original social philosophies. Among Romans, the most outstanding author is Cicero who, in his book De Officus (On Justice), transmitted to the western world the treasures of Greek learning in philosophy, politics, law and sociology.

The scholastic philosophy was a conservative philosophy. It gave theological interpretation to social attitudes. The scholastic propounded the Biblical thesis that man is a special creation of god. He is subject to no laws but those of god. The social system existing at the time was the divinely sanctioned one. There was not until the sixteenth century that clear cut distinction was made between state and society and there appeared writers who treated life's problems on a more realistic level.

Italian writers Vico and the French writer Montesquieu deserve special mention for their notable contribution towards the scientific investigation of social phenomenon. According to Montesquieu laws were an expression of nation character and the spirit which they exhibited was to be explained in the light of the social and geographical conditions under which men lived. Climate is the principal determinant of social life.

Sociology can be considered as one of the youngest as well as one of the oldest of social sciences. It came to be recognized as a distinct branch of knowledge only recently. From the beginning of civilization society has been a subject of inquiry and has agitated the restless and curious mind of man. For thousands of years men have reflected over the societies in which they lived. He wrote a series of books in which he has worked out a general approach to the study of sociology. In 1839, Comte used the word sociology in his book "Positive Philosophy".

According to August Comte, Sociology is a science of social phenomena subject to natural and invariable laws and their discovery is the object of investigation. Comte proposed the study of sociology in two main parts: 1. The social statistics, and 2. The social dynamics. In statistics, the subject of study is how societies are inter-related. Social dynamics deals with whole societies as the unit of analysis and explains how they developed and changed through time. Comte's important works are: 1. Positive philosophy, and 2. Positive polity.

Herbert Spencer lived between 1820 and 1903. He is considered as one of the most brilliant Englishman of modern times and he is the one who established sociology as a systematic discipline. His book principles of sociology in 3 volumes was published in 1877 and it deals with sociological analysis. According to him, family, politics, religion, social control and work (industry) are the fields of sociology. He stressed the importance of sociology in dealing with the inter-relations between different elements of history and it gives an account of how the parts influence the whole.

Emile Durheim, a French philosopher (1858-1917), was the first modern thinker who emphasized on the reality of society. According to him social facts are exterior and can be the subject of a general science because they can be arranged in categories. He studied division of labor as a social institution, a collective wherein the multiplicity of individuals secures social coherence. He introduced the concept of anomic which is product of–1. Separation of management of industry from labor;

2. Disregard to individual natural talent, and 3. Improper co-ordination of function activities. His main Works are: De La Division De Travail Social and Les Formes Elementariness de view Religious.

Max Weber, German sociologist the pioneering contribution of his theory was of social action, concept of bureaucracy and concept of ideal type. The ideal type, according to Max Weber, is not related to any type of perfection and has no connection at all with value judgements. It is purely a logical one, a methodical device which tries to render subject matter intelligible by revealing or constructing its internal rationality.

India, the study of sociology started in 1919 at the University of Bombay, but this was in 1930 that its study as a separate discipline was started. Now it was being taught at a number of universities and it is getting popular among the students. Some Indian writers like GS Ghurye, RK Mukerjee, and HT Mazumdar have also original contribution to sociological studies. These studies pertain to Indian villages, castes system, marriage, kinship and family.

HISTORICAL APPROACH (VIEW OF FOUNDING FATHERS)

Though the review of the development of modem sociology covers according to Prof Sorokin well over 1000 men whose work is important enough, Auguste Comte, Herbert Spencer, Emile Durkheim and Max Weber have been considered the central figures in sociology. Hence, we confine to explore the opinions of these four scholars about the subject matter of sociology.

Auguste Comte (1798-1857)

Auguste Comte, the French Philosopher, who gave sociology its name in his classic 'Positive Philosophy', was busy staking out claims of sociology then defining its subject matter. Yet, he did propose sociology to be studied under two heads namely social statics and social dynamics. These two concepts represent a basic division in the subject matter of sociology.

The social statics deals with the major institutions such as economy, family or polity. Sociology is conceived of as the study of inter-relations between such institutions. Comte says "the statical study of sociology consists in the investigation of the laws of action and reaction of the different parts of the social system. The parts of a society cannot be understood separately. As if they had an independent existence". Instead, they must be seen "as in mutual relation... forming a whole which compels us to treat them in combination".

The second major division of sociology which Comte proposed is social dynamics. It is the study of change. This part deals with societies they developed and changed through time. Comte said, "we must I, member that the laws of social dynamics are most recognizable when they relate to the largest societies". He was convinced that all societies involved through certain fixed stages of development, and that they progressed towards ever increasing perfection. Thus, according to Comte, comparative study of societies as whole was a major subject for sociological analysis.

According to Comte, all knowledge passes through three different stages. They are the theological stage, the metaphysical stage and positive stage.

During the first stage, phenomena were explained in terms of supernatural causation. For instance, rainfall, earthquakes, forest fire, flood, etc. were attributed to the will of God.

In the metaphysical stage, explanations were formulated in terms of abstract reasoning. Though there was a decline in the influence of supernatural factors, the explanation was not strictly scientific.

In the positive or scientific stage, man began to look for sequences of change, causal relationship and concomitant variations. In brief, this is Comte's famous "Law of three stages".

Comte also formulated a scheme of the "Hierarchy of Sciences". According to him knowledge develops from the simple to the complex. Even the complex knowledge can be hierarchically graded—Astronomy, Physics, Chemistry, Biology and Social Physics (later renamed as Sociology) coming in that order. Sociology was to be the Queen of all sciences.

Herbert Spencer (1820-1903)

Herbert Spencer, an Englishman, ranks high among the founders of modern sociology. Spencer was much more precise than Comte in specifying the subject matter of sociology. He did not have the advantage of university education and yet his contribution to the development of sociology is laudable.

In 1860, he published his "First Principles". This book was an outline of universal knowledge and was aimed at revealing the orderly structure of nature. He had hoped to extend this work to encompass all relevant knowledge on life, mind and society. The project was so encyclopedic in its scope that he could not complete it single-handed.

To the students of sociology his "Principles of Sociology", published in 1877, is the most important treatise. This three-volume work offers an exposition of sociology in a historical perspective.

According to Spencer, the study of sociology covers such fields as family, politics, religion, work and social control. He also emphasized the study of division of labor, associations, social stratification, sociology of knowledge and art and esthetics. Being influenced by Darwin, LF Ward and others, Spencer compared society with that of human organism. It is organic analogy, though rejected presently, is a worth noting contribution.

Spencer stressed the study of whole more than the study of parts. Institutions are inter-related and one can understand society through a close study of these inter-relations. His stress on the functional interdependence of parts continued to be influential. He stressed that the whole society should be considered as a unit of study. Comparative perspective, according to him, would better one's understanding of society at different stages of development. His approach was accepted and followed by several generations of sociologists.

Emile Durkheim (1858-1917)

Emile Durkheim, a distinguished French scholar, remarked that sociology should deal with society as a whole and carry on comparative study of societies.

It is recognized that while Comte was the first to bring home the necessity of scientific study of society, it was Durkheim who pointed out how sociologists should go about their business. Durkheim wanted sociology to emerge as a truly scientific discipline and towards this end, he formulated his 'Rules of Sociological Methods'.

Durkheim wanted sociology to take interest in a wide range of social institutions and social processes. Thus, according to him the discipline was to include general sociology as well as religion, sociology of law and morals, sociology of crime, economic sociology, and sociology of art and esthetics. Each of these branches was to be subdivided into narrower fields of specialization. For example, the sociology of law and morals was to include the subfields of political organization, social organization and marriage and family.

Durkheim laid stress on the relationships among institutions and their setting. His analysis of social facts is lucid. Social facts are nothing but the collective ways of thinking, feeling and acting which though coming from the individual are 'external' to him. They exert pressure on him. These have to be related to their specific social environment and to the type of society to which they belong.

Further, he emphasized the necessity of studying societies in a comparative perspective. He said, "comparative sociology is not a particular branch of sociology, it is sociology itself".

The study of collective representations, according to Durkhcim, forms a major part of the subject-matter of sociology. He believed that sociology could be understood by exploring collective representations. Men interact with one another and the various institutions in society provide ground for interaction. The symbolic level of interaction through language, norms, values, ideologics, etc. is as important as the groups and institutions. In every society individuals learn to look at the world much in the same way as the others. This common set of symbols that the individual members share in a group is called collective representations.

Durltheim also spoke on solidarity. He distinguished between two types of solidarity—mechanical solidarity and organic solidarity. The former is based on common assumptions, beliefs and sentiments like those found in traditional societies. The latter is based on the division of labor and inter connected and inter penetrating interests like the one found in industrial societies. When solidarity bonds break down the result is social disorganization. Thus, the study of solidarity forms an integral part of subject matter of sociology.

According to Durkheim, sociology has three main divisions or fields study. They are social morphology, social physiology and general sociology.

Social morphology is the study of the territorial basis of social life. It is concerned with the nature and extent of influence exercised by such factors as geographical location, size and density of population, on the social organization of social life.

Social physiology deals with the genesis and nature of various social institutions, etc. each of which may be the subject matter of a special discipline.

General sociology, regarded as philosophical part of sociology, attempts to discover general social laws. An attempt is made here to findout links that might exist among social institutions treated independently in social physiology.

The major works of Durkheim are—The Division of Labor in Society, The Rules of Sociological Method, Suicide, The Elementary forms of Religious Life. These speak of subjects Durkheim wanted to include in the scope of sociology.

Max Weber (1864-1920)

Max Weber's contribution to the discipline is indeed significant and covers many fields. Some of them were strictly historical and several others were concerned with methodology, philosophy and criticisms. Perhaps the most widely known are his studies in sociology of religion. He also wrote on general sociology, economy and society.

Weber defined sociology as "a science which attempts the interpretive understanding of social action in order to thereby arrive at a causal explanation of its course and effects". In his view, sociology is essentially a comprehensive science of social action.

Weber made a fundamental distinction between four types of action—Rational action in relation to a goal, rational action, in relation to a value, emotional action and traditional action. To Weber, a comprehensive study of social action meant understanding the meanings man gives to his acts.

Weber took great interest in explaining the special method of study called "the method of understanding". It meant putting oneself in imagination in the place of another and understanding his action. According to him, sociology should concern itself with the study of the parts of society and their mutual relations and also society as a whole. He was also concerned with comparative studies of different societies. His classification of authority into charismatic, traditional and rationalist is a significant contribution to sociology.

Weber confined himself to the analysis of concrete institutions. Lie wrote extensively on religion; various aspects of economic life, including money and division of labor; political parties and other forms of political organizations and authority; bureaucracy and other varieties of large scale organization, caste and class; the city and music. These and other topics, according to Weber, may be included in the subject matter of sociology.

Major works of Weber are—'Economy and Society', 'The Protestant Ethic and the Spirit of Capitalism', 'The Methodology of Social Sciences', 'Bureaucracy', 'The city'.

These pioneers of sociology broadly charted the course that it had to take in the decades to follow. They defined its scope and determined its contents. They also contributed towards the clarification of certain basic issues of method and perspective.

The four founding fathers, says Alex Inkles, seem to be in basic agreement about the proper subject matter of sociology. Firstly, all of them urge sociologists to study a wide range of institutions, from the family to the state. Secondly, all of them agree that a unique subject matter for sociology is found in the inter-relations among different institutions. Thirdly, there is consensus among them regarding society being taken as a distinctive unit of sociological analysis. It is the task of sociology to explain wherein and why societies are alike or different. Lastly, they were in favor of sociology focusing on social acts and relationships regardless of their institutional setting.

Pioneers of Sociology of Indian Society

Most of the pioneers of sociology from India were educated in India as well as in countries like UK, USA and Germany. The prominent among them were GS Ghurye, SV Ketkar, BN Dutta, KP Chattopadyaya, Brijendra Nath Seal, AK Kumaraswamy, Radha Kamal Mukherjee, DP Mukherjee, MN Srinivas, Iravathi Karve, AR Desai, MSA Rao, SC Dube and others.

Among them, contributions of GS Ghurye and MN Srinivas, in particular are very significant not only to the development of sociology of Indian society but also to the development of sociology in general. Govind Sadashiva Ghurye (1893-1984) wrote extensively on caste and races in India covering origin and geographical spread of caste, its features, impact of British rule on caste, role of caste in politics, etc. His other contributions are 'The Aborigines - 'so-called' - and 'Their Future', 'Social Tensions in India', 'Whither India?' India Recreates Democracy', 'Culture and Society', 'Occidental Civilization', etc.

Mysore Narasimhachar Srinivas, born in 1916, occupies a very significant place among the social scientists 'Sanskritization', 'Westernization' and 'Dominant Caste' are the conceptual tools devised by him to understand change in an immobile caste ridden Indian society. 'Religion and Society Among the Coorgs of South India', 'Caste in Modern India' , 'Remembered Village', 'Caste in Modern India and other Essays', 'Caste - Its Twentieth Century Avatar', etc. are his chief contributions.

Dr Irawathi B Karve, a student of Prof GS Ghurye and the first Indian lady sociologist is known to the students of sociology through her works on kinship. 'Kinship organization in India' published in 1953 is a significant proof of her contributions. Her contributions to the study of family are lucid.

KM Kapadia, also a student of GS Ghurye, is widely known for his contributions in the field of marriage, family and Hindu Kinship. His contributions include 'Hindu Kinship (1947), 'Marriage and Family in India (1955)', 'Rural Family Patterns'; A study in Urban-Rural Relations (1956).

AR Desai is known for his contributions to the study of socialmovements and also the study of rural society. His study of the Indian National Movement may be regarded as the first sociological study of social movement. His 'Social Background of Indian Nationalism', published in 1954 is a masterpiece both among sociologists and historians. 'Rural Sociology in India', edited by AR Desai, published in 1960 is a significant contribution' to the field of Rural Sociology.

SOCIOLOGY IS A SCIENCE

Sociology is a science, before proceeding precipitately to elaborate upon this state, it is necessary to know what science is. Some people look upon some specific subject matter as science, e.g. chemistry, engineering, etc.

Scientific Method

In the scientific method, the subject matter in a limited sphere is systematically studied. This method needs great patience, courage, diligence, a creative imagination and objectivity. Without this scientific attitude or spirit no person can profit by the scientific method. This scientific method processed ways of following steps:

1. **Observation:** The first or initial method step in the scientific method is a minute and careful observation of the subject matter of research. This observation often necessitates the use of apparatus, which must be accurate.
2. **Recording:** The second step of the scientific method is a careful recording of all the data obtained in the observation. This necessitates an unbiased objectivity.
3. **Classification:** Now the collected data have to be classified and organized. The classification is aimed to place the disintegrated facts into such relation that they exhibit a symmetrical pattern. In this way, the subject matter is systematically arranged on a logical basis.
4. **Generalization:** The fourth step in the scientific method is the extraction of general laws on the basis of the patterns exhibited by the classified material, or briefly generalization. This general law is known as scientific law.
5. **Verification:** The scientific method does not stop only at the formulation of general laws. The general principles must also be verified. The validity of scientific principles can be ascertained by examination. This validity is their essential condition, in the absence of which they forfeit their claim to the title of scientific laws.

Essential Elements of Science

From the preceding amount of the scientific method, it would be evident that certain elements are essentialy scientific, by virtue of which any study is a science. These essential elements or characteristics of science are as follows:

1. **Scientific method:** As has been stated before, a science is so called not because of its subject matter but because it employs the scientific method.
2. **Factual:** Science is the study of facts. Its subject matter is facts not ideals.
3. **Universal:** Scientific principles are universal. They hold true irrespective of the temporal and spatial order.
4. **Veridical:** Scientific law is veridical. Its validity can be examined at any time. It may be tested any number of times. It will prove true in every case.
5. **Discovery of cause-effect relationship:** Science searches for the cause-effect relationship in its subject matter and in this condition provides universal and valid laws.
6. **Prediction:** Science can make prediction on the basis of universal and valid laws relating to the cause-effect relationship, in any subject. The foundation of science is based upon a faith in casualty. The scientist believes that what will happen, can be predicted by basing this prediction upon what is, for the law of cause and effect, is universal and inevitable.

By examining sociology on the basis of the six foregoing essentials, it will be known that sociology possesses all the essential characteristics of a science.

Sociology

1. **Sociology employs scientific method:** All the methods of sociology are scientific. In them are employed among other such scientific apparatus as scales of sociometery, schedule, questionnaire, interview and case study, etc. In these methods, the first step is the collection of data through observation, which is then systematically recorded. Following this, data are classified, and finally laws are enunciated on the basis of accepted data. The validity of these laws is verified.

2. **Sociology is factual:** Sociology studies social relations and activities. As Reter and Hart have expressed it, the general problem that sociology gets for itself is a description of the social process. In this way, sociology makes a scientific study of facts and the general principles concealed in them.

3. **The principles of sociology are universal:** The law of sociology is proved true at all times and places. As long as the condition does not vary the law is devoid of any exceptions. For example, the principle that individual disorganization and social disorganization depends upon each other, is true for all times and at all places.

4. **Sociology principles are veridical:** In this way, the law of sociology proves true at every verification and re-verification. This validity can be examined by anyone. To make an example, one can consider the law that an increase in the number of divorces indicates acceleration of family disorganization. Now wherever the number of divorces is increasing family disorganization would be showing an upward trend. This principle can be examined anywhere statistics concerning divorces can be obtained.

5. **Sociology delineates cause-effect relationship:** In the foregoing example of divorces and family disorganization, divorces are an effect and family disorganization is one of its causes. Sociology has discovered a cause-effect relation between the phenomena of divorce and family disorganization. In this same way, sociology traces cause-effect relationship in social disorganization and other incidents, activities of relationships in society, and then formulates laws concerning them. In this way, sociology finds an answer to how as well as why.

6. **Sociology can make predictions:** On the basis of cause-effect relationship sociology can anticipate the future and make predictions concerning social relationships, activities, incidents, etc. If disorganization in the families becomes pronounced, it can make prediction concerning the number of divorces, illicit relationships, and many other things. Knowing cause-effect relationships, it can determine what will be on the basis of what is.

It is clearly evident from the foregoing description of sociology that it is a science. Sociologists think in terms of abstractions. And scientific study is possible only through abstract forms. The laws of these abstract forms determine the relations of concrete objects. In this way the laws of sociology are effectively universal and veridical. Sociology tries to discover cause-effect relations in social, familial and individual disorganization and other social maladies and relations, incidents and reactions, besides other social facts. Sociology has wrought a revolutionary change in man's assumptions and brought hope for a future harmony in human society.

SOCIOLOGY AND OTHER SCIENCES

Difference between Social Science and Physical Science

From the foregoing account the objections raised against sociology being called a science, it is evident that these objections do not take into consideration the difference between physical science and social science. A clarification of these differences too will have to show that these objections are unfounded. Roughly speaking, physical science and social science are different from each other in the following aspects:

Sl.No	Social science	Physical science
1.	Social science investigates laws related to man's social behavior	Physical science searches for physical laws in natural phenomena.
2.	Social science proceeds upon the assumption that man is the central figure.	There is no equivalent in physical science.
3.	The fundamental elements of social science are psychological related	The basic elements of physical science have a physical relation.
4.	The basic element of the social science cannot be separated analytically.	The basic element of the physical science can be separated by analysis.
5.	Being related to the study of society the social science has comparative less exactness.	Because they study physical elements the physical sciences possess greater exactness.
6.	Because of their lesser exactness, social science can make comparatively few predictions.	The physical sciences can make more predictions due to higher degree of exactness.
7.	For this reason objectivity is achieved with difficulty in social science.	Objectivity is attainted easily in physical sciences.
8.	Social science provides comparative lesser scope for measurement of subject matter.	There is greater possibility of measurement in the study of physical examination.
9.	It is difficult to construct laboratories for social sciences. Society is the laboratory.	Physical sciences have own laboratories because they can easily be made for studying physical objects.

Functions of Sociology

1. **Technical function:** India is a newly born democracy. Although it was at the peak of prosperity in ancient times, yet its condition deteriorated in the middle ages and there have been no improvements since, as a consequence of which the democracy is facing many obstacles and difficulties. In brief, the country's leader and the thoughtful citizens are faced with the problems of constructing the country. In this reconstruction will be the foundation of social reconstruction, problems concerning mores, traditions, institutions, classes, castes, etc. will have to be faced. Hence, the first step would be to know their meaning in the present context. This function is performed by the study of sociology.

2. **Introductory function:** Sociology will not only undertake to supply information concerning the meaning of these parts of the social system but will also acquaint one with their nature and their laws in order to facilitate the interaction of any change. Before any desired change can be made in a society, it is necessary to know the methods which can introduce this change into the various parts of it. These methods are scientifically studied in sociology.

3. **Informative function:** In this way the study of sociology would put the social worker and officers in India in possession of important information. A theoretical study can never be substitute for practical experience. The country can progress only by practical improvements, not by

theoretical study but a theoretical and scientific study of such problems of society as unemployment, poverty, prostitution, crime, social disorganization, individual disorganization, lack of food, etc. It is a good background for practical efforts at such improvement. Society is a complex structure the problems of which cannot be comprehensible to every individual. There must be a scientific study of them if they are to be understood. It is necessary to conduct sociological researches into special circumstances so that there can be proper guidance in practice.

4. **Tolerative function:** In India, one comes across people belonging to many different castes, races, tribes, religions and cultures. A sociological study would make a comprehensive survey of the customs and traditions of each of them. This would tend to enhance toleration and benevolence. For example, a person studying the customs relating to diet, living, clothing, marriage, etc. of one tribe would not compare them with his own and look at one or the other as superior but would be inclined to consider both from scientific view-point, an attitude of curious and speculative interest. As a result he would not restrict morality to thoughts of class segregation but would make an effort to recognize or discover its real universal nature or form. This would lead to the removal of narrow differences and would give the seed of nationalism a chance to strike roots and develop into a feeling of universal brotherhood, with the passage of time.

5. **Cultural function:** The development of society is impossible without cultural development. A scientific study of the various meanings of culture and principles of their activities, besides a study of their importance, would be added advantages, before trying to make any practical contribution to cultural development. As it is necessary to theoretically acquaint a person with machinery before he can be taught to repair motors, in the same way it is necessary for the pioneers of culture to be acquainted with the elements of culture.

6. **Democratic function:** The great benefit of the study of sociology lies in its democratic function. India has now become a republic but due to lack of any democratic sense in the masses social maladies like prejudice, selfishness, deceit, chicanery, etc., are very prevalent. The country's greatest need at the moment is character, as has been stressed repeated by national leaders. While on the other side this character implies a selfless tendency, it also on the other, does not lose sight of tolerance, benevolence, understanding, planning, etc. all of which are very important. In this direction the study of sociology can introduce a proper view point.

SOCIOLOGY AND OTHER SOCIAL SCIENCES

There are other sciences also, in addition to sociology, which study sociology. Among them are psychology, anthropology, history, and economics, etc. Comet considers these other sciences useless since society cannot be broken into parts and studied. In Comet's opinion, sociology is a totality and its study also should be as a whole. In this way, sociology is the sole social science according to Comet, but sociologist today does not agree with Comet's theory. Actually the structure of society is so vast and complex that a general science which studies in its entirety must be supplemented by special sciences which study the parts. Sociology synthesizes the other social sciences but it is at the same time an individual science having its own individual view-point. According to Ward, Sociology definitely does synthesize the other social sciences but it is a synthesis in which the individual social sciences lose their separate existence and form or create a novelty. Sorokin, too, looks upon sociology as an independent science.

SOCIOLOGY AND PSYCHOLOGY

Sociology studies society, psychology studies human behavior. In the words of Thouless, psychology is the positive science of human experience and behavior. In this way, the scope of sociology and psychology coincide to quite some extent and both are positive sciences. Both are factual and both employ the scientific method. Both have lesser capacity of prediction. And in both it is difficult to maintain objectivity.

Difference between Sociology and Psychology

1. **Difference in attitude:** MacIver written that "It is difference of attitude in regard to a common material". The attitude of psychology is individualistic, that of sociology social.
2. **Difference in units:** The unit of psychology is an individual while sociology regards society as a unit. In this way psychology studies man as an individual in interaction with culture and geographical environment. On other hand, the sociologist studies man as a part of society.
3. **Difference in methods:** The methods of sociology and psychology are not identical, they differ from each other.

Relation between Psychology and Sociology

Sociology and psychology have much in common and enjoy an intimate relationship. Without understanding human psychology it is more or less impossible to understand the interrelation and activities related to human being. In much the same way, many of the profound secrets of psychology remain secret unless there is knowledge of social relationships, behaviors and activities.

Sociology and Anthropology

AL Kroeber calls sociology and anthropology twin sisters. Social relations between sociology and anthropology are closer than those between anthropology and political science.

Three parts of anthropology:

1. **Physical anthropology:** This studies characteristics of human anatomy, from which is derived knowledge of human races and of the origin of human being. This study benefits sociology.
2. **Social and cultural anthropology:** According to the committee of the Royal Anthropological Institute, Great Britain, social anthropology deals with the behavior of man in social situations.
3. **Prehistoric archeology:** This studies cultures of prehistoric period. Using them as a standard for comparison, the sociologist facilitates his understanding of the present social structure.

Difference between sociology and anthropology

1. **Difference of subject matter:** The receptive subject matters of sociology and anthropology differ. Physical anthropology studies the subtle anatomical characteristics whereas sociology itself with their influence upon social relationships.
2. **Difference of attitude: Kluckhohn says:** "The sociological attitude has tended towards the practical and present, the anthropological towards pure understanding and the past."
3. **Difference of methods:** As a result of studying different subject matter from viewpoints, sociology and anthropology differ from each other in their respective methods. Sociology makes use of documents; statistics, etc., and makes survey. Social anthropology resorts in the main to the functional method, in which the person conducting the research actually goes to live in the society he is to study.

Relation between Sociology and Anthropology

Sl.No.	Sociology	Anthropology
1.	Mainly a study of modern communities.	Mainly a study of ancient communities.
2.	Makes use of documents and the statistical method.	Makes use of the functional method.
3.	In addition to study social problems, it makes suggestions for their solutions.	Studies social problems but does not make suggestions for their solution.
4.	Social science.	Natural science.
5.	Methods of social science.	Methods of natural sciences.
6.	Limited study of anatomical characteristics.	Detailed study of anatomical characteristics.
7.	Is concerned with influence of anatomical features upon social relationships.	Is not concerned with influence of anatomical features up on social relationships.
8.	Study of influence of races upon social relationship.	Profound study of races. No concern with their effect upon social relationship.
9.	Special individual study of various aspects and problems of society.	Study of society as a whole.
10	Besides discovering social facts, it also guides their change.	Does not guide.

Sociology and Economics

Defining economics, Farichild, Buck, and Slesinger write, economics is the study of man's activities devoted to obtaining the material means for the satisfaction of his wants. According to this definition, economics is the study of economic relations. Economic relationships bear a close relation to social activities and relationships. On the other hand, social relationship is also affected by economic relationships. Due to this close relation some sociologist have treated economics as a part of sociology.

Difference between Sociology and Economics

Sociology and economics differ from each other in respect of subject matter, scope, viewpoint, methods, etc. thus economics is an independent science whose relation to sociology is one of mutual assistances.

Sl.No.	Sociology	Economics
1.	Sociology studies social relationships.	Economics studies economic relationships
2.	Sociology comprehends the whole society in its scope.	The scope of economics is comparatively restricted.
3.	Scope has a comprehensive viewpoint.	Economics studies relations and activities only from the economic view-point.
4.	Sociology studies society. Its unit is group.	The unit of economics is an individual whose economic aspect it studies mainly.
5.	The method of sociology differs from those of economics.	In economics induction, deduction, etc. are used.

Sociology and History

History studies the activities of human race. Paul Barth has said that the history of cultures and institutions is of help in the understanding of sociology and in collection of its material. Sociology assists in the study of society. Nowadays history also is being studied from the sociological viewpoint. Philosophy of history is also proving very useful for sociology. In this way, sociology and history are closely related.

Difference between History and Sociology

1. **History is concrete and sociology is abstract:** According to Park, In the same sense that history is concrete, sociology is the abstract science of human experience and human nature. History presents a chronological description of incidents, cultures, etc. but sociology attempts to discover their cause and general principles.
2. **Sociology and history have different attitude:** As a general rule, history studies those incidents which are peculiar or unusual. Sociology studies those incidents which are frequently repeated. History describes incidents taking place at a definite place and time. Sociology strives to discover universal laws and is not related to particular spatiotemporal incidents.
3. History generally studies incidents which happened in the past. Sociology is interested in past incidents only in as much as they can render some assistance in understanding the present societies.
4. History emphasized the doing of the individual. Human group is the unit in sociological study.

Sociology and Political Science

Concerning the close relation of sociology to political science, Barnes has written, `The most significant thing about sociology and modern political theory is that most of the changes which have taken place in the political theory in the last thirty years have been along the line of development suggested and marked out by sociology'. Actually, knowledge of sociology is necessary for understanding the problems of political science because political problems also have a social aspect.

Problems Common to Sociology and Political Science

The law of the state has a profound influence upon society. It is by means of law that the government changes and improves society but it is necessary to keep in view the customs, traditions and racial norms of the country while formulating laws. The problem of deciding upon the form of government is best explained by having recourse to both sociology and political science. The problem of determining the government's policy also is common to both. Similarly the study of customs, behavior, institutions, values, etc. is common to both sociology and political sciences.

Difference between Sociology and Political Sciences

Sl.No	Sociology	Political science
1.	Science of sociology.	Science of government or political society.
2.	Social viewpoint.	Attitude of authority.
3.	Study of organized and disorganized communities.	Study of solely of organized communities.

Contd...

Contd...

Sl.No.	Sociology	Political science
4.	Study of all kinds of social relationships.	Study of political relationships only
5.	Study of all forms of society.	Study of the political society only
6.	Study of the means of social control.	Study only of government recognized means of control.

SOCIOLOGY AND BIOLOGY

According to Prof NG Muller, 'Our ideas of what sort of progress is possible or desired for man must depends in part at least upon our views of his nature, his manner of organization, the method by which he bears with the rest of nature. In this, study of biology is necessary for a study of sociology. It is not possible to determine the models and limits of man's social progress without being acquainted with man's physical capacities, qualities and short-coming and limitations. Biology presents us with this very knowledge. It studies man's original and biological development, describes his development, sexual, anatomical and personal peculiarities and formulates principles for his adjustments to the environment. Darwinian theory of evolution is just one such principles which has been used in sociology to good advantage. Human ecology is based upon biological ecology. Genetics, which is of major importance in sociology, is a branch of biology.

Limits of Biological Principles in Social Sphere

But biological principles can be applied in the social sphere only unto certain limits. Indiscriminate application beyond these limits can lead to drastic consequences. It is indicating towards this fact that Ginsberg has, however, resulted from the too facile application of biological categories to social facts and in particular, a tendency to over-emphasize the purely racial factors in social evolution or change.

MEDICAL SOCIOLOGY

Medical sociology is a specialized branch of sociology which studies health, healthy behavior and health institutions. Previously, disease and its treatment were considered only the problems of medical sciences, but medical sociologist declares that in diseases and health problems, the role of social and psychological factors is very significant. Similarly, it is very important to find out the role of behavioral and cultural factors in the causation of diseases.

Uses of Medical Sociology

1. To estimate the rural health status of individual and community.
2. To find out the social factors in the causation of communicable diseases like sexual diseases, TB, and AIDS, etc.
3. To find out the customs, traditions, beliefs and other cultural patterns which affect the health of a particular community.
4. To establish the interdependence of medical and social sciences.

The meaning of social pathology is to understand conditions like poverty, crime, and beggary, etc. The study of diseases and social factors responsible for the causation of diseases, also may be included in this. The study and survey of accidents, heart diseases, diabetes, asthma, cancer, etc. comes in the subject matter of social medicine.

HOSPITAL SOCIOLOGY

The study of hospital, patients, medical and nursing personnel and organizations of health care and services are included in hospital sociology. Hospital has become an indispensable part of society. In addition to the inpatients, a large section of the society is indirectly related to the hospital as outdoor patients. Hence, it is essential that the hospital should be studied in its entire social perspective. The following may be included in the subject matter of hospital sociology:

1. Social structure of hospital.
2. Medical and nursing professionals.
3. Hospital and nursing (as an industry).
4. Specialization in medical services.
5. Patient- doctor, nurse-patient, nurse-doctor, nurse-patient's relatives and other interpersonal relations within the hospital.
6. Medico-social work.
7. Consumer protection act.
8. Medical ethics, nursing code of conduct and social etiquette.
9. Role of patients and their relatives in the hospital.

SOCIO-CULTURAL AND ECONOMIC ASPECTS IN SOCIOLOGY

1. **Education:** It is an established fact that education improves health status, especially female education plays important role in the health behavior of people. Higher educated societies or states have low MMR and IMR.
2. **Political structure:** Policies, rules and regulation about health and their implementation depend upon the political structure of a particular country. Positive political system improves the health conditions of the citizen. Strong political will and democratic pattern always support the well-being of people.
3. **Occupation:** Financial position of any individual or family affects the health conditions. If an individual is unemployed, he or she cannot afford more on health prevention and promotion. Poor families are more susceptible to diseases. In illness, they feel stress due to lack of money.
4. **Economic status:** The nations, which have the sound economic ststus or financial strength, can spend more on health. So the citizens of developed countries have life expectancy and good health status.
5. **Demographic structure:** Demography is directly related to health conditions of the people. Male-female ratio, population of children, youth and older people, density of population, etc. affect and determine the health status.
6. **Cultural beliefs:** Cultural beliefs and values about food, living, housing, habits, personal hygiene, etc. affect the lifestyle of an individual and community. Lifestyle has greater impact on health. Healthy and positive lifestyle enhances the health promotion.
7. **Social environment:** It covers the wide area of social health. Social health is related to positive maternal environment and positive human environment.

METHODS OF SOCIOLOGY

The major methods of investigation in social phenomena used by sociology are following:

1. Questionnaire method.
2. Schedule method.
3. Interview method.
4. Case study method.

5. Participant observation.
6. Social survey.
7. Social research method.
8. Statistical method.

Questionnaire Method

In social research the questionnaire method is used comprehensively. In the questionnaire method, as it evident from the name, a list of selected question is compiled. These questions throw light upon the different aspects of the problem. Usually the questions are accompanied by `yes' and `no' as their answer and the informant has to reject the wrong answer. The questionnaire method has several difficulties. Often people, in answering the question, prevaricate. Sometimes the questions are so framed that they become ambiguous and are interpreted differently by the observer and the informant. Quiet often the questions are answered without their full significance having been grasped. Notwithstanding these difficulties the questionnaire method is by far the most popular method in social research.

Schedule Method

The schedule method resembles the questionnaire method to some extent, in as much as it, too, is a list of questions that answer to which supply the data. But these questionnaires are taken by the observer to the informant and filled in by this method are more valid, but compared to the questionnaire method, it involves more time, energy and money. This method achieves greater minuteness of detail.

Interview Method

In the interview method the observer, questions him across the table noting down the information which questions elicit. This certainly does not obtain much useful information but it simultaneously becomes plagued by the defect that much information which the informant can offer indirectly cannot be expected in a direct interview. Actually much of the success of the observer depends upon his individual ability. If the informant shows hesitation because the information is being transcribed, a tape recorder can be used.

Case Study Method

The case study is a form of qualitative analysis involving very careful and complete observation of a person, a situation or a person, a situation or an institution. The case study method may be defined as an all-inclusive and intensive study of an individual, in which the investigator brings to bear all his methods, or as a systematic gathering of enough information about a person to pursue one to understand how he or she functions as a unit of society. Burgess assigns the name of social microscope to his method. In this method, a scheduled or questionnaire of the questions relating to the problem of the people who are to be studied is prepared and laws are formulated by generalizing the answer to these questions. This method clarifies the learnt meaning of numerals and is therefore, complementary to a statistic study.

Participant Observation

As is evident from the name, in the participant observation method, the observer participates with the people whom he is observing. This gives him the opportunity coming into direct contact with the people who are to provide him with his information. This method provides much detailed information along with the faculty of its execution. But this method involves extensive use of time, money and energy. Yet in spite of these defects this method assists in a profound study of rural groups because other methods like the questionnaire method do not prove efficacious. This method finds an uninhibited use in all anthropologist studies.

Social Survey

Social survey is a process by which qualitative facts are collected about the social aspects of a community's composition and activities. It is evident from this definition that social survey is intended to be the study of social aspect of a community composition and activities. Social survey method also a fact finding study dealing chiefly with working class poverty and with the nature and problems of community.

Objectives of Social Survey

1. **Collection of data related to the social aspects of community:** Social survey studies individuals as members of society and in this way studies social circumstances and problems.
2. **Study of social problems, labor and problems:** In social survey, social problems and in particular problems of the labor class like illiteracy, poverty, insanitation, unemployment, drinking, crime, juvenile delinquency, prostitution, labor problems, etc. are studied.
3. **Practical and utilitarian viewpoint:** The studies of social survey are made a practical and utilitarian viewpoint in order that suggestions for collective program in solving different problems may be offered.

Subject Matter of Social Survey

1. **Direct or indirect survey:** Direct survey is one in which the facts can be qualitatively interpreted while on the other hand no such quantitative interpretation is possible in the case of an indirect survey. For example survey of the population is direct. On the other hand, the survey of the state of health or the level of nutrition is indirect.
2. **Census survey and sampling survey:** In the census survey the different parts of the entire area are individually studied and the figures are then compiled into one. On the other hand, in the sample survey instead of the whole area being studied, a part which will represent the entire area of it, is taken.
3. **Primary and secondary survey:** In the primary survey, the survey work is started right from beginning. In this survey he collects facts concurring with his objectives and thus primary surveys are more reliable and pure. The survey conducted under the circumstances is called secondary survey.
4. **Initial and repetitive survey:** If the survey conducted in the area is the first of its kind, it is called an initial survey while if some survey has been done in the past then the present survey is termed a repetitive survey. An initial survey involves comparatively greater effort and exertion and comparable data are not available. In repetitive survey the information obtained is more reliable and can be compared.
5. **Official, semi-official and private survey:** As the name indicates, official survey is the survey sponsored by the government; semi-official survey conducted by universities, district boards, municipalities and other similar semi-official intuitions; and the private survey is a survey attempted by individuals.
6. **Widespread survey and limited survey:** Surveys are given these names according to their extension or coverage. A survey covering a greater area is called widespread survey while one

more delimited or less extensive is known as limited survey. A limited survey is comparatively more reliable and less liable to mistakes but it carries with it the probability of some of the facts being omitted.

7. **Public and confidential survey:** It is evident that the public surveys are those in which the process and results of study are not concealed while the confidential surveys are those in which the processes and results are not revealed to people.

8. **Postal and personal survey:** Postal survey, as the term itself implies, is a method in which the surveyor obtains the answers by sending the questionnaire by post. If the survey is to be a personal one, then the surveyor has to move about in the areas to be surveyed and collect information. Postal survey certainly does economies upon time, effort and money but the information which it can obtain is very limited and lacks reliability.

9. **Regular ad-hoc survey:** Regular surveys are conducted after the lapse of a fixed period of time, as exemplified by the survey conducted by the state bank of India. The organizing made for an ad-hoc survey is temporary and is dissolved after the survey has been completed.

Major steps in the social survey:
1. Definition of the purpose or object.
2. Definition of the problem to be studied.
3. The analysis of this problem in a schedule.
4. The delimitation of the area or scope.
5. Examination of all documentary sources.
6. Field work.
7. The arrangement, tabulation and statistical analysis of data.
8. The interpretation of the results.
9. The deduction.
10. Graphic expression.

Social Research

Social research is the discovery of new truths about society. In the words of PV Yang, we may define social research as the systematic method of discovering new facts or verifying old facts, their sequences, interrelationships, causal explanations and the natural laws which govern them. In this way, social research or investigation discovers new facts about social activities, social circumstances, social assumptions, social groups, social values, social institutions, etc. and investigates the old facts on these subjects. It locates interrelationships or casual relations among social incidents. It verifies those natural laws which stimulate the different phenomena in social life. Objective of social research is to formulate general laws by collection, analysis, interpretation and generalization of facts, having studied social incidents and activities and to predict on the basis of these general laws as well as to indicate future changes and reactions. The aim of social research is obviously purely theoretical and scientific, lacking any direct relations with human welfare.

Major steps in social research:
1. Formulating hypothesis.
2. Observation and collection of data.
3. Classification and organization of collected data.
4. Generalization.
5. Verification of general laws and examination of their truth.

Statistical Method

The statistical method is widely used in sociology. In the words of Odum, statistic which is the science of numbering and measuring phenomena objectively is an essential tool of research. In the scientific method qualitative facts are collected, according to Bogardus, Social statistics is mathematics applied to human facts. This method is used in questions which involve measurement, numerical, etc. for example, this method is very much important in the study of the rates of birth and deaths, divorce, marriage, etc. This method can also used in the measurement of social situations and assumptions. This method helps to deduce averages and norms.

FIELDS OF SOCIOLOGY

The scope of sociology being wide, an effort has been made to divide its study into different fields. The main felids are:

Sl.No	Fields of sociology	Description
1.	Sociological theory	This includes the study of sociological concepts, principles and generalizations.
2.	Historical sociology	Under it we study the past social institutions and the origin of the present ones.
3.	Historical sociology	It studies the origin, growth, functions, kinds, nature of family and its problems like those of divorce, etc.
4.	Human ecology and demography	It studies the influence of population and geographical factors on society.
5.	Sociology of community	It is a study of community. It is divided into two parts: (a) rural sociology, (b) urban sociology.
6.	Special sociologies	Recently special sociologies have been developed to study different aspects of social relationships.

Other fields of sociology:

1. Sociology and family.
2. Sociology and community.
3. Sociology and demography.
4. Sociology and education.
5. Sociology and religion.
6. Sociology and economics.
7. Sociology and politics.
8. Sociology and social stratification.
9. Sociology of anthropology.
10. Medical sociology.
11. Sociology of law.
12. Military sociology.
13. Sociology of criminology.
14. Social psychology.
15. Social disorganization.

16. Sociology of ecology.
17. Sociology of rural and urban society.
18. Cultural sociology.

IMPORTANCE OF SOCIOLOGY

1. **Sociology makes a scientific study of society:** Scientific knowledge about society is pre-requisites to any marked improvements in the state of human affairs. Sociology studies roles of the institutions in the development of the individual: Sociology studies about social institutions and the relation of the individuals to each being made. The home and family, the school and education, the church and religion, the state and government, industry and work, the community and associations these are the great institutions through which society functions.

2. **The study of sociology is indispensable for understanding and planning of society:** Society is a complex phenomenon with a multiple of intricacies. It will be impossible to understand it and to solve its various problems without study of sociology. A certain amount of knowledge about the society is necessary before any social policies can be carried out. For example, that a policy of decreasing this goal cannot be determined in exclusively economic terms because matters of family organization, customs and traditional values must be taken into account and these require a sociological type of analysis.

3. **Sociology is of great importance in the solution of social problems:** The present world is suffering from many problems which can be solved only through scientific study of the society. It is obvious that social evils do not just happen and everything has its due cause. It is a task of sociology to study the social problems through the methods of scientific research and to find out solution for them.

4. **Sociology has drawn our attention to the intrinsic worth and dignity of man:** Sociology has been instrumental in changing our attitude towards human beings. In a huge specialized society, we are all limited as to the amount of the whole organization and culture that we can experience directly.

5. **Sociology has changed our outlook with regards to the problems of crime, etc:** Again, it is through the study of sociology that our whole outlook on various aspects of crime has changed. The sciences of criminology and penology and social work and social therapy which are rendering commendable service in understanding social situations and solving individual problems are but handmaids of sociology.

6. **Sociology has made great contribution to enrich human culture:** Human culture has been made richer by the contribution of sociology. It has removed so many cobwebs from our minds and knowledge and enquiry. Sociology also impresses egoistic, ambitious and class hatred. In short, its finding stimulates every person to render a full measure of service to every other person and to the common good.

7. **Sociology is of great importance in the solution of international problems:** The progress made by physical sciences has brought the nations of the world left behind, by the revolutionary progress of the science. We live in twentieth century world that is politically divided in terms of eighteenth century conditions. The consequences are that stresses within and between political units lead time to time to war and conflict. Given the workshop of the nation-state, men have failed to bring in peace. The study of sociology of war will help in understanding the underlying causes of war and remove all such causes which promote tensions between nations and ultimately lead to war.

8. **Sociology is useful as a teaching subject:** In the view of its importance. Sociology is becoming popular as a teaching subject also. It is being accorded an important place in the curriculum of colleges and universities.

9. **Sociology as profession:** The value of sociology lies in the fact that it keeps us up-to-date on modern situations; it contributes to making good citizens; it contributes to the solution of community problems; it adds to the knowledge of the society; it identifies good government with community and it helps one to understand causes of things and so on.

CONCLUSION

The field of sociology is fast expanding and its practical utility is widely recognized. Applied sociology is assuming importance day by day. In social work, social welfare, social planning, social reform and social reconstruction, the guidance of sociology is always sought. The growth has reached new heights under the favorable conditions in which it is finding itself today. Sociology will help the doctors and nurses to know the culture and social life of the patient. In country like India where people have their affiliation with different religious, caste, tribes and communities. It is essential to know the culture of the patients. The study of sociology helps nurse to identity the socio-psychological problems of the patient, which helps to improve the quality patient care.

BIBLIOGRAPHY

1. Adam Kuper, Jessica Kuper (Eds). The social science/Encyclopedia, Routledge, London, 1989.
2. Alvin W. Gouidner. The Coming Crisis of Western Sociology, Heinernann, London, 1963.
3. Barney Glaser, Anslem Stauss. Awareness of dying, Whitefield and Nicolson, London, 1967.
4. David Dressier, William M Wills. Jr. Sociology: The study of Human Interaction, 3rd edn. Alfred A. Knoff, New York, 1975.
5. Ely Chinnoy. Sociology, Random House, New York, 1961.
6. Ewing Goffman. Asylum: Essays on Social Situation of Mental Patients and Inmates, Double day, Garden city, NY 1961.
7. John J. Macionis and Ken Plummer. Sociology: A Global Introduction, Prentice Hall Europe, New York, 1998.
8. Kenneth Plimmer. "Organizing AIDS" in Peter Aggleton and Hilary Homans, Social Aspects of AIDDS;' Falmer Press, London, 1988.
9. Meluin L Defleur, et al. Sociology: Human society, 2nd edn. Scott, Foresman and Co, Glenview, Illinois, 1976.
10. Philip Strong. The ceremonial order of the clinic, Routledge, London, 1979.
11. Richard Chever Wallac, Wendy Drew Waliac. Sociologically and Bocon, MC, Boston, 1985.
12. Theodore Caplow, et. al. Recent social Trends in the United States, 1960-1990, McGill-Queen's University Press, Montreal, 1991.

24

Sociology and Nursing

DEFINITIONS

1. **Nursing process:** The nursing process is the core and essence of nursing; it is central to all nursing actions, it is applicable in all settings. There is a basic theme that underlies the process; it is organized, systematic and deliberated. Nursing process which is applied to solve the problem of the individual (patient) is termed as individualized nursing process. This is the most common nursing practice used in hospital care settings/institutional nursing.

2. **Assessment:** Assessment is the first step of nursing process which provides basis for other phases. Assessment is the organized, systematic and ongoing process of collecting data or information from a variety of sources. As a component of nursing process, assessment is an independent nursing function that depends upon the skill and discretion of nurses.

3. **Diagnosis:** Diagnosis is a process of analysis. Today the term diagnosis is not restricted to one particular profession or it is not the exclusive property or domain of physicians only.

4. **Nursing diagnosis:** A nursing diagnosis is a clinical judgment about individual, family or community responses to actual or potential health problems/life processes. Nursing diagnosis provide the basis for selection of nursing interventions to achieve outcomes for which the nurse is accountable.

5. **Planning:** Planning begins with the review of nursing diagnosis. Planning involves the development of strategies designed to prevent, minimize or correct the problems identified in the nursing diagnosis. It sets the priorities for nursing actions. The main objective of planning care is to make the best possible use of resources to help the person achieve the desired outcomes.

6. **Implementation:** Implementation phase of the nursing process is nursing intervention. It is also termed as nursing actions, nursing activities, nursing approaches and nursing orders.

7. **Evaluation:** Evaluation is the final phase of nursing process. The word evaluation refers to judgment or appraisal. It is examining the outcomes of the nursing actions or extent to which the expected outcomes or goals were achieved. Evaluation is an ongoing process in caring that is related to the previous phases of nursing process.

8. **Community:** Community is defined as "a locality-based entity, composed of systems of formal organizations reflecting societal institutions, informal groups and aggregates that are interdependent, and whose function or expressed intent is to meet a wide variety of collective needs.

9. **Community health:** Concept of community health in the community health nursing process is; meeting the collective needs through identifying problems and managing interactions within the community itself and between the community and the larger society.

10. **Community participation:** The goal of community health nursing practice aims at change in the community behavior for the promotion or wellness of community. Most changes need the community participation: That is also equated with partnership. All interventional or planning strategies require the partnership of the community. Participation should be active, informed, flexible and negotiable at every stage of the change process. Participation or partnership is very much important because health is not given but rather it is generated through lay-professional collaboration.

INTRODUCTION

The term sociology is derived from two words; the first word 'Socius' from Latin and second word 'Logas' from Greek language. Socius means *society* and logos mean *science*. Thus, sociology is the science of society, sociology defined as the study of society, social relationship, groups and social interactions. Sociology is the science of human relationship. Sociology studies man as a social animal. It deals with human groups evolve customs and behavior patterns that are handed down from generation to generation by personal contact.

The primary goal of sociology and nursing is promotion of health and prevention of illness and injury. Health promotion and illness prevention in the population may be achieved through interventions directed at the total population or at the individuals, families and groups that constitute its members.

Public health nursing is the practice of promoting and protecting the health of populations using knowledge from nursing, social, and public health sciences. The practice is population-focused, with the goals of promoting health and preventing disease and disability for all people through the creation of conditions in which people can be health (American Nurses Association, 2007). Community health nurse is a partner in a health team who provides nursing care, treatment to the sick, health counseling and does work in different places such as home, school and health center. She also responsible for family centered care.

During the middle ages, nursing was carried out by religious or military groups whose prime function was other than nursing care. They cared for the poor and destitute. Also the nursing needs of the sick at home were met by members of the family. With the evolution of medicine, surgery and public health, complicated technical dimensions requiring many procedures to be performed by specialized persons. However, the crimean war made the establishment of nursing as collectively organized and institutional resources were linked to its military basis. The wars and other social changes at the mid-century also brought the nurse into close association with the physicians, giving them control and jurisdiction over nursing activities—not only over curative actions but also over those which involved the patient's comfort, sanitary needs and all other conditions associated with the patient status.

SOCIOLOGICAL ASPECTS OF NURSING

Sociology has several branches like social psychology, industrial sociology, sociology and medicine, sociology of religion, sociology of education, sociology of family, rural sociology, etc. the importance of sociology in nursing is widely accepted. Sociology demystifies the nature of health and illness, highlights the social causes of disease and death, exposes power-factors and ethical dilemmas in the production of health care, and either directly or indirectly helps to create a discerning practitioner who then becomes capable of more focused and competent decision making. There has to be a fair and realistic balance between how much social science, biological science and pure nursing is taught in the education of nurses. Morever, the tendency for sociologist to lay to waste the factual and essential basis of every phenomenon is both unhelpful and ludicrous. While sociology does provide legitimate, tangible and abundant insight into the organization and shaping of matters relating to health and illness, much of what purports to be social science to the everyday experiences of nurses.

Consider the patient as a person is a precept given as the introduction to the special aspects of nursing care and nursing education. The relationship between social conditions and factors that influence health or development of disease is now established. Health problems tend to be accepted from the perspective of particular societies and cultures and as a result people have usually responded to the threat of disease in predictable ways. Knowledge about norms, values, beliefs, social structures and life styles has provided insight not only about the social organization and human resources designed to cope with health problems but the very nature and cause of illness. Knowledge of sociology will help nursing students to understand and appreciate the social factors of health and illness, mortality and fertility, problems of the aged, the social milieu of the most vulnerable group in the society, children and expectant mother, the social functions of health institutions, the relationship of systems of health care delivery to other social system and the social behavior of health personnel and those people who are user of health care systems.

Individual is composed of biophysical, psychological, spiritual and sociocultural elements. An individual develops through life cycles and stages. They have varying abilities to meet hierarchical needs as they strive toward health, growth, and self-actualization. Culture is viewed as the context within which self-care behavior is learned. Society composed of individuals, groups and communities. It is dynamic and shares a reciprocal relationship with integrated patterns of human behavior. Nursing is a dynamic practice discipline whose focus is caring for individuals, groups and communities using a holistic approach social education provides the foundation for the nurse to understand the biophysical, psychological, spiritual and sociocultural aspects of individuals, groups or communities. Nursing is composed of actions and roles involving human services, interpersonal process and technology. Actions and roles are deliberately selected and performed by nurses to help individuals, groups or communities under their care maintained or change their self-care practices.

NEED OF SOCIOLOGY IN NURSING

Sociology is a body of thought about man's inter-human life. To know how sociology illuminates the human experiences, one must first understand what sociology is. Sociology studies the general characteristics common to all classes of social phenomena of the relationship between these classes and of the relationship between social and non-social phenomena. He chooses interaction as the unit into which the phenomena should analyzed. The disease and cures differ according to habits, social and economic, climatic variations and ways of life. Those concerned with health care must reckon both the general importance of human biology and socioeconomic and environmental diversities of health problems. Such as constant and unavoidable exposure to stimuli of urban and industrial civilization, impact of technological advancement, physiological disturbances, emotional trauma and disruption of set patterns of community and society.

In the words of Jones & Jones (1975), sociology is concerned with the study of human relationships and more specifically the formulation and perpetration of these relationships and of the individual who enact them, within the broad context of human society. Sociology seeks to explain how it is that human system and organizations exist overtime in a recognizable and ordered fashion. Nursing services meet the needs of the society and any major change in social structure and dynamics will bring about changes in nursing too.

The need of nurses to study sociology:

Sl.No	Concepts	Areas
1.	Cultural values	Cultural aspects of health services, health institutions, health problems, health practices prevailing.
2.	Prediction	Modes of prediction
3.	Social structure	The nurse needs to know the social structure of the society based on that she can plan the nursing process.
4.	Distribution of power	The nurse should provide care to the community effectively by utilizing and distributing their power equally.
5.	Political organizations	The nurse needs to know various political organizations existing within the community and nation to help the people to avail health care facilities.
6.	Mobilization	Mobilization of resources and pattern of their uses within the community in the context of cultural perception and cultural meaning of the health problems.

IMPORTANCE OF SOCIOLOGY IN NURSING

Sociology plays an important role in the area of health sciences medicine and nursing have common goals, for example, prevention and restoration of health. The primary role of medicine comprises diagnosis and treatment the cure process. In contrast the primary role of nursing lies in the care process-consisting of caring, comforting and guiding. Nurses plays role in health care profession. Nurses are the key persons who have significant influence over the group members within the society. Nurses have to work for maintenance of healthier life styles and high standards of living.

Sociology is closely related to personal and community health. Specialized branches of sociology as medical sociology and hospital sociology have came to existence, which emphasize the importance of sociology in the area of health. Study of sociology is important for nurses due to following:

1. Through sociology the nurse get information about the sociocultural life of the patient. This is important for the planning and implementation of treatment.
2. With the help of sociology, we can study the structure of family, community and society, on the basis of which health organizations are made and services are distributed. Thus, medical sociology is useful for comprehensive health services.
3. With the help of sociology, nurses can understand the characteristics of social relationship, its complexities and its impact on health care.
4. Sociology helps in the understanding and eradication of social problems.
5. By the study of sociology, nurse learns the technique of adjustment which can be used in nursing.
6. Sociology helps to understand those forces and pressures which affect adversely.
7. Study of sociology helps the nurses to understand the behavior, conflicts, interpersonal relationships, hierarchy, groups, and adaptation, etc. of different people working in the hospital or health institutions.

1.	Quality care	To provide total patient care in a comprehensive manner and render loving care to meet the total needs of the clients either in the hospitals or in the community.
2.	Holistic care	To understand and meet the needs of the individual, family and social needs in a holistic manner thereby nations development can be achieved.
3.	Understand the human behavior	To broaden the view of nursing students to understand human behavior in relation to the society.
4.	Planning nursing process	To understand the cause and meaning of many kinds of patient behavior top make them comfortable and treat them all alike for improving of client care. In relation to the society.
5.	Continuity of care	To suggest the ways to work with families. Community agencies and groups of persons to provide health counseling in planning for continuity of care.
6.	Interpersonal relationship	To provide right motivation, treatment and physical, medical, vocational, psychosocial rehabilitation basing on attitudes and responses of others by understanding their behavior through good interpersonal relationship.
7.	Professional development	To understand emotional reaction pattern (e.g. level of perception, attitudes of people towards medical care, barriers of communication, individual differences, social distance, prejudice, change, emotional interpersonal components of disease process, the growth and decline of population in a special area, sociopsychological factors, etc.) to understand herself and others and the nurse has to make more effective use of her professional skills.
8.	Understand human problems	To gain greater insight into the human problems as related to the illness.
9.	Cultural value identifications	To identify some of the sociocultural barriers and promotes, the activities related to treatment, prevention, of disease and promotion of health.
10.	Community promotion	To develop a plan of operation of involving local people and plan of operation by involving local people and other engaged in community development keeping in mind the social realities.
11.	Innovative health care	To analyze health conditions of people and brining about changes and innovation in health care based on research.
12.	Social interactions	To plan social interactions and to establish good interpersonal relationship with superiors, subordinates, class IV employees, clients, students, visitors and community.
13.	Preventive and remedial approaches	To study the social problems related to behavior and suggest preventive remedial approach to tackle the problematic situations in the community in efficient manner.
14.	Analyzing social situations	To identify and analyze different social situations which are responsible for the incidence and prevention of morbidity and mortality.
15.	Effective liaison	To act an effective liaison between the client and the health team members.

USES OF SOCIOLOGY IN NURSING

Sociology is very useful science especially for the nursing profession. It will help the nurses to know the culture and social life of patients. In countries like India, where people have their affiliation with different religions, castes, tribes and communities, it is essential to know the culture of these groups. The customs, traditions, folkways, mores and values of the patients must be known before treating them, so as to make the medical and nursing services more effective. For this, study of sociology is necessary. In treatment of diseases, mental or physical, is a cooperative venture in which a united effort of various medical, paramedical and even nonmedical personnel are required. Usually, it is the nurse who acts as a key person in the hospital situation. Knowledge of sociology helps her to maintain congenital relationship between different personnel at different level. Nurses are working not only in the hospitals; a large number of nurses are working outside the hospital. In program like public health, industrial health, school health, military nursing, and so on, the nurse has to work in very close proximity with different sections of the society.

Knowledge she/he has about society is extremely useful. Technological progress has successfully eliminated many diseases, but it has brought new problems and challenges to nurses. The problems of aged, patients suffering from AIDS or persons suffering from permanent disabilities due to industrial or other types of accidents. Deep understanding of human behavior relationships and sociology can be very useful in handling such situations.

Nursing care is a primary and essential component of a nurse. To meet the needs of her patient adequately, it is essential that the nurse develops self-understanding. She must strive constantly to become emotionally, mentally, morally and socially mature. The study of sociology along with sociological and religious training is very useful in this process. Today, nursing is not simply an effect to cure illness. Preventive services and promotion of health are also equally important aspects of nursing. To be an effective agent of health promotion, knowledge of the community and facilities and resources available therein are essential.

The study of sociology helps nurses to identify the psychosocial problems of patients, which helps to improve the quality of treatment. The study of sociology also helps nurses to support the government in various schemes of social planning: for example, the family planning of the government can be successfully implemented only with the active participation of the nurses. The study of sociology helps the nurses to improve the quality of family welfare program and the community health services of the government. Sociology also helps the nurses to interact with wide spectrum of persons whose behaviors are varied: for example, patients, doctors, other family members, management, government and society at large. The study of sociology will assist in understanding these behavioral patterns, which will in turn help to improve health care.

CONCLUSION

Sociology is the science of human relationship. The word relationship is the key. Sociology studies man as a social animal. It deals with human groups and products of their activity. The group evolves customs and behavior patterns that are handed down from generation to generation by personal contact. Society is held together by these customs and patterns. The relationships between human being are determined by these elements that together comprise the social heritage. Sociology seeks additional insight into the nature of this relationship and the beliefs that define them. Nurses are the key person in proving care on the basis of preventive, promotive and rehabilitative cares in the hospital and community. She initiates and interacts with various people and professionals in health care delivery system. So it is very essential to study sociology in nursing.

BIBLIOGRAPHY

1. DW Johnson. Reaching Out, Prentice Hall, NJ, 1972.
2. E Adamson Hebel, Evereth 1. Forest. Cultural and Social Anthropology, TMH ed. New Delhi, 1979.
3. EH Erikson. Childhood and society, Norton, New York, 1963.
4. Francis E Merrill, Wentworth Eldredge H. Society and Culture, An Introductions to Sociology, Precentice Hall Inc., NJ, 1957.
5. Frank Lorimer et al. Cultural and Human Fertility, UNESCO, Paris, 1954.
6. Martin Marcus, Alan Ducklin. Success in sociology, John Murray, London, 1998.
7. NJ Brill. Working with people—The Helping York, 1973.
8. PR Carkhuff, et al. "The Art of Helping" Human Resource Development Press, Arnterst Mass, 1977.
9. Ronald C. Federico. Sociology (2nd edn) Addison Wesley Pub. Co. Reading, Mass, 1979.
10. William A. Havilland. Cultural Anthropology (4th edn) Hott, Rinehart and Winston, New York, 1983.

Man, Society and Environment

25

DEFINITIONS

1. **Education:** It is an established fact that education improves health status, specially "female education" plays important role in the health behavior of people. Higher educated societies or states have low MMR and IMR.

2. **Political structure:** Policies, rules and regulation about health and their implementation depends upon the political structure of a particular country. Positive political system improves the health conditions of the citizen. Strong political will and democratic pattern always support the "well-being" of people. In the well-being, health aspect is included first.

3. **Occupation:** Financial position of any individual or family affects the health conditions. If an individual is unemployed, he or she cannot afford more on health prevention and promotion. Poor families are more susceptible to diseases. In illness, they feel stress due to lack of money.

4. **Economic status:** The nations, which have the sound economic status or financial strength, can spend more on health. So the citizens of developed countries have high life expectancy and good health status. Per capita income and GNP reflects the well-being of people. Economic status also affects the: (i) health planning (ii) health service resources, and (iii) health organizations.

5. **Demographic structure:** Demography is directly related to health conditions of the people. Male-female ratio, population of children, youth, and older people, density of population, etc. affect and determine the health status.

6. **Cultural beliefs:** Cultural beliefs and values about food, living, housing, habits, personal hygiene, etc. affect the lifestyle of an individual and community. Lifestyle has greater impact on health. Healthy and positive lifestyle enhances the health promotion.

7. **Social environment:** It covers the wide area of social health. Social health is related to positive material environment (i.e. housing and economic matters) and positive human environment (i.e. social network). Social environment has a greater influence on the health status of community. Health service utilized is also concerned with social environment.

8. **Adaptation:** Adaptation is the process by which an organism makes itself suitable to live in a particular environment. Human beings are the most indifferent, all organisms, and due to his high degree of intelligence, and other spacities, he is able to make better adaptation to the environment.

9. **Physical adaptation:** By physical adaptation is meant adjustment to the physical environment. This adaptation is not voluntary, because, physical conditions are inevitable and organism

has to make adjustment in order to survive. For example, if there is hot sun, one has to protect oneself from it. In cold season, warm clothes are needed. It is rightly stated that "whatever the conditions are, whether wilderness or city, poverty or prosperity, whether in the eyes of men they are favorable or unfavorable, good or evil, this unconditional physical adaptation remains with all its compulsions".

10. **Biological adaptation:** Every organism is adapted to live in a particular environment. If they are taken out of the environment, life or even survival may be difficult. For example, a fresh water fish cannot survive in sea-water. Human beings are capable of making adaptation in this area also. For example, a person adapted to hot climate will try to make adjustments even in cold climate by making adaptations.

INTRODUCTION

Man everywhere lives in social groups and in society. Society has become an essential condition for human life to arise and to continue. The sociality of man is virtually the central problems of sociology. The essential fact is that man always belongs to a society or a group of one kind or the other, and without it, he cannot exist. Man is not only social but also cultural. It is the culture that provides opportunities for man to develop the personality. Development of personality is not an automatic process. Every society prescribes its own way and means of giving social training to its newborn members so that they may develop their personality. This social training is called socialization.

Human society is made of individuals. Every human being has a personality of his own, and he exhibits considerably variation from anybody around him. We are not ruled by instincts alone, but have learnt to modify our instincts according to our needs and the needs of the society in which we live. This is highly complex process, the mechanism of which is not clearly known till now. Even with individuality, man is essentially social and without society he has on existence. For his emotional, intellectual and even physical development, society is an absolute necessity. Man's social nature is not a new development. Probably, we are born with it, and it existed with us all throughout.

Aristotle recognized this fact when he proclaimed man is a social animal. This social necessity of man may be proved by various means. Two little girls, aged two and eight, were rescued from the cave of a wolf. Amana, the little girl, died within a few months, but kamala, the elder girl, survived for several years. Kamala had no human behavior. She used to move, eat and make sounds just like the wolf. In the nine years she survived, she gradually picked-up human habits, and started speaking a few words. In another case, a six months old illegitimate American child, Anna, was kept locked up in a room from the age of six months to five years. She was given only milk during this period, and she was kept away from all human contact. When brought out, Anna could not walk or talk. She avoided people. She lived for four more years. Social skill like wearing cloths, talking and eating she learnt gradually. There are several more examples of this type. But these cases show very clear that human nature is not inherent, but it develops only in association with other human beings.

Man becomes human only when he lives in the society. Summer and Keller have held that we do not believe that man was outfitted with any innate quality of sociability implanted in his gremplasa, but that the tendency to associate is acquired rather than inherited and that man's association with his kind is a product of social, rather than of organic evolution.

THEORIES OF MAN AND SOCIETY

Organism Theory

1. Nicholson, Spangler, Spencer and others are the major proponent of this theory.
2. Just like a body is made of individual units (cells), the society is made up of units (human beings).
3. Further, the society also goes through the same cycle of individual life that is, birth, growth, maturity, decline and death.
4. Both have system of control. In an individual, it is the nervous system which controls the activities of the entire body, and in the society, it is the government and other agencies of control.
5. Just as the individual body has a circulatory system, the society too has a system of transportation and communication.

Limitations of Organismic Theory

Sl.No	Body system	Society
1.	The brain is a concrete organ in the human being which is capable of thinking, acting, and controlling	But in a society, the mechanism is something very different and these two cannot be compared.
2.	In the case of an organism or individual, birth and death are two distinct incidents	But this is not so in the case of society.
3.	The cell unites to form organs	In society, this does not happen. Individual remain as separate units and they may be dispersed over different places.
4.	The organisms have a definite life cycle	But society has no such definite cycle. It is an ever-charging entity.

Group Mind Theory

1. This related to the organismic theory. Plato in his republic and Hegel in his political philosophy have mentioned about this. Others like TH Green, FH Burdle, Emerson, Wundt and Durkheium have supported this view.
2. William Mc Dougall in his book of group mind has elaborated this theory. According to him, every group has elaborated this theory. According to him, every group has a mind of its own, and in this mind is its culture, tradition and values.
3. The life of the individual in group is facilities and directed by this. The group of mind is not a collection of the minds of the individuals of the group. It has an existence of its own, and has the power of influencing the minds of the individuals.
4. It is because of this that the individual thinks and acts differently when he is part of the group. The behavior of man in crowd proves the influence of group mind.
5. Sociologists like McIver do not subscribe to this theory. He do not agree with the view that the society has a brain of its own and it is common for all its members. Thus, to him, group mind is a myth.

Social Contact Theory

1. According to Locke, Hobbes, and Rousseau, society is an entity created by man voluntarily in order to achieve his ends. To Hobbes, the primitive man was solitary, brutish, selfish and nasty and because of this evil nature, he had to live in constant fear of his neighbors.
2. To be free from fear, he made compromise with others, and made society. To Locke, the primitive man lived in a state of ideal freedom. He was absolutely happy and lived in complete harmony with his neighbors.
3. To preserve this freedom and happiness, he made contract with his neighbors and formed society.
4. To Rousseau, the primitive man was a noble savage, peaceful and unsophisticated. But when the number of people increased, quarrels and conflicts arose.
5. This necessitated the formation of contract by which he had linked himself with others, but preserved individuals freedom.
6. Through this contract, a general will evolve with represented the will of everyone and was sovereign in nature. If conflicts arise between individual will and common will, the individual will was subjected to the common will.
7. The main criticism against this theory is that theory considers society as an artificially created system. This is not the case at all. The social system grows spontaneously and cannot be artificially created.

RELATION BETWEEN SOCIETY AND INDIVIDUAL

The conception of social mind is doubtful. The social contract and organic theories contradict each other. According to the first theory there is no synthesis between society and individual and according to the second there is no different between the two. All the theories bear witness to the intimate relation between society and the individual but apart from this each is one-sided. In this word of MaIver and Page, No one can really be an absolute individualist any more than anyone can be an absolute socialist. For the individual and society interact on one another and depend on one another.

BRIEF REVIEW OF GROWTH AND DEVLOPMENT

Environment has influences from birth of the child to death either positively or negatively and person cannot stay away from the environment.

Effects of Environment on Childhood

As soon as the baby comes out from the womb of the mother he has to adjust to the environment for the existence and survival. The main tasks are breathing, sucking milk and the excretory activities. If the environment is favorable he develops and positive attitude towards all and vice versa. If the result is positive child starts to laugh, cry, smile and recognize others and slowly he will be able to understand other peoples. Through expression and language he communicates positively and thus be becomes an important part of environment. As the body grows he has to achieve new tasks such as eating different types of food, toilet training, adjustment, etc. in this entire activities environment plays a major role. He spend majority of his life in school and home so they also have a great influence on him. According to the environment he learns good or bad habits. The child's environment is the basis of socialization. The childs environment determines his personality.

Piaget, a social psychologist has explained the growth of child in six stages.

Sl.No	Stages	Description
1.	Stage-I	Develops reflexes such as sucking.
2.	Stage-II	Develops motor habits and perception.
3.	Stage-III	At the stage of six months, the infant grasps what he grasp, what he observes, uses its sensory perceptions such as seeing, hearing, touching and smelling.
4.	Stage-IV	9th to 10th month, he learns to search for objects that it has seen.
5.	Stage-V	11th to 14th month, takes account of changes of position.
6.	Stage-VI	15th to 16th month, the child has the ability to internalize objects and develops what is called primary identification.

Effects of Environment on Adolescence

Adolescence is commonly viewed as a period of preparation for adulthood. During this time they reach physical maturity, develops more sophisticated understanding of roles and relationships, acquired refine skills needed for successful performance of adult work and family roles. The developmental tasks during this period is coping with physical changes and emerging sexuality, developing interpersonal skills for opposite sex relationships, acquiring a set of values for successful functioning in adulthood. Adolescence are given increased freedom to choose to varying degrees, employment and family life, friends, etc. This age is also regarded as highly sensitive and delicate, this age is also called as age of tensions, emotions, problems and relations.

Persons are highly influenced by the people out their own family such as teachers, friends and peer groups. He also influenced by the environment in which he is living, if it is positive it lead to creative ideas and if negative it may lead to constructive alternatives. They may be selected person as their role model. Thus, environment has a great role in the development of the person in the adolescent stage and help to shape his personality.

Effects of Environment on Adult Age

The adulthood is characterized by both change and stability in many basic physical, psychological and social processes. Adults are molded more easily then children because of three reasons.

1. Adults are motivated to work towards a goal.
2. The new role to be internalized has similarities.
3. He can communicate easily through speech.

In adult change takes place in the individual body, mental capacities, views about life, emotionality's, work, political attitude and feeling about the self or sometimes changes may be due to life events such as marriage, birth of child, new job, illness, divorce, etc. They have to adjust themselves to the new environment if not they develops depression, disorganization and tension, etc.

Effects of Environment on Old Age

Due to decrease in the birth rate and life expectancy going up majority of the population belongs to the old age. This age is considered as the last segment of life but at this time also environment has its influences on the people, it may be due to divorce, behavior of children, death of spouse, retirement, loneliness or physical disabilities, etc. causes mental tension. There will be anxiety about the future and failure of the past becomes important part of social environment of the old person.

RIGHTS AND RESPONSIBILITIES OF INDIVIDUAL

Right takes place in determining the way in which one's country is governed and it in respect of the possession of these by into citizens that a form of state is called democratic. The definition of rights of the individual is power or securities of a kind such that the individual can rightly demand of others that they should normally not interfere with them. The society is a collection of status and roles of its members. The members of the society have certain rights and duties. The definition of rights of the individual which we should suggest is powers or securities of a kind such that the individual can rightly demand of others that they should normally not interfere with them.

Types of view concerning to rights:

Sl.No	Concept	Description
1.	Natural law	The view that according to constitution of their nature or the will of god all individuals have certain definite rights which it is always wrong to violate.
2.	State contract	The view that the state is based on a kind of contract and that therefore, the individual retains those rights, and those only, which he could not be conceived as contracting away.
3.	State law	The view that the individual has no rights except those which the state gives him, rights being created by the recognition of the state.
4.	Utilitarian view	The utilitarian view that what rights an individual possesses depend solely on the general good.

The republic of India is a federal, parliamentary democracy. The natural Government of India is officially headed by an indirectly elected president, but the president must follow instructions of the council of ministers. The Prime Minster heads the council of ministers, which is chosen or approved by the house of the people (Lok Sabha) the lower house of Parliament. The upper house (Rajya Sabha) the council of states is mostly composed of represents, elected by state legislatures with a dozen prominent people appointed by the president, it has few powers. The Lok Shaba is elected from single member's districts in which the candidate with the plurality of votes wins. Each State Government has Governor, Chief Minister, and State Legislative Assembly.

Fundamental rights are provided to all individuals to develop their personalities and attain their goals in life. In the world all the constitutions provide protection of fundamental rights. The World Human Rights Commission has made citizen concerns about human rights. In part (3) article 12 to 36 of Indian constitution seven fundamental rights are mentioned.

Fundamental Rights

The fundamental rights are:
1. Right to equality.
2. Right to liberty.
3. Right against exploitation.
4. Right of freedom of religion.
5. Right to property.
6. Cultural and educational right.
7. Right to constitutional remedies.

Concept	Description
Right to equality	It is the important basis of democracy. It provides equal rights to all the citizens of India. It includes: 1. Discrimination on the basis of religion, castes, sex, etc. is abolished. 2. It is promised that every individual is equal before law and in services controlled by the State at all will be given equal opportunity without any discrimination.
Right to liberty	It can be classified into: 1. Freedom of expression. 2. Freedom to assemble together peacefully (without arms, weapons, etc.). 3. Liberty to form groups and organizations. 4. Liberty to travel and stay anywhere in India. 5. Liberty to follow any occupation or professional and to earn livelihood, to start and trade or industry. 6. Protection of life and body. For the interest of the society and safety of the nation some restrictions are also applied. It does not given complete liberty.
Right against exploitation	Employing a child below 14 years is punishable offence. This is defined as traffic in human being.
Right of freedom of religion	The constitution protects religious freedom but reserves the government the right to regulate economic, financial and political activities connected with religion and to constitute certain reforms. It provides freedom to accept and propagate any religion.
Cultural and educational rights	In this every individual has the right to perpetuate his language, script or culture. Minorities are given right to start educational institutions on the basis of their religion or language. The state cannot discriminate against such institutions.
Right to constitutional remedies	If the state is denying any fundamental rights to any individual he may request judiciary to protect his right.

Rights of Individuals

Generally, the rights are two types 1. Civil right and 2. Political right. Civil right enables an individual to lead a normal life. The important civil and political rights are:

Civil Rights

1. Right to life.
2. Right to liberty.
3. Right to work.
4. Right to education.
5. Right to property.
6. Right to speak and press.
7. Right to association.
8. Right to equality.
9. Right to free movement.
10. Right to family.

Political Rights

1. Right to vote.
2. Right to contest for election.
3. Right to public office.
4. Right to petition.
5. Right to criticize government.

Fundamental Duties and Responsibilities of Individual

An individual as a citizen of a country must think positively and act positively. When he enjoys certain rights, he must know the he has certain obligations or duties to be performed for the good of society and for good of nation. In the 42nd amendment the fundamental duties/responsibilities of individual were added. After fourth chapter of constitution a new chapter 4 (a) was added. In Indian constitution only rights the individual were recognized. Realizing the importance of duties or responsibilities of the individual. The rights and duties are closely related. Infect they are two sides of the same coin. Some rights of the individuals become the duties of others. Some duties of individuals become the rights of others. The fundamental rights of the citizens are:

1. Follow the constitution; respect its ideals, institutions, national flag, and national anthem.
2. Remember the high ideal which motivates the freedom struggle and follower.
3. Protect the sovereign, unity and integrity of India.
4. Protect the nation and serve it, when called upon.
5. Establish equality and fraternity among all citizens rise above all discriminations on the basis of religion, language, area, or color. Leave all customs which are against honoring women.
6. Understand the proud traditions of our culture and protect it.
7. Protect the natural environment compressing of forest, lake, river and wild animals—be kind to animals and all living being.
8. Along with scientific attitude, humanism and attainment of knowledge, add the sentiment of reformation.
9. Protect public property and avoid violence.
10. Try to go towards progress, in all personal and social activities, so that the nation will go forward and may attain great heights.

Responsibility of Health

World today is accepting health as a fundamental right, but we cannot neglect individual duty in this respect. Under this good habits, nourishment, recreation, exercise, care of skin, eyes and ears, immunization and such personal responsibilities may be included.

PROCESS OF SOCIALIZATION

The social order is maintained largely by socialization. If they violate the rules of the social group socialization is not possible. It is said that process of socialization starts long before the child is born. The social circumstances preceding his birth lay down to a great extent the kind of life he is lead. Socialization is a process of learning to perform skills and to perform social roles. The term socialization refers to all the processes by which, how an infant acquires skills roles, norms, values and personality patterns.

Definitions

1. Socialization is a process of adaptation by the individual of the conventional patterns of behavior is described as his socialization, because it occurs on account of his integration with others and his exposure to the culture which operates through them—*VV Akolar.*
2. The development of 'we' feeling in association and the growth in their capacity and will to act together is called socialization of the individual—*EA Ross.*
3. Socialization is the process whereby persons learn to behave dependably together on behalf of human welfare and in so doing experience social self-control, social responsibility and balanced personality—*Bogardus.*
4. Socialization is the process by which the individual learns to conform to the norms of the group—*WF Ogburn.*
5. Socialization as a process of transmission of culture, the process whereby men learn the rules and practices of social groups—*Petter Worsley.*
6. Socialization as learning that enables the learner to perform social roles. He further says that it is a process by which individual acquire the already existing culture of groups they come into—*Harry M Johnson.*
7. Socialization consists of the complex processes of interaction through which the individual learns the habits, beliefs, skills and standards of judgment that are necessary for his effective participation in social groups and communities—*Lundberg.*

Kingsley Davis defines socialization as the subtle alchemy by which a human organism is transmuted into a social being. The process of training the child to develop its capacities is a difficult task. In all societies, primitive or modern we find difficult ways of training younger generations. The study of such a process of development of individuals from its childhood to adult is called socialization. Thus, a person becomes social person through the process of socialization. It is the learning process by means of which the individuals acquired the existing culture of groups.

Socialization is the process whereby an individual learns to behave in accordance with social traditions and mores. The human child possesses a tendency towards imitation. The child develops according to the environment in which he lives. The individual tries to win the praise of the group in which he lives. Man is a social being. He of his own nature tries to adopt the culture of society. Man becomes what he is by socialization and it is by virtue of this that he is believed to be superior to animals. Socialization brings balance to his personality because the social aspects of personality are also very important. Through socialization the individual learns to control himself in the interest of society and realizes his responsibility towards others. Socialization develops in him the community feeling and he learns to cooperate with others.

Individuals influence each other by means of imitation, suggestions and sympathy. In addition to these, social institutions and associations also carry out the individual's socialization. The individual is influenced by many processes in society, praise and blame, cooperation and conflict, submission and ascendancy. These help to form his personality and individuality.

Agencies of Socialization

Sl.No	Concept	Description
1.	Family	The family plays perhaps the most dominant role in the individual's socialization. The child finds much to learn in the behavior of the family members, parents, relatives, and friends. He imitates them in their mannerisms, behavior, clichés, etc. He tries to avoid such activities which result in punishment or which are considered bad in the family.
2.	School	The child in the school is, in addition to the effect of education, vulnerable to the influence exerted by the personalities of his teachers and friends. In much the same way, young men and women learns to conduct themselves and to give expression to their views, such as a person being an outcome of education and constant association with teachers, the unique environment, fellow collegiate, etc.
3.	Occupation and marriage	Following college education, the individual's occupations and marriages are strongly influenced by the personality of their life partner, and their future depends upon this to a large extent.

Need for Socialization

Socialization is not an exclusive but a prominent source of the individual's development, because hereditary also has its importance. The development of the individual, with the spread of culture through socialization is impossible. The self of the individual develops only due to socialization. Every social relationship of the individual contributes to his process of socialization. The problem of man's socialization is very complex and it has not yet been completely solved in any human society.

Factors influence socialization:

Sl.No	Concept	Description
1.	Imitation	It is copies by an individual of the actions of another. Mead defines, it as self conscious assumption of another's acts or roles. Thus, when the child attempts to walk he try to walk as his father does he may be conscious or unconscious. In imitation the person imitating performs exactly the same activity as the one being performed before him.
2.	Suggestion	According to Mc Dougall, suggestion is the process of communication resulting in the acceptance with conviction of the communicated proposition in the absence of logically adequate grounds for its acceptance. It the process of communicating information which has no logical or self evident basis. Suggestion influences individual behavior. Propaganda and advertising are based on the fundamental psychological principles of suggestion.
3.	Identification	Child cannot make differentiation between his organism and environment. Most of the actions are random, as the age increases he comes to know the nature of things which satisfy his needs.
4.	Language	Language is the medium of social intercourse and cultural transmission. At first child uses random syllables which have no meaning but gradually learns his mother tongue. The language moulds the personality of the individual from infancy.

In brief, socialization is a process which begins at birth and continues unceasingly until the death of the individual. In the words of Davis, the improvement of socialization offers one of the greatest possibilities for the future alteration of human society.

INDIVIDUALIZATION

Individualization is process which tends to make the individual more or less independent to his group and to create in him a self conscious of his own. According MacIver individualization is the process in which men became more autonomous or self determining in which they advance beyond inner imitations or acceptance of standards which come to them only an outer sanction in which they become less bound by tradition and custom in the regulation of their views, less submissive to authority and dictation in matters of thought and opinion recognizing that each is a unique focus of being and can achieve the ends of his life only as these grow clear in his own consciousness and become the objectives of his own will. Individualization help the man to known him self and know his inner responsibility.

Socialization bring man into relation with others, individualization make him autonomous or self determining. Not only the individual himself but society as well as helps him in acquiring the inner sense of responsibility and knowing himself. Ideas are merely the mental expressions of the process of individualization. The development of the self is the most important results of the process of socialization. The child gradually distinguishes the familiar person from the unfamiliar person. Then it develops the perception of the self. The child constantly use the pronouns I and Me. Thus, the child learns to look upon himself as an object to himself. He begins to think of himself, his body, his behavior and appearance to other persons.

The child not only learns that others are important to him to satisfy his needs, but also learns that he is important to others. At this stage he develops acquisitive nature. He also develops conscience and develops internal restraints. Consequently, the child avoids doing mistake. He incorporates standards into his self structure and corrects his faults. Thus, as an individual he develops awareness about his own character. He thinks that he is distinct from others. He evaluates himself as superior to others. This is what we call self glorification.

Individualization is a kind of introspection and inwardness about the self. This is king of feeling about one's own personality. The individualization is shaped in different individuals based on the environmental conditions, family background, influence of community and his own wishes. So socialization is the process of developing one's own self. It makes him to take decisions by himself and began to act independently. In other words it is called self determination.

ENVIRONMENT AND HEALTH

The environment has been described as a global life support system. Human requires a viable environment that incorporates the local ecosystem, including the air, water and soil and the availability of safe and adequate food. In addition, a viable environment requires sustainable development, which has been defined as development that meets the needs of the present without compromising the ability of future generations to meet their own need.

Definition

The World Health Organization (WHO) has defined environmental health as, those aspects of human health and diseases are determinate by factors in the environment. It includes both direct pathological effects of chemicals, radiations, and some biological agents, and the effects on health and well-being of the broad physical, psychological, social, and esthetic environment, which includes housing, urban development, land use, and transportation.

Environmental Health

According to WHO data, approximately 25 to 33% of the global burden of disease is due to environmental exposure, and environmental preventable illnesses in the world. In recent years, greater attention has been given to the health risks posed by environmental conditions. This attention is evident in the number of national health objectives that focus on environmental health issues. Many environmental forces influence human health. Microorganisms such as bacteria, viruses and fungi cause communicable diseases and animals contribute to the spread of these diseases. Plants may contribute to accidental poisoning or to allergic reactions. Industry, vehicles and buildings add to air water pollution and excess noise.

Climate and terrain contribute to natural disaster; it may promote air and water pollution, which have long-term health effects. The environmental has been described as a global life-support system. Human health requires a viable environment that incorporates the local ecosystem, including the air, water, and soil, and the availability of safe and adequate food. In addition, a viable environment requires sustainable development, which has been defined as development that meets the need of the present without compromising the ability of future generations to meet their own need.

Components of the Human Environment

The environmental context that influences human health incorporates a number of components. These include the natural and constructed, or built, environment, as well as the social and psychological environments.

The Natural Environment

The natural environment consists of those features of the environment that exist in a natural state, unmodified in any significant way by human being. Elements of the natural environment include weather and climate, terrin (e.g. mountains, rivers, and oceans), natural flora and fauna (plants and animals), biological agents, natural resources (air, wood, water, and fuel). **Climate** has multiple effects on human health. For example, from 1979 to 1999, more than 8,000 deaths occurred in the United States as a result of exposure of heat. Consequently, from 1979 to 2002, hypothermia, primarily due to cold weather, accounted for an average of 689 deaths per year, mostly among elderly persons. In addition, poor weather conditions contribute to 28% of motor vehicle accidents.

Although there have always been deaths due to hypo- and hyperthermia and motor vehicle accidents caused by weather conditions, the potential for illness and injury due to temperature extremes and adverse whither conditions has increased recently as a result of global climate changes. Global climate change results from several inter-related mechanisms. These include ocean oscillations, greenhouse gases, and stratospheric ozone depletion that result in global warming. Polar meltdown, rising sea levels, and increased tectonic and volcanic activities.

Greenhouse effect

Greenhouse gases are collection of gases released naturally and as a by-product of human industrial processes that accumulate in the troposphere (the portion of the earth's atmosphere that reaches from the earth's surface to the tropopause, where the stratosphere begins). Greenhouse gases absorbs infrared radiation from the earth and trap solar heat, leading to increased tropospheric temperatures. Carbon dioxide (CO_2) is the primary greenhouse gas contributing to this phenomenon, and atmospheric CO_2 levels are expected to have increased by 66% between 1850 and 2050. Approximately, three-fourths of the CO_2 buildup results from the burning of fossil fuels.

The loss of ozone layers in the stratosphere also contributes to global warming. Stratospheric ozone forms a protective layer around the earth's atmosphere that prevents a significant portion of ultraviolet light from reaching the earth's surface. Although the production of chlorofluorocarbons (CFCs) responsible for the depletion of the ozone layer has been halted by international agreement, it is anticipated that it will take approximately 50 years for any noticeable benefit to occur. In the meantime, global temperatures continue to rise and exposure to increasing levels of ultraviolet radiation result in increased prevalence of skin cancers, particularly malignant melanomas, and cataracts.

The Build Environment

The built environment includes all buildings, spaces, and products that are created or modified by people. Elements of the built environment include homes, schools, workplaces, roads, and features such as urban sprawl and air pollution. The built environment has both direct and indirect effects on health. Direct effects derive from exposure to hazardous conditions arising of health: Room the built environment. Indirect effects are the results of the effects of the built environment on the natural environment (e.g. contamination of air and water) or on human health related behavior. Examples of direct health effects include lead poisoning arising from ingestion or inhalation of lead from older structures painted with lead-based paints or respiratory disease due to air pollution.

Environmental pollution and ill-effects of health
It is known fact that people's health depends upon quality of environment in which they live. But unfortunately the environment is deteriorating due to human deeds such as modernization, urbanization, population explosion, deforestation, etc. The health and safety environment is therefore not only the concern of environmentalists but also the health personnel. The environmental science is an age old science and its impact on health has been documented during ancient period in India. In Great Britain it was observed by Edwin Chadwick in 1842 and he gave a detailed report about the sanitary conditions. Similar conditions were observed and reported in America around the same time and also in other countries. Since than lot of measures were taken by the government of various countries to improve environment sanitation.

EFFECTS OF ENVIRONMENTAL HEALTH ON MAN

Environment is the sum of all natural and man-made living and nonliving, visible and tangible things that surround a given host at a given time. The relation of life and environment is extremely intimate. According to physical scientist the word environment means the nature and according to sociologist it means physical conditions. The concept of environment is broad. All human behaviors take place in an environment and everything around us is environment in sociology, the environment is fully studied and there are different aspects of the total environment according to the sociologist.

Definitions

1. Environment as any external force which influences us—*EJ Ross*.
2. Environment is anything immediately surrounding an object and exerting direct influence on it—*P Gisbert*.
3. The total environment includes physical and social aspects—*MacIver and Page*.

Classifications of Environment

Sl. No	Concept	Description
1.	Natural environment	In the natural environment are included all natural conditions, forces and objects which influence life, but not influenced by man.
2.	Social environment	In the social environment is included social organizations, institutions and relationships in the midst of which man lives from birth to death.
3.	Cultural environment	In the cultural environment are included customs, traditions, folkways, mores and values.
4.	Physical environment	The term physical environment is applied to nonliving things or physical factors which directly or indirectly regulate body mechanism and affect health.
5.	Biological environment	The biological environment is the universe of living things which surrounds man including man himself. The living things are the virus and other microbial agents. Insects, rodents, animals and plants.
6.	Psychological environment	The psychological environment includes a complex of psychological factors which are defined as those factors affecting personal health.
7.	Psychsocial environment	Psychosocial factors can also affect negatively man's health and well-being. For example, poverty, urbanization, migration, and exposure to stressful situations such as bereavement desertion, loss of employment, and birth of a handicapped child may produce anxiety, depression, anger and frustration.
8.	Microenvironment	Microenvironment refers to immediate environment or personal environment and usually include home environment, occupational environment and sociocultural environment.
9.	Macroenvironment	Macroenvironment refers to external environment which is outside the home environment.

Factors Affecting Environmental Health

Sl.No	Concept	Description
1.	Population explosion	The rapid increase in our population is having harmful and unfavorable effect on our environment. It is creating problems due to over crowding, depletion of natural resources and development of man made resources by industrialization and green revolution, etc.
2.	Industrialization	The industries have multiplied not only in magnitude but also in variety. All the industries generate loss of waste product such as gases, effluents, solid matters, thermal waste, etc. which causes harmful effects on human health.
3.	Urbanization	People from village migrate to towns and cities for employment, education, etc. resulting in over crowding and slums most of the time on unauthorized lands.
4.	Modern agricultural practices	Chemical fertilizer are used to increase agricultural production for meeting agricultural demands of ever increasing population, in addition insecticides are added and sprayed to destroy pests and microorganisms it also causes harmful effects of living organisms.

Contd...

Contd...

Sl. No	Concept	Description
5.	Deforestation	Deforestation refers to reducing/removing of forest. Deforestation also reduces the amount of water being transferred from the ground to the air because of reduced trees. This phenomenon is causing change in the climate. All these situations have adverse effect on the environmental health.
6.	Radioactive substances	The radioactive substances are used in the laboratories, hospitals and power plants, where nuclear bombs are manufactured.
7.	Natural calamities	Natural calamities are grave disasters of misfortune of great magnitude which occurs by nature cause, disruption of the environment. These calamities include floods, earth quakes, droughts, cyclones, volcanoes, landslides, avalanches and tidal waves in the seas.

Environment and Adaptation

Human being are the most intelligent of all organisms, and due to his high degree of intelligence and other capacities, he is able to make better adaptation to the environment. Fairchild has defined adaptations as a process of acquiring fitness to live in a given environment.

Levels of Adaptations

Sl.No	Concept	Description
1.	Physical adaptation	Physical adaptation is meant adjustment to the physical environment. This adaptation is not voluntary, because, physical conditions are inevitable and organism has to make adjustment in order to survive. For example, if there is hot sun, one has to protect oneself from it. In cold season, warm cloths are needed.
2.	Biological adaptation	Every organism is adopted to live in a particular environment. If they are taken out of the environment, life or even survival may be difficult. For example, a fresh water fish cannot survive in sea-water. A person adapted to hot climate will try to make adjustments even in cold climate by making adaptations.
3.	Social adaptation	Social adaptation is the process of adjusting to sociocultural environment. This adjustment is peculiar to human society because culture and organized society are limited to human being. Social adjustments are not inherited, but learned.

PROTECTING HEALTH FROM CLIMATE CHANGE

Introduction

World Health Day, on 7th April, 2008, makes the founding of the World Health Organization and is an opportunity to draw worldwide attention to a subject of major importance to global health each year. In 2008, World Health Day focuses on the need to protect health from adverse effects on climate change. The theme "Protecting health from climate change" puts health at the center of the global dialogue about climate change. WHO selected this theme in recognition that climate change is posing ever growing threats to global public health security? Through increased

collaboration, the global community will be better prepared to cope with climate-related health changes world wide.
1. Collaborative action in strengthening surveillance.
2. Control of infectious diseases.
3. Ensuring safer use of diminishing water supplies.
4. Coordinating health action in emergencies.

Meteorological Environment

Meteorological environment includes temperature, humidity, wind and rainfall. These factors keep on changing between different places at the same time or at the same place at different times. The behavior of meteorological factors at a particular time of a place denotes the weather of the place.

Climate has a profound influence on all aspects of life patterns of populations. Climate shapes the physical, biological and social environment of places. Climate affects the health and nutritional status of populations and also the spectrum of diseases to which they are exposed.

Types of Climate

1. **Tropical type of climate:** In the tropical region, the sun is always shining vertically overhead and the temperature is uniformly high all round the year.
2. **Desert type of climate:** Desert climate is very dry, the temperature is very high during the day and the evaporation is excessive. The afternoons are characterized by dust storms, but nights are cold and become very chilly during winter season.
3. **Mediterranean type:** This climate is usually characterized by short, wet and mild winters, and long warm and dry summers. Mediterranean region area situated near deserts has hot summers and areas near sea coasts have cool summers.
4. **European type of climates:** Proximity to the ocean keeps the summers cold and the warm currents that wash the shores make the winter's warm and mild rainfalls through the year.
5. **Monsoon type of climates:** Monsoon lands have typically winter, summer and rainy seasons. The winter is relatively cold and dry; the summer is hot and dry.

Elements of Climate

The meteorological factors like temperature, humidity, wind and rainfall keep on changing between different places at the same time or at the same place at different times.

1. **Atmospheric pressure:** The atmospheric pressure at the surface of earth, close to sea level, averages 760 mm Hg per square inch of earth's surface. The greater the humidity of a place in a particular day, the lower the weight of the air column as indicated by the reading of the atmospheric pressure. A depression in atmospheric pressure is obviously an indicator of ensuring rainfall.
2. **Air temperature:** Several geographical factors such as altitude, latitude, direction of wind and proximity to sea influence the air temperature of a place. Air temperature does not remain the same even at the same places; it undergoes seasonal as well as diurnal variations in response to various metrological factors.
3. **Air humidity:** Moisture content in the air is expressed in terms of absolute or relative humidity. Absolute humidity is the weight of water vapor per unit volume of air and relative humidity is the percentage of moisture present in the air, complete saturation being taken as 100% humidity.

4. **Air movement:** Air movement is initiated by disturbance in the atmospheric equilibrium. Constant changes occurring in the temperature and humidity of air produce variations in the density of air columns.
5. **Climate influences:** The indoor and outdoor life activities and determines food, shelter and clothing of people. Climate affects the health and nutritional status of populations and also the spectrum of diseases to which they are exposed.

Environmental Health and Nurses Role

Community health nurses are most likely to become aware of environmental health problems. Protection of the environment is one of the essential functions of public health, and the participation of community health nursing activity related to environmental health nurses in this function is critical. Community health nursing activity related to environmental health issues occurs at both the level of the individual / family clients and the population. Community health nurses can make use of the dimensions models of community health nursing to address environmental problems. Use of the model focuses on assessment, intervention, planning and evaluation of environmental interventions. World Health Day, 2008 (on April 7) will be devoted to the theme of protecting health from the impact of climate change. Major activities are being planned around the world, in a concerted effort by the World Health Organization and its partners to bring home the fact that global warming is more than just an environmental issue, and that it will affect the health and well-being.

PROMOTING MAN'S HEALTH FORM HEAT WAVES

Climate Change

Climate change is a significant and fastest emerging threat to public health. There is growing evidence that global climate changes will affect the health and well-being of human beings. Intergovernmental panel on climate change in global climate. Climate variability and change has and will cause further death and disease through natural disasters, such as heat waves, floods and droughts. In addition to these disasters, many diseases are highly sensitive to changing temperatures and precipitations. These include common vector borne diseases like malaria and dengue. It also adds up to the global burden of disease.

As per WHO media release, health and well-being of populations must become the defining measures of the impact of climate change and our efforts to address it effectively. Climate change is gradually becoming a central part of planning future projects and top on the international agenda and it is becoming clearer that sustainable development leads to healthy environments and enhanced public health. There is an immediate need is to strengthen surveillance and control of infectious diseases, safer use of diminishing water supplies, and take action on health emergencies. But more focus as always should be on prevention as the old saying goes "prevention is better than cure".

Environmental Health

Socioeconomic developments of countries in the western pacific region are affected by globalization of trade and industry development, information and communication, and associated population movement. Rapid urbanization and rural to urban migration is also taking place in developing countries of this region. Such socioeconomic developments and continuing urbanization have recently introduced more modern environmental risks such as urban, industrial and agrochemical pollution and technological emergencies to developing countries of the region. However, these developing countries still suffer from traditional environment risks, such as inadequate water supply and sanitation, and indoor smoke from domestic cooking and heating, using solid fuels. Resolving the double burden of environment risks to health is a major challenge in these developing countries.

Climate Change and Public Health

There is widespread scientific consensus that the world's climate is changing. Some of the effects of climate change are likely to include more variable weather, heat waves, heavy precipitation events, flooding, droughts, more intense storms such as hurricanes, sea level rise, and air pollution. Each of these changes has the potential to negatively affect health. While climate change is recognized as global issues, the effects of climate changes will vary across geographic regions and populations.

Although scientific understanding of the effects of climate change is still emerging. There is a pressing need to prepare for potential health risks. This public health preparedness approach is applied to other threats in the absence to complete data, such as terrorism and pandemic influenza. A wide variety of organizations (federal, state, local, multilateral, private and nongovernmental) is working to address the implications of global climate change. Despite this breadth of activity, the public health effects of climate change remain largely unaddressed.

Sl. No	Weather event	Health effects	Populations most affected
1.	Health waves	Heat stress	Extremes of age, athletes, people with respiratory diseases.
2.	Extreme weather events (rain, hurricane, tomado, flooding)	Injuries, drowning	Coastal, low-lying and dwellers.
3.	Droughts, floods, increased mean temperature	Vector, food- and water-borne diseases	Multiple populations at risk.

How Climate Change will Affect Our Health

Climate change will affect our health in profoundly adverse ways, some of the most fundamental pillars of health: Food, air and water. The warming of the planet will be gradual, but the frequency and severity of extreme weather events, such as intense storms, heat waves, droughts and floods could be abrupt and consequences will be dramatically felt. The most severe threats are to developing countries, with direct negative implications for the achievements of the health-related millennium developmental goals, and for health equity.

The health risks posed by climate change are global, and difficult to reverse. Recent changes in climate in the South-East Asia (SEA) region have had diverse impacts on health. According to IPCC eighteen heat waves were reported in India between 1980 and 1998. A heat wave in 1998 caused 1300 deaths, while another one in 2003 caused more than 3000 deaths. Heat waves in South-east Asia cause high mortality in rural populations, and among the elderly and outdoor workers. Examples are the reported cases of heatstroke in metal workers and in rickshaw pullers in Bangladesh.

In 2007, for moon son depressions double the normal number caused severe floods in Bangladesh, India, and Nepal, but also in the democratic people's republic of Korea causing death, loss of livehood and displacement of millions. In November 2008, tropical cyclone made landfall in Bangladesh, generating winds of up to 240 km/h and torrential rains. More than 8.5 million people were affected and over 3300 died. Nearly, 4.7 million people saw their houses damaged or destroyed, most of them belonging to the poorest of the poor.

Many risk factors and illness that are currently among the most important contributors to the global burden of diseases are sensitive to climate, notably to temperature changes. These include malnutrition (estimated to kill 3.7 million people per year, globally), diarrhea (1.9 million) and malaria (0.9 million). Warmer temperatures will have adverse effects on food production, water availability and the spread of disease vectors.

The main outcomes threatened by climate change:
1. Meeting increasing energy demands by greater use of fossil fuels will add number of respiratory disorders, such as asthma.
2. Human-induced climate change significantly amplifies the likelihood of heat waves increasing the possibility of heat strokes, cardiovascular and respiratory disorders.
3. More variable precipitation patterns are likely to compromise the supply of fresh water, increasing risk of water-borne diseases like cholera and out breaks of diarrhea diseases.
4. Raising temperatures and variable precipitation are likely to decrease the production of staple foods in many of the poorest regions, increasing risks of malnutrition.
5. The increase in frequency and intensity of extreme weather events will translate into loss of life, injuries and disability.
6. Changes in climate are likely to lengthen the transmission season of important vector-borne diseases (like dengue and malaria) and to alter their geographic range, potentially reaching regions that lack either population immunity or a strong public health infrastructure.
7. Rising sea levels increase the risk of coastal flooding, and may lead to displacement of population. The most vulnerable areas in SEA are the Ganges-Brahmaputra, Delta in Bangladesh and small islands, for example, in the Maldives and in Indonesia—as well as the entire coastline of the Indian Ocean.
8. Loss of livelihood will increase psychological stress in the affected populations.

WHO is Protecting Health from Climate Change?

Since global climate change began to emerge as a major issue in the late 1980's WHO has guided and coordinated the research agenda on this threat, and contributed to major assessments, such as those of the UN Intergovernmental Panel on Climate Change (IPCC). WHO has also assembled and reported the evidence of the links between climate change and human health, quantified past and projected future impacts and identified vulnerable populations. WHO has worked with member countries around the world to raise awareness of the impacts of climate change on health and to give guidance on assessing risks and developing national and local response to specific threats, such as heat waves, floods and vector-borne diseases.

NURSES ROLE AFTER LEARNING ABOUT MAN, SOCIETY AND ENVIRONMENT

1. Study of man and society help the nurses to learn about the nature of different human behaviors in the society.
2. To understand the basic nature of society.
3. To gain knowledge about different sociological views and its influence on society and man.
4. To know about normal adjusting mechanism of human minds in the society.
5. To differentiate and gain knowledge about the normal growth and development of human in various stages from birth till death.
6. To know about the normal socialization process.

7. To identify the abnormal such as isolated behaviors of man in the society, reaction of society towards an abnormal behavior.
8. To understand the basic human rights and responsibilities and to create awareness among people in the society.
9. To guide each human in the society to become a responsible citizen.
10. To differentiate and gain knowledge about the uniqueness of each human behavior and appreciate the individuality in the society.

CONCLUSION

Individual is the unit of society. Society is the necessary environment in which individual is nurtured and developed his personality. So society belongs to individuals, individuals belong to society and both are interdependent. The sociological view is that every individual is part of society and that society is composed of interacting individuals, each having an influence on other and each being influenced others. Socialization is carried out in many different ways by different people and in different social settings. Parents, playmates, people in the neighborhood, teachers, peer groups, fellow students, co-workers, friends, leader's political party, religious leaders, spouses, all contribute to socialization.

The measurement of the impact of climate change on health can only be very approximate. A WHO qualitative assessment concluded that the effects of climate change since the mid-1970s may have caused at least 160 000 additional deaths annually by the year 2000. Globally, people at greatest risk include the very young, the elderly and the medically frail. Low income countries and areas where malnutrition is widespread, the level of education is poor and with weak infrastructures will have the most difficulty adapting to climate change and related health hazards. The populations considered to be greatest risk are those living in small islands, mountainous regions, water-stressed areas, mega cities and coastal areas, particularly the large urban and periurban agglomerations in delta regions in the SEA region, as well as poor people and those unprotected by health services.

BIBLIOGRAPHY

1. Anthony Giddens. Sociology—Polity Press, UK, 1997.
2. Barnes. An Introduction to the History of Sociology. The University of Chicago Press.
3. Cyyde Kluckhon, Henry A Murray (Eds). Personality in nature society arid culture, Alfred A Knop Mc, New York, 1953.
4. E Melford Spiro. "Culture and personality" psychiatry 14 (Feb), 1951.
5. Frank Lorimer et al. Cultural and Human Fertility, UNESCO, Paris, 1954.
6. Harry M. Johnson. Sociology—A Systematic Introduction, Allied Publishers, New Delhi, 1981.
7. Introduction to Sociology—Stewart and Glynn. Tarn McGraw Hill Co. Ltd, Delhi, 1981.
8. John J Honigrnann. Culture and personality, Harper and Brother, New York, 1954.
9. K Davis. Human Society. Surjeet Publications. New Delhi, 1981.
10. Karen Homey. The neurotic personality of our time, w.w. Norton. and Co, New York, 1937.
11. Leonard Schatzman, Anselm Strauss. "Social class and modes of communication" American Journal of Sociology, 60 (Jan), 1955.
12. Maclver and Page. Society—An Introductory Analysis, McMillan India Ltd., 1998.
13. NJ Smelser. Sociology, Prentice Hall, India Ltd., 1993.
14. Ogburn, Nimkoff. A handbook of Sociology. Eurasia Publishing House, New Delhi.

15. P Gisbert. Fundamentals of Sociology-Orient Longman.
16. RN Sharma. Principles of Sociology, Rajahasa Prakasliana, Meerut.
17. Robert Bierstedt. The Social Order, Tata McGraw-Hill, 1970.
18. Ronald Fletcher. The Making of Sociology Vol 1 and 11. Rawat Publication.
19. Samuel Koening Barnes, Noble. An Introduction to the Science of Society, 1968.
20. TB Bottomore. Sociology—A Guide to Problems and Literature, Blackie and Soms (India) Ltd.
21. Vilhelrn Aubert Heineirian. Elements of Sociology—Educational Books Ltd. London, 1969
22. Alex Inkles. What is Sociology? Prentice Hall India Ltd, 1991.
23. Young and Mack. Systematic: Sociology—East-West Press, New Delhi, 1972.

Primary Concepts in Sociology

26

DEFINITIONS

1. **Society:** Society may be defined as groups who have lived long enough to become organized and to consider themselves and to be considered as a unit more or less distinct from other human units.

2. **Community:** Community may be defined as a permanent local aggregation of people having diversified as well as common interests and served by a constellation of institutions.

3. Association is an organization deliberately formed the collective pursuit of some interest or set of interests, which the members of it share, is termed as association.

4. **Institution:** Institution is a definite organization pursuing some specific interests or pursuing general interests in a specific way.

5. **Organization:** Organization means an arrangement of persons or parts. Thus, family, church, college, factory a play group, a political party, a community, an empire, United Nations all are examples of organization.

6. **Social structure:** Social structure is concerned with the principal forms of social organizations, i.e. types of groups, associations and institutions and the complex of these which constitute societies.

7. **Social system:** Social system is an orderly and systematic arrangement of social interactions. It is a network of interactive relationships; it may be defined as plurality of individuals interacting with each other according to shared cultural norms and meanings.

8. **Community sentiment:** Physical locality by itself is not enough to create a community. A mere collection of human beings in a physical locality is not a true community. A community is essentially an area of common living with a feeling of belonging together. Inhabitants develop a sense of identification with the entire pattern of life that evolves in and around a given geographical area. The individual identifies his interest with the larger interest of the group. A sense of dependence develops in him. This sense of belonging together and the feeling of unity is called "Community Sentiment".

9. **We feeling:** We feeling refers to the feeling of oneness and the sense of participation. For example, rich and poor, Brahmin and Shudra, Kannadiga and Tamilian, Hindu and Muslim—all feel and act as members primarily of the Indian community. This feeling of oneness or we feeling is more evidently expressed when a community faces a crisis. For instance, during Pakistani war Indians despite the differences in caste, color, creed, etc. stood like a firm rock, as one body forgetting all the differences.

10. **Role feeling:** Every individual in society holds a social position. By virtue of the position held by him, he is expected to perform certain roles. Thus, the expectations of social position are called roles. The feeling present in an individual that he has a role to play is called role feeling. No matter what office a person occupies, he must have a sense of duty. Every role that the individuals play is essential and valuable for the community. Thus, he looks upon himself as a specific and inseparable part of the community.

SOCIETY

Sociology makes a scientific study of society. Society is an organization, a system or a pattern of relationships among human being. Persons have written, society may be defined as the total complex of human relationships in so far they grow out of action in terms of means-end relationships, intrinsic or symbolic. Society cannot be limited within any space or time. But a society is demarcated by geographical limits. In this way, the societies of people who live in India, Russia, China and other countries are differentiated from each other whereas the name, human society or merely society would apply to all people of all countries in the world.

Society consists, not of individuals, but in their mutual interactions and mutual inter-relations. It is a complex structure formed by these mutual relations; it is a system, a pattern. Individuals or people do not merit the name society but a society is sometimes used to denote people. Some sociologist have viewed society is a web of social relationships. These social relationships are not of one kind. Some of them are simple and some complex, some are permanent and some temporary—these includes behavior, usages, customs, modes of operations, authority, assistance and other types of relations.

Definitions

1. A society is a collection of individuals united by certain relations or modes of behavior which mark them off from other who do not enter into these relations or who differ from them in behavior—*Ginsberg*.
2. Society is a system of usage and procedures of authority and mutual aid, of many groupings and divisions, of controls of human behavior and liberties—*MacIver and Page*.
3. Society is the union itself, the organization, the sum of formal relations in which associating individuals are bound together—*Giddings*.
4. A society is the larger group of which any individual belongs—*Green*.
5. Society is any permanent or continuing group of men, women and children, able to carry on independently the process of racial perpetuation and maintenance on their own cultural level—*Harkins*.
6. A society may be defined as a group of people who have lived long enough to become organized and to consider themselves and be considered as a unit more or less distinct from other human units—*John F Cuber*.
7. Society is the complex of organized associations and institutions within the community—*GDH Cole*.
8. Society is not a group of people; it is the system of relationships that exists between the individuals of the group—*Prof Wright*.
9. Society includes not only the political relations by which men are bound together but the whole range of human relations and collective activities—*Leacock*.
10. Society may be defined as the total complex of human relationships in so far as they grow out of action in terms of mean-end relationship, internsic or symbolic—*Parson*.

Characteristics of Society

1. **Society is abstract:** Thus, while describing the nature of society; it is necessary to keep in mind the prominent difference between society and a society. In this way society is abstract because it is constituted of the social relations, customs and laws, besides other elements. In the words of Odum, in another aspect society may be visualized as the behavior of human being and the consequent problems of relationship and adjustments that arise.

2. **Society is not a group of people:** Some sociologist have viewed society as a group of people. Hankins writes, we may for our purpose here define society as any permanent or continuing group of men, women and children, able to carry on independently the process of racial perpetuation and maintenance on their own cultural level.

3. **Society is an organization of relationships:** Society is an organization, a system or a pattern of relationships among human being. Parsons has written society may be defined as the total complex of human relationships in so far as they grow out of action in terms of means-end relationships, intrinsic or symbolic.

4. **Psychic element in social relationships:** According to MacIver and Giddings and some other sociologist, social relationships invariably possess a psychic element, which takes the form of awareness of another's presence, common objectives, common interest, etc. There is neither any society nor any social relationship without this realization. Society exists only where social being behaved towards one another in a manner determined by recognition of each other.

5. **Liberty: Human society is dynamic:** In society the individual given liberty in respect of many kinds of changes. In all civilized societies of the world people have the freedom to get educated, choose a desired profession, marry and beget children, think independently and to express their thoughts in an appropriate manner.

6. **Many group and divisions:** In this way there are many groups and divisions in each society. Some of these groups are natural while other are constituted intentionally. Keeping in view some specific objectives. Both primary groups like family and neighborhood, and secondary groups like unions, labor unions, etc. are extremely important for the development of social life.

7. **Mutual assistance:** In society, even inequality is based upon mutual relationships. People possessing diverse characteristics often assume complementary roles. People of opposite sexes are able to achieve more intense and intimate relations than individuals of the same sex because each fulfills the deficiency of the other. In the same way, people who differ from one another in respect of income, status, wealth, education, etc. help and assist each other.

8. **Usage and customs:** Man is a social being. His very existence and development is impossible in the absence of society. He has to establish relations with other members of society to fulfill his own needs. These relations lead to mutual behavior. This behavior becomes progressively complex and takes on the form of usage or custom.

9. **Modes of action or procedure:** MacIver has used the word procedures for institutions. In this way procedures or institutions like marriage, inheritance, education, religious beliefs, political parties, etc. play an important part in society.

10. **Authority:** Authority is indicative of that relation who regulates or controls the related individuals or classes in such a way that one evinces a sense of respect, faith, and subordination towards the other. The cause of authority is the inevitable inequality in society. There is greater similarity than dissimilarity in society but even then inequality is found in every society in some form or other.

11. **Organization:** Every society has its own individual and unique organization in which there is division of labor of one kind or the other. People who are completely disorganized cannot be said to be consisting a society.

12. **Assistance:** Dukheim has expressly said that, due to division of work, there is greater evidence of dissimilarity. The life of society depends upon mutual assistance.
13. **Independence:** An important element in the organization of society is independence. Man cannot satisfy his needs if he leads a solitary life. So he needs society, and stay in society because it is his nature. The members of society are dependent upon each other for the fulfillment of their needs.

Difference between Society and Association

Sl. No	Society	Association
1.	Society is a system of social relationships	Association is a group of people.
2.	Society is abstract	Association is concrete.
3.	Society is almost permanent	Association is temporary.
4.	Society is natural	Association is established.
5.	There are both cooperation and conflict in society	Association is based upon cooperation alone.
6.	It is not established for society to be organized	Association must be organized.
7.	Society comprehends all conscious and unconscious relations	The basis of association consists of conscious feelings and thoughts.
8.	The objectives of society are not completely determined	The objectives of an association are predetermined.
9.	Society is inevitable	Association is a matter of violation. It is voluntary.
10.	Society is an end in itself	Association is merely a means.

Society Involves Both Likeness and Differences

1. **Likeness in society:** Social relationship is based upon a similarity of interest, objectives, mores, and needs, etc. men do not form a society in association with animals because their interests, mores, objectives, etc. are dissimilar and widely divergent. Human society can be comprised only of human being because they share many characteristics in common and many features of nature, interest, anatomy, mind, etc. the fundamental elements of human psychology vary with very small limits at all times and places. For example, men and women of all ages and all countries has experienced and exhibited a very natural attraction for each other, and even in the future one cannot imagine this attraction losing its intensity; the edifice of human society, the family, rest upon this mutual attraction. Human society is divided into many societies. These different societies have vast differences in interests, traditions, behaviors, so that individuals in one society look upon an individual from another as a stranger.
2. **Difference in society:** Differences in society but similarity alone is not adequate for social organization. The economic structure of society is based upon division of labor in which the professional and economic activities of people are different or dissimilar. The social structure of humanity is based upon the family at the base of which is the mutual attraction between

individuals of different sexes, viz. men and women. The culture of society prospers with the difference in thoughts, ideas, viewpoints, etc. father-son, man-women, husband-wife, brother-sister, ruler-ruled, in brief, in all relationships in society the rights and duties of individuals differ and for this reason are supplementary to each other.

3. **Likeness and difference in society:** In this way, both likeness and differences are found in human society. Both these elements are essential for the existence, organization and development of society. Despite the fact that there are different races, nations and countries in the world today there is a growing consciousness of one universe and universal government is no longer an inconceivable impossibility. But this unity of the world cannot be achieved by abolishing the differences of the various cultures. One in the many is a profound truth of universal existence. Only by establishing unity through a synthesis of differences can a prosperous would be society created.

COMMUNITY

Definitions

1. By community is to be understood a group of social being living a common life including all the infinite variety and complexity of relations which result from that common life or constitute it—*Ginsberg*.
2. Wherever the members of any group, small or vast, live together in such a way that they share, not this or that particular interest but the basic conditions of common life, we call that group a community—*MacIver*.
3. By a community I mean a complex of social life, a complex including a number of human being, living together under conditions of social relationships, bound together by a common, however constantly changing stock of conventions, customs and traditions and conscious to the some extent of common social objects and interests—*GHD Cole*.
4. Community is a human population living with in limited geographic area and caring on a common interdependent life—*Lundberg*.
5. Community is any circle of people who live together and belong together in such a way that they do not share this or that particular interest only. But a whole set of interests—*Mannheim*.
6. Community is a social group with some degree of we feeling and living in given area—*Bogardus*.
7. A community is a collectivity of actors sharing a limited territorial area as the base for caring out the greatest share of their daily activities—*Joe Berg Giddon*.
8. A human community is a functionally related aggregate of people who live in a particular geographic locality at a particular time, share a common culture, are arranged in a social structure, and exhibit an awareness of their uniqueness and separate identity as a group—*Blaire E Merca*.
9. A community is that collectivity the members of which share a common territorial area as their base of operation for daily activities—*Talcott Parsons*.
10. Community comprises the entire group sympathetically entering into a common life within a given area, regardless of the extent of area or state boundaries.
11. A community is cluster of people, living within a contiguous small area, who share a common way of life—*Green, Arnold*.
12. A community may be defined as a permanent local aggregation of people having diversified as well as common interests and served by a constellation of institutions—*FL Lumley*.

13. Community is a unit of territory within which is distributed a population which possesses the basic institutions by means of which a common life is made possible—*Dawson and Gettys*.
14. A community is local area over which people are using the same languages, conforming to the same mores, feeling more or less the same sentiments and acting upon the same attitude— *Sutherland*.

Essential Elements of Community

Defining community Bogardus has written, a community is a social group with some degree of we feeling and living in a given area. The essential characteristics of community is:

1. **Definite locality:** The first condition of the community is a definite locality, since without it the relation between human being cannot be established and the we feeling cannot evolve. In the words of Sample, Man is a product of the earth's surface.
2. **Group of human being:** Community is a group of human being. It cannot even be imagined without a group of human being.
3. **Community sentiment:** According to Sutherland, Woodward and Maxwell, A community is a local area over which people are using the same language, conforming the some mores, feeling more or less the same sentiments and acting upon the same attitudes. In this way, this community sentiment is extremely essential in the people belonging to a community.
4. **Likenesses:** According to Green, A community is a cluster of people, living within narrow territorial radius, who share a common way of life. In this way the community exhibits similarity and concurrence in language, customs, mores, traditions, etc. besides many other things.
5. **Permanency:** A community is not transitory and temporary like a crowed. For, it is essentially a permanent life in a definite place.
6. **Natural:** Communities are not made or created by an act of will but are natural. As individual is born in a community. It is by virtue of community that he develops.
7. **Particular name:** Every community has some particular name, which is expressive of the individuality or personality of its locality. In the words of Lumley, it points to identify; it indicates reality; it points out individuality; it often describes personality and each community is something of a personality.
8. **Wider ends:** In communities the people associate not for the fulfillment of a particular end. The ends of a community are wider. These are natural and not artificial.
9. **No legal status:** A community is not a legal person. It cannot sue, nor can it be sued. In the eyes of law, it has no rights and duties.

Difference between Community and Socity

Sl. No.	Community	Society
1.	Community consists of a group of individuals	Society is a web of social relationships.
2.	Community is concrete.	Society is abstract.
3.	A definite geographical area is essential for a community	A definite geographical is not necessary.
4.	They cannot be more than one society in a community.	There can be more than one community in a society.
5.	Community sentiment is indispensable for a community.	Community sentiment or a sense of unity is not essential in a society.

Contd...

Contd...

Sl. No.	Community	Society
6.	In a community the common objectives are comparatively less extensive and coordinated.	In society the common objectives are extensive and coordinated.
7.	In a community a common agreement of interest and objectives is necessary.	In a society common interests and common objectives are not necessary.

Constituents of Community Sentiment

1. **We feeling:** The most important element in community sentiment is that we feeling. As a result of it an individual, instead of regarding himself as separate from other, believes himself to be identified with them. All the people look upon the pain or pleasure of any member of community as their own pain or pleasure. This kind of we feeling can be seen among people of one sector, of one village and among those of foreign strands who hail from the same town or country. The fundamental cause of this feeling is a similarity of interests of people who live in the same place.
2. **Role feeling:** In the community, every individual has his own status and he should make his contribution towards the working of the community in accordance with this status. The community sentiment inevitably induces this desire of contribution because this is part of the community sentiment. As a result of his feeling, an individual looks upon himself as a specific part of society and shoulders his responsibility accordingly.
3. **Sense of dependence:** The third element of community sentiment is the sense of dependence, which means that an individual believes him to be dependent upon community and denies his existence apart from community. Due to this feeling of dependence he does not object to any designs which society has upon him always tries to work in its favor.

Difference between Community and Neighborhood

Sl. No.	Community	Neighborhood
1.	Community is extensive.	Neighborhood is limited.
2.	The circle of personal acquaintance is wide.	The circle of personal acquaintance is narrow.
3.	Community is a unity of society.	Neighborhood is a unity of community.
4.	Prominent importance of community sentiment.	Main importance of sentiment of local unity.
5.	Community sentiment is caused by definite locality, common life, etc.	Sentiment of neighborhood is comparatively less strong.
6.	Community sentiment is stronger.	Sentiment of neighborhood is comparatively less strong.
7.	Community is more organized and controlled.	There is no particular organization of a neighborhood.

ASSOCIATION

An association is a group of people organized for a particular purpose or a a limited number of purposes. According to MacIver, an association is an organization deliberately formed for the collective pursuit of some interest or set of interests, which its members share. An association is a rationally constituted organization of human being, for the fulfillment of objectives, which has its own rule and its own modus, operandi (mode of operation). According to Bogardus, association is usually a working together of people to achieve some purposes. To constitute an association there must be firstly, a group of people. Secondly, these people must be organized ones, i.e. there must be certain rules for their conduct in the group and thirdly, they must have purpose of specific nature to pursue. Thus, family, church, trade, union, music club all are the instances of association. The elements of association are: A group of people, common interest, organized, spirit of cooperation, set or rules and code of ethics.

Definitions

1. An organization deliberately formed for the collective pursuit of some interest or set of interests, which the members of it share, is termed as association—*Malver*.
2. A group of social being related to one another by that fact they possess or have instituted in common an organization with a view to securing a specific end or specific ends—*Ginsberg*.
3. By an association I mean any group of persons perusing a common purpose by a course of cooperative action extending beyond a single act and for this purpose agreeing together upon certain methods of procedure, and laying down, in however rudimentary a form, rules for common action—*GDH Cole*.

Difference between Association and Community

Sl.No	Association	Community
1.	Association is voluntarily constituted.	Community comes into existence of itself.
2.	Membership of an association is voluntary.	Membership of a community is compulsory.
3.	As association have some definite objectives.	Community fulfills all the needs of its members.
4.	Association is comparatively more unstable.	Community is comparatively more stable.
5	An intimate community sentiment is not found in association.	Community is based upon an intimate community sentiment.
6.	Association has its own property, etc.	Community does not have any property of its own.
7.	Association has a legal status.	Community has no legal status.
8.	Association has its own special rules which maintain its harmony.	This function is performed by custom and traditions in the community.
9.	Association is made for specific interests.	Community is formed for common interest.
10.	In this way, association is a part of community. There can be many associations in one community.	Community employs an association as means to the fulfillment of its special of specific need.
11.	An individual takes part in an association because of particular interests.	Man is born in a community, and he also dies in a community.
12.	There are invariable some workers to perform the functions of an association.	Workers are not indispensable for community.

INSTITUTION

Definitions

1. Institution is a definite organization pursuing some specific interest or pursuing general interests in a specific way—*MacIver*.

2. A social institution is a structure of society that is organized to meet the needs of people chiefly through well established procedures—*Bogardus*.
3. An institution is the organization of several folkways and mores (and most often but not necessarily laws) into a unit which serves a number of social functions—*Green*.
4. An institution consists of concept (idea, notion, doctrine or interest) and a structure—*Sumner*.
5. In sociological parlance, an institution is a net of folkways and mores that center in the achievement of some human end or purpose—*Woodward and Maxwell*.

Characteristics of Institution

It is evident from the foregoing definitions of institution that an institution has some definite aims by virtue of which it is beneficial to society. Institution is not only an organized from of racial customs, dogmas and rituals or methods. The following characteristics of institution further clarify form of an institution.

1. Institution has some definite objectives.
2. There is a symbol of an institution which can be either material or nonmaterial.
3. Every institution has some rules which must be compulsorily obeyed by individuals.
4. The institution has definite procedures which are formulated on the basis of customs and dogmas.
5. Institution depends upon the collective or group activities of man.
6. Institutions are means of controlling individuals.
7. Institution is more stable than other means of social control.
8. Institutions are formal for the fulfillment of primary needs.

Social Importance of the Institutions

In connection with the social importance of the institution MacIver has written that it transfers cultural elements from one generation to another, introduces unity in human behavior, controls their conduct and guides man according to circumstances. The following considerations deserve mention with regard to social importance of the institution.

1. In society moral ideals, knowledge and forms or modes of behavior are transferred from one generation to another through the medium of an institution. This helps the younger generation in its solution of the problems confronting it.
2. Institution indicates the right path to man and imposes control upon his activities.
3. The society by means of the institutions compels people, collectively, to work in conformity with social culture.

Difference between Institution and Association

Sl. No.	Institution	Association
1.	Formless and abstract	Concrete.
2.	Evolved	Constituted.
3.	Permanent	Comparatively impermanent.
4.	Procedure of working	Organized group.
5.	Indicative of a method of working	Indicative of membership.

Contd...

Contd...

Sl.No.	Institution	Association
6.	Comprised of laws and system	Comprised of human being.
7.	Aims at primary needs	Aims at other kinds of definite objectives.
8.	Dependent upon human activities.	Based upon mutual cooperation.
9.	Has a definite structure	Has no specific structure.
10.	Laws based upon racial customs and dogmas.	Laws formed after rational considerations.
11.	Compulsory observance of laws	Observance of laws is limited only as long as membership remains.
12.	A symbol, not a name	Definite name.

Difference between Institution and Community

Sl.No.	Institution	Community
1.	Fulfils primary needs.	There is no such definite aim
2.	Dependent upon collective activity.	Dependent upon mutual relations.
3.	A particular type of behavior.	No particular type of behavior
4.	The structure of institution encompasses workers, festivals and rituals besides social relations.	The structure of community is inclusive of group of human being, community sentiments and social relations.
5.	Indicative of procedures.	Indicative of organization.
6.	Draws its life breath from association and communities.	It is of spontaneous birth.
7.	Abstract.	Concrete.
8.	One institution is related to one particular sphere of life.	It is related to the community life in its entirety.

ORGANIZATION

Organization means an arrangement of persons our parts. Thus, family, church, college, factory, a play group, a political party, a community, an empire, united nations all are examples of organization. There are many kinds of organizations. A state is called political organization because it is concerned with political matters. A factory is called an economic organization because it is concerned with production and distribution of wealth. A church is a religious organization. A bank is a financial organization. A college is an educational organization. But all these organizations are also social organizations that are organization of society. Thus, in sociology the term social organization is used in a wide sense to include any organization of society.

Essential Elements of Organization

1. **A goal:** The members of an organization of an organization are inter-related to each other for the pursuit of a common goal. They have unity of interest. In the absence of such unity they would fall apart and the organization will come to an end.

2. **Preparedness:** To accept one's role and status: Organization is an arrangement of persons and parts. By arrangement is meant that every members of the organization has an assigned role, a position and status. Man enjoys status in proportion to the social value of his role. In an organization all the members have an assigned role and status. They should be prepared to accept their role and do acts which the role assigned to them expects of them.

3. **Norms and mores:** Every organization has its norms and mores which control its members. Norms are the socially approved ways of behavior. The norms define the roles of an individual. An organization can function smoothly if its members follow the organization norms. A family has its norms. The father and mother and the children have their assigned roles and are expected to behave according to family norms.

4. **Sanctions:** Every organization has a system of sanctions which support the norms. If a member does not follow the norms, he is compelled to follow them through sanctions which may range from warning to physical punishment.

SOCIAL STRUCTURE

Social structure is the basic concept in sociology. Herbert Spencer was the first thinker to throw light on the structure of society, but he could not give clear cut definitions. Spencer's evaluation of structure as the maintenance of component parts as independent units was indeed a positive step in the development of structural studies. Thus, units were considered independent structures and the adequate functioning of these units was a preliminary requirement of the maintained of the total whole.

Social structure studies are of special and basic interest to the social anthropologist since most of the complexities in preliterate societies and their peculiar customs can be understood in their basic structural terms. Thus, the whole structure of many primitive societies can be understood only in relation to their kinship structure which extends its tentacles in all directions. Starting from the elementary family, various peculiar terminologies and their implications can be understood only in kinship terms.

Definitions

1. The various modes of grouping together comprise the complex pattern of social structure. In the analysis of the social structure the role of diverse attitudes and interests of social beings is revealed—*MacIver*.

2. The components of social structure are human being, the structure itself being an arrangement of persons in relationship institutionally defined and regulated—*Radcliffe Brown*.

3. Social structure is concerned with the principal forms of social organizations, i.e. types of groups, associations and institutions and the complex of these which constitute societies—*Ginsberg*.

4. Social structure is the web of interacting social forces from which have arise the various modes of observing and thinking—*Karl Mannheim*

5. We arrive at the structure of a society through abstracting from the concrete population and its behavior, the pattern or network (or system) of relationship obtaining between actors in their capacity of playing roles relative to one another—*SF Nadel*.

6. Social structure is the term applied to the particular arrangement of the inter-related institutions, agencies and social patterns as well as the statuses and roles which each person assumes in the groups—*Tolcott Parsons*.

Social System

A social system is an orderly and systematic arrangement of social inter-actions. The word system signifies patterned relationship among the constituent parts of structure which is based on functional relations and which makes these parts active and binds them into unity. It is a network of interactive relationships; it may be defined as a plurality of individuals interacting with each other according to shared cultural norms and meanings. The constitute parts of social system are individuals. Each individual has a role to play. He participates in interactive relationship. He influences the behavior of each individual and is influenced by their behavior. The behavior of individuals and groups in society is controlled by social institutions. The various groups do not act in an independent and isolated manner.

Special Feature of a System

1. System is not a unitary concept. A system is made of different parts which together constitute a system.
2. Mere collection of these parts does not make a system these parts must be arranged in a systematic manner. There must be systematic relationship between them.
3. The arrangements of these parts should create a pattern. The parts of a watch should be so arranged that it may create a specific pattern called a watch.
4. There is a functional relationship among the parts of a system. Each part has a function to perform. The system is related with every part and every part is related to the system.
5. The plurality of parts creates unity. Although the parts perform different functions. in a system the parts do not lose their existence. They continue to exist and perform their specific functions. It may also be noted that a defect in any part may affect the working of the system.

Types of System

1. **Natural system:** The natural system is created by nature. It is independent of man's will. It is of two types: (a) inorganic and (b) organic. The inorganic relates to nonliving things and the organic relates to biological things like human body.
2. **Man made system:** The man made system which is created by man. It may be of four types: (a) mechanical system, (b) personality system, (c) cultural system, (d) social system.

Characteristics of Social System

1. **Social system is based on social interaction:** Social system is based on the interaction of plurality of individuals. When a number of individuals act and interact, the interaction produce a system which is called social system.
2. **The interaction should be meaningful:** Social system is an organization of meaningful interactions. Aimless and meaningless interactions do not produce social system.
3. **Social system is a unity:** Social system is a state or condition where the various parts are arranged in an integrated manner. A social system implies order among the interacting units of the system.
4. **The parts of social system** are related on the basis of functional relationship.
5. **Social system is related with cultural system:** Culture determines the nature and scope of inter-relations and interactions of the members of society.
6. **Social system has environmental aspects:** A social system is related to a particular age, a definite territory and a particular society.

BIBLIOGRAPHY

1. An Introduction to Sociology. Vidya Bhushan and Kitab Mahal, Allahabad, 1997.
2. Anthony Giddens. Sociology—Polity Press, UK, 1997.
3. Broom Selznick, Harper, Row. Publishers Company Ltd.
4. G Subramanya. Principles of Sociology, Sapna Books, Bengaluru, 2003.
5. Harold A Philips. Contemporary Social Problems (3rd edn) Prentice Hall, Mc, New York, 1947.
6. K Davis. Human Society. Surjeet Publications, New Delhi, 1981.
7. Karl A Meanninger. Man against Himself Harcourt, Brance and Co. New York, 1938.
8. Maclver and Page. Society—An Introductory Analysis, McMillan India Ltd., 1998.
9. Minendra Nath Basu. Sociology, The World Press, Kolkata, 1975.
10. NJ Smelser. Sociology. Prentice Hall India Ltd., 1993.
11. P Gisbert. Fundamentals of Sociology, Orient Longman.
12. Paul H Landis. Social Policies in the Making. DC Health and Co, Boston, 1947.
13. Robert Bierstedt. The Social Order, Tata McGraw-Hill, 1970.
14. Ronald Fletcher. The Making of Sociology Vol I & II. Rawat Publication
15. Ronald Freedman, et al. Principles of Sociology, New York, 1956.
16. TB Bottomore. Sociology—A Guide to Problems and Literature. Blackie and Sons (India) Ltd.
17. UNDP. Human Development Report, 1999.
18. Young and Mack. Principles of Sociology. Eurasia Publishing House Ltd, New Delhi, 1965.

27 *Social Process*

DEFINITIONS

1. **Social process:** Social processes means various modes of interaction between individuals or groups including cooperation, and conflict, social differentiation and integration, development, arrest and decay.
2. **Conjunctive processes:** These are the interactions which bring persons together. These are called positive processes and reflect mutual altruism and justice or associative processes. Conjunctive processes of interactions are cooperation accommodation and assimilation.
3. **Disjunctive processes:** These are the interactions which push people apart. These are called negative processes or dissociative processes that reflect hostility. The disjunctive processes of interactions are conflict and competition.
4. **Cooperation:** Cooperation is a form of social process in which two or more persons or groups act jointly in the pursuit of a common goal. Cooperation is a reciprocal relation. Generally, cooperation means working together in pursuit of common interests.
5. **Primary cooperation:** It is a type of cooperation in which individual interests are merged in group interests. This type of cooperation is found in family, where cooperation is highly valued.
6. **Secondary cooperation:** It is a characteristic of modern society. Each individual devotes only a part of his life to the group. For example, factory.
7. **Tertiary cooperation:** It is found in certain groups, in which these groups mutually adjust and adopt on certain issues. For example, political parties.
8. **Accommodation:** Accommodation is forms of social process in which two or more persons or groups interact in order to prevent reduce or eliminate conflict. Accommodation refers to termination of rivalries interaction. It avoids conflict and competitions. Accommodation is a process which makes the individuals to adjust and adapt themselves to each other. The main objective of accommodation is living peacefully and in co-existence with one another. It avoids hostility and based on give and take policy. Thus accommodation alters the behavior patterns of the individuals or groups.
9. **Assimilation:** Assimilation is a process of interpretation and fusion in which persons and group acquire the memories, sentiments, and attitudes of other persons or groups and by shaping their experiences and history are incorporated into a common cultural life.
10. **Conflict:** Conflict may be defined as a process of seeking to monopolies rewards by eliminating or weakening the competitors.

11. **Competition:** Competition is the striving of two or more persons for the same goal, which is so limited that all cannot share it.

INTRODUCTION

Society is a system of relationships between two or more individuals and also between different groups. The contents of social relations are actions between persons, who are acting towards and responding reciprocally. Social interactions are social processes where by two or more persons are in meaningful contact and exert reciprocal on each other. The term social relationship refers to the relationship that exists among people. We may witness such relationships between father and son, employer and employee, teacher and student, merchant and customer, leader and follower, or between friends and enemies, between children, etc. Such relationships are among the most obvious features of society.

Social relationships represent the functional aspects of society. Analyzing and classifying social relationships is a difficult task. Social relationships involve reciprocal obligations, reciprocal statuses and reciprocal ends and means as between two or more actors in mutual contact. They refer to a pattern of interaction between these individuals and this is why the school of sociology which has attempted to systematize its thought in relationship terms has been called the formal school. Thus, social relationships may be studied by the kind or mode of interaction they exhibit. These kinds or modes of interaction are called social process. Social processes are the fundamental ways in which men interact and establish relationships.

DEFINITIONS OF SOCIAL PROCESS

1. Social process is the manner in which the relations of the members of a group, once brought together, acquire a distinctive chapter—*MacIver*.
2. Social processes are merely the characteristic ways in which interaction occurs—*AW Green*.
3. Social processes mean the various modes of interaction between individuals or groups including cooperation, and conflict, social differentiation and integration, development, arrest and decay —*Ginsberg*.
4. The term social processes refer to the repetitive forms of behavior which are commonly found in social life—*Horton and Hunt*.

FORMS OF SOCIAL PROCESSES

The society contains hundreds and perhaps thousands of socially defined relationships. These relationships are beyond measurement. It is humanly impossible for any individual to make a detailed study of each and every social relationship. Instead they must be classified and dealt with as general types. For this reason social relationships have been classified and discussed in terms of the kinds of interaction they manifest. The forms of social interactions are two types:

1. **Conjunctive processes:** These are the interactions which bring persons together. These are called positive processes and reflect mutual altruism and justice or associative processes. Conjunctive processes of interactions are cooperation accommodation and assimilation.
2. **Disjunctive processes:** These are the interactions which push people apart. These are called negative processes or dissociate processes that reflect hostility. The disjunctive processes of interactions are conflict and competition. Both conflict and competition are basic processes that are disintegrative in nature. Both are the forms of non-cooperation and opposition. But they also

differ from each other in considerable respects. The fundamental differences between conflict and competition can be understood from the following table.

Sl.No.	Competition	Conflict
1.	Continuous	Intermittent.
2.	Impersonal	Personal
3.	Unconscious	Conscious.
4.	Based on non-violence	Violence employed
5.	Both combatants gain	Both combatants suffer loss.
6.	Productive	Non-productive
7.	Encourages hard work	Discourages hard work.
8.	Separates into very small	Divides into large division
9.	Observes social laws	Discourages social law
10.	Achievement of aim the primary object	Prevention of damage the prime consideration
11.	The aim is self-interest with loss to opponent	The aim is self-interest

COOPERATION

Cooperation is that form of social interaction in which two or more persons works for the achievement of a common end. For example, the aim of all the teachers in a college is maintenance of a high stranded of education and creating and maintaining a respectable position of the college in social cycles. Hence, they all cooperate with each other. If any one teacher does not care for maintaining a high level of education in the college or its honors and respect in sociology or desires to cause indiscipline and disorder in the institution then he does not cooperate with the other teachers. The government of a state runs successfully only when the administer and administered extended their full cooperation to each other.

Meaning of Cooperation

Cooperation is one of the most basic, pervasive and continuous social process. It is the very basis of our social existences. Cooperation generally means. Working together for the pursuit of a common goal. The term cooperation is derived from the two Latin words: Co-meaning together and Operai meaning to work; literally, cooperation means joint work or working together for common rewards. Cooperation is a form of social process in which two or more persons or groups act jointly in the pursuit of a common goal. Cooperation is a reciprocal relation. Generally, cooperation means working together in pursuit of common interests. Thus cooperation refers to group effort to realize certain common goal.

Cooperation consists of two elements namely: (1) Common goals, (2) An organized effort. The social life depends upon cooperation. We cooperate several ways with others daily in our social activities. For example, we play together, worship together, the farmers till their fields together, the agricultural activities are generally carried on the basis of cooperation. Cooperation is a significant interactional process, because the basic social activities are carried on smoothly by cooperation. So, cooperation is necessary for our existence. For example, cooperation results in procreation and in rearing of children and in socialization. Cooperation requires sympathy and identification. We cannot have cooperation without the development of sympathy. Sympathy depends upon the capacity of an individual to imagine himself in the place of another, particularly when the other person is in difficulties.

Definitions

1. Cooperation is the progress by which individuals or groups combine their effort, in a more or less, organized form, in the attainment of common objective—*Fairchild.*
2. Cooperation is a form of social interaction wherein two or more persons work together to gain a common end—*Merrill and Eldredge.*
3. Cooperation is the continuous and common endeavor of two or more persons to perform a task or to reach a goal that is commonly cherished—*AW Green.*

Types of Cooperation

1. **Direct cooperation:** Individuals involved do the identical function. For example, playing together, working together, tilling together, people do work in company with other members. Performance of a common task with joint efforts brings them social satisfaction.
2. **Indirect cooperation:** In this case, people work individually for the attainment of a common end. People here do unlike tasks towards a similar end. This is based on the principle of division of labor and specialization.
3. **Primary cooperation:** It is found in the primary groups such as family, neighborhood, friends group, children's playing group and so on. In this group cooperation in which individual interests are merged in group interests. Every member works for the betterment of all. There is an interlocking identification of individuals, group and the task performed. The group contains all or nearly all, of each individual's life. The rewards for which everyone works are shared, or meant to be shared, with every other member in the group. Means and goals become one for cooperation itself is a highly prized value.
4. **Secondary cooperation:** It is the characteristic features of the modern civilized society and is found mainly in secondary groups. It is highly formalized and specialized. Here, cooperation is not itself a value; attitudes are more likely to be individualistic and calculating. Most members of the group feel some loyalty toward the group. Each performs his tasks, and thus helps others to perform their tasks, so that he can seperatately enjoy the fruits of his cooperation.
5. **Tertiary cooperation:** In this cooperation may be found between bigger groups also. It may be found between two or more political parties, castes, tribes, religious groups and so on. It if often called accommodation.

Importance of Cooperation

The importance of cooperation is made abundantly clear by the simple reflection that the very existence of society depends on the mutual cooperation between the male and females of the species. It is by mutual cooperation that man and women procreate and bring up their offspring. The cooperation of the members of the members of family is essential for the socialization of the child and the development of his various potential capacities. Outside the family the child is influenced by his contacts with his teachers and his colleagues at school. Cooperation is important in the life of an individual that according to Prince Kropokin, it is difficult for man to survive without it. He calls it Mutual Aid. In rearing of progeny and in the provision of protection and food, cooperation is inevitable. The continuation of human race requires the cooperation of male and female for reproduction and upbringing of children. Cooperation has its origin in the biological level.

Cooperation helps society to progress; progress better is achieved through united action. Progress in science and technology, agricultural, and industry, transport and communication, etc. would not have been possible without cooperation. Person who co-operate may generate unbounded enthusiasm. It is the main spring of our collective life. It gives strength to union. It builds, it conserve. In democratic countries, cooperation has become a necessary condition of people's collective life and activities. The growth of the role of cooperation is seen in the increase in the size of communities. Cooperation is an urgent need of the present-day world. It is needed not only among the individuals, associations, groups, and communities but also among nations.

ACCOMMODATION

Accommodation is the first step from conflict to reconciliation and cooperation. Man cannot always be conflicting with and struggling against his environment and all the people who surround him. Even if he sometimes fails to agree with them, he usually has to tolerate or to suffer them. This understanding or common agreement is accommodation. This is an unconscious process that is forever active in some or the other sphere of life. The life of adolescent in the family is an interesting and instructive example of accommodation. This process of accommodation is to seen in every sphere of life. The people from the rural areas accommodate themselves when placed in an urban situation. A person must accommodate himself, be it a new country, a new society, new caste, social circle, neighborhood, or any other sphere.

Accommodation is forms of social process in which two or more persons interact in order to prevent reduce or eliminate conflict. Accommodation refers to termination of rivalous interaction. It avoids conflict and competitions. Accommodation is a process which makes the individuals to adjust and adopt themselves to each other. The main accommodation is living peacefully and in co-existence with one another. It avoids hostility and based on give and take policy. Accommodation also a condition. It is condition or state of mental and social understanding and peace. Every individual is born under a particular set of circumstances some of which are good and some bad.

Definitions

1. As a process of accommodation is the sequence of steps by which persons are reconciled to changed conditions of life through the formation of habits and attitudes make necessary by the changed conditions themselves—*Reuter and Hart*.
2. In one sense, accommodation is the basis of all formal social organizations—*Biesanz*.
3. In one sense, accommodation may be said to the agreement to disagree—*Jones*.
4. The term accommodation refers particularly to the process in which man attains a sense of harmony with his environment—*MacIver and Page*.
5. Accommodation is the natural issue of conflicts. In an accommodation the antagonism of the hostile elements is for the time being regulated and conflict disappear as over action, although it remains latent as a potential force—*Park and Burgess*.
6. Accommodation is a term used by the sociologist to describe the adjustment of hostile individuals or groups—*Ogburn and Nimkoff*.
7. The word accommodation has been used to designate the adjustments which people in groups make to relieve the fatigue and tensions of competition and conflict—*Lungberg*.

8. The term accommodation denotes acquired changes in the behavior of individuals which help them to adjust to their environment—*JM Baldwin.*

Needs of Accommodation

1. It is clear from the above that accommodation assumes various forms, without accommodation social life could hardly go on. Since conflicts disturbs social integration, disturbs social order and damages social stability; in all societies, efforts are made to solve them at the earliest.
2. Accommodation checks, conflicts and helps persons and groups in maintain cooperation.
3. It enables persons and groups to adjust themselves to changed functions and statutes which are brought about by changed conditions.
4. It helps the carry on their life activities together even with conflicting interests.
5. It is a means of resolving conflict without the complete destruction of the opponent.
6. It makes possible cooperation between antagonistic or conflicting element or parties. Hence, it is often called antagonistic cooperation.

Difference between Accommodation and Adjustment

Sl.No.	Accommodation	Adjustment
1.	Unconscious activity	Conscious activity
2.	Both external and internal	Only external
3.	Is later stage after adjustment	Is the first step towards accommodation.

Difference between Accommodation and Adaptation

Sl.No.	Accommodation	Adaptation
1.	Social process	Biological process
2.	Outcome of conflict	Natural results of competition
3.	A process of learning	Ultimate results of the process of biological evolution.

Characteristics of Accommodation

1. **Accommodation is the natural results of conflict:** Since conflicts cannot take place continuously they make room for accommodation. When parties or individuals involved in conflict do not relish the scene of conflict they sit down for its settlement.
2. **Accommodation may be a conscious or an unconscious activity:** Man's adjustment with the social environment is mostly unconscious. The newborn individual learns to accommodate himself with the social order which is dictated by various norms such as customs, morals, traditions, etc. accommodation becomes conscious when the conflicting individuals and groups make deliberate and an open attempts to stop fighting and start working together.
3. **Accommodation is universal:** Accommodation as a condition and as a process is universal. Accommodation is found in all societies and in all fields of social life.
4. **Accommodation is continuous:** The process of accommodation is not confined to any particular stage in the life of an individual. It is not limited to any fixed social situation also. On the country, throughout one's life one has to accommodate oneself with various situations.

5. **The effects of accommodation may very with the circumstances:** It may act to reduce the conflict between persons or groups. It may serve to postpone outright conflict for a specific period of time, and may permit groups marked by sharp sociopsychological distance to get along together.

Forms or Methods of Accommodation

Gillin and Gillin have mentioned methods of adjustment.

1. **Yielding to coercion:** Coercion involves the use of force or the threat of force for making the weaker party to accept conditions of agreement. This can take place when the parties are of unequal strength. It implies the existence of the weak and the strong in any conflict.
2. **Compromise:** When the contending parties are almost equal in power they attain accommodation by means of compromise. In compromise each party to the dispute makes some concession and yields to some demand of the other.
3. **Toleration:** Toleration is another form of accommodation in which the conflicts are avoided rather than settled or resolved. Toleration or tolerant participation is an outgrowth of the live and let live policy. It is a form of accommodation without formal agreement. Here is no settlement of difference but there is only the avoidance of over conflict.
4. **Conversion:** This form of accommodation involves a sudden rejection of one's beliefs, convictions and loyalties and the adaptation of others. This term is ordinarily used in the religious context to refer to one's conversion into some other religion. The concept is now used in the literary, artistic, economic, political and other fields.
5. **Sublimation:** Adjustment by means of sublimation involves the substitution of non-aggressive attitudes and activities for aggressive ones. It may take place at the individual as well as the group level.
6. **Rationalization:** This involves plausible excuses or explanations for one's behavior. One is not prepared to acknowledge one's failures or defects for it may indicate guilt or the need for change. Hence, one blames others for one's own defects, one can retain self-respect.

ASSIMILATION

Assimilation is the process by which when persons and groups come into contact with other cultural groups, in a long run acquire its ways of life. Assimilation is one from of social adjustment. In its process the individual or group begins to absorb slowly and gradually, somewhat unconsciously, the new circumstances in which it finds itself. It results in the modification of social attitudes. For example, in many parts of India, the Hindus and Muslims have become so intimate and well-acquainted with each other that they have assimilated many points of each other's cultures in to their own and made them integral part of their own social conduct.

Assimilation is both a process and a stage or state. It is a cultural process. When different cultures come into contact, originally it is the sentiment of mutual conflict that is most prominent but they gradually synthesize with each other and assimilate any element from each other, they develop a more tolerant approach towards each other. This is the process of assimilation. When different cultures get the opportunity of combining with each other promoted by feeling of kindness and tolerance of each other, each absorbs many features of the other within itself. In this process of assimilation is evident in the relations between individual and society, husbands and wife, members of the family, social institutions, association and communities, etc.

Definitions

1. Assimilation denotes conformity and uniformity in respect of culture—*Dawson and Getty's*.
2. Assimilation is a process of interpenetration and fusion in which persons and group acquire the memories, sentiments and attitudes of other persons or groups and, by shaping their experience and history, are incorporated into a common cultural life—*Park and Burgess*.
3. Assimilation is the process whereby individual or groups once dissimilar become similar, that is become identified in their interests and outlook—*Ogburn and Nimkoff*.
4. Assimilation is a process whereby attitudes of many persons are united and they thus develop into a unified group—*Bogardus*.
5. Assimilation is the social process whereby individual and groups come to share the same sentiments and goals—*Bissanz and Biesanz*.

Factors Promoting Assimilation

1. **Toleration:** Intimates and close relationships are essential for assimilation to occur and these are impossible if there is no tolerance. It is only when people who believe in one culture are prepared to tolerate the proximate existence of people who uphold the cause of different culture that they can be influenced by the culture the other upholds. It is here that the process of assimilation finds its roots.
2. **Intimate social relationships:** The next factor after toleration that helps the process of assimilation is intimate and close social relationship and contacts. The process of assimilation progresses in direct proportion to the growth of the social relationships.
3. **Amalgamation:** Assimilation is further encouraged by amalgamation, since amalgamation leads to the creation of blood relationships. Blood being thicker than water, these relationships are more intimate and strong and they wield their influence upon people by making them impress each other, thus accelerating process of assimilation.
4. **Cultural similarity:** If two cultures resemble each other in some vital respects, then the intimacy and toleration between their members for each other is of a higher order. This too, encourages assimilation.
5. **Equality of opportunity for economic progress:** Economical inequalities lead to jealousy, hatred and conflict. If people get the same opportunities for economic progress as the neighbors, social intimacy increases and assimilation progresses.
6. **Education:** Education is another conductive factor for assimilation. For immigrant people public education has played a prominent role in providing cultural conduct.

Factors Hindering Assimilation

1. **Strong feelings of superiority and inferiority:** People have nothing but hatred and disgust for each other if they harbor strong feelings of superiority and inferiority. They even decline to establish any relationship among themselves. The outcome of this that they learn little if anything from each other, avoiding mutual contact and influence, as they do. This naturally hinders assimilation.
2. **Isolation:** Just as intimacy helps to promote assimilation, isolation helps to hinder it. Living in isolation does not lead to the formation of social contacts and relations. Hence, the very question of mutual influence is precluded from the field of practice.

3. **Difference in color and physiological characteristics:** People distinguish between themselves on the basis of the skin and their physiological characteristics. One can see differences and discrimination between the white and black or Negro races almost everywhere in the world. There are very few occasions for mutual contact between the Whites and negroes. This discrimination leads to the white considering themselves somehow superior to the black people and looking upon all social contact with them as degrading. This naturally becomes an obstacle to assimilation.

4. **Cultural differences:** Just as cultural similarity or identify promotes assimilation, cultural dissimilarity tends to accelerate and hinder the process of assimilation.

5. **Domination and subordination:** If some people manage to dominate others, they come to think themselves superior to the people dominate and do not consider on equal footing. The Aryans who came to India as victors looked upon the native races as inferior, whom they abhorred. In this way, when people lose their independence and of this hatred for their persecutors and ruler is but a corollary. Thus, social relations do not grow in either condition, and assimilation becomes difficult.

6. **Social persecution:** Social persecution, exploitation and injustice only lead to increased conflict between the exploiters and the exploited. Whatever the justification for this conflict, it prevents the growth of social intimacy and consequently that of assimilation.

Difference between Assimilation and Accommodation

Sl.No.	Assimilation	Accommodation
1.	Assimilation is a slow and a gradual process. It makes time. For example, immigrant takes time to get assimilated with majority group.	Accommodation may take place suddenly and in radical manner. Example, working after having talks with the management may decide to stop their month-long strike all on a sudden.
2.	Assimilation normally provides a permanent solution to inter-group disputes and differences.	It may or may not provide permanent solution to group differences and disputes. It may only provide a temporary solution.
3.	It is mostly an unconscious process. Individuals and groups involved in it are often not aware of what actually happens within themselves or in their group.	It may be both conscious and unconscious process. It most of the instances it takes place consciously. Example, labor leader who come for talks are sufficiently aware of the fact that they are purposefully seeking out a solution to their dispute.

CONFLICT

Conflict is an ever-present process in human relation. It is one of the forms of struggle between individuals or groups. Conflict takes place whenever a person or group seeks to gain a reward not by surpassing other competitors but by preventing them from effectively competing. Conflict and cooperation are universal interactional process in human life. Conflict is expressed in numerous ways in our daily activities. Conflict occurs when crude hostility and more intense forms of struggle become common between individuals or groups to realize certain common objectives. The best examples for this are armed warfare, riots, revolution, street fight, etc. in which large groups of persons combat with the intension of destroying one another. So conflict refers to all rivalries interactions between individuals and groups.

Competition gradually changes into rivalry which, in turn, changes into conflict. Hence, Kingsley Davis is corrected in observing, it is thus a modified form of struggle. The basic differences between competition and conflict have already been discussed. According to Gillin and Gillin, conflict is the social process in which individual or groups seek their ends by directly changing the antagonist by violence or the treat of violence. Moreover, the desire for revenge is also found in conflicts and is one of its ingredient.

Definitions

1. Conflict is the deliberate attempts to oppose resist or coerce the will of another or others—*Green.*
2. Conflict may be defined as a process of seeking to monopolise rewards by eliminating or weakening the competitors—*Horton and Hunt.*
3. Conflict is a process in which individuals or groups seek their ends by directly challenges the antagonist by violence or threat of violence—*JG Gillin and JA Gillin.*
4. It is thus a modified form of stugle—*Kingsly Davis.*
5. It takes the form of emotionalized and violent opposition, in which the major concern is to overcome the opponent as a means of securing a given goal or reward—*Young and Young.*
6. Conflict may be defined as a process of seeking to monopolize rewards like eliminating or weakening the competitors—*Horton and Hunt.*
7. A process situation in which two or more human beings or groups seek activity to thwart each others purpose to prevent each other's interests even to the extent of injuries or destroying the others—*Sociology Dictionary.*

Nature of Conflict

1. Conflict as a process, is the very antithesis of cooperation. The functions of a person or group of persons are hindered by ways of conflict.
2. Sometimes, individuals try to destroy their opponents by resorting to means of violent action. But it is not essential that violent action should always be associated with the conflict.
3. Sometimes, the conflict carries a legal sanction and occurs peacefully. For example, Indian national army employed violent measures to fight against the British government under the guidance and leadership of Netaji.
4. Conflict arises due to contradictory aims. For example, the primary aims of Indians were to strengthen the country while the British people arose conflict.
5. Contradictory methods also lead to conflict. There is a conflict between the different political parties of India mainly due to their contradictory methods.

Characteristics of Conflict

1. **Conflict is universal:** Conflict or clash of interest is universal in nature. It is present in almost all the societies. Karl Marx, the architect of communism, has said that the history of the hitherto existing human society is nothing but the history of the class struggle.
2. **Conflict is a continuous action:** Individuals and group who are involves in conflict are aware of the fact that they are conflicting. As Park and Burgess have pointed out conflicts is always conscious and evokes the deepest emotions and strong passions.
3. **Conflict of personal interests:** When competition is personalized it leads to conflict. In the struggle to overcome the other persons or group. The goal is temporarily relegated to a level of secondary importance.

4. **Conflict is not continuous but intermittent:** Conflict never takes place continuously. It takes place occasionally. No society can sustain itself in a state of continuous conflict.
5. **Conflict is conditioned by culture:** Conflict is affected by the nature of the group and its particular culture. The objectives of conflicts may be property, power and status, freedom and action and thought or any other highly desired value.
6. **Conflicts and norms:** Not only culture modifies conflict and its forms but also controls and governs it. When conflict is frequent and when no adequate techniques have been worked out, more violent and unpredictable sorts of conflict such as race riots arise.
7. **Conflict may be personal or impersonal and open and subtle:** Conflicts may assume a variety of forms. We may observe conflicts between two individuals, families, classes, races, nations and groups of nations. It may take place between smaller or larger groups.
8. **Ways of resolving conflict:** Conflict can be resolved in two main ways: (a) accommodation and (b) assimilation.
9. **Frustration and insecurity promotes conflicts:** Sometimes, factors like frustration and insecurity promote conflicts within the same society. Individuals feel frustration if they are thoroughly disturbed in their attempts to reach their goals. Insecurities like economic crisis, unemployment, the fear of deprivation of love and affection may add to the frustration. A society marked by widespread insecurity is one in which conflict is potential.

Functions of Conflict

1. Conflict results in new consensus.
2. Conflict stiffness the morals and improves the solidarity of the group.
3. Conflicts alter the relative status of the parties involved.
4. At the end of the conflict the victor group enlarges.
5. Conflict provides opportunity to work out non-violent techniques for resolving crisis.
6. Conflict results in redefinition of value system.

Difference between Competition and Conflict

Sl.No.	Competition	Conflict
1.	Competition is a process of seeking to monopolise a reward by overtaking all rivals.	Conflict is a process of seeking to posses a reward by weakening or eliminating all rivals.
2.	Competition may be conscious or unconscious.	Conflict is always a conscious activity.
3.	Competition is universal as well as continuous.	Conflict is universal nut not continuous. It is intermittent.
4.	Here, the attention of an individual is concentrated on the object or the gcal. It is mostly impersonal in nature.	Here, the concentration is on the person rather that the object. Hence, it is mostly personal in nature.
5.	Competition may lead to positive as well as negative results. Healthy competition even contributes to progress.	Conflict mostly brings negative results. Its negative results outweigh its positive results.
6.	Competition when becomes rigorous, results in conflict.	Competition when becomes personalized, leads to conflicts.

Difference between Cooperation and Conflict

Sl.No.	Cooperation	Conflict
1.	Cooperation refers to joint activity in pursuit of common goals or shared rewards.	Conflicts is a process of seeking to monopolise a reward by weakening or destroying the other competitions.
2.	Cooperation may be conscious or unconscious. It may not be a deliberative act always.	Conflict is mostly conscious in nature. It is mostly a deliberate act.
3.	Cooperation requires sympathy and identification, kindness and consideration for others.	But conflict is always associated with the deepest emotions and strongest sentiments. In it there is no regard for others.
4.	Cooperation is universal and continuous in nature.	Conflict is universal no doubt. But it is not continuous, it is intermittent.
5.	Cooperation brings mostly positive results; it builds, conserves, and leads to progress.	Conflict brings mostly negative results. It harms, destroys and retards progress.
6.	Cooperation is basic to group life. There can be no society without cooperation.	Conflict is not fundamental to the group life of man. Society can persist without it.
7.	Cooperation assumes different forms—primary, secondary and tertiary cooperation, direct and indirect cooperation.	We may speak of class conflict, international conflict, conflict of interpersonal ideas, religious, cultural, racial and caste conflicts.

Forms or Types of Conflict

1. **Corporate conflict:** Corporate conflict, which is often known as group conflict, occurs among the groups within a society or between two societies. When one group tries imposing its will on the other conflict takes place. Example, race, communal upheavals, religious persecutions, labor-management conflicts and war between nations, etc.
2. **Personal conflict:** It takes place within the groups. It is more severely restricted and disapproved than the conflict between the groups. The group as a whole has nothing to gain from internal conflict. Personal conflicts arise on account of various motives, envy, hostility, betrayal of trust and so on. Violence occurs much less often though not always, in personal conflict than in corporate conflict. Husband may be quarrel with the wife, student with the teacher, friend with the friend, but they may not start fighting.
3. **Latent and overt conflict:** Conflicts may be overt or latent. In most cases, long before conflict erupts in hostile action; it has existed in latent from in social tension and dissatisfaction. Latent conflict becomes overt conflict when an issues is declared and when hostile action is taken the overt conflict takes place when one side or the other feels strong and wishes to take advantages of this fact. For example, the latent conflict between democratic and communist countries becomes overt at the time of war between them.
4. **Class conflict:** It arises between social classes which have mutually hostile or opposite interests. Karl Marx has spoken much about the conflict between the social classes: The rich and the poor or the capitalists and proletariats.
5. **Racial conflict:** Racial conflict is mostly due to the physiological differences which are apparently seen among people. One race may claim superiority over the other and start suppressing the other resulting in conflicts. Example, conflicts between whites and negroes.

6. **Caste conflicts:** A sense of highness and lowness of superiority and inferiority, of holy and unholy which some caste groups have developed have been responsible for caste conflicts. The so called upper castes or Savarna Hindus conflicting with the so called harijans or lower castes (untouchables) has become a common feature in India.

7. **International conflicts:** It refers to the conflict between two or more nations or groups of nations. It may take place for political, religious, economic, imperialistic or ideological or for any other such reasons.

Negative Effects of Conflict

1. Conflict is the most vigorous form of social interaction and evokes the deepest passions and strongest emotions. It disrupts social unity. It is a costly way of settling disputes. The results of intragroup conflict are largely negative in that such a struggle lowers the morale and weakens the solidarity of the group.

2. Conflict causes social disorder, chaos and confusion, war as a form of conflict may destroy the lives and properties of countless individuals. It may bring incalculable damage and immeasurable suffering to number of people. Human history is a monumental evidence in this regard. The modern modes of welfare which can destroy millions of people and vast amount of properties within a few minutes, has brought new fears and anxieties for the mankind.

3. Conflict does a lot of psychological and moral damage also; it spoils the mental peace of man. Conflicts may even make the people to become in human. Lovers of conflict have scant respect for human and moral values. Conflicts between the labors and the management have resulted in material losses. Due to the labor strikes productivity decreases and men and machines become idle.

Positive Effects of Conflict

1. A limited amount of internal conflict may indirectly contribute to group stability. An occasional conflict within the group may seek its leadership alert and its policies up-to-date. If there is no scope of occasional expression of conflict, and if it is deliberately suppressed, the accumulated discontent may explode and cause irreparable loss.

2. External conflict brings about social unity and oneness among the members. During the Indo-Pak War, all the political parties joined together forgetting their differences and supported the Government of India in facing the challenges.

3. Personal conflicts also have their advantages. It is through constant struggle only that individuals can rise to a higher level. The opposition of one individual by the other is the only way in which the continued relationship can be made personally tolerable.

COMPETITION

Competition is the most fundamental form of social struggle. It is a natural result of the universal struggle for existence. It is based on the fact that all people can never satisfy all their desires. Competition takes place whenever there is an insufficient supply of things that human being commonly desire. Whenever and wherever commodities which people want are available in a limited supply, there is competition. Competition is a modified struggle. It is a social process in which two or more individuals or groups are striving to achieve some mutually desired goal. The desire wants of the persons are unlimited. The objects are short in supply and of high value. If they are available in abundance, then no competition tales place. For example, people do not compete for air and water. Food products are essential for the continuation of life. Since they are short in supply, to secure food, human being engage in competitive endeavor. The degree of competitive process is expressed more in modern society than in simple society. Though it is a disjunctive process, it is a kind of game, must be played fairly and involve certain conscious or unconscious rules of the game.

Competition is a process of struggle between people for scarce goods, goals, money, rewards, status, values, or love. In it the attention of the competitors is not upon each other so much as upon the goods, the goals, the status and recognition that they are seeking. Competition may take place on a conscious level. Individual complete to achieve their objectives unaware of the competitive character of their activities, example, a large number of students in Metric or Higher secondary, compete unaware of the competitive character of each one of them. Competition may be personal as in election to an office. In business field one can observe the competition between merchants, which takes place in the absence of coercion or physical force. In society we find competition to secure higher status. Competitive opportunities are provided in all cultural systems. For example, educational opportunities are provided in which the members can strive hard to achieve their common goal.

Definitions of Competition

1. Competition is the striving of two or more persons for the same goal, which is so limited that all cannot share it—*Biesanz and Biesanz*.
2. Competition is a contest to obtain something which does not exist in a quality sufficient to meet the demands—*Bogardus*.
3. Competition is an impersonal, unconscious, continuous struggle between individuals or groups for satisfaction which, because of their limited supply, all may not have—*Sutherland*.
4. Competition is the struggle for possession of rewards which are limited in supply, goods, status, power, love anything—*Horton and Hunt*.
5. The form of social action in which we strive against each other for the possession or use of so limited material or non-materials goods—*Anderson and Parker*.

Nature of Competition

1. **Competition is an unconscious action:** It is concerned with the subject and not the individual. Therefore, besides the knowledge of the subject, it is an unconscious action.
2. **Competition is an impersonal action:** The only difference between competitions is always impersonal whereas struggle is always personal. In other words of Ogburn and Nimkoff, struggle is personal competition.
3. **Competition is continuous activity:** Competition never ends. It always tends to increase like competition in the acquisition of wealth.
4. **Competition is universal action:** Competition is found in each society as people everywhere wishes to procure the things are limited in supply. Moreover, competition is found in every class of people, viz students, procedure, laborers, artists, etc. It enables the development of both the individual and the action.

Forms of Competition

1. **Economic competition:** It is found in production, exchange and distribution as well as consumption in the field of economic activities.
2. **Cultural competition:** Cultural competition is found in different cultures. Taking the history of any country, it can be seen that there was a great difference in the cultures of the natives and the invaders.

3. **Social competition:** To get a high status in society, everybody seems to be engaged in competitive activity.
4. **Racial competition:** In South Africa, there is an intense competition between the black and white races.
5. **Political competition:** All countries competition is obvious between the various political parties and even between the different members of a political party to obtain political power. Similarity, in the international circle too there is always diplomatic competition between different nations.

Importance of Competition

1. Competition plays an important role in the life of persons, society and group. It increases efficiency. As Biesanz and Biesanz put it, we are convinced that while cooperation gets things done, competition assures that they will be well done. Social status and competition are very closely associated.
2. In words of Bernard, thus altogether we may speak of economic, social and political competition. In all cases competition for status is present. In fact, competition has an important hand in causing an amazing development of individual and society as the chief aim of competition is to move towards progress.
3. In other words of Eldredge, competition between individuals and groups aims largely towards the objective of preserving their respective status rather than survival. But however advantageous the competition may be, it should not be left uncontrolled, because then its disadvantages will overcome the advantages and the result will be harmful to the society. Bogardus is correct is saying that competition logically develops into conflict.
4. Competition may be impersonal. The individual competitor may be aware that others are competing with him. But the competitors have no personal contact with each other. The farmer is not in contact with other farmer with whom he is competing, in determining the price of rice or wheat.
5. Through competition the distributive and ecological order of society is created (Park and Burgess). Competition determines the distribution of population territorially and vocationally. The division of labor and all the vast organized interdependence of individuals and groups, characteristics of modern life are a product of competition.

Characteristics of Competition

1. **Scarcity as a condition of competition:** Whenever there are commonly desired goods and services, there is competition. In fact, economics starts with its fundamental proposition that while human wants are unlimited the resources that can satisfy these wants are strictly limited. Hence, people complete for possession of these limited resources.
2. **Competition and affluence:** Competition may be found even in circumstances of abundance of affluence. In a time employment competition may take place for the status of the top class. There is competition not only for food, shelter and basic needs, but also for luxuries, power, name, fame, social position, mates and so on.
3. **Competition is continuous:** Competition is continuous. It is found virtually in every area of social activity and social interaction. Particularly, competition for status, wealth and fame is always present in almost all societies.
4. **Competition is universal:** Modern civilized society is marked by the phenomenon of competition. Competition is covering almost all the areas of our social living. Business people complete for customers, lawyers for clients, doctors for patients, students for ranks or distinctions, athletes

and sportsman for trophies, political parties for power, young men and women for mates and so on. Still no society can be said to be exclusively competitive or cooperative.

5. **Competition is dynamic:** It stimulates achievement and contributes to social change. It lifts the level of aspiration from the lower level to a higher level. A college student who competes with other to get selected to the college cricket team, after becoming successful may later struggle to get selected to the university cricket team, to the state team. To the national team and so on.

6. **Competition—a cause of social change:** Competition is a cause of social change in that, it cause persons to adopt new forms of behavior in order to attain desired ends. New forms of behavior involve intentions and innovations which naturally bring about social life. It is an effect of social change also, because a changing society has more goals to open than a relatively static society.

7. **Competition may be personal or impersonal:** Completion is normally directed towards a goal and not against any individual. Sometimes, it takes place without the actual knowledge of other's existence. It is impersonal as in the case of civil service examination in which the contestants are not aware of one another's identity. Competition may also be personal as when two individuals contest for election to an office. As competition becomes more personal it leads to rivalry and shades into conflict. Competition in the social world is largely impersonal. The individual may be vaguely aware of, but has no personal contact with other competitors.

8. **Competition may be constructive or destructive:** Competitions may be healthy or unhealthy. If one of the or more competitors tries to win only at the expense of the others, it is destructive. Sometimes, big industries or capitalists resort to such a kind of competition and make the small petty businessmen to become virtually bankrupt. But constructive competition is mutually stimulating and helpful. It contributes to the welfare of all at large. For example, farmers may compete to raise the best crops, workers in a factory to maximize production, student in a college to get distinctions and so on.

9. **Competition is always governed by norms:** Competition is not limitless nor is it unregulated. There is no such thing as unrestricted competition. Such a phrase is contradiction in terms. Moral norms or legal rules always govern and control competition. Competitors are expected to use fair tactics and not cut-throat devices.

10. **Competition may be unconscious also:** Competition may take place on an unconscious level. Many times individuals who are engaged in competition may be oblivious of the fact they are in a competitive race.

Special Functions of Competition

1. **Assigns status to the individuals:** Competition assigns individuals their respective place in the social system. Social status and competition are always associated. Some people compete with others to retain their status; others compete to enhance their status.

2. **Source of motivation:** Competition is a source of motivation for the individuals. It makes the individual to show his ability and express the talents. It increases individual efficiency.

3. **Provides for social mobility:** As far as the individual is concerned, competition implies mobility and freedom. The spirit of competition helps the individual to improve his social status.

4. **Competition contributes to social economic progress:** Fair competition is conductive to economic as well as social progress. It even contributes to general welfare because it spurs individuals and groups on to exert their best efforts. When the competition is directed to promote the general interests of the community as a whole, it can bring about miraculous results.

5. **Provides for new experiences:** As Ogburn and Nimkoff have pointed out competition provides the individuals better opportunities to satisfy desires for new experiences and recognition. As far as the group is concerned, competition means experimental change.

Difference between Cooperation and Competition

Sl.No.	Competition	Cooperation
1.	Competition is a form of social interaction wherein the individuals try to monopolize rewards by surpassing all the rivals.	Cooperation refers to a form of social interaction wherein two or more persons work together to gain a common end.
2.	Competition can take place at the level of the group and also at the level of the individual.	Cooperation is always based on the combined or the joint efforts of the people.
3.	Thorough competition can bring about positive results; it can cause damages or losses to the patients and persons involved.	Cooperation normally brings about positive results. It rarely causes losses too.
4.	Competition has its own limitations. It is bound by norms. Limitless or unregulated competition can cause much harm.	Cooperation is boundless. It has no limitations. One can go to any extent to help others.
5.	Competition requires qualities such as strong aspirations. Self-confidence, the desire to earn name and fame in society, the spirit of adventure and the readiness to suffer and to struggle.	As CH Cooley has pointed out cooperation requires qualities such as kindness, sympathy, concern for others, mutual understanding and some amount of readiness to help others.
6.	But the competition may cause satisfaction as well as dissatisfaction, anxiety, indefiniteness and uncertain.	Cooperation brings people satisfaction and contentment.

CONCLUSION

The individual in a society are undergoing strains of mutual conflict or competition or cooperation in their various contacts. This interaction is usually based on social processes. Social interaction depends on two fundamental factors—social contact and communication. In this process of human interaction, the first phase is a social contact. Society is based on social interactions and naturally we can understand their importance in the growth of social process. Hence their study is essential for understanding social relations.

BIBLIOGRAPHY

1. Clyde Handrick. Perspectives in Social Psychology, Lawrence Elbaum Association, Publishers, New Jersey, 1977.
2. Cohen E. Human Behavior in the Concentration Camp. Jonathan Cape, London, 1954.
3. Cooper and McGangh. Integrating Principles of Social Psychology. Eurasia Publishing House (Pvt) Ltd, New Delhi, 1970.
4. Coser L. The Functions of Social Conflict. Free Press, New York, 1956.
5. Coutu W. Emergent human nature, Alfred A. Knopf, Inc. New York, 1949.
6. Cyril S Belshaw. The Condition of Social Performance. Rontledge and Kegan Paul, London, 1969.
7. Daniel Katz, Robert L Khan. The Social Psychology of Organizations, Wiley Eastern Private Ltd., New Delhi, 1970.
8. Drucker PF. The Concept of the Corporation. Mentor (c. 1946), New York, 1964.
9. Dubin R. Human Relations in Administration Prentice-Hall, Englewood Cliffs, NJ 1951.
10. Dunlap K. Religion: Its functions in Human, McGraw-Hill Book Co., Inc., New York, 1946.
11. Edgar Vinkacke W, Warner R Wilson. Dimensions of Social Psychology, DB Taraporevala Sons and Co Pvt Ltd, Mumbai, 1973.

28 *Culture*

DEFINITIONS

1. **Culture:** Culture as the cumulative creations of man. He also regards culture as the handiwork of man and medium through which he achieves his ends. Culture has accumulation of thoughts, values and objects. It is the social heritage acquired by us from proceeding generations through learning, as distinguished from biological heritage which is passed on to us automatically through genes.
2. **Dionysian culture:** The Dionysian culture is marked by high emotionalism, aggressiveness, individualism, superficiality, prestige and Competitiveness.
3. **Apollonian culture:** The apollonian culture characterized by qualities such as self-control, even-temperedness, moderation, mutual understanding, mutual assistance and cooperativeness.
4. **Cultural change:** Cultural change embraces all changes occurring in any branch of culture including art, science, technology, philosophy, etc., as well as change in the forms and rules of social organization.
5. **Cultural diffusion:** Cultural diffusion is the process by which the cultural traits invented and discovered in one society will spread directly or indirectly to other societies. In the course of transmission of this, it may be difficult to trace the origin of the cultural trait.
6. **Civilization:** Civilization refers to those devices and instruments by which nature is controlled. It includes material and technological equipment like printing press, locomotive, and machine-gun, television, teleprinter, typewriter, aeroplane. It also includes the whole apparatus of economic and political organization like our schools, colleges, currency, banks, parliament, insurance schemes, etc.
7. **Acculturation:** Acculturation is a process whereby an individual or a group acquires the cultural characteristics of another through direct contact and interaction. From an individual point of view, this is a process of social learning similar to that of adult socialization in which linguistic communication (language) plays an important role.
8. **Social telesis:** Social telesis is a planned progress and purposeful use of natural and social forces. It is a total process of cultural transformation, e.g. adult education, satellite programs, free education are a powerful indicator for quality of life, social change, social development and positive social change. Bogardus describes it as an economic development, regional development, and rural development.
9. **Enculturation:** When a growing child learns to confirm to his own cultural tradition, it is known as enculturation It involves numerous means of cultural transmission. Some of these are explicit.

Adults and peer groups teach children the beliefs they are to hold and act out the appropriate ways to behave. Children also learn facts of a culture in many ways. They identify with adults, unconsciously picking up appropriate behavior patterns, ways of thinking and feeling. Enculturation includes more than the process of growing up. Cultural learning continues throughout a person's life.

10. **Cultural lag:** The strain that exists between two correlated parts of culture that change unequal rates of speed may be interpreted as a lag in the part, this is changing at slower rates for the one lag behind the other. We accept the material aspects of another culture without any difficulty, but our values, beliefs, norms, morality, etc. will change only very slowly.

INTRODUCTION

Culture is a basic concept in sociology, anthropology because culture is what makes humans unique in the animal kingdom. Man is an animal with culture. Human social structure from the simplest family to the most complex corporations depends on culture for its existence. But although societies cannot exist without cultures, the two are not the same thing. Culture consists of commonly accepted and expected ideas, attitudes, values and habits of individuals which they learn in connection with social living. For the individual in the early years of life, culture is of enormous aid in learning to get on more effectively in the world. An understanding of human culture, says Stuart Chase, enlarges one's perspective. He shows us how all people have similar needs, but meet those needs by habits, customs and beliefs which are peculiar to each group.

Culture has been defined in a number of ways, some thinkers include in culture all the major social components that bind men together in a society. Culture is that knowledge which a new generation subjectively derives from the previous one. Culture is an essential intergradient of human society. The essential point in regard to culture is that it is acquired by man as a member of society and persists through tradition. These points of acquisition and tradition have been emphasized by Tylor and Redfield in their definitions. The essential factors in this acquisition through tradition are the ability to learn from the group. A man learns his behavior and behavior which is learnt denotes his culture. Singing, talking, dancing and eating belong to the category of culture. Moreover, the behaviors are not his own but are shared by others. They have been transmitted to him by someone, be it his school teacher, his parents or friend.

DEFINITIONS OF CULTURE

1. Culture is that complex whole which includes knowledge, belief, art, morals, law, custom and any other capacities and habits acquired by man as a member of society—*Tylor*.
2. An organized body of conventional understanding manifested in art and artifact which persists through tradition characterized human group—*Redfield*.
3. Culture is the quintessence of all natural goods of the world and of those gifts and qualities, while belonging to man, lie beyond the immediate sphere of his needs and wants—*Joseph Piper*.
4. Culture is a symbolic, continuous, cumulative and progressive process—*White*.
5. Culture is the product of artifacts (products of industry) agrofacts (products of agriculture) sociofacts (social organization) and mentifacts (language, religion, etc.)
6. Culture refers to a social heritage that is all the knowledge, beliefs, customs and skills that are available to the members of a society—*Clyde Kluckhohn* (1951).
7. Culture is the socially transmitted system of idealized ways in which knowledge and practice produce and maintain as they change in time—*AW Green*.

8. Culture is the expression of our nature in our modes of living and thinking; intercourse in our literature, in religion, in recreation and enjoyment—*MacIver.*

9. Culture is the sum total of human achievements, material as well as non-material, capable of transmission, sociologically, i.e. by tradition and communication, vertically as well as horizontally—*Mazumdar HT.*

10. Culture is the entire accumulation of artificial objects, conditions, tools, techniques, ideas, symbols, and behavior patterns peculiar to a group of people possessing a certain consistency of its own, and capable of transmission from one generation to anther—*Cooley, Argell and Carr.*

11. Culture includes those general attitudes, views of life, and specific manifestation of civilization that give a particular people its distinctive place in the world—*Sapir.*

12. Culture is the complex whole that consists of everything we think and do and have as members of society—*Bierstedt.*

13. Culture is the total content of the physico-social, bio-social and psycho-social products man has produced and the socially created mechanisms through which these social products operate—*Anderson and Parker.*

14. The culture of a people may be defined as the sum total of the material and intellectual equipment whereby they satisfy their biological and social needs and adapt themselves to their environment—*Ralph Piddington.*

15. Culture is totally of group ways of thought and action duly accepted and followed by a group of people—*AF Walter Paul.*

16. Culture is the sum total of integrated learned behavior patterns which are characteristics of the members of a society and which is, therefore, not the result of biological inheritance—*EA Hoebel.*

17. Culture refers to the social mechanisms of behavior and to the physical and symbolic products of this behavior—*Lungberg.*

18. Culture is the sum total of man's efforts to adjust himself to his environment and to improve his modes of living—*Koenig.*

19. Culture is the expression of our nature in our modes of living and our thinking, intercourse, in our literature, in religion, in reaction and enjoyment—*MacIver.*

20. Culture is the embodiment in customs, tradition, etc. of learning of a social group over the generation—*Lapiere.*

21. Culture is the handiwork of man and the medium through which he achieves his ends—*Malinowski.*

22. Culture is an organized body of conventional understanding manifest in art and artifact, which, persisting through tradition, characteristics of a human group—*Redfield.*

23. Culture consists in the instruments constituted by men to assist him in satisfying his wants—*CC North.*

24. Culture is the super organic environment as distinguished from the organic or physical, the world of plants and animals—*Spencer.*

25. Culture is an accumulation of thoughts, values and objects, it is the social heritage acquired by us from preceding generalities through learning, as distinguished from the biological heritage which is passed on to us automatically through the genes—*Graham Wallas.*

26. Culture is the embodiment in customs, tradition, etc. of learning of a social group over the generation—*Lapiere.*

CLASSIFICATION OF CULTURES

An American anthropologist Ruth Benedict in her patterns of culture published in 1935 has classified cultures into two types on the basis of their ethos or distinctive feeling tones. Sumner defines ethos as the totality of characteristics traids by which a group, i.e. a society is individualized and differentialed from others. She has made a comparison of three tribal cultures—the Zuni, the Dobuan and the Cacti Indian and shown how each has its own unique impact on personality. The two types of cultures which she has mentioned are: 1. The Apollonian culture; 2. The Dionysian culture.

Apollonian Culture

It is characterized by qualities such as self-control, even-temperedness, moderation, mutual understanding, mutual assistance and cooperativeness. As Ruth Benedict has pointed out the Zuni tribe of the southwestern USA represents the Apollonian culture. In the Zuni tribe or society which represents the Apollonian culture; the members reveal characteristics which are peculiar to their culture. The Zuni people dislike individualism, violence and power. They respect moderation and modesty, co-operation and mutual understanding. They are emotionally undisturbed. The spirit of competition is virtually absent in them.

Dionysian Culture

It is marked by high emotionalism, aggressiveness, individualism, superficially, prestige and competitiveness. According to Ruth Benedict, the Dobuans of Melanesia and the Kwakiutl Indians represent the Dionysian culture. In the Dobuan and Kwakiutl societies, which are Dionysian in character, members existing traits common on their culture. The Dobuans make virtues of ill-will and treachery. They fight against one another for possession of good things in life. Suspicion, cruelty, animosity and malignancy are traits of almost all Dobuans.

The Kwakiutl Indians of the Pacific Northwest coast define everything that happens in terms of the Pacific Northwest coast, define everything that happens in terms of triumph or shame. For them, life is a constant struggle to put one's rivals to shame. They destroy the material possessions of the defeated. The defeated resort to sulking or to acts of desperation. Benedict has tried to show that it is possible to identify the influence of the total culture on personality. She has tried to establish that each culture will produce its special type or types of personality. It is true that her study reveals the mutual interplay of culture and socialization in conditioning personality. Culture provides for the way in which personality is to be developed. But personality as such is developed through the process of socialization. It may also be argued that different ways and means of socialization may produce different personalities. Individuals try to develop their personalities in accordance with their cultural ideas and expectations.

CHARACTERISTICS OF CULTURE

1. **Culture is an acquired quality, not innate:** Traits learnt through socialization, habits and thoughts are what is called culture. Man acquires the cultural behavior because he has the capacity of symbolic communication.
2. **Culture is social, not individual:** Every individual takes some part in the transmission and communication of culture, but culture is social rather than individual. It is inclusive of the expectation of the members of groups. Man cannot create or generate culture while existing apart from the group.

3. **Culture is idealistic:** In culture are included those ideal patterns or ideal norms of behavior according to which the members of society attempt to conduct themselves. Society accepts these ideals, norms and patterns.
4. **Culture is communicative:** In this way culture is communicated from one generation to the next. As a result of this, culture is constantly accumulating. The new generation benefits by the experiences of the older generation through the communicability of culture. In this way culture becomes semi-temporary and remains unaffected by the extinction of a group or an individual.
5. **Culture fulfills some needs:** Culture fulfills those ethical and social needs which are ends in themselves. Social habits are included in culture. Habits can be formed of these activities only which tend to fulfill some needs. Without fulfilling these needs culture cannot exist.
6. **Culture has the characteristic of adaptation:** Culture is constantly undergoing change in concurring to the environment and due to this transformation it is constantly being adapted to external forces but once it is developed, the influences of the natural environment begin to decrease. Besides, the various aspects of culture are also undergoing development and some internal adaptation among them consequently being necessitated.
7. **Culture has the quality of becoming integrated:** Cultural possesses an order and a system. Its various parts are integrated with each other and any new element which is introduced is also integrated. Those cultures which are more open to external influences are comparatively more heterogeneous but nevertheless some degree of integration is evident in all cultures.
8. **Culture evolves into more complex forms through division of labor** which develops special skills and increases the independence society's members.
9. **Language is the chief vehicle of culture:** Man lives not only in the present but also in the past and future. This he is enabled to do because he possesses language which transmits to him what was learnt in the past and enables him to transmit the accumulated wisdom.

According to Hames and Joseph (1980):

1. Culture is a group's blueprint for acceptable ways of thinking and behaving.
2. Though culture is universal in man's experience, it is unique for each group (Alfred Weber–Culture is unique and civilization is universal).
3. Culture is transmitted from generation to generation.
4. Culture is stable, but continuously adapting.
5. Culture is affected by the environment including such variables as climate, geographical location, food resources and natural resources.
6. Culture does not affect man's basic physiological needs (such as need for food or water) but people from different cultural groups may vary genetically.
7. All cultures have four components in common: Art, forms, language, institutions and technology.

RELATION OF CULTURE AND CIVILIZATION

Civilization is the Developed Form of Culture

1. JL Gillin and JP Gillin, "Civilization is a more complex and evolved form of culture".
2. AW Green has written, "A culture becomes civilization only when it possesses written languages, science, philosophy, a specialized division of labor and a complex technology and political system".
3. Ancient culture did not posses all these elements and would consequently be considered as having no civilization.

4. Franz Boas, Ogburn and Nimkoff also treated civilization as a state which follows culture.
5. Ogburn has written that civilization may be defined as the later phase of superior organic culture.

Weber's Opinion

According to Weber, civilization includes useful material objects and the methods of producing and using them whereas culture consists of the ideals, values and the mental and emotional aspects of a group. Murton, Richard, Thurnwald and many other sociologists have subscribed to this opinion. PA Sorokin has opposed it. But this is the opinion most widely prevalent among the sociologist today.

Opinions of MacIver and Page

1. According to MacIver and Page, civilization includes all those things by means of which some other objective is attained such as typewriters, press, lathe, motor, etc. in civilization are included both basic technology which means the authority of man over natural phenomena as well as social technology or model which controls man's behavior.
2. On the other hand, culture comprehends such elements as religion, art, philosophy, literature, music, etc. which bring satisfaction and pleasure to man.
3. In the words of MacIver and Page, it is the expression of our nature in our models of living and thinking, in our everyday intercourse, in art, in literature, in recreation and enjoyment.

DIFFERENCE BETWEEN CULTURE AND CIVILIZATION

To understand the term culture clearly, it would be described to distinguish it from civilization. Writes have many different concepts of civilization. Civilization is considered to have begun at a time of writing and advent of metals. As history beings with writing, so does civilization. Ogburn and Nimkoff conceived of civilization as the latter phase of the super organic culture. Some based civilization on civil organization as contrasted to clan or kinship organization. Since civil organization was found more commonly in large towns, so people living in these towns were called civilized. AA Goldenweiser used the word civilization as synonymous to culture and applied the term to non-literate peoples.

1. **Civilization has a precise standard of measurement but not culture:** The universal standard of civilization is utility because civilization is a means. Culture has no similar qualitative or quantitative standard of measurement because culture is an end in self. The elements, ideas, values and thoughts, etc. of culture change are accordance with the time and place.
2. **Civilization is always advancing but not culture**: The various constituents of civilization, example, machines, means of transportation, and communication, etc. are constantly progressing. But concerning culture, it cannot be asserted that the art, literature, thoughts or ideals of today are superior to those of the past.
3. **Civilization is passed on without effort, but not culture:** Objects comprehended by civilization have utility and are connected with the external life of man. Hence, they can be easily adopted from one generation to another or from one country to another but culture is not communicated and adopted with equal facility because it is related to an inner tendency and can be adopted only after the appropriate inner development.
4. **Civilization is borrowed without change or loss; but not culture:** When civilization is borrowed by a country or a generation other than its originator, it does not suffer any deterioration or loss or damage. Railway, motor cars, machines, etc. are borrowed as they are but the elements of culture such as religion, art, literature, ideas, etc. can never be borrowed in their original

character. For example, the Indian Christian is found to posses many elements, borrowed from the Hindu and Muslim religions which are not to be found in their western counterpart.

5. **Culture is internal and an end while civilization is external and a means:** Civilization is inclusive of external things, culture is related to internal thoughts, feelings, ideas, values, etc. civilization is the means for the expression and manifestation of culture. It is the body and culture is the soul.

6. **Civilization is always advancing, but not culture:** According to MacIver, civilization not only marches, it marches always ahead, provided there is no catastrophic break of social continuity in the same direction. Civilization shows a persistent upward trend. It is unlined and cumulative and trends to advance indefinitely. Since man invented automobile, it has continuously improved.

COMPONENTS OF CULTURE

1. **Cultural traits:** Cultural traits are the single elements or smallest units of a culture. They are the units of observation which when put together constitute culture. According to Hoebel, cultural traits are repeatedly irreducible unit of learned behavior pattern of material product thereof. Any culture can be seen as to include thousands of such units. Thus shaking hands, touching the feet, tipping hats, the kiss on the cheeks as gesture of affection, giving seats to ladies first, saluting the flag, wearing white saris at mourning, taking vegetarian diets, walking bare-footed, sprinkling water on the idols, carring kirpans, growing beard and hair, eating in brass utensils, etc. are cultural traits.

2. **Cultural complex:** According to Hoebel, cultural complexes are nothing but larger clusters of traits organized about some nuclear points of references. Culture traits as we known, do not usually appear singly or independently. They are customarily associated with other related traits to form cultural complex. The importance of a single trait is indicated when it fits into a cluster of traits, each one of which performs a significant role in the total complex. Examples are kneeling before idol and taking prashad from the priest.

3. **Cultural pattern:** A cultural pattern is formed when traits and complexes become related to each other in functional roles. Each culture complex has a role to play in society consists of a number of cultural complexes. Thus the Indian cultural pattern consists of Gandhism, spiritualism, joint family, caste system and ruralism.

Clerk Wissler Classification of Cultural Pattern

Sl.No.	Classifications
1.	Speech and language
2.	Material traits–Food habits, shelter, transportation, dress, utensils, tools, weapons, occupations and industries
3.	Art
4.	Mythology and scientific knowledge
5.	Religious practices
6.	Family and social system
7.	Property
8.	Government
9.	War

Kimball Young Classification of Cultural Pattern

Sl.No.	Classifications
1.	Patterns of communication: Gestures and language
2.	Methods of objects for providing for men's physical welfare: Food-getting, personal care, shelter, tools, etc.
3.	Means or techniques of travel and transportation of goods and services
4.	Exchange of goods and services, barter, trade, commerce, occupations
5.	Forms of property: Real and personal
6.	The sex and family pattern: Marriage and divorce, forms of kinship, relation, guardianship, inheritance
7.	Social control and institutions of government: Mores, public opinion, organized state: laws and political officers
8.	Artistic expression: Architecture, painting, culture, music, literature, dancing
9.	Recreational and leisure time interests and activities
10.	Mythology and philosophy
11.	Religious and magical ideas and practices
12.	Science
13.	Cultural structuring of basic interactional process.

Universals, Alternatives and Specialties

Linton has pointed out that some culture traits are necessary to all members of the society, while other traits are shared by only some members. The traits which are followed by all members are called universals. As a matter of fact, these traits are so widely shared that, without them, one is obviously different or an outcast. Man must clothe certain parts of the body. One must be monogamous, one should drive on the left of the street, he must condemn free love and infanticides are the universals of Indian culture. Alternatives are different activities allowed and accepted for achieving the same end. It may be noted that alternatives in one society may be universals elsewhere or universals may be alternatives. Specialties are elements of the culture which are shared by some but not all groups within a society.

Subcultures

Subcultures are the cultural traits of a particular group or category. They are of course related to the general culture of the society. Yet are distinguishable from it. Thus, the cultures of occupational groups, religious groups, caste, social class, age group, sex group and many other are sub-groups. The Hindu culture is a sub-culture of Indian culture.

Cultural Relativism

The concept of cultural relativity states the standards of rightness and wrongness (values) and of usage and effectiveness (customs) are relative to the given of which they are a part. In this most extreme form, it holds that every custom is valid in terms of its own cultural setting. In practical terms, it means the anthropolists and sociologists learn to suspend judgment, to strive to understand what goes on from the point of view of the people being studied is, to achieve empathy, for the sake of humanistic perception and scientific accuracy.

Contracultures

The term contraculture is applied to designate those groups which not only differ from the prevailing patterns but sharply challenge them. Thus a group of dacoits has its own norms and standards which are compulsory for all the members of the group but these norms and standards sharply differ from conventional prevailing patterns. The people trained in these norms are influenced against the dominant cultural norms; hence the term contraculture.

Cultural Area

Culture as we have seen above is specified to a group or category of persons. The cultural traits and complexes of some societies may be similar. The societies having similar cultural traits and complexes constitute cultural area. Such societies are generally those which live in similar natural environment.

Cultural Lag

According to Ogburn, a situation in which one part of culture, i.e. non-material cultures lags behind the material and causes an imbalance or disharmony in the society. The strain that exists between two correlated parts of culture that change at unequal rates of speed may be interpreted as a lag in the part, that is changing at the slower rate for the one lags behind the other. We accept the material aspects of another culture without any difficulty, but our values, beliefs, norms, morality. etc. will change only very slowly.

Cultural Complex

The simple unit of culture is the cultural trait. These cultural traits develop concurrently and collect together like a branch of flowers and again their importance in terms of the degree of significance they have for the behavior of human being. This bunch of collected traits is called a cultural complex. These culture complexes are formed according to the various needs of life. In this way cultural complexes concerning food habits, the different occupations, etc. can seen in different cultures. Examples of culture complexes found in Indian culture are in the form of the caste system, joint family system, the principle of karma, etc. metallic utensils are indicative of the culture complex concerning food habits in Indian culture.

Cultural Diffusion

According to MacIver and Page, cultural diffusion is the most important cause of social development. All the great cultures developed as a result of the mutual contacts of various cultures. The culture which grew upon the banks of Nile influenced India. Indian thoughts reached China and they made important contribution to western civilization. Greek culture was influenced by the Egyptian culture. Rome was affected by Greek culture. In much the same way the modern cultures are adopting from one another. Ogburn and Nimkoff have written that the transference of culture parts from one sphere to another or from one part of culture to another is called diffusion.

Diffusion of this kind is evinced in most of the objects of the modern world such as railways, motor car, aeroplane, cinema, telephone, telegraph, television, etc. not only machines and tools spread from one country to another, but the same is true of thoughts which spread from one country to another. The following factors are influential in the process of diffusion: Relations and communications, need of and desire for new traits, competition with old traits and objections to them and the respect and recognition of those who bring new traits.

Cultural Growth

The developmental of culture is a continuous process. In this process while the experiences of proponents of one culture are accumulated and handled down from one generation to another on the one hand, new elements from other cultures are introduced through accommodation, cross fertilization and diffusion on the other hand, and culture progresses as a result of their unification. The existing development culture of any country is a result of this process carried out over a period of hundreds and thousands of years. In this development the rate of progress is not uniform. At times it is slow while at other times it is relatively fast: Sometimes it is moving towards progress, at other towards deterioration. In order to understand cultural growth properly, it is necessary to understand those processes of cultural growth. The processes of cultural growth are:

1. **Accumulation:** To begin with, individual experiments with an object about which he knows virtually nothing. Of the various experiments he makes, he discards those which have proved fruitless and adopts those for subsequent application which have been successful. In this way the experience gained in this experimentation is accumulated and passed on by one generation to its successor as the social heritage. The development of language has been of tremendous value in this accumulation. New experiments continue to be made, in addition to these experiments. Inventions increase along with the increase in needs. It has been said that necessity is the mother of invention. In this way, both the material and non-material aspects of culture progress through such accumulation.

2. **Diffusion:** Cultural growth results not merely from accumulation but also by the adaptation of novel concepts from other cultures. Accordingly, diffusion applies to the adaptation of new ideas by one individual or society from another individual or society. Almost all the cultures of the world are adopting innumerable new ideas and things from the modern western culture through diffusion.

3. **Accommodation:** The new ideas which have been acquired through diffusion have to be accommodated with the other features of the culture. It is only through having accommodated themselves with Indian culture that the numerous objects and various elements of western culture which have been acquired and adopted in India have become a part of its life and have added to its progress.

4. **Cross-fertilization:** The conjunction of two cultures is beneficial to both since it does not happen that one should borrow from the other exclusively. This process of mutual `give and take' is called cross-fertilization.

5. **Acculturation:** When such a conjunction of two cultures occurs, causing cultural growth, and they are intimately related rather than identified, the process of contraculturation also sets in. it is the opposite of the process of acculturation. For example, many English things were adopted in India but the Swedish movement and the development of nationalism abolished and condemned many things of Western origin.

6. **Assimilation:** In this process of cultural conjunction, when one culture becomes as intimate with another as to lose its individuality it is called assimilation.

EVOLUTION OF CULTURE

1. For the century and many archeologists have dug up the tools, weapons, pottery, idols, coins and other material things of peoples who have long since died out, in search of clues to their social life. Such evidences, however, do not reveal the origin of culture; they indicate its antiquity.

2. If they reveal something about the evolution of culture, it is only about its material aspects. To trace the origin of a specific cultural trait is difficult. It is lost in the mists of antiquity. However, the basic process valued in cultural development is discovery and invention. All cultural traits—material as well as non material—have been invented at some time and in some places by some person.

3. But no single invention contributes very much to development of a culture; it is only an addition to what already exists: Moreover, the invention though achieved by one individual, has itself been made possible by forces that grow out of the culture.

4. The inventor or a person is not, therefore, the cause of the invention, he is only the agent of cultural conditions that bring about a modification of the culture.

5. Although culture develops trait, a culture is actually a patterning of interdependent trait complexes. A trait does not evolve independent of the entire complex of which it is a part, not does it operate independent of the other traits. The existing cultural traits influence the invention of the new trait.

6. An invention, whether material or non-material is improvement over the existing cultural traits. It is only partly new. It is a new synthesis. Everywhere that has been the case. The compositions and combine them into what is considered to be a new song.

7. The inventor takes elements from a variety of old or existing modes of living and runs them together into a new mode of living. The importance of the inventor, however, may not be minimized. His invention, though may be regarded an improvement over or a synthesis of existing cultural traits, yet he does contribute purpose and endeavor to it.

8. Intent upon the creation of a new idea or a new mechanical device, he proceeds to try this or that combination of cultural element. This implies initiative and perseverance in him. Unless there are people in a society with the required initiative, there will be no new culture development and the society may stagnate.

9. It may also be noted that for cultural development men must become discontent with some of the many things as they are, and provoked by their discontent must be led to find a way out. They must feel that thing should not be the way they are. If they think that disease, famine, war, political corruption, rising prices, and moral depredation are acts of God that cannot be avoided the society will lose its vigor.

NEED OF CULTURE IN MAN

Man differs from animal species in that he lives in a world of ideas. He acts and reacts in terms of ideas about objects and organisms. The animals live only in the present. They lack language; their knowledge is limited to instincts plus what is learned by direct observation. Such learning can never accumulate. Only man simultaneously inhabits past, present and future. He possesses the capacity to vocalize, to respond, to represent, articulate and to learn from the stimulus-response relationship. These peculiar elements in the makeup of man provided a background against which culture arose. The rudiments of culture developed by one generation serve as foundation-stone to the next generation which makes its own addition. Man is born in the stream of culture and must continuously swim in it if he is to live as a member of society.

CULTURAL VARIABILITY

Culture is a distinctive character of a nation, of a group or a period of history. It is why we speak of the culture of India, of Japan or of America. A popular joke about members of different nations gives us an insight into different cultures of different societies. Once three students—Japanese, an Indian, and an American visited the Niagra falls. The Japanese boy was bewitched by the beauty of the grand spectacle, while the Indian student began to philosophize about the Supreme Being manifested in this phenomenon of nature. The silent communion of the two Orientals with the Niagara Falls was sharply interrupted as the American student asked: friends, how much horse-power is there in these falls. in India non-violence is considered to be a great virtue, while in Russia violence is a part of the Russian culture. Among certain groups men and women mix and move freely on the roads, whereas among other groups the free mixing of men and women is severely condemned. Thus we find group variations of cultural behavior among different peoples over the world and also among the same peoples at different periods of history. These variations are not to be interpreted as merely amusing and motivated. The factors influences the cultural variability are:

1. **Historical accidents:** Some of the customs whose origin is difficult to trace must have been originated due to some personal or group unconscious behavior. A man might have done unconsciously a particular action; others imitated him and through imitation by and large it becomes a custom, a part of culture.

2. **Geographical environment:** In India snake workshop is due to abundance of reptiles; the marriage dates according to the harvesting time and agricultural pursuits of the people. Geographical factors play very important part in individual and group living, these are chiefly limiting rather than directly causative. Cultures may vary even when the geographic conditions are the same.

3. **Mobility of human organism:** Man has always adjusted himself to his natural environment, to his group and his fellows and on account of his constant adjustment cultural behavior has shown great variability among the same people during periods of history.

4. **Inventions and discoveries:** Inventions and discoveries also bring about cultural variability. A country which is technologically advanced will have a culture different from the one which is technologically backward.

5. **Individual peculiarities or personal eccentricities:** Sometimes individual peculiarities or personal eccentricities also influence cultural behavior. Gandhi cap has come to our culture through individual peculiarity. Not very unoften the conscious efforts of an individual may change the current modes of behavior. The change to Khadi has also an economic significance.

6. **Change in the modes of production:** Karl Marx held that the mode of production is the sole determinants of the culture of a people—their art, morals, customs, laws, literature, etc. any change in the mode of production affects the culture.

7. **Dominant cultural themes:** The superiority of men over women is the main theme around which Indian culture is built. Egypt was organized about the world themes. The American society is organized around the themes of free enterprise and equality. Marxism is the dominant theme of Russian culture.

FUNCTIONS OF CULTURE

1. **Culture makes man a human being:** It is culture that makes the human animal a man, regulates his conduct and prepares him for group life. It provides to him a complete design for living. It teaches him what type of food he should take and in what manner, how he should cover himself and behave with his fellows, how he should speak with the people and how he should cooperate or compete with others.

2. **Culture provides solutions for complicated situations:** Culture provides man with a set of behavior even for complicated situations. It has so thoroughly influenced him that often he does not require any external force to keep himself in conformity with social requirements.

3. **Culture provides traditional interpretations to certain situations:** Through culture man gets traditional interpretations for many situations according to which he determines his behavior. For example, if a cat crosses his way he postpones the journey.
4. **Culture keeps social relationships intact:** Culture has importance not only for man but also for the group. Had there been no culture there would have been no group life. By regulating the behavior of the people and satisfying their primary drives pertaining to hunger, shelter and sex it has been able to maintain group life.
5. **Culture broadens the vision of the individual:** Culture has given a new vision to the individual by providing him a set of rules for the cooperation of the individuals. Culture teaches him to think himself a part of the larger whole. It provides him with the concepts of family, state, nation and class and makes possible the coordination and division of labor.
6. **Culture creates new needs:** Culture also creates new needs and new drives, for example, thirst for knowledge, and arranges for their satisfaction. It satisfies the aesthetic, moral and religious interests of the members of the group.

CONCLUSION

Man is not only a social animal but also a cultural being. Man's social life has been made possible because of culture. Culture is something that has elevated him from the level of animal to the heights of man. Man cannot survive as man without culture. It represents the entire achievements of mankind. Culture and society are interdependent. Culture possesses continuity and extends beyond the life-time of those who possess, create and utilize it. Culture is passed from the old to the new members. Culture provides knowledge which is essential for physical, social and intellectual existence of man. Society and culture and social culture are mutually related concepts. There is no culture without human society. There can be no society without individuals. Culture is human accomplishments acquired and passed on in terms of social inheritance. Culture is learned behavior acquired by man as a member of society.

BIBLIOGRAPHY

1. Abram Kardiner. The Psychological Frontier of Society. Columbia University Press, New York 1945.
2. Alfred R, Lindesmith, Anseim L Strauss. Readings in Social Psychology. Rinehart and Winston, Chicago Hort, 1969.
3. Allport GW. Personality: A Psychological Interpretation, Holt, New York, 1937.
4. Allport FH. Social Psychology, Houghton Mifflin, Boston, 1924.
5. Allport GW, Kramer BM. Some Roots of Prejudice, J of Psychol; 1946;22:9-39.
6. Allport GW. The Nature of Prejudice, Reading, Mass. Addison Wesley Publishing Co., Inc, 1954a.
7. Jack H Curtin. Social Psychology. McGraw-Hill Book Company, Inc, New York, 1960.
8. James W. The principles of psychology (Vol.1) Henry Holt & Co., Inc., New York 1890.
9. John W Kinch. Social Psychology, 1978.
10. Katz E, P Lazarsfeld. Personal Influence. The part played by people in the flow of mass communication, Free Press, New York 1955.
11. Kohier W. Gestalt psychology. Live Right Publishing Corp, New York , 1929.
12. Krech D, Crhuchfield RS. Elements of Psychology, Alfred A. Knopf, Inc, New York, 1958.

29 *Population*

DEFINITIONS

1. **Population health:** Population health can be defined as the attainment of the greatest possible biological, psychological and social well-being of the population as an entity and of its individual members. Health is derived from opportunities and choices provided to the public as well as the population's response to those choices.
2. **Population explosion:** Population explosion means very rapid and unprecedented growth of population. The problem of over population has become a world phenomenon today. Most of the developing countries of the world are experiencing this problem. The population of the world started increasing since 1650 and in the 20th century its growth gained momentum and reached aclimax between 1960 and 1970.
3. **Demographic process:** Demography as understood today is the scientific study of human population. It deals with five demographic process namely fertility, mortality, marriage, migration and social mobility. These five processes are continually at work within a population determining size, composition and distribution.
4. **Growth rate:** When the crude death rate is subtracted from the crude birth rate, the net residual is the current annual growth rate, exclusive of migration.
5. **Sex ratio:** Sex ratio is defined as the number of females per 1000 males. One of the basic demographic characteristics of the population is the sex composition. The sex composition of the population is affected by differentials in mortality conditions of males and females, sex selective migration and sex ratio at birth.
6. **Urbanization:** Increase in urban population has been attributed both to natural growth (through births) and migration from villages because of employment opportunities, attraction of better living conditions are availability of social services such as education, health, transport, entertainment, etc.
7. **Life expectancy:** Life expectancy or expectation of life at a given age is the average number of years which a person of that age may expect to live, demographers consider life-expectancy as one the best indications of a country levels of development and of the over all health status of its population.
8. **Fertility:** By fertility, it is meant the actual bearing of children. Some demographers prefer to use the world natality in place of fertility. A women's reproductive period is roughly from 15 to 45 years—a period of 30 years.

9. **Demography:** Demography is a branch of science which studies the human population.
10. **Population density:** Population density means number of persons living in 1 square kilometer. Density of population is continuously increasing in India. In 1951, India's density of population was 117 persons per square kilometer, which has increased to 324 persons/square kilometer in 2000.

Demography is the science of population. It studies the total number of people in a given area, the growth, decline, age composition, sex ratio and other demographic processes like fertility, morality and migration. Population of India is increasing rapidly. In spite of economic development, the standard of living is low. The increase in population has created a number of problems like poverty, unemployment, food and shelter problems, education and health problems. The growth of population adversely affected the economy of the country. Every year 17 million people are added to existing population. The rapidly growing population retards all our development efforts.

SOCIETY AND POUPLATION

The science of population called demography represents a fundamental approach to the understanding of human society. In a general sense, the task of a demographer is to ascertain the number of people in a given area, the changes that have taken place over the last years and to estimate on this basis the future trend. He takes into consideration the births, deaths and migration. The fertility, mortality and migration are of concern not only to a demographer, these are important to a sociologist as well. All these are to a greater extent socially determined and socially determining.

Fertility is the incidence of childbearing in a country's population. During her childbearing years, from the onset of menstruation to menopause a woman capable of bearing more than twenty children. Demographers gauge fertility using the crude birth rate, the number of live births in a given year for every thousand people in population. To calculate a crude birth rate, divide the number of live births in the year by the society's total population and multiply the result by 1000. A country's birth rate is described as crude because it is based on the entire population, not just women in their childbearing years.

Population size also reflects mortality, the incidence of death in a country's population. To measure mortality, demographer uses a crude death rate, the number of deaths in a given year for every thousand people in a population. This time we take the number of deaths in a year divided by the total population and multiply the result by 1000. The third useful demographic measure is the infant mortality rate, the number of deaths among infants under one year of age for each thousand live births in a given year. To compute infant mortality, divide the number of deaths of children under one year of age by the number of live births during the same year and multiply the result by 1000.

Population size is also affected by migration, the movement of people into and out of a specified territory. Movement into a territory or immigration is measured as an in-migration rate, calculated as the number of people entering an area for every thousands people in the population. Movement out of a territory or emigration is measured in terms of an out-migration rate, the number of people leaving for every thousand people. Both types of migration usually occur at once; the difference is the net-migration rate.

Population growth: Fertility, mortality, and migration all affect the size of a society's population. In general, rich nations grow as much from immigration as from natural increase; poor nations grow almost entirely from natural increase. To calculate a population's natural growth rate, demographers subtract the crude death rate from the crude birth rate.

Population composition: Demographer also studies the makeup of society's population at a given point in time. One variable is the sex ratio, the number of males for every hundred females in a nation's population. A more complex measure is the age-sex pyramid, a graphic representation of the age and sex of a population.

HISTORY AND THEORY OF POPULATION GROWTH

In the past, people favored large families because human labor was the key to productivity. Moreover, until rubber condoms appeared 150 years ago, the prevention of pregnancy was an uncertain proposition at best. But high death rates from widespread infectious diseases put a constant brake on population growth. Global population reached 3 billion by 1962 and 4 billion by 1974. In the rate of world population increase has slowed in recent years, but our planet passed the 5 million mark in 1987 and the 6 million mark in 1999. In previous century the world's population even double. In the twentieth century, it quadrupled. Currently the world is adding about 73 million people each year; 96 percent of this increase is in poor countries. Experts predict that the earth's population will reach up to 8 billion by 2050.

India is the world's second most populous country. According to the 1991 census India's population was 84.39 crore which has by the end of 1996 increased to 93.4 crore. According to projections made in a World Bank report, India's estimated population by 2150 will be over 1756 million against China's 1680 million. India will thereby overtake China and become the most populous country of the world. The world population report published by the United Nations population division revealed that world population estimated to be six billion in 1998 and annual addition to the world population in the next decade will average 97 million, the highest in history. Nearly all of this population growth will be in Africa, Asia and Latin America. Over half will reach 10 billion and in 2150 it is projected to be 11.6 billion.

Malthusian Theory

It was the sudden population growth two centuries ago that sparked the development of demography. Thomas Robert Malthus (1766-1834), an English economist and clergyman, warned that population increase would soon lead to social chaos. Malthus calculated that population would increase by what mathematicians call a geometric progression. Malthus concluded, world population would soon soar out of control. Food production would also increase, Malthus explained, but only in arithmetic progression because, even with new agricultural technology, farmland is limited. Thus Malthus presented a distressing vision of the future: People reproducing beyond what the planet could feed, leading ultimately widespread starvation. Malthus recognized that artificial birth control or abstinence might change the equation.

Fortunately, Malthus' prediction was flawed. First, by 1850, the European birth rate began to drop, partly because children were becoming an economic liability rather than an asset, and partly because people began using artificial birth control. Second, Malthus underestimated human ingenuity: modern irrigation techniques, fertilizers and pesticides have increased farm production far more than he would imagine. Some criticized Malthus for ignoring the role of social inequality in world abundance and famine. Karl Marx objected to viewing suffering as a law of nature rather than the curse of capitalism.

Demographic Transition Theory

A more complex analysis of population change is demographic transition theory, the thesis that population patterns reflect a society's level of technological development. It is explained as demographic consequences at four levels of technological development.

Stage-I: Very high birth rates because of the economic values of children and absence of birth control. Deaths rates are also high because of low living standards and limited medical technology. Outbreaks of disease neutralize births, so population rises and falls with only a modest overall increase. This was the case for thousands of years in Europe before the Industrial Revolution.

Stage-II: The onset of industrialization—brings a demographic transition as death rates fall due to greater food supplies and scientific medicine. But birth rates remain high, resulting in rapid population growth. It was during Europe's stage-2 that Malthus formulated his ideas, which explains his pessimistic view of the future. The world's poorest countries today are in this high-growth stage.

Stage-III: A mature industrial economy—the birth rate drops, curbing population growth once again. Fertility falls, first, because most children survive to adulthood and second, because high living standards make raising children from economic assets into economic liabilities. Smaller families, made possible by effective birth control, are also favored by women working outside the home. As birth rates follow death rates downward, population growth slows further.

Stage-IV: A postindustrial economy—the demographic transition is complete. The birth rates keep falling, partly because dual-income couples gradually become the norm and partly because the cost of raising children continues to rise. This trend, coupled with steady death rates, means that, at best, population grows only very slowly or even decreases. This is the case today in Japan, Europe and United States.

Critical evaluation of demographic transition theory suggests that the key to population control lies in technology. Instead of the runway population increase feared by Malthus, this theory sees technology reining in growth and spreading material plenty.

POPULATION CONTROL

Population Control Methods

Sl. No.	Methods	Description
1.	Family planning	In modern days family planning is considered as an indispensable method for population control. It highlights babies by choice and not by chance. It limits the size of the family.
1a.	Moral or self-restraint	This is self-control. It has many possible ways like celibacy, postponing marriage, raising age of marriage, etc.
1b.	Use of birth control	This method includes use of contraceptives, tablets, drugs, sterilization, tubectomy, vasectomy, abortion of unwanted child. Now-a-days family planning refers to this method.
2.	Rise in the age of marriage	Child marriages should be banned. Rise in the age of marriage will reduce reproductive span of woman. Minimum age for marriage for boys and girls should be increased if possible, from 21 to 24 and 18 to 21 years respectively.

Contd...

Contd...

3.	Improvement in status of women	This statement is proved true in the western countries. The educated and employed urban women exhibit a desire for small family. Social welfare schemes for couples going for permanent sterilization, tax benefits, educational help for two children, social security for the couple in their old age, etc. Incentives related to housing, jobs, loans, representation in civic bodies education for women help for the children, etc.
4.	Introduction of compulsory education	This develops a rational attitude towards life. It creates awareness among people.
5.	Internal migration	Population has to be equally distributed. Densly populated area and scarcely populated areas should be balanced. However, this is not an easy job.
6.	Change in tax structure	Dr S Chandrasekhar, a noted Indian Demographer, is of the opinion that a change in the policy of taxation can reduce the problem of population. Incentives to the unmarried and couples with limited children may lead to a desirable change.
7.	Provision of social security	It is necessary to introduce various social insurance and social security schemes to help the poor to develop confidence to face the future independently. Poor families have the tendency towards large family.
8.	Propaganda in favor of small family	Mass media are of great help in this regard. Public as well as private organizations should help the ignorant people realize the importance of family planning.
9.	Condoms	Another important consideration is that the condom is used for birth control, some protection from sexually transmitted diseases. This is especially relevant today in view of the advent of non-treatable conditions such as AIDS and Herpes.
10.	Cervical caps	These are similar to diaphragms in action as well but small and thimble shaped, fitting the cervical cap correctly within the vagina covering the cervix needs practice and experience.
11.	Mass education	This is one of the best ways to bring about a positive change in the attitude of people to medico-sociological issues be it to drink, smoking, drug addiction, high risk sexual behavior of family planning.

India requires a very effective population control policy which would launch a well-planned attack on over-population. During a population explosive period, when unemployment is looming large, the population control program should get the highest priority in our development plans. A national population policy should be immediately framed and effectively implemented. The important points to be noted while drafting a national population policy are:

1. Planning should be undertaken both for the existing and the future population. If proper care is taken, during the plan period the rate of economic growth is accelerated and the benefit of economic progress reaches a large number of people within a short time.
2. In addition to better public health and sanitation measures for controlling death rate, a concerted effort should also be made for an effective quantitative control of population growth.

3. A population planning commission consisting a demographer, sociologist, statisticians, etc. is an urgent necessity in a high population-growth potential underdeveloped country like India. This commission should evolve a population control policy and devise means for its implementation.

4. Family planning program should be integrated with the community development program. The people should be convinced that develop planning becomes ten times more successful with family planning. People should understand that family planning implies planned family which serves as the basic pillar of a planned economy.

5. The state should set up as many family planning centers as possible in rural areas. Finance should not come in the way.

6. Spread of adult education in rural areas is also essential in a backward country like India.

CAUSES OF POPULATION GROWTH

The population of the world is growing rapidly in the last hundred years. Industrialization increased the output and in a short span of time more food, more goods and more wealth can be provided to men. This led to increase in population. As more and more countries got industrialized death rate fell. Birth remained constant. So, there has been growth of population. The change in population is caused mainly either by an increase in birth rate or by decrease in death rate.

Sl. No.	Methods	Description
1.	Widening gap between birth and death rates	The average annual birth rate in India was 42 /1000 population in 1951-61 came down to 28.7 persons per 1000 in 1993. The death rate also came down from over 27/1000 population in 1951-61 to 9.3 in 1993 (The Hindustan Times, July 11,1995).Thus since rate has shown a small decline and the death rate has gone down rather sharply, the widening gap increased our population rapidly.
2.	Low age marriage	Child marriages have been very common in our country. According to the 1931 census 72% marriages in India were performed before 15 years of age and 34% before ten years of age. Since then, there has been a continuous increase in the mean age of marriage among both males and females. In 1994 the mean age marriage was estimated to be 23.1 years.
3.	Illiteracy	Family planning has a direct link with female education, and female education is directly associated with age at marriage, general status of woman, their fertility and infant mortality rate and so fourth. If both men and woman are educated, they will easily understand the logic of planning their family, but if either of them or both of them are illiterate, they would be more orthodox, illogical and religious minded.
4.	Environmental factor	The physical environment exerts an effect through the postulated effect of climate on reproductive span of women. Women become biologically sound with the onset of menstruation and her capacity to bear children ceases with the onset of menopause. It is generally believed that women in the tropic mature and grow old earlier than women living in cold or temperate climates.

Contd...

Contd...

Sl. No.	Methods	Description
5.	Religious attitude towards family planning	The religious orthodox and conservative people are against the use of family planning measures. They disfavor family planning on the plea that they cannot go against the wishes of God. There are some other women who argue that the purpose of a woman's life is to bear children. Indian Muslims have higher birth rate as well as fertility rate than the Hindu women.
6.	Other causes	1. Joint family system and lack of responsibility of young couples in these families to bring up their children. 2. Lack of recreational facilities. 3. Lack of information or wrong information about the adverse effects of vasectomy, tubectomy and the loop.

POPULATION EXPLOSION

Effects of Population Explosion

The growth of population not only affects the people economically but also social, religious living and health conditions also. The problems created by the over population is also called population explosion.

Sl. No	Methods	Description
1.	Pressure on land	Rapid growth of population increases the pressure on India, has only 2.4% of world's geographical area, but it is 16% of the world's population thus, when compared to other developing countries density of population in India is very high. According to 1991 census, it was 276 people living per square kilometer. The land is almost fixed and does not increase simultaneously with population. Thus growing numbers, density of population goes up, per capita availability of and comes down and available land falls.
2.	Unemployment	Employment is another area of serious concern on account of rapid population growth. It is estimated that about 3.3 million unemployed are added every year to existing labor force in India. The society finds it almost impossible to provide employment opportunities to the increasing population. This results in poverty and unemployment. We have already discussed the serious problems which both these social problems create.
3.	Poverty	Poverty is a condition of chronic insufficient. It is a condition in which a person is not able to lead a life according to the desirable standard of life. Even after 50 years of independence in India a major portion of population is found below the poverty line.
4.	Housing problem	Shelter or housing is one of the basic needs. As it affects health and character of inmates, abolishing houselessness becomes a serious problem. It is estimated that 25 million people are homeless. It becomes very difficult to provide houses to the ever-increasing population with the result that people begin to live in slums and shanties.

Contd...

Contd...

Sl. No.	Methods	Description
5.	Food problem	Rapid population growth gives birth to food problems. Food problem in India is both qualitative and quantitative. About 40 to 54% of rural population and 41 to 50% of urban population consume between 2100 and 2250 calories per day, which is less than the 2500 calories, the minimum prescribed to maintain normal health non-availability of nutritious diet affects the physical and mental health of people.
6.	High illiteracy	The number of school going children increases with an increase in population. It has been calculated that for every addition of about 10 crore people in our country, we will require 1.50 lakh primary and middle schools, 10 thousand higher secondary schools, 50 lakh primary and middle school teachers, 1.5 lakhs higher secondary school teachers. The need for educating them puts a heavy pressure on the natural resources.
7.	Health problems	Health is a condition of all-round well-being physical, mental, moral and spiritual, so that the members of society can lead a wholesome life. Fertility causes important health problems not only for the society but even for the mother and the child. In India there is an acute shortage of medical services due to rapid increase of population. Nation finds it almost impossible to provide adequate health facilities to the growing population. Thus the mass become lean, think weak and thus they become more a liability than as asset for the society.
8.	Law and order problems	Population explosion creates serious law and order problems because existing agencies which are responsible for maintaining law and order find it impossible to cope with the problem.

Other Problems of Population Explosion

1. When nation cannot provide facilities to the growing population, the result is that for getting whatever facilities are available, corrupt means is used. Thus corruption becomes wide-spread in the society.
2. When there is strain on every resource, it becomes difficult to develop talent. Thus the nation very much loses good talent, putting whole generation in the reverse gear.
3. It becomes difficult to maintain an even sex ratio which gets disturbed quite frequently, resulting in many social problems.
4. When vast majority lives in shanties then the problem of maintaining moral character arises. Moral usually becomes low and results in many social problems.

POPULATION DISTRIBUTION IN INDIA

According to the census of 1991, the population of the Indian union has been estimated at an increase of 23.50% over the 1981.

Sl.No.	State	Census
1.	Andhra Pradesh	66,304,854
2.	Assam	22,294,562
3.	Bihar	86,338,853
4.	Gujarat	41,174,060
5.	Jammu & Kashmir	7,718,700
6.	Kerala	29,011,237
7.	Madhya Pradesh	66,135,862
8.	Tamil Nadu	55,638,318
9.	Maharashtra	78,706,719
10.	Karnataka	44,817,398
11.	Nagaland	1,215,573
12.	Orissa	31,512,070
13.	Punjab	20,190,795
14.	Haryana	16,317,715
15.	Rajasthan	43,880,640
16.	Uttar Pradesh	138,760,417
17.	West Bengal	67,982,732
18.	Chandigarh	640,725
19.	Andaman & Nicobar	277,989
20.	Delhi	9,370,475
21.	Himachal Pradesh	5,111,079
22.	Lakshadweep	51,681
23.	Puducherry	789,416
24.	Dadra and Nagar Haveli	138,542
25.	Manipur	1,826,714
26.	Tripura	2,744,827
27.	Goa	1,168,622
28.	Meghalaya	1,760,626
29.	Mizoram	686,217
30.	Arunachal Pradesh	858,392
31.	Daman and Diu	101,439
32.	Sikkim	4,03,612

Population Distribution between Villages and Towns

According to the census of 1991, 25.2% of population lived in towns and cities, while the remaining 74.8% in villages. The data are mentioned as following:

Census	Rural	Urban
1872	91.3	6.7
1881	90.6	9.4
1891	90.5	9.5
1901	90.2	9.8
1911	90.6	9.4
1921	89.7	10.3
1931	89.0	11.0
1941	87.0	13.0
1951	82.7	17.3
1961	82.0	18.0
1971	80.09	19.91
1981	76.21	23.73
1991	74.8	25.20

Growth of Population in India

Population in India is very large and it is also growing rapidly. India stands second in the World, next to China. The pressure of population on land is very heavy. The per-capita acre of land is very less. Though India has made considerable development in the field of agriculture and industry, we are not able to improve the economic condition of the people, because of continuous increase in population. The density of population is also very high in India; the manpower is underfed, diseased, illiterate and unskilled. The following statistical figures show how the population of India is increasing rapidly.

Year	1941	1951	1961	1971	1981	1991	2001
Total population (in crore)	31.9	36.1	43.9	54.4	68.3	84.4	102.8

POPULATION HEALTH

The population groups that form the focus for community health nursing can be many and varied. Populations are groups of people who may or may not interact with each other. Population may refer to the residents of a specific geographic area, but can also include specific groups of people with some trait or attribute in common three other commonly used, similar, but different terms for these smaller sub-groups are aggregate, neighborhood and community.

Sl. No.	Population type	Characteristics
1.	Aggregates	Aggregates are subpopulation within the larger population who possess some common characteristics, often related to high risk for specific health problems.
2.	Neighborhood	A neighborhood is a smaller, more homogeneous group than a community and involves an interface with others living nearly and a level of identification with those others. Neighborhood is self-defined and although they may be constrained by natural or man-made factors, they often do not have specifically demarcated boundaries.

Contd...

Contd...

3.	Community	A community may be composed of several neighborhoods. Some authors define communities within geographic locations or settings. In addition to location, other potential defining aspects of communities include a social system or social institutions designed to carry out specific functions, identity, commitment, or emotional connections, common norms and values, common history or interest, common symbols, social interaction and intentional action to meet common needs.

Definition of Population Health

Population health can be defined as the attainment of the greatest possible biological, psychological, and social well-being of the population as an entity and of its individual members. Health is derived from opportunities and choices provided to the public as well as the population's response to those choices (*Wilcox & Knapp, 2000*).

Characteristics of Healthy Community

1. Foster dialogue among residents to develop a shared vision for the community.
2. Promote community leadership that fosters collaboration and partnership.
3. Engage in action based on a shared vision of the community.
4. Embrace diversity among residents.
5. Assess both needs among assets.
6. Link residents to community resources.
7. Foster a sense of responsibility and cohesion among residents.

Principles of Healthy Communities

1. Health must be broadly defined to encompass quality-of-life issues (emotional, physical, and spiritual) not just the absence of disease.
2. Community must also be broadly defined to encompass a variety of groups, not just populations defined by specific geographic boundaries.
3. Action related to community health must arise from a shared vision derived from community values.
4. Action must address the quality of life for all residents, not just a select few.
5. Widespread community ownership and diverse citizen participation are required for effective community action.
6. The focus of action should be on system change in the way decisions are made and community services are delivered.
7. Community health rests on the development of local assets and resources to create an environment and infrastructure that support health.
8. Effectiveness is measured on the basis of specific community indicators and outcomes and promotes accountability of residents.

Level of Population Health Care

Health care for population takes place at three levels, often referred to as the three levels of prevention. These three levels of care are primary prevention, secondary prevention and tertiary prevention.

Sl. No.	Levels of prevention	Description
1.	Primary prevention	Primary prevention was defined by the originators of the term as measures designed to promote general optimum health or.... The specific protection of man against disease agent. Primary prevention is action taken prior to the occurrence of health problems and is directed towards avoiding their occurrence. Primary prevention may include increasing people's resistance to illness (as in the case of immunization), decreasing or eliminating the cause of health problems, or creating an environment conductive to health rather than health problems.
2.	Secondary prevention	Secondary prevention is the early identification of existing health problems, and takes place after health problem has occurred. Emphasis is on resolving health problems and preventing serious consequences. Secondary prevention activities include screening and early diagnosis, as well as treatment for existing health problems.
3.	Tertiary prevention	Tertiary prevention is activity aimed at returning the client to the highest level of function and preventing further deterioration in health. Tertiary prevention also focuses on preventing recurrences of the problem. Placing a client on a maintenance diet after the loss of a desired number of pounds consistitutes tertiary preventions.

Objectives for Population Health

Healthy people 2010 incorporates a common structure for each focus area that includes:

1. Identification of the lead agency responsible for monitoring progress toward achievement of objectives.
2. A concise goal statement for the focus area that delineates the overall purpose of the focus area.
3. An overview of context and background for the objectives related to the focus area. This overview includes related issues, trends, disparities among population subgroups and opportunities for prevention or intervention.
4. Data on progress towards meeting related objectives.
5. Objectives related to the focus area. These objectives are of two types—measurable outcome objectives and developmental objectives. Measurable objectives include baseline data, the target for 2010, and potential data sources for monitoring progress toward the target. Unlike the year 2000 objectives, which set separate targets for subpopulation, a single target is set for the entire population.
6. A standard data table, including a set of population variable by which progress will be monitored. The minimum set of variables includes races and ethnicity, gender, family income, and education level. Additional categories of variable will be incorporated where relevant and include geographic location, health insurance status, disability status and other selected populations.

CONCLUSION

Human population is closely related to society and culture. The reality is that human population cannot survive without socio-cultural interaction. Population processes cannot be explained in biologist approach only. The processes of demography like fertility, mortality migration, procreation and survival of each new generation are determined by society and culture (Social controls over fertility taboos on the association of males and females, taboos on sexual intercourse, restraints on conception, abortion, infanticide, lower fertility rate).

BIBLIOGRAPHY

1. Alex Inkle. What is Sociology? Prentice Hall India Ltd., 1991.
2. Anthony Giddens. Sociology: Polity Press, UK, 1997.
3. Barnes. An Introduction to the History of Sociology. The University of Chicago Press.
4. Harry M Johnson. Sociology: A Systematic Introduction. Allied Publishers, New Delhi, 1981.
5. K Davis. Human Society. Surjeet Publications. New Delhi, 1981.
6. MacIver and Page. Society: An Introductory Analysis. MacMillan India Ltd, 1998.
7. NJ Smelser. Sociology. Prentice Hall-India Ltd, 1993.
8. Ogburn and Nimkoff. A Handbook of Sociology. Eurasia Publishing House, New Delhi.
9. P Gisbert. Fundamentals of Sociology, Orient Longman.
10. RN Sharma. Principles of Sociology, Rajahansa Pakistani, Meerut.
11. Robert Bierstedt. The Social Order. Tata Mc Graw Hill, 1970.
12. Ronald Fletcher. The Making of Sociology, Vol I and II. Rawat Publication.
13. Samuel Koening, Barnes and Noble. An Introduction to the Science of Society, 1968.
14. Stewart and Glynn. Introduction to Sociology. Tata Mc Graw Hill Co. Ltd, Delhi, 1981.
15. TB Bottomore. Sociology: A Guide to Problems and Literature. Blackie and Son (India) Ltd.
16. Vilhelm Aubert. Elements of Sociology. Heineuann Educational Books Ltd, London,1969.
17. Young and Mack. Systematic Sociology. East-West Press, New Delhi, 1972.

30 Social Group

DEFINITIONS

1. **Social group:** Social groups as masses of people in regular contact or communication as possessing a recognizable structure. A social group grows out of and requires a situation which permits meaningful interstimulation and meaningful responses between the individuals involved, common focusing of attention, common stimuli and interest and the development of certain common drives, motivations or emotions.

2. **Group cycle:** Group cycle or group dynamics helps to understand the nature of groups, their development and interrelations with individuals and other groups. Group dynamics aims at studying the mental and social forces associated with groups.

3. **Group:** The word group is used in a very general sense. It refers to any collection of persons who are bound together by a distinctive set of social relations. Group can be highly organized and stable or very fluid and temporary.

4. **Social categories:** People who have similar income or who are alike in other ways, such as age, occupation or reading habits, do not necessarily form social groups. Such classifications may be called statistical aggregates or social categories. They are important in sociological analysis because people who are similar in these ways often enter into social relationships and form groups.

5. **Associations:** Special purpose organizations, such as trade-unions, corporations and political parties are called parties. In this category are factories, where the main incentive to participation in money income, as well as voluntary association, such as clubs or veterans groups.

6. **Crowd:** A crowd is a gathering of considerable number of persons around a center or of common attention.

7. **Audience:** The audience is a polarized crowd which assembles in one place. Polarization provides an index of the mental unity of the crowd.

8. **Group cooperation:** Group cooperation is agreed-upon joint action. Such agreement may be based on similar group aspirations, e.g. organizations interested in preventing delinquency; groups may have a common enemy and thus have temporarily convergent interests; or they may agree upon a set of common rules to regulate their competition.

9. **Clan:** Clan refers to unilateral kin-group based on either matrilineal or partilineal descent.

10. **Tribe:** Tribal group was based on the need for protection, of common determination and on the strength of a common religion.

INTRODUCTION

Man lives in groups, groups are universal aspects of human life. The term group means a number of units are close proximity to one another, for example a group of trees, animals or collection of individuals. In sociology, we are considered with not mere groups of human beings, but we are interested in social groups. The simple meaning of social group is human being in reciprocal relationships. Social group is a collection of interrelated individuals who are involved in interactional processes. In sociology where ever we use the term group, it refers to social group. It is the pivotal concept of sociology.

Social group is a collection of human being. In its elementary sense, a group is a number of units of anything is close proximity to another. Thus, we may speak of a group of houses on a street, of trees in a forest or of buses in a bus stand. In the human field, by group we mean any collection of human beings who are brought into social relationships with one another. A group of social unit which consists of a number of individuals who stand in (more or less) definite status and role relationships to another and which possesses a set of values or norms of its own regulating the behavior of individual members at least in matters of consequences to the group.

Social group has been defined in a variety of ways by sociologist and social psychologist. Each of those definitions emphasizes someone or other features of the social groups, according to the viewpoint of the scholar who has advanced the particular definition. An analytical description and discussion of the definitions of the social group will bring out its nature.

DEFINITIONS OF SOCIAL GROUP

1. Social groups as masses of people in regular contact or communication as possessing a recognizable structure—*Moris Ginsberg*.
2. Groups as any collection of human being who are brought into social relationships with one another—*MacIver*.
3. A group is any number of human being is reciprocal communication—*Cuber*.
4. A social group grows out of and requires a situation which permits meaningful interstimulation and meaningful response between the individuals involved, common focusing of attention, common stimuli and or interest and the development of certain common drives, motivations or emotions—*Gillin and Gillin*.
5. Whenever two or more individuals come together and influence one another, they may be said to constitute a social group—*Ogburn and Nimkoff*.
6. A group is a number of people in definable and persisting interaction directed towards common goals and using agreed upon means—*Bennet and Tumin*.
7. A group may be defined as a plurality of individuals who are in contact with one another, who take one another into account, and who are aware of some significant communality—*Michael S Oemsted*.
8. A social group may be thought of as a number of persons two or more, who have some common objectives of attention, who are stimulating to each other, who have common loyalty and participate in similar activities—*Bogardus*.
9. A social group is a given aggregate of people, playing inter-related roles and recognized by themselves or others as a unit of interaction—*Williams*.
10. Groups are aggregates or categories of people who have a consciousness of membership and interaction—*Horton and Hunt*.
11. A group is an aggregate of individuals which persists in time, which has one or more interests and activities in common and which is organized—*Green and Arnold*.

12. A social group may be defined as two or more persons who are in communication over an appreciable period of time and who act in accordance with a common function or purposes—*Eldredge and Merrill.*
13. A group always consists of people who are in interaction and whose interaction is affected by the sense that they constitute a unit—*Turner and Killian.*
14. A social group is constituted by the fact that there is some interest which holds its members together—*Edward Sapir's.*
15. Social group may be defined as a number of persons whose relationship are based upon a set of interrelated roles and statuses who share certain beliefs and values and who are sufficiently aware of their shared or similar values and their relations to one another to be able to differentiate themselves for others—*Ely Chinoy.*
16. By group, we mean small or large collection of people among whom such relationship exists that they may be identified as a united unit—*Small.*
17. Social group is two or more people between whom there is an established pattern of interaction—*Marshal Jones.*

DIFFERENCE BETWEEN GROUP AND SOCIETY

Sl.No	Group	Society
1.	A collection of human being	A system of social relationships.
2.	An artificial creation	A natural growth.
3.	Membership is voluntary	Membership is compulsory.
4.	Group is always organized	Society may be unorganized.
5.	A specific purpose	General purpose.
6.	Marked by cooperation	Marked by both cooperation and conflict.
7.	Group may be temporary	Society is permanent.

DIFFERENCE BETWEEN GROUP AND INSTITUTION

Sl.No	Group	Institution
1.	Group is a collection of human being	Institution is a set of folkways and mores.
2.	Group is an artificial creation	Institution is a natural growth.
3.	Group may be temporary	Institution is comparatively permanent.

DIFFERENCE BETWEEN GROUP AND COMMUNITY

Sl.No	Group	Community
1.	Group is an artificial creation	Community is a natural growth.
2.	Group is formed to realize some specific purpose or purposes	Community includes the whole circle of social life.
3.	Membership of group is voluntary	Membership of community is compulsory.
4.	Group is comparatively temporary	Community is comparatively permanent.
5	Group is a part of community	Community is a whole.

CHARACTERISTICS OF SOCIAL GROUPS

The main characteristics of social groups are as follows:

1. **Reciprocal relations:** The members of a group are interrelated to each other. A gathering of person forms a social group only when they are interrelated. Reciprocal relations form an essential feature of a group.

2. **Sense of unity:** The members of the group are united by the sense of unity and a feeing of sympathy.

3. **We-feeling:** The members of a group help each other and defined their interests collectively.

4. **Common interests:** The interests and ideals of a group are common. It is for the realization of common interests that they meet together.

5. **Similar behavior:** The members of a group behave in a similar way for pursuit of common interests.

6. **Group norms**: Every group has its own rules or norms which the members are supposed to follow.

7. **Collection of individuals**: Social group consists of people. Without individuals there can be no group. Just as we cannot have a college or a group or a university without students and teachers.

8. **Interaction among members**: Social interaction is the very basis of group life. Hence more collection of individuals does not make a group. The members must have interaction. The limits of social groups are marked by the limits of social interaction.

9. **Influence on personality**: Social groups directly or indirectly shape the personality of their members. They also provide opportunities for the expression of individuality.

10. **Stability**: Groups are stable or unstable, permanent or temporary in character. Some groups like the crowd, mob, audience, spectator's groups, etc. are temporary and unstable.

11. **Size of the group**: Every group involves an idea of size. Social groups vary in size. Size will have its own impact on the character of the group.

12. **Group dynamics**: Social groups are not static but dynamic. They are subjected to changes whether slow or rapid. Old member die and new members are born. Whether due to internal and external pressures or forces, groups undergo changes.

CLASSIFICATIONS/TYPES OF SOCIAL GROUP

Classification on Various Bases

Sl.No.	Types	Description
1.	On basis of number of members	Small groups like family or friendship group. Large groups, like nation and religion.
2.	On the basis of interest	Formal group: there is lack of intimacy in this group, e.g. political party, college. Informal group: there is an intense, we feeling among members, e.g. wardstaff, neighborhood.
3.	On the basis of permanency	In group: our family, our nation, etc. Out group: those group which are not ours, e.g. other nation.

Contd...

Contd...

Sl.No.	Types	Description
4.	On the basis of function	Voluntary group: like club, music group, etc. In voluntary group: trade union.
5.	On the basis of performance	Reference group: is formed on this basis. Merton has said that group as a reference group. In which person is not member but aspires to be member. This aspiration influences his attitude, values and behavior.
6.	On the basis of relationship	Primary groups. Secondary groups.

Classification-based on Various Sociologists

Sl.No.	Types	Description
1.	Coolys	Primary and secondary groups.
2.	FH Gidding	Genetic and congregate.
3.	George Hasen	Unsocial, pseudosocial, antisocial or prosocial.
4.	Miller	Horizontal and vertical
5.	Charles	1. Involuntary and voluntary groups. 2. Institutional or non-institutional groups. 3. Temporary and permanent groups.
6.	Leopold	Crowds, groups and abstract.
7.	Park and Burgess	Territorial and non-territorial groups.
8.	Lewis Gillin and Philip Gillin	Blood relationship, bodily characteristics, physical proximity and culturally derived interests.
9.	Sumner	In-group and out-group.
10.	Giddings's	Public and private group.
11.	Elwood's	Sanctioned and unsanctioned group.
12.	Ward's	Voluntary and involuntary.

GROUP CYCLE, GROUP BEHAVIOR AND GROUP MORALE

Group Cycle

Group cycle or group dynamics helps to understand the nature of groups, their development and interrelations with individuals and other groups. Group dynamics aims at studying the mental and social forces associated with groups. It makes us to understand the principles of group life and group activities. When head of the family dies, the family changes. When new political party comes into power, changes take place. So, the fundamental problems studies in group dynamics.

Essential Features of Group Cycle

1. Although one's life, a person always remains member of social groups. The characteristics and objectives of these groups may be different.

2. At the time of birth, a person is the member of his family, but after marriage he establishes his own family.
3. Even after establishing his new group, his membership in the old group continues. Like this a person can be member of several primary groups at the same time.
4. One being dissociated from one group, he gets associated to other group. Hence, a person keeps on forming or dissolving the groups on the basis of his age, objectives, culture, professional interest, family interest and for the lifetime this cycle continuous.
5. Because of social nature, the utility and absolute necessity of group cycle for man is, undisputed.

Group Morale

The group of the members of different apart social groups is regulated by norms. Norms are controls, found in all human societies from the beginning. Norms include the does and does not. There are the moral codes prescribed to lead a good life, free from sin and evil. Thus group norms are shared acceptance of a rule. The group norms give some regularity to social events and the social relationships. As individuals each person has his own individual norms. When individuals are put in a group, they share the group morals.

Essential Features of Group Morale

1. With the formation of group, group leadership also starts developing. In every group the burden of leadership falls on some member. For group solidarity, unity and proper behavior, this leadership is responsible. This element is responsible for group morale.
2. The group structure includes definite program and purposes. There is similarity in thought, experience and similarity in thought, experiences and actions of group members. Thus, many of the problems of the group are solved automatically. These achievements raise the morale of the group.
3. Group morale is also influenced by the initiative of group leadership and the ideal, they establish.
4. The programs and procedures of the group also influence the morale of the group.
5. The satisfaction that participating members feel and their happiness over its achievements also increase group morale.

Functions of the Group Morale

Group morale is advantageous to the group as a whole. Group norms or morals provide stability and orderliness to the group. In the absence of group morale the members may behave in their own way, and there will not be uniform behavior patterns. Without group norms life will be chaotic and unpredictable. Another group norm functions is it facilitate interaction between the members.

Group Behavior

Group behavior or collective behavior is unorganized, unpredictable and plan less in its course of development. It develops on interstimulation among the participants. It includes group behavior like riots, protest movements, strikes of students or laborers, public revolts, etc.

Essential Features of Group Behavior

1. Group behavior, like group morale, is a subject matter of the study of social psychology.
2. In group behavior, we study about the behavior of people in groups, mobs (crowd), audience and other social situations.

3. Man is associated with society from birth to death. Hence many social situations determined group behavior.
4. Through social interactions, individuals develop attitudes regarding different subjects, persons, thoughts, etc. these acquires attitudes naturally influence group behavior.
5. At the root of person's attitude regarding child marriage, family planning, abortion, divorce, etc. are social interactions, which in turn in exhibiting in group behavior.
6. The participants in such crowds may behave in the noble or heroic way or in the most savage and destructive manner.
7. The group behavior may be expressed in two distinguish crowd such as mob and audience.

Factors Affecting Individual Behavior
1. Group into which person is born.
2. Traditions and culture.
3. Rules, regulations and ideals.
4. Art and literature.
5. Science and technology.
6. Social institutions.

Role of Social Interactions
1. **Inter-relations of persons:** An individual acquires a large number of thoughts, facts fro his parents, teachers and friends. This interaction between individuals influences group behavior.
2. **Intra-group relation:** An individual is the member of some group or the other and he follows the tradition of that group. In India, intercaste marriage is not popular because of intra-group pressure.
3. **Reference group behavior:** In reference group behavior, a person is striving to act as a member of group superior to him, thought he is not a member of that group.

PRIMARY AND SECONDARY GROUPS

One of the most important classifications of social group is that of American sociologist's distinction between primary groups and secondary groups. The concept of primary group is introduced by CH Cooly in his book Social organization in 1909. Secondary group are many in modern industrial society. MacIver and Page have called them the great associations. Secondary groups are also known as special interest groups. Secondary groups are inevitable in modern society.

PRIMARY GROUPS

Primary groups are small and intimate groups. Primary groups are very important in the society. They are foundation and nucleus of social structure. The development of the personality of an individual depends upon primary groups. They play a vital role in the socialization process. The primary group helps a person to increase his efficiency.

Definitions of Primary Group

1. Primary groups are those characterized by intimate face-to-face association and cooperation. They are primary in several senses and are fundamental in forming the social nature and ideals of the individuals. The simplest way of describing these groups is that they involve a sort of sympathy and mutual identification, for which we is the natural expression—*CH Cooly.*

2. Primary group means two or more persons behaving in relation to each other in a way that is intimate, cohesive and personal—*George Lundberg*.

Characteristics of Primary Group

1. **Physical proximity:** The members of the primary group have close physical contact. Physical closeness provides face to face interaction and intimacy.
2. **Smallness of the group:** Primary groups are smaller in size. In small group members can know each other personally and participate directly in all group activities.
3. **Duration of the relationship:** The relationship is durable because the groups remain together for a longer period.
4. **Relationships are primary:** In primary group the relationships are personal, spontaneous, sentimental and inclusive.
5. The members are stimulated to pursue their interest.
6. The members are governed by norms.
7. The members directly cooperative with each other and one can see the functional unity.

Importance of Primary Group

1. Primary group are very importance in the society. They are the foundation and nucleus of social structure. The development of personality of an individual develops upon the primary groups. They play vital role in the socialization process.
2. Primary groups satisfy many psychological and physical needs of the individuals. A person gets benefits of companionship, love and sympathy.
3. The primary groups provide a sense of contentment and security. They insist the individuals to behave in accordance with group norms and act as means of social control.
4. Primary groups satisfy many psychological and physical needs of the individuals. A person gets benefits of companionship, love and sympathy. Primary groups provide a sense of contentment and security. They insist the individuals to behave in accordance with group norms and act as means of social control.
5. Primary groups teach individuals high ideals like freedom, loyalty, love, sacrifice, patriotism and justice.
6. All important functions of the society such as reproduction, sex satisfaction, emotional security and social control are fulfilled in primary groups.
7. Primary groups are responsible for maintaining social order. In fact, social organization depends upon the members of the primary groups.

SECONDARY GROUP

Secondary groups are important to the modern society. A secondary group is one which is large in size such as a city, nation, party, corporation, international cartel and labor union. Secondary group are also known as special interest groups. Secondary groups are inevitable in modern society. Secondary groups are opposite to the primary groups in all respect.

Definitions of Secondary Group

1. Secondary groups are those that are relatively casual and impersonal in their relationships, relationships in them are usually competitive rather than mutually helpful—*PH Landis*.
2. The groups which provide experience lacking in intimacy are called secondary groups—*Ogburn*.

3. Secondary groups can be roughly defined as the opposite of everything already said about primary groups—*Davis*.
4. When face-to-face contacts are not present in the relations of members, we have secondary group—*Mazumdar HT*.
5. Secondary groups are those that are relatively casual and impersonal in their relationships. Relationships in them are usually competitive rather than mutually helpful—*Landis*.
6. Secondary groups are larger in size. Formal and specialized groups in which members possess secondary relationship. For example, state, labor union, college, university, political party, banks, rotary club, etc.—*FD Watson*.
7. Secondary groups mean two or more persons behaving towards each other in a way that is impersonal, concerned with specialized interests and guided by consideration of efficiency—*George Lundberg*.
8. Secondary groups can roughly be defined as the opposite of every thing already said about primary groups—*Kingley Davis*.

Characteristics of Secondary Group

1. The relations of the members are limited in scope and arrived at by much trial and error and in terms of self-interest calculations of the members.
2. The members exert only indirect influences over the other. He knows personally only a very few of the other members and functions as one among almost countless members.
3. The relations of the members in a secondary group are of a formal and impersonal type. It does not exercise primary influence over its members.
4. The secondary groups are large in size; they might be spread all over the world, e.g. Red Cross Society.
5. The membership is not compulsory. It is not essential to become the member of Rotary International or Red Cross Society.
6. The large group has less intimacy. Due to the absence of intimate relations some members of the group become inactive while some become quite active.
7. Members of a secondary group hardly meet face-to-face, are scattered throughout the country and throughout the world. They communicate with each others by direct means.
8. Status of the individual depends on his role in the secondary group.

Important of Secondary Group

1. A secondary group is marked by clear cut division of labor. There are set rules to regulate it. A formal authority is set up with the responsibility of managing the organization effectively.
2. A secondary group broadens the outlook of its members. The members of a secondary group are widespread. It is wide in outlook and crosses the boundaries, of localism, provincialism, regionalism, castesism and communalism.
3. The secondary groups are playing a very important role in the modern civilized and industrialized societies. For a long-time the primary groups could meet the essential requirements of people. Due to the growth of cities and population, complexity of social structure and differentiation of interests secondary groups have become a necessity. Particularly, the process of industrialization and urbanization has added to the unprecedented expansion and growth of societies.

Characteristics of Primary and Secondary Group

Sl.No.	Primary Group	Characteristics
1.	Family	Smaller number.
2.	Play group	Personal.
3.	Traditional	Face-to-face relationship.
4.	Neighborhood	Intimacy, informal, spontaneous, general goals, permanency and stability. We feeling, members are interact with one another as total personalities, not as segmental personalities.

Sl.No.	Secondary Groups	Characteristics
1.	Large groups	
2.	School	Impersonal.
3.	Factory	Formal.
4.	Army	Utilitarian.
5.	City, Neighborhood	Specialized goals.
6.	Clubs	Focus on skills and interests, not personality. Communication rational and purposeful. Role expectations precisely defined. Members are together for a purpose and not because they like each other.

Difference between Primary and Secondary Group

	Primary Group	Secondary Group
Physical characteristics	Physical proximity, Small size closeness of relations	Absence of physical proximity, large size, limited responsibility, interest based on relations.
Mental characteristics	Similarity of objectives Relationship end in itself Personal relation Develops spontaneously More controlling power Emotional attachment Intimacy Face-to-face relation, we feeling Mental security	Infirmity. Absence of intimacy Formal or special reasons No emotional attachment Competition Artificially made Absence of face-to-face relationship
Examples	Family, neighborhood Play group, ward staff, Small community, Friendship group, etc.	Military, political party Trade union, College, hospital, Religion, national, etc.

IN-GROUP AND OUT-GROUP

In-group and out-group relationship are very simple and direct. WG Sumner and AG Keller first introduced the concept of in-group and out-group in there work, The Science of Society- there is a sense of solidarity, a feeling of brotherhood, loyalty, sacrifice, etc. in an in-group. But their attitudes towards outsiders are hostility contempt and hatred. In-group and out-group are found in all societies through the interest which they develop vary from society, in India with thousands of tribes, castes, sub-castes, religions and races. In-group life, there may be conflict among individuals and also between different groups.

According to Horton and Hunt, there are some groups to which I belong- my family, my church, my clique, my profession, my race, my sex, my nation- any group which I precede with pronoun, my. These are in-groups, because I feel I belong to them. There are other groups to which I do not belong- other families, cliques, occupations, races, nationalities, religious, the other sex these are out-groups, for I am outside them. The members of an in-group feel that their personal welfare is in someway or other found up with that of the other members of the group.

Ethnocentrism is a feature of the in-group. According to Sumner, this means one's own group is the center of everything and other are scaled and rated with reference to it. A conviction of values, the ways of life, the whole culture of one's group is superior to those of others. Ethnocentrism involves a double moral standard, one inside and the other outside. Every group thinks that the other group is not with them. We are Indians, they are Americans. We are south Indian, they are north Indians. We are Christians and they are Hindus.

In-groups and out-group are found in all societies through the interests around which they develop vary from society to society. The in-group and out-group attitudes are very striking. One has to make adjustments and develop a sense of tolerance and co-existence; otherwise there will be conflicts, tension and disturbances. In-groups and out-groups are important because they affect behavior. From fellow members of an in-group we expect recognition, loyalty and helpfulness. Between them there is always a considerable degree of sympathy. In their relationships towards each other display cooperation, goodwill, mutual help and respect for one another's right.

CLAN/SIB

A clan is the group of individuals who belies themselves to be descendents of a common ancestor real or mythical ancestor. Mazumdar writes, a clan or sib is after the combination of few lineages and decent traced to a mythical ancestor. Clans are exogamous in nature. It also helps in maintain peace and other within the clan. The disputes among the members of a clan are settled by the heart of the clan. Group of families whole members to be the common descendants of a real of mythical ancestor. It is that exogamous combination of unilateral families, whose members are related by some common ties.

A clan is constituted of all the relatives of either the patriarchal or matriarchal. The ancestor is considered to be the founder of the family. All the descendents of the family are known by his name. The clan and sib is an important part of the tribal organization. A clan is constituted by including all the relatives of either the mother's or the father's lineages and all offsprings of ancestors in such a lineage.

According to Majumdar and Madan, A sib or clan is often the combination of few lineages and descendants who may be ultimately traced to a mythical ancestor, who may be human, human like, animal, plant or even inanimate. A committee has defined the clan thus "Clan is an exogamous division of a tribe, the member of which are held to be related to one another by some communities, it may be belief in descent from a common ancestors, possession of a common totem or habitation of a common territory.

The term Sib and Clan are often used in sociological and anthropolical literature to mean more or less the same thing. Sib refers to a group of two or more lineages claiming common ancestry, whether the founder can be traced or not. European usage favors the term clan instead of sib, while Americans use clan in a special way. The term Sib was proposed by George P Murdock in place of the less precise clan to signify a consanguineal unilateral kin group whose ancestry is too old for all the members of the group to trace all the links.

Definitions of Clan

1. Clan refers to a unilateral kin-group based on either matrilineal or part lineal descent—*William P Scott.*
2. A clan is that collection of unilateral families whose members believe them to be the common descendants of a real of mythical ancestor—*RN Sharma.*

Characteristics of Clan

1. **Exogamous group:** The clan is an exogamous group since all the members of a clan believe themselves to have descended from one ancestor. Consequently, they do not marry any member of their clan. Marriage is contract only out one's own clan.
2. **Common ancestor:** The organization of the clan is based on the conception of a common ancestor. The ancestor can be real or mythical.
3. **Unilateral:** The nature of the clan is unilateral, viz., in one clan there is either the collection of all families on the mother's side or of all families on the father's side.
4. **Clans having their own name:** Clans may have their own names. Example of some Indian clans: Shandiya, Kaundiya, Bharadwaj, Kunjam, Naagsori, Jaunpuriya, Mahanadiya.
5. **Totemic worship:** Members of a clan normally worship a totemic object or god. Members of a clan believe in some totemic object.

Types of Clan

1. **Matrilineal clan:** In this all the offspring of one woman are held to be members of one clan. At the same time the sisters and brothers of the woman are also members of his clan. In this way a matrilineal clan includes of the woman, her offspring's, her sisters and their children. But it does not include the children of the brothers.
2. **Patrilineal clan:** In this clan are included the man, his children, his brothers and sisters and the children of the brothers but not of the sister.

Functions of Clan

1. **Mutual assistance and production:** The members of a clan possess a we feeling because of their belief in descent from a common ancestor. They are prepared not merely to assist one another but even to lay down their lives fro each other.
2. **Control over members:** Individuals including in anti-social act are extradited from the clan. In this way, the conduct of clan members is controlled. Extradition from the clan provides more effective and disastrous than even a death sentence from the members.
3. **Legal function:** It is the universal legal function of the clan to punish miscreants and maintain peace and order in this manner.
4. **Exogamy:** With the help of the law of exogamy the clan arranges marriages from outside the group. This on the one hand avoids conflicts within the clan between a man or a woman and on the other services to increase cordiality and friendship with the members of the other clans.
5. **Governmental function:** The clan performs all the governmental (administrative) functions for its members. The heads of the various clans meet and form a committee for the tribe which serves to mediate in the conflict between clan members and takes political decision in war and peace time.
6. **Property:** In the villages where agriculture is carried on it is the clan which arranges for agricultural land. The head of the clan distributes the land. When a person is deprived of the membership of the clan he is also deprived of this land. Members can only rent the land.

7. **Religious responsibilities:** The clan and particularly, its leadership is given the responsibility of protecting the sanctity of the totemic object. Since, the head of the clan is also its chief priest, he takes the responsibility of consuming the religious undertaking of all the members.

Difference between Clan and Caste

1. Clan is well-organized group based on a mythical ancestor. Caste is a real, actual, organized group.
2. Clan is an exogamous and caste an endogamous group. Members of the clan marry outside the clan. Members of the caste cannot marry outside the clan. Members of the caste cannot marry outside the caste.
3. In the clan individual possess the same status. In the caste individual possess higher and lower social status.

Difference between Clan and Tribe

The clan and tribe are different and distinct from each other on the following counts:
1. Clan has no definite topographical area whereas members of a tribe generally live a definite geographical location.
2. Clan has no definite language; the tribe has a common language.
3. Clan is an exogamous group. The members of the clan do not wed a member of their own clan. The tribe is commonly an endogamous group although, with increasing contact among neighboring tribe's consequence upon an increase in the means transportation, the tribe has now lost some of its endogamous character.

TRIBE

Tribe is a social group in which there are many clans, nomadic bands, villages or other subgroups which usually have a definite geographical area, a separate language, a singular and distinct culture and either a common political organization or at least a feeling of common determination against the strangers. Tribe is a community occupying a common geographic area and having a similar language and culture.

Definitions of Tribe

1. Defining the tribe in dictionary of sociology, George peter Murdock has stated that it is social group in which there are many clans, nomadic bands, villages or other subgroups which usually have a definite geographical area, a separate language, a singular and distinct culture and either a common political organization or at least a feeling of common determination against strangers.
2. According to Bogardus, the tribal group was based on the need for protection, of common determination and on the strength of a common religion.
3. According to another view, two essential elements of the tribe are a common dialect and common topography.

Characteristics of Tribe

1. **Definite common tomography:** The tribe inhabits and remains within a definite and common topography. In the absence of a common topography the tribe would also lose its other

characteristics features as community sentiments, common language, etc. for this reason a common habit at is essential for a tribe.

2. **Sense of unity:** But any group of people living in a particular geographical area cannot be called a tribe as long its member does not possess a mutual sense of unity. This mental element is an invariable and essential characteristic of the tribe.

3. **Common language:** The members of a tribe speak a common language. This also helps to generate and evolve a sense of communal unity among them.

4. **Endogamous group:** The members of a tribe generally marry into their own tribe but now due to increased contact with other tribes the consequences of an increase in the means of transportation, the system of marrying in the tribe is also changing.

5. **Ties of blood relationships:** A major cause of the sense of communal unity in the tribe is the tie of blood relationships between its members. The members of the tribe believe in their having descends from a common, real or mythical ancestor and hence believe in blood relationships with the other members.

6. **Experience of the need of protection:** The members of a tribe always experience of the need for protection. Keeping this need in view the political organization of the tribe is established and all authority for administration is vested in one person. This leader employs his mental power and his skill in protecting the entire tribe.

7. **Political organization:** In this way each tribe has its own political organization which maintains harmony and avoids notes of discord among its members and protects them.

8. **Importance of religion:** Religion of great importance in the tribe. The tribe political and social organization is based on his religion because social and political laws become inviolable once they are granted religious sanctity and recognition.

9. **Common name:** The tribe has a common name.

10. **Common culture:** A common culture resulting from a sense of unity, common language, common religion, common political organization, etc. is found to exist in a tribe.

11. **Organization of clans:** Tribe is constituted of many clans. There exists law of mutual reciprocity among its members.

Distinction between Tribe and Horde

A nomadic horde is a group of small number of people. When the member of the nomadic horde increase to a very sizable figure it is characterized a tribe. A very strong community feeling exists in both horde and tribe, which differ from each other mainly in respects of size. In both, such economic activities as collection of fruits, animal hunting, animal husbandry, fishing, etc. are carried on. In both, there is a conglomeration of families. The chief is well respected and obeyed in both. In spite of such a great similarity, the horde and the tribe differ from each other in the following respects:

1. According to Bogardus, in the tribal group which an advance was over the horde, the need of protection stands out prominently.

2. The tribe is bigger in size than the nomadic horde.

3. Being of a larger and more cumbersome size the tribe possesses a weaker sense of unity than does the horde.

4. In the tribe, religion is more developed and evolved than in the horde because in the latter a greater solidarity and strength of political and social laws is to be expected.

5. The tribe is divided into many smaller groups but the horde has no such divisions.

6. Agricultural occupations is an accepted mode of life in the tribe whereas in the horde agriculture is not included into any large extent.
7. The tribe inhabits a definite place. Instead of staying at a definite place the horde wanders over a definite geographical area.

Distinction between Tribe and Caste

Marriage within the clan is forbidden both in tribe as well as in the caste. Both generally condemn marriage outside the group. The modern development in the means of transport and communication has induced increased contact between members of various tribes and castes and has weakened the laws of endogamy in both. The two do exhibit considerable similarity, yet they also differ in the following respects:

1. According to Risley, the convention of endogamy is not rigidly enforced in tribe whereas such is the case in a caste.
2. Max Weber writes in social structures when Indian tribe's losses in territorial significance it assumes the form of an Indian caste. In this way, the tribe is a local group whereas the caste is a social group.
3. The caste was originated, in ancient Hindu society, with a view to division of labor on the basis of professions and occupations. The tribe came about because of the evolution of community feeling in a group inhabiting a definite geographical area.
4. According to Dr DN Majumdar the tribe looks upon Hindu ritualism as foreign and extra-religious even though indulging in it and in the worship of Gods and Goddesses whereas in the caste there are necessary parts of religion. The tribes of Madhya Bharat which are called Hindu and Kshatriya tribes are better acquainted with their own Bonga than with the Hindu Gods.
5. According to Max Weber the Status of all people is similar in the caste, whereas there is much difference of status and rank in the tribe. The view of Max Weber does not apply to all castes. Difference of rank and status can be found in many castes also.
6. There is greater consciousness of difference in status and rank in the caste than in the tribe.
7. The caste is never a political association whereas the tribe is a political association.

CROWD

Human being always belong to groups, in associations and institutions, group life is organized by social norms.

Definitions of Crowd

1. A crowd is a gathering of a considerable number of persons around a center or a point of common activities—*Kimball Young*.
2. A crowd is transitory group spontaneously formed as a result of some common interests. The crowd is a collection of individuals gathered temporarily whose object may be different. Crowd is quickly created and quickly dissolved—*RH Thouless*.
3. A crowd is a temporary collection of people reacting together to a stimuli—*Horton and Hunt*.
4. A crowd is transitory contiguous group organized with completely permeable boundaries, spontaneous formed as a result of some common interest—*Thouless*.
5. Crowd is a congregate group of individuals who have temporarily identified themselves with common values and who are expressing similar emotions—*Contrill*.

6. A crowd involves a temporary physical gathering of people, experiencing much of the same reaction from the same stimuli—*Britt.*

Characteristics of Crowd

1. **Crowd is a gathering:** Individuals are physically present in a definite place responding to a particular object of attention.
2. **Temporary group:** Crowd is a short-lived social group. It is transitory. It is quickly dissolved.
3. **Unorganized group:** A crowd is an unorganized group. It has no definite goals, no aims, social norms and crowd has no leaders and has no social contacts.
4. **Anonymity:** Crowd is a anonymous group. The members of a crowd do not know each other. Among the members of a crowd there is a lack of personal contacts and individual identity.
5. **Narrow attention:** Crowd directs its attention only to a particular thing or object.
6. **Highly irrational:** Members of a crowd are highly emotional. They do not see any reason in the agreement of others.
7. **Crowd behavior is a part of culture:** Crowd behavior may appear to be spontaneous and unpredicted, but actually, it is not entirely may appear to be spontaneous and unpredictable but actually, it is not entirely so.

PUBLIC

Public represents other kind of unorganized groups, the term public is used in several sense. In popular use, the public is synonymous with the people or with practically everybody.

Definitions of Public

1. A public is a scattered group of people who shared an interest in a particular topic—*Harton and Hunt.*
2. Public are inclusive interest group usually with different opinion concerning social issues.
3. Public is a substantial number of people with a shared interest in some issues on which there are differing opinions—*Ian Robertson.*
4. The word public refers to an unrecognized aggregation of persons who are bounded together by common opinions, desires, but are too numerous for each to maintain personal relations with others—*Morris Ginsberg.*
5. The term public is used to refer to a group of people who are confronted by issue, who are divided in their ideas as to how to meet the issue and who engage in discussion over the issue—*Herbert Blumer.*
6. The public is a group of individuals who are united together by common interest or objective—*Schettler.*
7. Public are inclusive interest groups, usually with divergent opinion concerning social issues—*Ogburn.*
8. Public is a group of people interested in and divided about an issue, engaged in discussion of the issue, with a view to registering a collective opinion which is expected to affect the course of action of some group or individual—*Killian.*
9. The public is an interaction of many people not based on personal interaction but no reaction to the same stimuli, a reaction arising without the members of the public necessarily being physically near to one another—*JS Eros.*

Characteristics of the Public

1. **A dispersed group:** Public is a dispersed group. It never meets together. The interaction of the public takes place through the media of mass communications.
2. **A deliberate group:** Public is a deliberate collectively. It is not marked by emotional intensity. There is an interchanging idea, decision between the members of the public.
3. **A definite issue:** Public centers around a specific issue. The issue may be economic, political, religious, local, national or international. A public comes into existence only when an issue arises.
4. **Lack of organization:** The public do not have definite status and role. A public does not have any form or organization.
5. **Disagreement:** The public is marked by discussion and disagreement.
6. **Self-awareness:** The members of public are aware of themselves and their own interest. The members take interests in the issue and discuss it.

Sl. No.	Public	Crowd
1.	The public is not based on physical proximity	The crowd is based on physical proximity.
2.	One can be a member of several publics simultaneously	One can belong to only one crowd at a time.
3.	Ideas cannot be communicated quickly	Ideas can be communicated very quickly.
4.	There is less suggestibility and more rationally. There is scope for debate and discussion and disagreement	The crowd is highly suggestible, emotional, rational and impulsive. There is no scope for discussion.
5.	The public is bound by norms. If forms various organization. Hence, the behavior of people is more regular and predictable	The crowd is bound by no norms. It behaves impulsively. Hence, people's behavior is irregular and unpredictable. It may even become violent.

AUDIENCE

Audience is a group, almost in the nature of a crowd. In audience, the members are less stimulated for any action which is found in a mob or crowd. The members who constitute an audience are aware of the presence of others with whom there is no interaction. An audience is ritualistic by certain materials devices like chairs, platforms or dais, stadium, lecture hall, public parks. Intensity of interaction among the members of an audience is usually low because members of the audience are usually conscious that others are viewing them and hence they modify their behavior to some or more extent.

Definition

An audience is a number of persons in physical contiguity (that is the same place at the same time) all of whom are subject to same stimulus—*Young and Mack.*

Characteristics of Audience

1. The stage or screen provides an audience to listen or witness the performance of the actors in music, dance, drama, and other cultural activities.

2. There are stadiums for athletic performance and games for the assemblages of audience. There are audience in public venues and platforms to listen to speeches by leaders, scholars and persons of eminence.
3. Audience expects some standard in performance.
4. Emotional response in terms of appreciation or dislike is noticed among audience.
5. In audience ritualized behavior is found that it takes the form of institutionalized behavior in cultural pattern.

Sl.No.	Audience	Crowd
1.	Audience is temporary, but gathers at a definite places and time. Soon after the realization of the purpose disperse	Crowd is temporary. Quickly formed and quickly dispersed no definite place.
2.	Audience is invited	It is formed on its own.
3.	No stimulation and no emotion	Based on stimulation and emotion.
4.	Controlled and organized	Uncontrolled and unorganized.
5.	Preference of rationality	No rationality.

CONCLUSION

Social group is called social relations may be friendly or unfriendly, intimate or non-intimate, inclusive or non-inclusive, specialized or non-specialized in character. A social group is a collection of individuals, two or more, interacting on each other, which have some common objects of attention and participate in similar activities. Social group is determined by the habit system of persons and of society. Every person is born and lives till death in the inherited need or urge and characterize it as an instinct. The overall experience of every individual is characterized by his association with his fellow-being. Social group is deliberate and purposive.

BIBLIOGRAPHY

1. Barnes. An Introduction to the History of Sociology. The University of Chicago Press.
2. Bierstedt Robert. The Social Order. Tata McGraw Hill, 1970.
3. Davis K. Human Society. Surjeet Publications, New Delhi, 1981.
4. Gisbert P. Fundamentals of Sociology. Orient Longman.
5. Koening Samuel. An Introduction to the Science of Society. Barnes and Noble, 1968.
6. Murphy G, Murphy LB. Experimental Social Psychology. Harper & Bos, New York, 1931.
7. Murray, HA. Explorations in Personality. Oxford University Press, New York, 1938.
8. Newcomb TM. Personality and Social Change. The Dryden Press, New York 1943.
9. Newcomb, TM. Personality and Social Change Attitude Formation in a Student Community, The Dryden Press, New York, 1943.
10. Newcomb TM. Social Psychology, Dryden, New York, 1950.
11. Ogbrun WF. Social Change with Respect to Culture and Original Nature, Huebsch, New York, 1922.
12. Ogburn and Nimkoff. A Handbook of Sociology. Eurasia Publishing House, New Delhi.
13. Otto Klineberg. Social Psychology, Holt, Rinehart and Winston, New York, 1954.
14. Fletcher Ronald. The Making of Sociology, Vol I and II. Rawat Publication.
15. Sharma RN. Principles of Sociology, Rajahansa Pakistani, Meerut.
16. Smelser NJ. Sociology. Prentice Hall of India Ltd. 1993.
17. Vilhelm Aubert. Elements of Sociology. Heineuann Educational Books Ltd., London, 1969.
18. Young and Mack. Systematic Sociology. East-West Press, New Delhi,1972.

31 *Marriage and Family*

DEFINITIONS

1. **Marriage:** Marriage is a socially sanctioned union of male and female or as a secondary institution devised by society to sanction the union and mating of male and female, for purpose of: (a) establishing a household, (b) entering into sex relations, (c) procreating, and (d) providing care of the offspring.
2. **Family:** The family is a group defined by a relationship sufficiently precise and enduring to provide for the procreation and up bringing of children.
3. **Patriarchal family:** Under the patriarchal family the meal-head of the family possessed all powers. He is the owner and administrator of the family property and right, to him all persons living in the family are subordinates.
4. **Matriarchal family:** In matriarchal family the authority vests of the women as head of the family with the males being subordinate. She is the owner of property and rules over the family.
5. **Monogamy:** When a male marries with a single female, the marriage is called monogamous type. Almost all civilized societies regarded this type marriage as an ideal one. Hindu religion, lays great importance having a male issue. Due to this fact a Hindu male is allowed to commit bigamy or even polygamy.
6. **Polygamy:** In polygamous marriage; a man marries with more than one woman. These types of marriage are prevalent amongst these societies when number of member of one sex is greater than that of other. This, marriage by a male with more than one female is called polygamy.
7. **Polyandry:** Polyandry marriage of women with more than one man is called polyandry.
8. **Group marriage:** Group marriage is the type of marriage in which whole group of men is married to a whole group of women. Each man of male groups is considered to be the husbands every women of female group.
9. **Endogamy:** Endogamy is the rule that one must marry within one's own caste or other group. However, it seldom permits marriages of class kin. Endogamous marriage is that which is controlled within the group.
10. **Child marriage:** Child marriage is mostly prevalent among the lower castes of Hindus. It can be defined as a marriage which is performed before the attainment of puberty of husband and wife.

MARRIAGE

Marriages are usually arranged within social units according to customs and traditions and for this societies at all times in history have formulated rules for marriage. In every society it is found that men and women are aware of the rights and duties of the husband and wife, much before they enter into any relations and these rights and duties from a part and parcel of the whole of whole marriage complex in any society.

Marriage involves the social sanction, generally in the form of civil or religious ceremony, authorizing the persons of opposite sex, to engage in sexual union and other consequent or correlated socioeconomic relations with one another. Marriage is an institution which admits men and women to family life. It is a stable relationship in which a man and a woman are socially permitted to have children implying the right to sexual relations.

All living being, including human beings, has to satisfy their instincts and desires for their survival and continuity. The most important desires to be satisfied by these living being are hunger and sexual instinct in the natural environment. Human beings fulfill their desire and instincts according to established norms of their society. The sex instinct among human being is regulated through institutionalized pattern called marriage.

Definitions

1. Marriage as the more or less durable connection between male and female, lasting beyond the mere act of propagation till after the birth of offspring—*Edward Westermarck*.
2. Marriage as a public confession and legal registration of an adventure in fellowship—*Ernest R Groves*.
3. Marriage as a relatively permanent bound between permissible mates—*Lowie*.
4. Marriage as a contract for the production and maintenance of children—*Malinowski*.
5. Marriage consists of the rules and regulations which define the rights, duties and privileges of husband and wife, with respect to each other—*Lundberg*.
6. Marriage is the approved social pattern whereby two or more persons establish a family—*Horton* and *Hunt*.
7. Marriage as a socially sanctioned union of male and female, or as a secondary institution devised by society to sanction the union and mating of male and female, for purposes of a. establishing a household, b. entering into sex relations, c. procreating and d. providing care for the offspring—*Marumdar HT*.
8. Marriage is the sanctioning by a society of a durable bond between one or more males and one or more females established to permit sexual intercourse for the implied purpose of parenthood—*Anderson* and *Parker*.
9. Marriage as an institution which establishes stable relationship in which man and a woman are socially permitted to have children—*Harry M Johnson*.
10. Marriage is a relatively permanent bond between permissible mates—*Robert H Lowie*.

Functions of Marriage

1. Marriage is an institution which initiates a man and woman to establish family life and to play the role of husband and wife.
2. Marriage provides essential arrangements for permanent human meeting and enduring relationships between male and female.

3. Husband and wife are socially permitted to have children. The right to have children implies the right to sexual relations.
4. Marriage provides appropriate controls, order and stability to relationships by regulating sexual relationships.
5. Marriage and family are responsible for survival of society by procreating and providing care of offsprings.

Rules of Marriage

1. Marriage in general is a social, legal or religious contract between one or more male and one or more female for the purpose of procreation, sex enjoyment and satisfaction of psychophysical needs.
2. In some communities people have to avoid seven degrees from the father's side and five degrees from the mother's side. Each society has got its own prohibited degree of relations.
3. Marriages are usually arranged with social units according to customs and traditions and for this societies at all times in history have formulated rules for marriage.
4. The incest taboo prohibits marriage between certain close relatives. Universal incest parallel cousins, parent and child, between father-in-law and daughter-in-law: Mother-in-law and son-in-law.
5. Virginity is usually considered as an absolute prerequisite for marriage, among the orthodox and conservative people, throughout the world.
6. Modern societies have legislative measures to avoid child marriage and ensure that the partners are mature enough to enter into matrimony for which minimum age is prescribed.

Forms of Marriage

1. **Monogamy:** When a male marries with a single female, the marriage is called monogamous type. Monogamy appears to be the most popular form of marriage in all societies. Among Christians monogamy is the rule.
2. **Polygamy:** Polygamy is a type of marriage that permits a man to marry two or more wives at a time. The principle followed in polygamy is one husband several wives. Plurality of wives is more frequent and more generally practiced among the pastoral and agriculturalists.
3. **Polyandry:** Polyandry is a type of polygamy. In this kind of marriage a woman is permitted to have two or more husbands at a time. Polyandry is found among the Today's of Nilgiri Hills of Tamil Nadu; the inhabitants of Jaubsar Bawar in the Siwalik Hills of Uttar Pradesh; the Tibetans and people of Sikkim.
4. **Endogamy:** Endogamy means marriage within one's own group. The best example for this is caste endogamy. The basic rule followed in caste is to marry within the caste group, that too with in the subgroups.
5. **Exogamy:** Exogamy means to marry outside the group. It is the process by means of which group ties are expanded. People also believed that to marry within their nearest kin is not a healthy practice. Exogamy is advantageous from the biological point of view. This is beneficial in the reproduction of healthy and intelligent offsprings.
6. **Group marriage:** Group marriage, two or more women married to the same two or more man, but this arrangement is rare. This type of marriage is found only in polyandrous societies. Group marriage is not a marriage at all but a kind of sexual communism.

ENDOGAMY

Endogamy is the rule that one must marry within one's own caste or other group—*Folsom*.

Forms of Endogamy

1. **Divisional or tribal endogamy:** In which no individual can marry outside own tribe or division.
2. **Caste endogamy:** In which marriage is contracted within the caste.
3. **Class endogamy:** In which, marriage can take place between people of only one class or of a particular status.
4. **Subcaste endogamy:** In which choice for marriage is restricted to the subgroups.
5. **Race endogamy:** In which, one can marry in the race. People of the Veddah race never marry outside the race.
6. **Tribal endogamy:** In this type of endogamy no one can marry outside his own tribe.

Causes of Endogamy

1. **Policy of separation:** Meaning thereby the will to live in separation from others.
2. **To keep wealth in the group:** When any women of a group marries into another, her children also being to the other group and in this way the numerical force of the first group suffers.
3. **Religious difference:** Generally, marriage between people of dissimilar religious is not considered good.
4. **Racial or cultural difference:** Racial exogamy does not take place due to racial and cultural differences.
5. **Sense of superiority or inferiority:** At the root of caste endogamy and racial endogamy is the sense of superiority or inferiority.
6. **Geographic separation:** People who are separated by long distance naturally do not prefer to marry on another.

Advantages of Endogamy

1. It tends to maintain the sense of unity within the group.
2. Women are happier within their own group.
3. Other people do not gain authority over the groups wealth.
4. The business secrets of the group are kept in tact.
5. Purity in the group is maintained.

Defects of Endogamy

1. The scope for choice of a life partner is limited due to which malpractices such as unsuitable marriages, polygamy, dowry system, bride price, etc. are fostered.
2. It generates hatred and jealousy for other groups. This is the main cause of the root of castism in India. It shatters the national unity.

EXOGAMY

Endogamy is conservative while exogamy is progressive, exogamy is approved from the biological viewpoint—*Sumner* and *Keller*.

Exogamy means to marry to marry out side the group. It is the progress by means of which group ties are expanded. People also believed that to marry with in their nearest kin is not a healthy practice.

Forms of Exogamy

1. **Marriage outside gotra:** Among the Brahmins the prevailing practice is to marry outside the gotra. People who marry within the gotra have repent and treat the woman like a sister or mother.
2. **Marriage outside pravar:** Parvar is a kind of religious and spiritual relation. Besides forbidding marriage within the gotra the Brahmins also forbid marriage between persons belonging to the same pravar. People who utter the name of a common saint at religious functions are believed to belong to the same pravar.
3. **Marriage outside gotras among the Kshatriyas and Vaishyas:** Among Kshatriyas and Vaishyas it is the gotra of the purohit which is taken into consideration. In these the ancestry is carried on not through the saint but some follower.
4. **Marriage outside the totem:** In most tribes of India it is customary to marry outside the totem. Totem is the name given to any specific vegetation or animals with which a tribe believes it has some specific relation.
5. **Village exogamy:** Among many Indian tribes there is the practice to marry outside side village. This restriction is prevalent in the munda and other tribes of chhota Nagpur of Madhya Pradesh.
6. **Panda exogamy:** In Hindu society marriage within the panda is prohibited. Panda means common parentage. According to Brahaspati, offspring from five maternal generations and seven paternal generations are sapinda and they cannot intermarry.

Causes of Exogamy

1. The most important cause of exogamy is the absence of the erotic feeling or the presence of sexual indifference between near related persons—*Westermark.*
2. Incest taboos exist because they are essential to and form part of the family structure. In the absence of incest taboos, the different statuses and relationships in the family would become confused and thereby the organizational and functional efficiency of the family would be lost.
3. In India till recently sagotra marriages were held invalid, which were legal in 1948. It seems that in ancient time's people living in one household were not permitted to intermarry; but when the household broke up, the prohibited range of marriage was also contracted.

POLYGAMY

Causes of Polygamy

1. **Enforced celibacy:** In the uncivilized tribes men did not approach the women in the period of pregnancy and while the child was being breastfed. Thus, due to this long period of enforced celibacy, a second marriage was constricted.
2. **Earlier aging of the female:** In the uncivilized tribes man remarried a number of times because the women aged earlier.
3. **Variety:** Upon being questioned as to the polygamy a Muslim of morocco replied that a person cannot live for ever on a diet of fish. In this way the desire for variety is also a cause of polygamy.
4. **More children:** A son has much utility in the uncivilized society, agriculture, war and conflicts, etc. where numerical superiority is an important factor. Secondly, in these tribes the birth rate is low while the rate of infantile mortality is high.
5. **Social prestige:** In leaders of uncivilized tribes in Congo exaggerate the number of their wives in order to prove their superiority. A single marriage is constructed a sign of poverty. In this

way where the number of spouse is accepted as a sign of prestige and prosperity, a custom of polygamy is natural.

6. **Economy necessity:** In Hindu of Human marriage Westermarck writes that when a zulau is asked why he has married a second time he is apt to reply that will cook when my only wives, if she is the only one, falls ill? In this way one cause of polygamy is economic necessity. In the Himalayan tribes of India the men marry many times in order to increase their property and in order to obtain help in their agriculture activities. In this way they get a cheap and reliable laborer in the form of a wife.

Forms of Polygamy

1. **Polygamy:** In this one man marries many women. The above mentioned causes are causes of this form of polygamy.
2. **Bigamy:** In this one man marries two women.
3. **Polyandry:** In this one woman marries many men and lives as their wife.
4. **Group marriages:** In this many young men and women are gathered together at some special occasion and married collectively.

Advantages of Polygamy

1. **Superfluous and powerful offspring:** The practice gives a greater number of strong children because powerful men can beget children from more than one woman.
2. **Less corruption:** Cases of sexual infidelity are few because the husband finds the desired variety in his numerous wives.

Disadvantages of Polygamy

But more disadvantages than advantages are the outcome of polygamy. For this reason it is not considered good in any of the civilized societies.

1. The status of women suffers.
2. Jealousy hatred, etc. among the women increase and the full development of their respective personalities is hindered.
3. The financial burden is much increased and the children cannot be brought up well.

POLYANDRY

Polyandry is the marriage of one woman with several men. It is much less common than polygamy. The practice of polyandry is to be seen in many parts of the world. In India, the tribes such as Tiyan, Toda, Khasa and Bota of Ladakhi. The Nairs of Kerala were polyandrous previously.

Types of Polyandry

1. **Fraternal polyandry:** In this one woman is regarded as the wife of all brothers who have sexual relations with her. The resulting children are treated as the offspring of the eldest. This practice is found in Punjab, Malabar, Nilgiri, Ladakh, Sikkim and Assam. It also exists in Tibet.
2. **Non-fraternal polyandry:** In this one woman has many husbands with whom she cohabits in turn. It is not necessary that these husbands be brothers. If a child is born then any husbands is elected its social parent by a special ritual. This practice once prevailed among the Nayars of Malabar but is now almost completely defunct.

Causes of Polyandry

Although polyandry depends to a large extent upon local conditions yet its causes can, to some extent, be generalized. The following are these causes:

1. Shortage of women as compared with the number of men.
2. Extreme poverty due to which one man cannot support even one wife.
3. Desire to limit the population.
4. Disutility in society from the economic viewpoint.
5. Desire to maintain the strength of the joint family.
6. Generally polyandry is found is such areas as are situated far away from the centers of culture and progress.
7. Polyandry has also been considered a means to check the growth of population in some societies.
8. When in a society bride price is high on account of the lesser number of women, polyandry develops.

POLYGYNY

Polygyny is a form marriage in which one man marries more than one woman at a given time. Polygyny is more popular than polyandry. Since, it is not as universal as monogamy. Polygyny is practice among the Nagas, Gonds, and Baigas in India. It is permitted in the Muslim community and various tribal communities of the world.

Causes of Polygyny

1. **Enforced celibacy:** Men do not approach the women during the period of pregnancy and while the child is being breastfed. Due to this long period of enforced celibacy, a second marriage was contracted.
2. **Earlier aging of the female:** In the uncivilized tribes men remarried a number of times because the women aged earlier.
3. **Variety:** The desire for variety is also the cause of polygyny.
4. **More children:** Polygyny is also a practice to obtain more children.
5. **Social prestige:** In some tribes the leaders have more wives in order to prove their superiority. A single marriage is considered a sign of poverty.

Advantages of Polygyny

1. It checks prostitution because man can satisfy his sex desire in a better way by keeping himself within the confines of marriage.
2. It gives healthy children to society because rich people only can affords to maintain several wives.
3. Children are better looked after because there are several women to look after them.

Disadvantages of Polygyny

1. It increases economic burden on the head of the family because he has to support many women and children.
2. The children cannot be looked after properly because too many of them are to be looked after.
3. It creates jealousy among the wives and their children.

4. It destroys family happiness.
5. Two women possess lower position.

Types of Polygyny

1. **Sororal polygyny:** It is type of marriage in which the wives are invariably the sisters. It is often called sororate. The Latin word soror stands for sister. When the several sisters are simultaneously or potentially the spouses of the same man, the practice is called sororate.
2. **Non-sororal polygyny:** It is a type of marriage in which the wives are not related as sisters. For social, economic, political and other reasons both types are practiced by some people.

MONOGAMY

Monogamy is a form of marriage in which one man marries one woman. This is the most popular form of marriage found among the primitive as well as the civilized societies.

Advantages of Monogamy

1. **Universally practicable:** In almost all the societies, only monogamy can provide marital opportunity and satisfaction to all the individuals.
2. **Economically better suited:** No man of ordinary income can think or practicing polygyny only. Monogamy can adjust itself with poverty.
3. **Promotes better understanding between husband and wife:** Monogamy produces the highest type of love and affection between husband and wife. It contributes to family peaces, solidarity and happiness.
4. **Contributes to suitable family and sex life:** Monogamous family is more stable and long lasting. It is from conflicts that are commonly found in polyandrous and polygynous families. There is no scope for sexual jealousy also.
5. **Helps in better socialization:** Since husband and wife have better understanding, they can give greater attention to the socialization of their children.
6. **Aged parents are not neglected:** It is only is monogamy that old parents are protected and looked after property.
7. **Provide better status for women:** In monogamy women enjoy better social status. In the modern families they enjoy almost equal social status with men.

Reasons for Monogamy

1. The sex ratio most societies is almost equal and hence monogamy is the natural form.
2. There is everywhere sets of rules governing division of labor among the sexes, so that for practical and economic reasons monogamy is often the best form.
3. Strong feelings of affection and loyalty often develop between one man and one woman, even if not present at the beginning. Jealousy and passiveness could be cited as another reason.
4. Monogamy probably offers the best environment for the rearing of children.
5. May be as a result of the influence of Christian and Jewish teaching; monogamy has been widely accepted.
6. Economic conditions of many societies, forced people to be monogamous.

INTERCASTE MARRIAGES

Intercaste marriage means the union of a man and woman belonging to different castes. According to sociologists, intercaste marriage existed in very ancient India. The strict laws of endogamy came into force only when the Varna system was transformed into the caste system. This led to difficulties in finding a bridegroom as a consequence of which such mal practice. The sole means to putting an end to such malpractices is the encouragement of intercaste marriages. Two forms of intercaste marriages have been accepted, anuloma and protiloma marriages.

MARRIAGE LEGISLATION AND FAMILY PROBLEMS IN INDIA

In India, according to traditional Hindu Law, marriage is a sacrament and not a civil contract. It is a sanskara or purificatory ceremony obligatory for every Hindu. The Hindu religious books have enjoined marriage as a duty because an unmarried man cannot perform some of the most important religious rites. Accordingly, marriage in India is a holy performance of religious duties. Among Hindus marriage is compulsory. It is a sacrament. An indestructible and secret union. Second marriages, especially for women, are abhorred.

Hindu Marriage Act, 1955

The Hindu Marriage Act of 1955 has now regulated the marriage among Hindus. Section 5 of the act lies down. A marriage may be solemnized between any two Hindus, if the following conditions are fulfilled:
1. Neither party has a spouse living at the time of the marriage.
2. Neither party is an idiot or a lunatic at the time of the marriage.
3. The bridegroom has completed the age of eighteen years and the bridge the age of fifteen years at the time of marriage; it has now been raised to twenty-one and eighteen years respectively.
4. The parties are not within the degrees of prohibited relationship, unless the custom or usage governing each of them permits of a marriage between the two.
5. The parties are not sapindas of each other, unless the custom or usage governing each of them permits of a marriage between two.
6. Where the bride has not completed the age of eighteen years, the consent of her guardians in marriage, if any has been obtained for the marriage.

Divorce in India

The Hindu shastras regarded marriage a bond indissoluble in life. The wife was to worship her husband as a God. To Hindu Law there was no such thing as divorce. The custom of divorce existed only among the lower castes. The Hindu Marriage Act of 1955 has recognized the right of the Hindu woman to divorce her husband. Under section 13 of the Act any marriage solemnized, whether before or after the commencement of this Act, may on a petition presented by either the husband or the wife, be dissolved by a decree of divorce on the ground that the other party.
1. Is living in adultery?
2. Has ceased to be a Hindu by conversion to another religion?
3. Has been incurably of unsound mind for continuous period of not less than three years immediately preceding the presentation of the petition?
4. Has, for a period of not less than three years immediately preceding the presentation of the petition, been suffering from a virulent and incurable form of leprosy?

5. Has, for a period of not less than three years immediately preceding the presentation of the petition, been suffering from disease in communicable form?
6. Has, renounced the world by entering any religious order.
7. Has not been heard of as being alive for a period of seven years or by those persons who would naturally have heard of it, had that party been alive or.
8. Has not resumed cohabitation for a space of two years or upwards after the passing of a course for judicial separation against that party.
9. Has failed to comply with a degree for restitution of conjugal rights for a period of two years or upwards after the passing of the degree.

Social Legislation before and after Independence of India

Sl.No.	Act/Law	Details
		BEFORE INDEPENDENCE
1.	The Hindu Widow Remarriage Act of 1856	The Hindu institution of marriage was established on the ethical foundations provided by religion. Therefore, the wife was not permitted to contact the second marriage after the death of her husband. The suffering of the Hindu widows attracted the attention of many social reformers like Iswarachandra Vidya Sagar, Raja Ram Mohan Roy. As a result of the efforts of these social reformers in 1856, the Hindu widow re-marriage act was passed and from that day widow re-marriage received legal validity.
2.	The Special Marriage Act of 1872	Abolish the endogamous restrictions on the selection of mates for marriage; the British government enacted the special marriage Act in 1872. This Act permitted a man to contract legal marriage with a woman not belonging to his own endogamous group.
3.	The child Marriage Restraint Act	This act is also called as a Sharada Act of 1929. According to this act the minimum marriage age of boys and girls was fixed at 18 years and 15 years respectively. To put end to the practice of child marriage the British government and the Indian social reformers made hard efforts. As a result, Arivils Sharada presented a bill in this direction in 1929 and the child marriage restraint act was passed.
4.	The Hindu Women's Right to Property Act of 1937	The Hindu Women's Right Property Act of 1937 recognized a widow of a deceased person as his surviving personality with the same right as his in the joint family property. Here it is quite clear to us that the British courts of law set into motion the tendencies disintegrating the joint family of the Hindus.
		AFTER INDEPENDENCE
1.	The Special Marriage Act of 1954	The Special Marriage Act was passed by the Government of India in 1954. This Act is also known as the Civil Marriage Act. In fact, this Act is an amended from the special Marriage Act of 1872. This act fixed the minimum age of marriage at 21 years and 18 years for boys and girls respectively.
2.	The Hindu Marriage Act of 1955	The Hindu Marriage Act of 1955 applies to all the members of Hindu society. According to this act, the word Hindu includes a Jain, Buddhist or Sikh by religion and any person who is not a Christian, Muslim, Paris or Jew. This Act has recognized the equal right of a women and man to divorce. Section 13 of this Act has laid down the grounds of divorce.

Contd...

Contd...

Sl.No.	Act/Law	Details
3.	The Hindu Succession Act of 1956	Hindu Succession Act, which has affected very much our property and family relations in the Hindu Succession Act of 1956. This act passed to recognize equal rights for women in the matter of inheritance of property. Before the enactment of this Act, under the provision of Hindu law, a woman has no right to inherit property. This Act property of a man after his death is equally divided among his widow, sons and unmarried daughters.
4.	The Dowry Prohibition Act of 1961	This Act has affected very much the marriage among the Hindu is the Dowry Prohibition Act of 1961. The main object of this act is to abolish giving and taking dowry at the time of marriage. The provision of this Act was enforced since, July 1st, 1961. The Dowry Prohibition Act of 1961 extends to the whole of India except the state of Jammu and Kashmir. According to this Act giving and taking dowry before, during and after marriage is a crime. This Act prescribes the punishment for the persons who are giving and who accepting dowry. The punishment is the imprisonment for six months or fine of Rs. 5000 in special circumstances, both types of punishment can be imposed.

Marriage and Family Problems in India

Sl.No.	Problems	Description
1.	Present lower status of women	In considering the marriage and family problems in India we have first to consider the status of women in Hindu family. Critics of the Indian family system say that Indian women do not enjoy equal rights with men in the social, political, religious and economic fields; that they are ill treated and that they cannot claim any share in the family property. Before marriage a woman depends on her father, after marriage on her husband and in old age on her sons.
2.	Reform movements	Women in large numbers began to take part in the freedom movement. The part they played amazed the world. The Hindu Marriage Act of 1955, the Hindu Succession Act of 1956, the Dowry Prohibition Act 1985 and the Commission of Sati Act 1987 are fresh efforts to remove most of the disabilities from which Indian women are suffering. The department of women and child development in the Government of India has been given the main responsibility of coordinating and executing the Welfare Program for Women in India. A national commission of self-employed women has also been appointed. However, there is much to be done especially for the womenfolk of the villages where old prejudice and customs still hold deep roots in the family life.
3.	Dowry system	Another problem that is to be considered regarding marriage problems in India is the commercial aspects of the marriage. By it we mean the dowry system. It needs no mention with what evils the system is fraught. The father of the girl commits suicide because he has not been able to manage for the dowry demanded by the parents of the boy. Sometimes the girl herself commits suicide on that account. The parents often commit theft, forgery or misappropriation to manage for dowry.

CHILD MARRIAGES

Child marriage is mostly prevalent among the lower castes of Hindus, it can be defined as a marriage which is performed before the attainment of puberty of husband and wife. In the Vedic literature, we do not find any evidence about child marriages. But this state later got mitigated. As the father was the head of the patriarchal family, therefore, there was no voice of woman. In the house of her father; she was under his tutelage, at marriage she passed into the tutelage of her husband, and after his death into that of her son or male next of kin, thus a complete subjection of womanhood remained. Later the Mohammedan rule in India enhanced the custom of child marriage.

Causes of Child Marriage

1. **Lack of education:** Child marriage is mostly prevalent in those Hindu castes, where there is illiteracy.
2. **Agricultural assistance:** It is a noticeable fact that India is an agricultural country. Here peasants generally like to marry their sons in an early age so that an additional member may be available to assist in domestic and agricultural work.
3. **Lower status woman:** After Vedic period, we find that womanhood was degraded. It was recognized that a woman should always remain under control. Before marriage, father is her guardian. After marriage, husband is considered her guardian and after death of husband her sons or any other male member of the family is her guardian. This attitude of Hindu community helped in the enhancement of child marriage system.
4. **Restrictions of intercastes marriages:** Restriction on intercastes marriages is another factor, which has encouraged child marriages. It is well recognized fact in human psychology that the mutual attraction of youth never considers the bondage of caste and creed. To avoid such a state, parents marry their daughter's and sons in an early age of ignorance.
5. **Joint family system:** Joint family is also powerful factor for child marriage. In such family, the patriarchal head is responsible for all the important affairs of his family. Therefore, he tries his best either to avoid the burden of a daughter or to bring an additional member for work by marrying his soils.
6. **Religious attitude:** It is a general belief among all uneducated and orthodox, Hindus that a daughter should be married before her puberty.
7. **Foreign invasions:** In the Muslim period, the entire Hindu community was suppressed by some orthodox Muslim rulers. Therefore, to protect the chastity of a virgin and in order to retain their racial purity and religious sacredness, Hindus began to marry their daughters in an early age.
8. **Legal reforms:** Child marriage is a curse to Hindu society as well as the incumbent of marriage. Therefore, various legislations relating to this evil has been passed. In this direction, the earliest measures were initiated by Lord Williams Bentick. Raja Ram Mohan Roy created an atmosphere for those measures by the Reformation Movement.
   Regulation No. 17 of 1929 prohibited the custom of 'Sati in Bengal'.

Child Marriage Restraint Act, 1929 or Sarda Act

The Child Marriages Restraint Act which is also known as Sarda Act was passed in 1929. The following are some of its main features.

1. The act fixed the age of marriage for boys at 18 and girls at 15 years.
2. It penalized the performance of marriage under the prescribed age with a view to check the evils of child marriage but the marriage itself remains valid.
3. All principal persons or parents who perform child marriage are liable to be penalized.
4. Court on receiving information is authorized to issue orders for checking a child marriage which may likely be solemnized.

WIDOW MARRIAGE

The second problem concerning Hindu marriage is widow marriage. It is one of the main restrictions of Hindu marriages that a woman cannot remarry after her husband's death.

The following are the main reasons which prohibited widow marriages.

1. **Ideas of kanyadan:** According to this concept, the girl are donated to a suitable candidate. One who acts kanyadan cultivates punya for his next birth.
2. **Idea of sacredness:** According to Hindu religious text "A women can retain faithfulness to her husband in all aspects namely by her mind, body and intellect". Therefore, a Hindu widow cannot render her body to another man.
3. **Emphasis on racial purity:** After the Mohammedan settlements in India, Hindus recognized the necessity of maintaining their racial purity. This feeling strengthened the restrictions upon women.
4. **Concept of eternal relationship:** A Hindu marriage is not only a social contract but it also recognizes that marriage relations are eternal. Therefore, almost all Hindu widows never accept to remarry.
5. **Economic dependency:** One of the most important factors in the hindrance of widow marriage lies in economic dependency of women. Their economic dependency is the main factor which discourages them for taking a step towards this direction.

Reformation Movements

On late, social reforms and various organizations have striven to remove the ban on the remarriage of widows; Arya Samaj has a great contribution in this direction. This organization among their other activities has started a widow remarriage society. Though there is strong opposition from the higher caste Hindus but the social attitude is changed.

Legal Steps

The following are some of the legal measures adapted to 'widow marriage'.

1. **The Hindu Widow Remarriage Act:** This Act was passed in 1856. It is an enabling measure which legalises the 'widow marriage' and offspring's of such marriages.
2. **Hindu Marriage Act, 1955:** It extends to the whole of India except the state of Jammu and Kashrnir, and applies also Hindus domiciled in the territories to which this Act extends who are outside the said territories.

FAMILY

Man's social life begins with family. It is the most important primary group. It is the oldest social institution known to man. Family is the mother of social institutions. It is the first social environment to which a child is exposed. It is a place where most of the people spend more than one half of their lifetime. Family is the center of our life activities. It gives shape to our personality and provides us inspiration. Family is in the center of the social system. All other system has a close bearing with the family. Family contributes to their strength. Any major change in the family will have repercussions throughout the social system.

Family has regulated the sexual relations to avoid promiscuity, by prescribing customary sex morals. It is a permanent organization, which has provided stable family life. It is the shelter where man is fed, clothed, and housed from the beginning. It has upheld and inculcated the traditions and customs of the group. Thus, family is the foundation stone on which the cultural heritage is built. Family as a unit of sociological inquiry is dealt with in various ways by sociologists. It is studied as an institution, as an association, as an organization. It is also referred to as a subsystem because it is regarded as one of the parts of the society.

The study of the Indian family system deserves special attention, not only because they are born in Indian families but also for here the family system differs in material respects from the Western family system. The family in India does not consist only husband, wife and their children but also of uncles, aunts and cousins and grandsons. This system called joint family or extended family system is a peculiar characteristic of the Indian social life. The family in India is based on partilineal descent. Children are identified by name and allegiance with the father's family.

Meaning of Family

The origin of the English word, Family is traced to the Roman word Famulus or to the Latin word Familia meaning a household comprising or servants or workers and of slaves along with other individuals having marriage or blood relations. The word denotes group of procedures, consisting of slaves, servants, and members connected by common descent or marriage. Thus originally, family consisted of a man and woman with a child or children and servants. This meaning of family has changed over the years.

Definitions

1. Family is a more or less durable association of husband and wife or without child or of a man or woman alone, with children—*MF Nimkoff.*
2. Family is a group of persons united by ties of marriage, blood or adaptation consisting a single household interacting and intercommunicating with each other in their respective social roles of husband and wife, father and mother, son and daughter, brother and sister, creating a common culture—*Burgess* and *Locke.*
3. Family is the biological social unit composed of husband, wife and children—*Eliot* and *Merrill.*
4. Family is a group defined by sex relationship sufficiently precise and enduring to provide for the procreation and upbringing of children—*MacIver.*
5. Family is a system of patterned expectations defining the proper behavior of persons playing certain roles, enforced both by the incumbents own positive motives for conformity and by the sanction of others—*Parsons.*
6. Family is a recognized and established usage governing the relations between individuals and groups—*Ginsberg.*
7. Family is a habitual way of living together which have been sanctioned, systematized and established by the authority of communities—*Ellwood CA.*
8. Family is a group of two or more persons related by blood, marriage, or adaptation and residing together, all such persons are considered as members of one family—The American Bureau of the census.
9. Family is a socially recognized unit of people related to each other by kinship, marital and legal ties—*Andersons* and *Parker.*
10. Family is a system of relationships existing between parents and children—*Clare.*
11. Family is the institutionalized social group charged with duty of population replacement—*Green* and *Amold.*

12. Family is a miniature social organization, including at least two generation and is characteristically formed upon the blood bond—*Sumner* and *Keller*.
13. Family is a group of persons whose relations to one another are based upon consanguinity and who are, therefore, kin to another—*Davis*.
14. Family is a group of persons united by the ties of marriage, blood or adaptation; consisting of a single household, interacting and inter-communicating with each other in their respective social roles of husband and wife, mother and father, son and daughter, brother and sister creating a common culture—*Burgess* and *Locke*.
15. The family may be described as women with a child, and a man to look after them—*Biesanz* and *Biesanz*.

Characteristics of Family

Sl.No.	Functions	Description
1.	Social unit	Family is a basic kinship unit, in its minimal form consisting of a wife, husband children. In its widest sense it refers to all relatives living together or recognized as a social unit including adopted persons.
2.	Emotional basis	The love, affection, sense of belonging and intimate relationship and concern show the emotional basis of the family. Between the family members, love and affection is established. It works as a fuel to run the family.
3.	Formative influence	The family moulds the character and personality of the individual by impressing them the organic and mental habits.
4.	Basic needs	Family is responsible to provide minimum basic needs, including those of food, clothing and shelter for its members.
5.	Limited size	Family is a small group. Smallness of the group affords greater relationship. It is the smallest of the organizations that makes up the social structure.
6.	Sexual transmission	Family came into being to satisfy sex needs and instincts of the couples. Sex is also needed to human being. Thus, family is a biological unit allowing institutionalized sex relationship between wife and husband.
7.	Cultural transmission	Family respected, religious traditions, mores, customs, values and beliefs and society worship the respected social customs.
8.	Nuclear position in the social structure	Family is the basic unit of social organization. It is also a center of all social organizations and possesses a close relation with them. Besides, it is an agent of both social control and socialization.
9.	Social regulation	Family is a very important agency of social control. Socialization and personality development take place in the family.
10.	Permanent and temporary in nature	Family as an association is temporary and transitional. People composing of family perish in due course of time. Family is an institution or a stable procedure of performing certain activities which are permanent.
11.	A system of name	Each family is recognized by some name. The system of naming differs from group to group. The naming can be done on the basis of geographical area or occupation or caste or religion or ancestral origin.
12.	Social regulation	Family is a very important agency of social control socialization and personality development take place in the family. The discipline that is learnt and followed in the family is the foundation of control.

Essential Characteristics of Family

1. **Permanent relations between husband and wife:** the family is constituted of the husband and wife and their children. Thus, a permanent relation of some kind between men and women is the main characteristic of the family. Marital relations in different countries may be more or less permanent, but the relations between men and women have some degree of permanency in all cultures.
2. **Permanent sexual relationship:** The family rests on permanent marital relations because one object of it is the establishment of permanent sexual relationship. Without marriage, there can be no family even though there may be sexual relations.
3. **Attachment of blood relations:** Another necessary characteristic of the family is the existence of blood relationship among the members. These blood relationships can be real as well as imaginary. The members of the family are generally the descendants of the same ancestors. The relation between adopted children and their parents is accepted as legal but blood relationship means no more than that among the members of a family there should exist an attachment of the degree of blood relationship.
4. **Financial provisions for the sustenance of the members:** In a family there is financial provision for the upkeep of its members, senile folk, children, women folk, etc. the earning members of the family arrange for substance of the other members. In this way the members of the family are enmeshed in the ties of duties and rights. In different cultures the burden of earning may fall on different members.
5. **Common habituation:** It the members of a family reside at different places, it would be difficult to call them a family in spite of there being blood and other relationships. It is a different matter for a member to leave temporarily or for the entire family to change its habitat but generally all the members of a family live in one residence be it one room or an entire palace, rented or the ancestral home of the family.
6. **Nomenclature:** Among the essential characteristics of the family it is a distinct nomenclature which serves to identify the family.

In this way, the family is a group of individuals in which men and women have the permanent sex relations of husband and wife, which is distinguished by a name, in which there is adequate financial provision for the relations among the members and who live in common habitual.

Classification/Types of Family

Sl.No.	Types	Classification
1.	Basis of authority	1. Patriarchal family—the father is the most powerful and unquestionable authority (supreme authoritarian). 2. Matriarchal family—mother plays dominant role in the family.
2.	Basis of residence	1. Matrilocal family—the husband lives in the wife home. 2. Patrilocal family—the wife lives in the husband's home. 3. Changing residents—husband and wife alternate continuously change between each others residence.
3.	Basis of ancestry	1. Matrilineal family—mother is the basis of ancestry. 2. Patrineal family—father is the basis of ancestry.

Contd...

Contd...

Sl.No.	Types	Classification
4.	Basis of marriage	1. Polygamy family—one man marries many women and lives in a family with his wives and children.
		2. Polyandryous family—woman marries many men and lives in a family with all of them or with each of them.
		3. Monogamous family—one man marries only one woman and establishes a family.
5.	Based on dominance	1. Nuclear family—husband and wife with their offspring live together.
		2. Joint family—couple with their children family lives together.
		3. Extended family—husband, wife, children and other dependents like brothers, sisters stay together.

Family as a Social Institution and Basic Unit for Health Services

Family is a group defined by relationship sufficiently precise and enduring to provide for the procreation and upbringing of children. Family is the first institution in the history of man. It is a fundamental unit of human society. Its foundations rest upon man's biological and psychological needs. In the modern age many functions of the family have shifted to other institutions. Psychologists have proved that the absence of family affection has serious impact upon the child's development.

Family as a social institution, which are essential for smooth functioning of the society? It functions through a complete structure of reciprocal roles that prescribes the individuals behavior in his institutional capacity. Institution has its followers; it has an inseparable part of our collective life. Thus, institutions are structured processes through which people carry on their activities. The structure of social institution refers to the way human being behave and mechanism they employ in the process of fulfillment of the basis social function and the realization of social values.

The social institution structure includes

Sl.No.	Types	Description
1.	Personnel	The members of society as they play the social roles related to the various institutional functions. Example, in the institution of family the social role like siblings and grand parents will exist.
2.	Equipments	All the apparatus through which the personnel functions.
3.	System	It refers to the pathway in which the personnel and equipment are arranged under a set of organizing principles which give direction to their behavior.

Family as a Unit for Health Services

1. Family is a primary socializing agency and basic institution which moulds the personality of the child. Family fulfills the basic needs of total family members which includes health needs also.
2. Family is a fundamental unit of society where the psychological, emotional, social needs of child will be met through family members.
3. To protect the health and welfare of family members the elders in the family will be working.
4. Sacrifice, affection, binding, caring, looking after welfare, etc. are the some of the basic functions of the society.
5. As a social institution family performs the functions of socialization it teaches the accepted ways of behavior for its members. If health personnel wants to bring awareness about health

in the society and community, first identify the families who are in need and identify the influencing personalities, provide situational support who can motivate the individuals to inculcate healthier habits, family should encourage the blossoming of the intelligence of children, provides opportunities for the expression of joy, desires, pleasures, urges, and familiar with the factual life, religious, ethical educational, and character training and intellectual development of the child.

6. The health of the family members is affected on account of early marriage, frequent pregnancies, high mortality of children and mothers, large size of the family, poverty, illiteracy, ignorance, and lack of food, shelter, clothing and employment.

Basic Needs of the Family

In order to restore and maintain health, the basic needs of the family must be fulfilled. These basic needs are:

Sl.No	Types	Description
1.	Physical needs	Food, shelter, clothing, and safe physical environment.
2.	Biological needs	Safe biological environment, free from communicable diseases, controlled reproduction.
3.	Psychosocial needs	A happy home, work for husband, wife and children, basic social securities for old, disabled and health care for all. Psychological security.

Health Care Provided for Family

The important health services are provided by the nurse and community health worker to the family:

Sl.No.	Types	Description
1.	Child rearing and caring	The health workers and nurses need to educate mothers about breast-feeding, nutrition, cleanliness, clothing, habit formation and hygiene.
2.	Socialization	Teaching the young the values of society and acquire different roles and cultural patterns.
3.	MCH care	Care of women during the pregnancy period and child birth.
4.	Preventive care	Care must be taken to prevent the communicable diseases.
5.	Follow-ups	Regular care given to main the health condition of the family members and care of sick and old people.

Functions of Family

Sl.No.	Functions	Description
1.	Psychological function	The psychological function includes affection, sympathy, love, security, attention, and emotional satisfaction of responses. The affectional activities in the family include the care of offspring, sexual relationship, companionship, intimacy and romantic fulfillments.
2.	Educational function	Home is the first institution of the child and mother is the first teacher, who gives primary care. Child receives the earliest knowledge and experience in the family, which lay foundation for the child's personality and character formation.

Contd...

Contd...

Sl.No.	Functions	Description
3.	Protective function	It has to protect the interest of the child. It gives security in all the dimensions of healthy behavior.
4.	Recreational function	The family provides entertainment for its members.
5.	Religious function	The family has to provide some religious instructions to child to develop thoughts kind natredness are fulfilling fellow feeling.
6.	Cultural function	Family keeps the culture of the society alive. It moulds its members accordingly to the social culture. Family serves as an instrument of cultural continuity of the society. It transmits ideas, ideologies, folkways, mores, customs, traditions, beliefs and values from one generation to another. Thus, it helps to maintain status of family.
7.	Social function	To establish status. It is a socializing agency maintains social control. Accumulation and transmission of social heritage and social contract with all members is established.
8.	Stable satisfaction of sex	Sex drive is powerful in human being. Man is susceptible to sexual stimulation throughout his life. The sex need is irresistible also. It motivates man to seek an established basis for its satisfaction. Family regulates sexual behavior of man by its agent, the marriage.
9.	Reproductive and procreation	Reproductive activity is carried on by all lower and higher animals. But it an activity that needs control or regulation. The result of sexual satisfaction is reproduction. The process of reproduction is instutionalized in the family.
10.	Provision of home	Family provides the home for its members. The desire for home is strongly felt in men and women. Though children are often born in hospitals, clinics, maternity homes, etc. they are ultimately nurtured and sustained at home. Even the parents who work outside are dependent on their home for comfort, protection and peace.
11.	Status ascribing function	The family also performs a pair of functions- status ascription for the individual and societal identification for the individual.
12.	Affectional function	Man has his physical, as well as mental needs. He requires the fulfillment of both of these needs. Family is an institution which provides the mental or the emotional satisfaction and security to its individual members. It the family which provides the most intimate and the dearest relationship for all its members.
13.	Economic function	The family fulfils the economic needs of its members. This has been the traditional function of family. Previously, the family was an economic unit. Goods were produced in the family. Men used to work in family or in farms for the production of goods. Family members used to work together for this purpose.
14 .	Governmental function	The role of family in controlling its members is limited to childhood years. In areas of control and administering justice, secondary agencies like the state, laws, regulations and legislations, police, court, etc. are the main agencies.

Family Education: Pre-Marriage, Marriage and Parenthood

Education is an important aspect of human life, because man feels the necessity to train his young according to his values and cultural traditions. Every society has some system by which it can transfer its culture to the coming generations. Education for marriage and family life is essential; in order to overcome the problems of family life the younger generation should be trained for the responsibilities of marriage and parenthood. The family problems are multiple and solutions to these problems are not simple. Maladjustments and misunderstanding in family are multiple, their causes are also many. So to promote harmony and stabilization in family life, the most important requirements is education for social life. But the study of curricula from schools to colleges, we find the study of social life is insignificant in our educational system.

Educating younger generation before marriage, make them to understand the ideals of marriage, and family, pre-marriage guidance helps them to know the prerequisites of happy family life. Youngsters should not jump into family life without proper education. Before marriage, they select their partners after careful thinking and understanding each other. Though individuals are free to select their partner, they should not rely upon only love, but they must give priority to parents consent, chastity, economic competence, etc. both the partner must develop confidence and cooperation. They must be prepared to cherish in joy and sorrow, in health and sickness in prosperity and adversity. Strict scrutiny of application of marriage licenses to wed is a must. State control in prescribing the age at marriage, regulation of divorces through family courts is very essential to prevent instability in family life.

Family Cycle

Family cycle or the various stages in the development of the family vary from culture to culture. MacIver and Page indicates certain stage in the family cycle.

Sl.No.	Types	Description
1.	Formative pre-nuptial stage (pre-marriage)	It is marked by an increasing intimacy of men and women. An exploration and understanding of personality of each other.
2.	Stage of formation (the nuptial stage) marriage	This phase begins with marriage when the young man and woman begin to form their family. The couple starts to form the family before the arrival of their offspring. It involves the couple to live together, promotes conducive environment to live at home and creates new experiences, establishing positive attitudes towards each other.
3.	Childbearing stage (parenthood)	It fulfills the family proper linking the parents to one another through child, introduce newer growing responsibilities.
4.	Growth stage	The children are born and the family size increases. The average size in India is 4-5 compared to about 3 in USA.
5.	The maturity stage	Parents have been fulfilled their responsibilities and children are no longer requires parental care.
6.	Stage of retraction	The children grow up and leave the family of origin and form their own families. The parents are left alone.

Description/Types of Family

Sl.No.	Types	Description
1.	Nuclear family	The nuclear family or elementary family is universal in all human societies. It consists of the married couple and their children. They occupy the same house called home. The husband plays a dominant role in the family.
2.	Joint family	The joint family or extended family is a kind of family grouping which is common in India. It consists of number of married family couples and their children who lives together in the same household. All the men are related by blood. The property is held in common. The senior male member controls the internal and external affairs of the family.
3.	The three generation family	This is a household where there are representatives of three generations, the grandfather, father and grand children. It occurs continue to live with their parents and have their own children.

JOINT FAMILY

Joint family consists of males having a common male ancestor, female offspring not yet married, and women brought into the group by marriage. All of these persons might live in a common household or in several households near to one another. In any case, so long as the joint family holds together, its members are expected to contribute to the support of the whole and to receive from it a share of the total product.

Definitions

1. Joint family as a group of kinds several generations, ruled by a head, in which residence health of property, and whose members are bound to each other by mutual obligations—*RN Sharma*.
2. Joint family is a group of people who generally live under one roof, who eat food cooked at one hearth, who hold property in common and who participate in common family worship and are related to each other as some particular type of kindred—*Smt. Iravathi Karve*.
3. The Hindu joint family is a group constituted of known ancestors and adopted sons and relatives related to these sons through marriage—*Henry Maine*.
4. In joint family not only parents and children, brothers and step-brothers live on the common property, but it may sometimes include ascendants and collaterals up to many generations—*Jolly*.
5. We call that household a joint family which has greater generation depth than individual family and the members of which are related to one another by property, income and mutual rights and obligation—*IP Desai*.

Characteristics of Joint Family

Sl.No.	Characteristics	Description
1.	Large size	A joint family consists of parents, children, grand children and other near relatives along with their women. It is a group of which several basic families live together at one and the same time.
2.	Combined habitation	The most striking feature of the joint family is living of several families in one house, it facilitates combined habitation.

Contd...

Contd...

Sl.No.	Characteristics	Description
3.	Depth of generation	The joint family consists of people, three or more generations including at least grand parents, parents and children. Some times other with and kin such as uncles, aunts, cousins and grandsons leave in the joint family itself.
4.	Common roof	Members of the joint family normally reside together under the same roof. Because of scarcity of accommodation or due to educational and employment problems members of the joint family may reside separately.
5.	Joint property	In a joint family, the ownership, production and consumption of wealth takes place on a joint basis. It is a cooperative institution. Similar to a joint stock company, in which there is joint property. The head of the family is like a trustee who manages the property of the family for the material and spiritual welfare of the family members.
6.	Cooperative organization	The basis of joint family system is cooperation. A joint family consists of a large number of members and if they do not cooperate with one another it is not possible to maintain the organization and structure of the joint family.
7.	Common religion	Generally the members of a joint family believe in the same religion and worship similar deities. They perform jointly the religious rites and duties.
8.	Exercise of authority	In the patriarchal joint family usually the eldest male members exercise the authority. The superordination of the eldest members and the subordination of all the other members of him in keynote of the joint family.
9.	Identification with obligation towards the family	The members tend to identify themselves with their family. Every member has its own duties and obligation towards family. The family is turn protects the interest and promotes the welfare of all. The senior most member of the family acts as the guide for other members.
10.	A productive unit	This feature of joint family is found among agricultural families. All the members work at one and the same field. The rural agricultural joint families were mostly self-reliant.
11.	Self-sufficiency	There was a time the joint family was mostly self-sufficient. It uses to mean the economic, recreational, medical, educational and other needs of the family.

Advantages of Joint Family

Sl.No.	Advantages	Description
1.	Economic advantage	The joint family system has proved to be a very advantageous institution from the economic viewpoint. It prevents property from being divided. Land is protected from extreme subdivision and fragmentation. Land, when divided in to many small pieces, becomes an uneconomic holding. Besides keeping the land intact, the joint family also assists in economic position. In a joint agriculturist family the male members do such work as furrowing, sowing, and irritation. Women assist at the harvest. Children graze the cattle and collect fuel and manure. In this way, the cooperation of all the members helps to save money which would otherwise be paid to a laborer.

Contd...

Contd...

Sl.No.	Advantages	Description
2.	Protection of members	Praising the joint family system Shri. Jawaharlal Lal Nehru had said that the system of joint family is insurance for the family members which has carried a guarantee for those who are mentally and physically weak. In times of crisis the joint family can provide assistance to the children, the old, the insane, the widow and the helpless. The joint family is capable of providing much assistance at such times as pregnancy, sickness, etc.
3.	Means of recreation	The joint family is one of the best means of recreation. A stimulating atmosphere is created by cumulative effect of the stammered talking of the children, love between brother and sister, mother's love, the reproach of the elders and the fun and frolic of the other family members. In this way the joint family also naturally takes over the role of a club.
4.	Development of good habits	In this way the joint family system makes possible the ideal development of the good qualities of man. In the care of elders the undesirable and antisocial tendencies of the young and checked, they are prevented from staying from their path and they learn to exercise self-control. In the joint family, young men and women learn the lesson of generosity, patience, service, cooperation and obedience.
5.	Cooperation and economy	The joint family fosters cooperation and economy to extent achieved by few, if any, other institutions. A sense of cultural unity and an associational feeling exists among the members. There can be much economy in expenditure since a large saving can be made in the payment of rent and in cooking for a large family unit.
6.	Socialism in wealth	According to Jather and Bery, everyone in a joint family earns according to his capabilities but obtains according to his needs and in this way to a large extent achieves the socialistic order. From each according to his ability to each according to his needs.

Disadvantages of Joint Family

Sl.No.	Disadvantages	Description
1.	Hindrance in the development of personality	The most glaring defect of the joint family system is the hindrance in the development of the personalities of its members. In the joint family, the head is the absolute ruler-administrator. This head is usually the oldest member of the family who looks upon men and women as children even when they attain adulthood and behaves towards them accordingly. In the way, there is very little opportunity for the fostering of individual autonomy of self-dependence.
2.	Bad condition of women	The bad condition of women is also a major defect of the family system and is at the same time an important factor in its disintegration, in the joint family the brides of the sons do not get an opportunity to develop their personality. They serve the entire family like slaves not getting the time to look after even their own children. They hardly ever meet their husbands during the day and even when he returns late at night he either falls asleep or gratifies his sexual impulse with them. In some cases this oppression becomes so inhuman and unbearable that women become fed up and commit suicide. Any natural love between the husband and wife or between the mother and children is prevented from blossoming by these artificial circumstances.

Contd...

Contd...

Sl.No.	Advantages	Description
3.	Strife	If the brides contradicts this oppression or if their husbands choose to speak in their favors the house becomes strife-born and a center of conflict. When the brides talk back to their mother-in-laws they are abused and even beaten by their husbands who are provoked by their mothers. Hearted and jealousy between the wives of brothers can lead to a conflict between brothers, which can assume dangerous proportions. There is a continuous strife and fighting over the doing of children.
4.	Laziness	Due to common responsibility many people take their minds of their work and become completely lazy. In this state, the conditions of those who literally break their backs and those who are very lazy more or less, the same. Hence laziness is encouraged. When a person can eat comfortably without exerting himself he is unlikely to indulge in any strenuous activity. And the wives of the hard working people tell them to desist from such toil as they do not benefit from it mostly, in the joint family it happens that some people have exhaust themselves while others lead a life of utter lethargy.
5.	More reproduction	In a joint family the responsibility for the upbringing and education, etc. of children is shared. Thus, no individual considers is necessary to lay stress upon controlling procreation. In the family, no distinction in the status of the family members is made on the basis of their respective earning and the corresponding number of children. The offspring of one member will be treated the same as that of there irrespective of the high level of his earning and the fewer children.
6.	Poverty	As a consequence of almost daily strife, the bad condition of women, absolute rule, lack of responsibility and blind procreation, the economic condition of the joint family becomes very unenviable. If the conflict is strong enough to bring about division and land and property the condition becomes even worse.
7.	Other defects	In addition to the aforemention major shortcoming the joint family system is further blemished by many other minor defects. Family strife leads to litigation. Customs and traditions are strictly adhered to in the joint family and superstition reigns supreme because the guiding hand is that of the oldest members. Due to the strict administration of the old men the younger people do not gain-confident and they fail to adopt new currents of thought.

Effects of Present Legislation on Joint Family

1. The foregoing Acts of legislation have influenced the solidarity of the joint family. As a consequence of the Hindu Marriage Act the number of divorces is increasing. Previously, the women silently suffered many injustices and outrages.
2. The status of women was extremely low in joint families. Sometimes the mother-in-law behaved inhumanly towards them. Their husbands also treated them as they wished and yet the joint family did not disintegrate. Now, having got the support of the law, women have initiated a strong revolt against the oppression which is leading to a disorganization of the joint family.

3. With the enactment of laws providing for their separate maintenance and residence, the women no longer need submit to oppression in the joint family due to financial considerations. Upon being mal treated they can now leave their husbands and live separately and can demand money from them in order to carryout on their expenditure.

4. The Hindu Succession Act has influenced in adversely. Now the women have the right to sell her property and the girls to share equally in the property of their father it is almost impossible to maintain the family property conjointly. Hence, the result is that the joint families are disorganized at a rapid rate.

5. Modern legislation has put an end to male ascendancy. This too has profoundly influenced the organization of the joint family. The wives in the joint family come from other families. Thus, it is only natural that they should resent having to sacrifice their own pleasure for the well-being of the family.

New Social Legislation
Joint family has been every much influenced by certain new social legislation in India.

1. **Hindu Married Women's Right to Separate Residence and Maintenance Act:** This legislation was enacted in 1946, according to it, under specific conditions a wife can demand alimony while living separately from her husband.

2. **Hindu Marriage Act:** According to Para 13 of this Act, any husband and wife, who have been married either before or after the enactment of this legislation can, under specific conditions apply to the court for divorce. This law was enacted in 1955.

3. **Hindu Succession Act:** This Act became law in 1956, according to it, the daughter was given equal rights to the property of the father and the women also got the right to dispose of, mortgage and use their property in any manner they pleased.

Changes in Hindu Joint Family
In modern India joint family is changing structurally and functionally. The factors that are responsible for the changes in joint family system are:

1. Economic changes and political ideologies released by the British government.
2. Science and technology.
3. Modern means of transport and communication.
4. The introduction of new legal system.
5. Modern education.
6. Industrialization and urbanization.
7. Democratic ideals of equality and liberty.
8. Emencipation of women.

MODERN FAMILY

The modern family is more individualized and democratic where women enjoy a high prestige and position. About hundred years back the family was more of a community. Today it has become an association. It has completed the transition from institution to association. The functions of modern family are very limited. The role and status of men and women have very much changed. The economic liberalization of women has resulted in equal status for them.

Modern family MacIver says, changed from a production to consumption unit. The changing modern family equation of women in the family has transferred family into a new kind of partnership and created new problem for the family of the present and of the future.

Features of Modern Family

1. The traditional patriarchal family began to crumble after 18th and 19th centuries. The new social, economical and technological forces affected the character of patriarchal family.
2. Industrialization, urbanization process, democratic ideals of liberty and equality, the decline of authoritarian mores have affected the social significance of the family.
3. Women are employed in factories and offices. They are economically independent. The family changed from production to consumption unit. Various home appliances for cooking, baking, washing and the use of readymade food products provides lot of leisure to women.
4. The life partners are selected freely by the youngsters freely and marriage is based on individual romantic love. Parental control and authority is lessened.
5. The modern family woman is not devoted to man but considered as an equal partner in life with equal rights.
6. Both men and women have ample opportunities for their frequent contact, which may lead to laxity of sex relationships, resulting in premarital and extramarital relationships.
7. The modern family is a smaller family. It is not a joint family. There is a tendency to have a smaller family and contraceptive are in large use.
8. The modern family is secular in character. There is little religious control. The authority of religion over marriage and divorce, has markedly declined.
9. In modern family physical punishment is rarely given to children. The children themselves decide as to which school will study in, what cloths they will wear, what food will be cooked and to which movie they are to go. It has become a felocentric family.

Changes in the Modern Family

In the modern period, the institution of family is undergoing rapid change and modification. The main changes, in this connection are the following:

Sl.No.	Change in modern family	Description
1.	Reduction in the economic functions of life	In the modern age, many of the economic functions which were previously being performed by the family, are now being performed by the schools, factories, government aid and other associations.
2.	Reduction in other activities of family	Many of other functions of the family have now been taken over by other agencies. The work of looking after and bringing up children is now being performed in crèches, children parks, and kindergarten schools and by baby sitters. Hospitals undertake the work of delivering children and of treatment. Restaurants prepare food for thousands of families.
3.	Increase in family recreation	Modern families have been transformed into centers of recreation with the invention of radio and television, and the advent of indoor games.
4.	Laxity in martial and sex relationships	The rigidity traditionally associated with marital and sexual relationships no longer characterizes the modern family.
5.	Changes in relationship of men and women	Now that the women have gained equal rights with men, their mutual relationships have undergone many changes. Moreover has correctly written of the modern women, she is no longer the drudge and solve of older days.

Contd...

Contd...

Sl.No.	Change in modern family	Description
6.	Increase in importance of children.	In the modern family the importance of children has increased. They are now physically maltreated or punished only rarely but are instead taught lovingly. The modern families tend to become filiocenric families.
7.	Decrease in importance of blood relationships	In the modern families there has been a continuous decrease in the importance of blood relationships. The family is now constituted of a husband, a wife and their children.
8.	Disorganization of joint family	The modern family is no longer joint. The joint family is rapidly being disorganized.
9.	Smaller family	Due to the prolific use of contraceptives and the tendency to regard children as an obstacle in the progress and enjoyment of life, the birth rate in continuously falling and the modern families are becoming smaller.
10.	Family disorganization	The process of disorganization is quiet apparent in the modern family. The number of divorces is on the increase. The control which the family exercises over the individual is being lessened.
11.	Instability	The modern family is no longer a permanent association. It is precarious and can be rendered violent any time. Marriage has reduced to a mere social contract which it is not difficult to break in the event of even the slightest function.

New Problems Confronting the Modern Family

Sl.No.	Problems	Description
1.	Problems of adjustment of the husband wife relationship	In the modern family the most difficult problems is that of the mutual adjustment of husband and wife. The educated and enlighten women of today wants to be the equal of her husband in every sphere of life. But the husbands have not yet adjusted to this situation. Hence a conflict between the two is inevitable. Laxity in sexual relations and the instability of marital relations also tend to create conflict between the husband and wife and to spoil their relationship.
2.	Problems of sexual adjustment	The modern family is also faced with the problem of sexual adjustment, it being outcome of changes in sexual value. Today much importance is attached to the gratification of sexual drives. Some people have gone so far as to declare variety in sex relationships not only desirable but necessary. This tends to encourage premarital and extramarital sex relationships. All the factors have the effort of creating sexual disharmony between husband and wife and as a result numerous families are disorganized.
3.	Marriages based on romantic love	The third major problem that confronts the family is that of marriages being based on romantic love. After marriages of this nature when the dreams of the husband and wife do not materialize in the family they are seriously frustrated. They start blaming each other and either live in a state of perpetual strife or break the ties of marriage.

Contd...

Contd...

Sl.No.	Problems	Description
4.	Problem of broken marriage	A major problem faced by the modern family is an increase in the number of broken marriages has been reduced to a mere social contract. Materialism, individualism, rationalism are the cause of paucity of such of such feelings as benevolence, love, etc. greater stress is laid on sexual pleasure. The women are far less dependent upon men. The laws of divorce are also not very stringent. All these cause have the cumulative effect of increasing the number of divorces.
5.	Problem of working women	Nowadays there are more women are employed outside the precincts of the home. They consequently do not get sufficient time to look after their children. Returning exhausted from their work they do not have the energy left to attend to their husband or their children. This hinders the development of children and increase conflict and misunderstanding between husband and wife.
6.	Laxity in family control	A major problem has been created for the modern family by the decrease in the control exercised by the family over its members. This has undermined the administration of the family. Boy-girl, husband-wife, brother-sister each wants to pursue his own course and does not relish and interference, be it advice or be it rebuke.
7.	Family conflict and strife	Changes in the values of life and a reduction of the family control in the modern family have led to increased conflict between husband and wife as well as between parents and children. This conflict is usually not apparent but it does disturb the peace of the family, destroy the faith in one another and remove the sense of psychological security.
8.	Lower birth rate	The birth rate is falling constantly due to late marriages, frequent use of contraceptives and a tendency to consider children a burden. This tends to accentuate the instability of the family since the absence of children reduces the sense of responsibility in the husband and wife, besides preventing intimate family relations.

Causes of Instability of Modern Family

The modern family is instable. An increase in the number of desertions, separations and divorces, etc. are a proof of this. The main causes of this instability are the following:

Sl.No.	Causes of instability	Description
1.	Less social protection in family crises	Previously, a family crisis of the nature of a maladjustment between husbands and wife was overcome by the constraining influence of the elders, kinsmen, and social mores and traditions and the family was served from disintegration but with the existing loss of respect for the power of these modes of social control the husband and wife are deprived of any guide or mediator and in a fit of temper or even vengeance they destroy the delicately and lovingly nurtured sapling which is the family, no matter how much remorse they may experience when they have cool down. At some places extreme laxity of divorce laws has led to very great instability and impermanence of the family.

Contd...

Contd...

Sl.No.	Causes of instability	Description
2.	Replacement of domination by cooperation	According to MacIver and Page, the basis of husband-wife relationship in the family is no longer domination but cooperation. Previously, everywhere, be it the east or the west, the wife was dominated by the husband and hence, the family stability survived despite the husband's domination. But the removal of this dominance, in the modern time, the stability of the family can be maintained only by benevolence, sympathy and cooperation.

Effects of Modern Civilization of Family Diorganization

Many factors of modern civilization have major hand in the disorganization of the family. The main causes are the following:

Sl.No.	Causes	Description
1.	Industrialism	In the modern industrial system women and children work in factories along with the men. This reduces the unity of the family and increase disorganization.
2.	Ideal of romantic love	Modern marriages are based on the ideals of the romantic love. When the dreams of the two partners do not materialize in the family, conflict increases and is gradually transformed into enmity.
3.	Hedonism	Modern civilization is hedonistic. In this, people pay more attention to their rights than to their duties. This increase selfishness and the occasions for conflict.
4.	Individualism	Modern civilization is also individualistic. No one wants to consider the interests of the family. Everyone is engaged in the consideration of solely his own interest. No one is prepared to sacrifice this smallest interest to benefit another. As a result of this, conflict in the family increases.
5.	Lack of control in sexual relationship	Another consequence of modern civilization is a change in the values concerning sex. This tends to diminish control in sex relationships, to reduce fidelity in marital relations and also to increase chances for family disorganization.

CONCLUSION

The family is a social institution found in all societies that unite people in cooperative groups to oversee the bearing and raising of children. Family ties are also called kinship, a social bond based on blood, marriage or adaptation. Throughout the world, families form around marriage, a legally sanctioned relationship, usually involving economic cooperation as well as sexual activity and childbearing, that people expect the enduring.

BIBLIOGRAPHY

1. Bingham WV. Aptitude and Aptitude Testing, Haper & Brothers, New York, 1937.
2. Brown JF. Educational Sociology, Prentice Hall, New York, 1960 (5th Printing).
3. Brown JF. The Psychodynamics of Abnormal Behaviour, Asia Publishing House (Indian Reprint), New Delhi, 1969.

4. Hull CL. Aptitude Testing, Youkers, World Book Co, New York, 1928.
5. Korman AK. The Psychology of Motivation, Englewood Cliffs, Prentice Hall, NJ, 1974.
6. Murphy G, Murphy LB. Experimental Social Psychology. Harper & Bos., New York, 1931.
7. Murray HA. Explorations in Personality. Oxford University Press, New York, 1938.
8. Newcomb TM. Personality and Social Change Attitude Formation in a Student Community, Dryden, New York, 1943.
9. Newcomb TM. Personality and Social Change. The Dryden Press, New York, 1943.
10. Ogburn and Nimkoff. A Handbook of Sociology. Eurasia Publishing House, New Delhi.
11. Seashore CE. Seashore, Measures of Musical Talents, Psychological Cooperation, New York, 1960.
12. Sharma RN. Principles of Sociology, Rajahamsa Pakistani, Meerut.
13. Vilhelm Aubert Heineuann. Elements of Sociology. Educational Books Ltd. London, 1969.
14. Young and Mack. East Systematic Sociology. West Press, New Delhi, 1972.

32 *Rural Community*

DEFINITIONS

1. **Village:** The village community consists of a group of the related or unrelated persons larger than a single family occupying a large house or a number of dwellings placed closed together, sometimes irregularly, sometimes in a street and cultivating, originally in common a number agreeable fields, dividing the available meadow land between them and pasturing their cattle upon surrounding waste land over which the community claims rights as far as the boundaries of each community.
2. **Community feeling:** Even when a group of person lives on a specified geographical area and has a common way of life. It does not assume the form of a community unless the community feeling is there. Because of this community feeling this group separates itself from other groups. It has a sense of "We feeling". It is prepared to make sacrifices for that group.
3. **Rural community:** Rural community is based on ruralism. Ruralism is nothing but a way of life which is different from urbanism. There are two ways of life in one. It is the agriculture that dominates while in the other, it is the industry that dominates.
4. **Common life:** Common life means that they have more or less common occupation, similar religious, believes, customs, traditions, etc. these things are to be found in a typical manner in Indian villages.
5. **Panchayat Raj:** Panchayat Raj system is parallel to this official structure of administration; there are institutions of local self government rural areas. This refers to Panchayat Raj system.
6. **Community development:** Community development is defined as a movement designed to promote better living for the whole community with the active participation of the community and to stimulate it in order to secure its active responses.
7. **Indian village:** Villages emerged when nomadic men settled down with agricultural operations for their subsistence. The typical Indian village has its central residential site with an open area for corn and cattle shed.
8. **Social processes:** Social process is the social interactions of groups and individual with one another. They are mainly competition, conflict, cooperation and accommodation.
9. **Specific geographical area:** The village community is the members of the village community generally live in a specified geographical area. Persons belonging to the village community are not necessarily related.
10. **Centralization:** Centralization is the integration of human being and facilities around pivotal points at which school, economic and cultural integration occurs most frequently.

INTRODUCTION

Rural sociology is the branch which studies the life of rural people. It is considered with rural society, its social structure, social institutions and their relationships. It studies the life of rural people and analysis their attitudes and beliefs. India is a land of villages; the majority of the people are living in villages. So villages are the significant aspect of Indian society. Indian villages are considered unique and distinct from villages of other countries. Generally a village refers to a small group of people living permanently in a definite geographic area who depend mainly on farming activities.

DEFINITIONS OF RURAL COMMUNITY

1. The village is unit of rural society. It is the theatre where in the quantum of rural life unfolds itself and functions—*AR Desai.*
2. The rural community comprises of the constellation of institutions and persons grouped about a small center and sharing common primary interest—*Elridge and Merrill.*
3. A village as a unit of compact settlement varying in size, smaller than a town—*Anthony Giddens.*
4. The village communities are little republics, having nearly every thing they can want with in themselves and almost independent of any foreign relations….. dynasty after dynasty tumbles, communities remain the same—*Sir Charles Met Calfe.*

CHARACTERISTICS OF RURAL COMMUNITY

Sl.No.	Characteristics	Description
1.	Village is a primary institution	The development of villages is influenced considerably by the life of the village is a primary institution.
2.	Group feeling	In the life of the villagers group feeling occupies an important place. They respect the judgment and obey the orders of their elders and panchayat.
3.	Occupation	The main occupation of the rural community is agricultural and allied activities like animal husbandry, poultry and small enterprises like apiculture and fishing.
4.	Size	The village community is small in size. There may be few household or small number of people.
5.	Environment	Villages have natural set-up. Animals, birds, river, ponds and other natural things are found in the village. This natural atmosphere enables the rural people to have simple and natural lifestyle.
6.	Population density	Population density refers to the number of people living per square mile or Km area. As the villages have large areas of land for cultivation the number of inhabitants is surely small. Therefore, the village community has low density population.
7.	Low mobility	Mobility refers to movement or transition of people from one place to another or from one social status to another. Example there is physical as well as social mobility. Both are limited in villages, especially in Indian villages. Economic class mobility is also not much in rural community.

Contd...

Contd...

Sl.No.	Characteristics	Description
8.	Simplicity	The village people lead a simple life. They are far away from evils of modern civilization. They are simple and plain people into believe in God. Their behavior is natural and not artificial. They live a peaceful life.
9.	Faith in religion	The people in the villages have deep faith in religion. Their main occupation is agriculture which largely depends upon nature. The farmers acquires a feeling of fear towards natural forces and starts worshiping them.
10.	Joint family	Though in cities the joint family system is breaking down yet in the villages it still retains its hold. The agricultural occupation requires the cooperation of all the family members. The men plough the field, the women harvest the crops and the children graze the cattle.
11.	Role of neighborhood	In a village neighborhood is of great importance. The village people assist each other and thus they have close neighborhood relationship both during joy and sorrow.
12.	Community consciousness	The village dwellers have sense of community. The relations between the village people are intimate. They personally know each other. Their customs, convention and culture are common. They jointly take part in religious celebrations. Structurally and functionally the village is a unit.
13.	Homogeneity	The village life has much homogeneity. People of a village have common occupation and common style of life.
14.	Less education	A most of the villagers are engaged in agriculture, advanced education and specialization are not needed. So there is less education in village. Even the rate of literacy is low especially in Indian villages.
15.	Less political consciousness	Political consciousness and participation are less in villages. The people are engaged and interested in day-to-day activities of their life and there is no time or interest for politics.
16.	Stable public opinion	Public opinion is not easily changeable in villages due to the rigidity of customs, traditions and values, education, transportation and communication and new ideas and ideologies are however changing the public opinion in our villages too.
17.	Low status of women	Women are not considered to be worthy to take decisions in family matters. Men consult other male members in different types of work. The rate of literacy and education is also relatively less among women.

CHARACTERISTICS OF INDIAN VILLAGE

1. **Family:** In village community, family is still the basic and most important unit. The whole of the village community structure is dependent on the family. Joint family structure in Indian villages, family as the center of production and consumption in village community, the family is an independent unit, so far as the production and consumption is concerned.

2. **Social stratification:** An order of ranking the individuals based upon relative position in society. Caste and class system are the two major types of social stratification in society. Caste status is and ascribed one while class status is achieved. Certain characteristics or attributes influence the position of individual in stratification system.

3. **Social process:** Social process is the social interactions of groups and individuals with one another. They are mainly competition, conflict, cooperation and accommodation.
4. **Caste system:** Membership of caste, caste restrictions social distance, disabilities and even untouchablity are still found in Indian villages. Mostly Indian villages are multi caste villages, even though we have hundreds of different castes in India, the caste composition of villages differ from region to region.
5. **Education:** The inadequate physical facilities of the village school, poorly trained and disinterested teacher and inefficient and corrupt administration of the schools contribute much for the problems of village education. Introduction of new educational schemes without proper equipment, facilities, guidance and supervision affect the secondary education in village areas.
6. **Agriculture:** In Indian rural society, there joint family structure, because of agriculture economy. Agriculture is such a job in which a large number of people have to involve.

SOCIOLOGICAL IMPORTANCE OF VILLAGES IN INDIA

1. **A village is a unit of a society:** In India there are more than half a million villages. According to Max Weber, the German scholar, India has always been a country of villages. Eighty percent of the Indian population lives in villages. India is predominantly an agricultural country. Thus, in every respect the future of India depends upon the villages.
2. **Intensity of primary and family relations:** The relations between the primary groups and families in the villages are intense. The family fulfils the needs of its members in all aspects of their life and exercises control over them. It is through the family that the new members are initially introduced to the customs, conventions and cultures of the society. In this way the village people hold family as an institution having revered status, but the results is that individuality does not develop properly in the members of a family. Due to limited contact with the external world their viewpoint is narrow and they are aggressively opposed to violent change. In the village the relations among the people are direct and intimate so that the entire village is often organized like a family.
3. **Simple and economical life:** The life of the villagers is simple and economical. They have very limited needs. The spirit of ambition and competition is generally absent and they are not constantly devoured by a consuming desire for progress as is the case with their urban counterparts.
4. **Preserves of the ancient culture of the society:** From the sociological viewpoint the villagers are also important because they preserve the ancient culture of society. India is a religious country. The life of the villagers depends considerably upon natural forces due to their occupations, which is agriculture, and thus they worship natural forces like the sun, rain, etc. the villages in India still exhibit faith in the doctrine of karma, a fundamental principle in Indian culture, and lead a simple and natural life dominated by sacrifice, theistic tendency and the important of religion in every aspect of life.
5. **Ideal democracy:** In ancient times the Indian villages were an ideal democracy. Life in a village is self-dependent. Most of the people are agriculturalist, and besides farming the farmer is quiet capable of handling the work generally done by carpenter, black-smith, mason, veterinary surgeon, woodcutter and sometimes even a weaver. In some developed villages these occupations are carried on by different people, but whatever the conditions, all the needs of villages are generally fulfilled in the village itself.

FACTORS IN THE GROWTH OF VILLAGE COMMUNITY

The growth of village community is not caused by any one factor. Various factors like geographic, economic and social factors have been active participants in this growth. A brief survey of the important factors in the growth of village community will explain the growth of village communities.

Topographical Factors

Sl.No.	Factors	Description
1.	Land	The most important topographical factor with respect to permanent village community land. In this both the fertility and the layout of the land are important. It is difficult to carry on agriculture on land which is rocky and uneven. If the land is completely unfertile and sandy then villages cannot easily develop there.
2.	Water	The facility of water has much to do with the growth of a village community at any particular locale. It is almost inconceivable that villages can come up where water is not available. Besides its need for the daily recurring needs of man like drinking, bathing, etc. the village must use it for irrigating the farms. As the rivers are a perennial source of this extremely useful commodity the village's communities which exist on river banks are particularly prosperous and well developed. In India the villages along the banks of the Ganga are in a much better condition than those which are seeking out a miserable existence in the deserts and hills. If the water scarce, not much use can be made of even the most fertile and cultivable land. In the desert, where water is not easily available, the villages are scattered far and wide. In the oasis where water can be found, some palm trees and grass grow and the villages crop up. The greatest cultures of the world have grown and developed along the banks of the mightiest rivers.
3.	Climate	The climate of a place is also an important factor in the growth of village communities. A temperate climate is most favorable to the health of man as well as agriculture. Thus, the village communities of these areas are the most prosperous, cultured and developed. Man cannot lead a natural and proper life in areas of extreme climate. In a warm climate people become supine and lazy. In India there is another operative factor which has been the cause of the low living standard in the village communities. The village communities of Europe are in a far better condition than their counterparts in India.

Economic Factors

Sl.No.	Factors	Description
1.	Conditions of agriculture	Even today mainstay of the village communities is agriculture and thus their growth depends upon the state of agriculture. The phrase state of agriculture means the state of production by farming. If farming yields a fair amount of produce then the village communities will be prosperous and they will have more time at their disposal to engage in cultural activities. In India the village communities in state like Punjab are more developed due to the greater production in agriculture than in any other part of the country. On the other hand, the village communities in hilly or unfertile area are in a very poor, disintegrated and at times precarious condition.

Contd...

Contd...

Sl.No.	Factors	Description
2.	The economy	In the growth of village communities, besides agricultural production, the village economy is another important economic factor. In agriculture if greater production is to be achieved then animal of good breed and proper implements like good ploughs, good seeds, and good manure will have to be acquired by the farmer, for which he needs money. Secondly, besides greater agricultural production, there is also the need for adequate consumption. It is necessary that the farmers should have the facility of being able to raise loan in times of need. In India institutions like cooperative banks. Cooperative seed stores, cooperative warehouse and community projects have led to an improvement in the conditions of agriculturists. In a village community, a prosperous and organized economy is essential for the growth and development of the occupations and cottage industries.
3.	Cottage industries	Cottage industries are very important economic factor in the growth of the village community. In village the cottage industries are concerned with the manufacture of handspun cloth, robe and baskets, toys, gur and molasses, etc. while on the one hand these cottage industries provide a means of livelihood to landless people they also offer means of utilization of the leisure of the farmers and feminine labor in productive activities. In India the farmers is completely unoccupied for a very long period in the years.

Social Factors

Sl.No.	Factors	Description
1.	Peace	For a permanent and healthy development of a village community it is essential that there should be external and internal peace. In countries where there exists an atmosphere of perpetual unrest and dark clouds of war are always hovering an atmosphere of perpetual unrest and dark clouds of war are always hovering on the horizon, the development of village communities is hampered.
2.	Security	Peace is based on security, the permanent growth of village communities being impossible in the absence of the later. Security includes various kinds of security like security from want, security in business, security of agriculture, security of property, security from diseases and security in the areas where there is unceasing strife, looting and murder because the destructive forces will obviate at constructive plans. Agriculturists and villagers also need security from natural catastrophes like famine, epidemic, excessive rain, floods, etc. in this regard the government shoulders a very heavy responsibility.
3.	Cooperation	Community development is difficult to achieve when there is no cooperation. The inhabitants of the villages are so close to each other that they cannot make progress without cooperation. There are many activities in a village which depend upon the collective cooperation of the whole community and cannot be entrusted to the responsibility of any one individual. Such activities are public health, security, peace, and proper use of public property as well as the other allied activities.

Contd...

Contd...

Sl.No.	Factors	Description
4.	Intelligence and labor	The biggest single social factor responsible for the growth of a permanent village community is the labor of people. Ultimately, the development of the village communities depends upon the intelligence and the labor of the villagers. Lacking this they cannot face natural exigencies of the problems concerning agriculture, etc. they cannot increase agricultural output nor profit by the neither scientific discoveries nor can conditions of village communities must go to the business and intelligence.

RURAL HEALTH

Health of the individual or group affects its work output and efficiency. Good health is not only essential for a normal life and activities, but it is the basic factor for a happy life. The health survey and development committee (1946) rightly points out that the term health implies more than absence of sickness in the individual and indicate a state of harmonious functioning of the body and the mind in relation to his physical and sociological environment, so as to enable him to enjoy life to the fullest possible extent and to reach his maximum level of productive capacity. Thus, we find that health is a condition of all-round well-being, physical, mental, moral, and spiritual so that the members of society can lead a wholesome life. There are several causes of ill-health in our villages.

Rural Problems

1. Higher birth and death rate.
2. Social problems: Day-to-day rural population increase, problems of employment, some rural families migrate to urban area, the become bonded labor.
3. Poor health knowledge, occurrence of communicable disease and infection. Child deaths, much rural area PHC not working and also poor health awareness for the rural people.
4. In time of disease or ill health people prefer to go to places of worship witch craft than to a medical official leading to poor utilization of health care.
5. Low mobility of social status and less social differences and stratifications.
6. Lack of communication and transport, many villages still has very poor transport mass Medias.
7. Child marriages: child marriages are still rampant in Indian villages. Lack of education and the force of customs and values help them to have child marriages.
8. Unemployment/under employment.
9. Untouchables and discriminations.
10. Problems of sanitation (insufficient drinking water, lack of sewage disposal system).
11. Casteism and group conflicts.
12. Indebtedness.

Causes of Ill-health in Rural Community

Illiteracy, unemployment, poverty, increase in population, lack of awareness, etc. are some of the common reason for ill-health in rural community. Some important factors are mentioned here:

1. **Bad habits:** Bad habits like alcoholism, smoking, consumption of intoxicating substances, etc. are causing ill-health in rural population.

2. **Lack of medical facilities:** Because of the unequal distribution of health facilities, limited number of health care institutions and facilities are found in villages. Protection and care of the patients are affected due to this, which affect the health status of villages.

3. **Lack of proper housing:** In villages, kaccha houses, temporary structures and unhealthy dwelling places are commonly found. They do not have facilities like toilet or bathroom, latrine, kitchen, lighting and ventilation. In addition to this, many people are homeless. Therefore, lack of housing or improper housing is a major reason for ill health in village community.

4. **Lack of healthy or hygienic environment:** Lack of safe drinking water or lack of availability of sufficient water for daily necessities. Lack of sanitation people is not careful about personal hygiene or public sanitation in villages. No latrine and sewage disposal system. Due to this reason, the possibility of infection is higher in village community and the villagers have to face serious health problems.

5. **Low resistance:** Imbalanced diet and absence of proper nourishment reduces the availability to resist diseases and due to this, the person falls easy prey to diseases.

6. **Social and cultural beliefs:** Many superstitions, customs and tradition harmful to health are found in the villages:
   a. **Food restrictions:** It includes vegetarian/nonvegetarian and avoidance of some fruits and vegetables also, e.g. Jain community do not eat potato, tuber and some fruits of root origin.
   b. Occupational and social restrictions like having separate sources for water, sanitary work and considering the cleaning is the responsibility of a particular caste.
   c. Purdah and eating from a common plate with the bride.
   d. Religious restriction on the use of contraceptives.
   e. Prevalence of child marriage and prohibition of widow re-marriage.
   f. Poor status ascribed to women.

7. **Lack of health education:** Because illiteracy and very low education, most villages in India are unaware of the common facts regarding health. Due to this, personal health and public sanitation are neglected. Their health status is adversely affected due to lack of knowledge regarding health.

Measures of Promoting Health in Rural Community

In order to improve the health status of rural community, we have to eradicate the factors causing ill health. By adopting the following measures, the health status of the villagers can be improved.

1. Reasonable distribution of medical care facilities and making health facilities available at the grass-root level. Equip and strengthen the health care institutions existing in the villages.
2. Improve the educational standard of the village community with special care to girl child education. Provide facilities for informal education.
3. Provide clean drinking water and also enough water for other daily needs.
4. Improve housing facilities in villages. By using locally available material and technology, encouraging the construction of cheap and healthy houses.
5. Accept meaningful methods of population control. Encourage the use of contraceptives.
6. Better cooperation with village panchayat or other local self government to improve the health care facilities in villages.
7. Effective management of primary health centers, subcenters and community health centers.
8. Population education by making effective use of communication facilities, create health awareness among villagers.

9. Better health management and health information system to be developed in villages, so that in time of emergency (plague, cholera, natural calamities, etc.) health care can be provided immediately.
10. Strengthen reproductive and child health and school health services in villages.

Difference between Rural and Urban Society

Sl.No.	Criteria	Rural society	Urban society
1.	Size of population	Rural population is limited	Urban population is large.
2.	Environment	Natural environment, more close to nature	Artificial environment and more problems of environmental pollution.
3.	Family	Trend of joint family is found	Nuclear family is more common.
4.	Occupation	Agriculture and agriculture based occupations	Industry, trade and different occupations (education, medical, administration, engineering, management, etc.).
5.	Social uniformity	More uniformity found	Heterogeneity and differences are found.
6.	Stratification	More based on castes, otherwise stratification is simple	More based on class. Stratification is complex.
7.	Mobility	Physical and social mobility is limited	High rate of physical and social mobility.
8.	Density of population	Less density	High density
9.	Means of recreation	More natural and cultural Social ridicule is natural	Professional and complex. Media is relatively more powerful.
10.	Political awareness	Relatively less, increasing now	Political awareness is more.
11.	Marriage and divorce	Marriage is traditional and permanent. Divorce is negligible	Love marriages are also found. Divorce is more common. Marriage institution is in more danger.
12.	Condition of social change	Change is less	Changes are fast and more political.
13.	Education	Less literacy	Changes are fast and more political.
14.	Social problems	Unsociability, child marriage, superstitions, etc. found more	Problems are based on class, economy, power, etc.
15.	Social interaction and relationship	Personal and more cordial	Indirect and formal relationship is found more.
16.	Interaction	Social contacts are limited. Primary contacts, relationships are personal, durable, human relationships	Wider contacts, secondary in nature, relationships are impersonal, indirect, short lived-superficial and touch and go relationships.

Contd...

Contd...

Sl.No.	Criteria	Rural society	Urban society
17.	Social organization families	Family ties are stronger joint family system more parental control sense of we feeling, neighborhood is important, divorces cannot escape from means of social control like customs, traditions, mores, etc.	Wider contacts, secondary in nature relationships are impersonal indirect, short lived-superficial and touch and go relationship.
18.	Attitudes	Rural people are frank, open and conservative	Artificial, cosmopolitan, hide and secret, more progressive.

CHANGE IN THE VILLAGE LIFE

Actually, the villagers everywhere are at present passing through a transitional period. The relations, bounds and ties have fallen into disfavor and they cannot be reinstated in the original form. Even now the village can be given equally simple, if not simpler, plainer and higher life by improving the conditions in these villages, through the establishment of Panchayats, spread of education, economic reform in agriculture, etc. rural reconstruction through scientific methods is very essential for this. Change is the law of nature and need of life. The village community is less susceptible to change than the urban community. The change in village community may be based in different ways:

1. **Caste system:** British rule in India gave a serious blow to the caste system in the villages. The economic policy and the laws of British rulers induced the different castes restrictions on food, dress, mode of living and other matters imposed under caste system to be removed. Even untouchability was weakened.
2. **Jaimani system:** Jajmani system a feature of village community in India has now weakened due to the governmental efforts to raise the status of the lower casters and the impact of urbanization. The occupations adopted by the village people are not entirely hereditary or based on caste system nor the payment for services rendered by the lower castes is in kind, any more as it is now mostly cash payment.
3. **Family system:** The joint family system is no longer the peculiar characteristics of the village community. Nuclear families have formed. The family control over its members in matters of diet, dress, and marriage are weakened. The family is no longer economic unit. The education of the village girl has raised the status of rural women.
4. **Marriage system:** Change can also be seen in the institution of marriage, although intercaste marriages are rare and parents continue to dominate the mate-choice, yet boys and girls are consulted by the parents in the matter of mate-choice. The individual qualities like education, economic status, beauty and appearance of the parents are given preference over the old family status.
5. **Living standards:** The standard of living in the village community is gradually going higher. The rural diet now includes vegetables, milk, bread, tea, ghee, etc. the dress is getting urbanized. The youth there paints and the girls were stitched dresses like urban girls. There are now well ventilated, well furnished, electrified houses with sanitary latrines in some villages. Mud houses are replaced with concrete cement houses. Gobar gas plants have been installed in some houses.
6. **Health services:** The primary health center has made people health conscious. The immunization services, MCH services, family planning services, school health services and other health

services provided to villages and ensure good health and prevention of epidemics. Agriculture I institutes and social welfare institutes have also been opened in some villages.

7. **Economic system:** Change has also taken place in the economic field. The education rural youth seeks jobs in the cities rather than in agriculture. The utilization of modern technologies in agriculture has started. The farmer is taught new methods to raise their production. The rural cooperative societies have lessened the villagers in getting seeds, fertilizer and credit. The per capita income of villagers has increased as they get good price for their products.

8. **Political system:** The development of Panchayats has led to the growth of political consciousness among village people. The media like TV, radio, newspaper, etc. have added to the political knowledge of villagers.

9. **Modern means of transportation and communication:** Better transportation and communication facilities are being extended to rural areas. Roads are constructed and railway lines are extended. This provides more opportunities for villagers to around and also to establish better connection with urban centers. With the advent of Radio, even the illiterate masses could hear things and learn slowly. The government has extended television facilities to most of the rural areas and this is going to be a powerful agent of social change.

10. **Education:** Education is a catalyst to change. Education broadens one's outlook and makes one open to change. After the attainment of independence of India, many schools are established in rural area and rural children are also receiving education. The educated ruralities are migrating to cities for higher education and employment. Along educated children their parents and relatives also migrate to urban areas. Thus education is responsible for many changes in rural India.

RURAL RECONSTRUCTION PROGRAM

After independence, union government has realized the need for rebuilding the rural life by improving their economic and social problems. Mahatma Gandhi during the freedom movement often emphasized the deteriorating conditions of villages and emphasized the need for rural reconstruction programs for all development of villages. Its aim is to usher new life of prosperity and total change. The government of India gave importance to rural planning to improve the rural life the government of India generated change by implementing certain measures. Some of the measures adopted can be classified into following categories:

1. Introducing scientific method of agriculture. Use of improved seeds, fertilizer, insecticides, improved agriculture tools, construction of major and minor irrigation projects.
2. Land reforms: to improve the conditions of tenants by providing rights over the land.
3. To protect the farmers from the clutches of money lenders.
4. Introduction of community development project, encourage cottage industries, to establish co-operative societies.
5. To educate the mass.
6. To provide better health facilities.

In spite of such rural development programs adopted by the government, has failed to uplift the poor laborers and in providing employment opportunities. So, the results have not reached to the poor and the weaker sections. So, to identify the rural development and change the following new programs and policies have been implemented by the government through five years plan.

1. Community development program (1952)
2. Twenty-point programs (1975).

Special Programs
1. DPAP— Drought prone areas program.
2. SFDA and MFAL—The small farmer's development agency marginal farmers and agricultural laborers development agencies.
3. IRDP—Integrated rural development program.
4. TRYSEM—Training of rural youth for self-employment.
5. Introducing Panchayat Raj.

COMMUNITY DEVELOPMENT PROGRAM

India after independence has to face many vital economic and social problems. Food production was the lowest in the world. Cottage industries were on decline. Literacy was very low, death rate was very high. People suffered from various epidemic and other general diseases. Health care facilities were very meager. So many felt that political freedom has no meaning unless we improve the social and economic conditions of the people.

Community development is a purposive attempt induced and directed towards all around development of villages. This program was sponsored by the government of India in their first five years plan in 1952. The planning commission initiated this program as a process of transformation of the social and economic life of the villages.

Definitions
1. Community development is defined as a movement designed to promote better living for the whole community with the active participation of the community and to stimulate it in order to secure its active response.
2. Community development project is a method initiated through five years plan to bring out change in social and economic life of the villages by self help and cooperation of villagers—*AR Desai*.
3. Community development program is a systematic and planned integrative method of reconstruction of rural India by self help and participation of villagers.

Aims and Objectives of Community Development Program
1. To develop agricultural production, transport and communications, rural health, sanitation and rural education.
2. To bring over all change in the outlook of people and to rise the standard of living by modernizing agriculture and to develop rural industries.
3. To develop rural leadership, to improve the status of women in villages.
4. To provide education to rural illiterates and compulsory education.
5. To provide better housing facilities to the poor and the weaker sections.
6. To provide employment opportunities to rural youth.
7. To provide better health facilities, by starting public health centers. To protect the villagers from epidemic diseases, prevention and curative measures to improve the health at the village level.
8. To provide health education, maternity and child health welfare, family welfare programs.

20-POINT PROGRAM

Unfortunately the community development programs through five year plans did not reach the poor and weaker sections. The social and economic life of the people did not improve. Realizing this

Smt. Indra Gandhi initiated certain bold and progressive measures with the sole objective of eradicating poverty. She was instrumental in nationalizing banks and abolished royalty given to kings. On 1st July 1975, she implemented 20-point programs. This program opened a new chapter in the country.

1. To provide more and more irrigation facilities, to encourage dry land agriculture.
2. To increase the production of pulses and oil seeds.
3. IRDP and NREP.
4. To distribute the land to landless.
5. To fix the minimum wages to agriculture labors.
6. Removal of bounded labor and their rehabilitation.
7. Special emphasis to SC/ST development.
8. To provide drinking water to all villages.
9. Free site distribution to houseless.
10. To increase the electric production.
11. Afforestation program.
12. Women and child welfare, protection to mother and child.
13. Universal primary education.
14. Important to girls education.
15. Spread of literacy.
16. Public health facilities, control of TB, eradication of leprosy and blindness.
17. To open more and more fair price shops.
18. Development of industries, particularly handlooms and handy crafts.
19. Family welfare programs.
20. Control of black marketers and tax evaders.

PANCHAYAT RAJ (DEMOCRATIC DECENTRALIZATION)

Panchayat raj is a three tire structure of the rural local self government. It is a complex system, which represents the local inhabitants, possessing a range or degree of autonomy. The panchayat raj institutions are accepted as agencies public welfare. All development programs are channeled through these bodies. Balwantrai Mehta study team which evaluated the community development program realized the necessity for democratic decentralization of administration so as to create institutions of democratic administration at the village level. It recommended a tree-tire system of decentralization. At the grass root village level village panchayats, panchayat samathis at the Block level and Zila Parishads at District level.

The village panchayats are elected bodies of village people. All adults- men and women- vote to elect the members of the village panchayat. The village panchayats send their elected representative to Block panchayat samitis. A few coopted members' representation women, depressed and scheduled castes are also included in the Samitis. The Samiti elects its president and vice-president of the panchayat samiti, along with MPs and MLAs of the district. The national development council approved the scheme of the Balwantrai Metha committee regarding the establishment of Panchayat Raj on January 1958.

Panchayat Raj system is parallel to this official structure of administration; there are institutions of local self government rural areas. This refers to Panchayat Raj system. This system is introduced since 1957 to link to the district, to have people's participation and strengthen the administration at the gross root level.

Panchayat Raj at Village Level

Sl.No.	Types	Description
1.	Gram Sabha	It is comprised of all the adult men and women of the village. This body meets at least twice in a year and discusses important issues and considers proposals pertaining to various development aspects including health matters.
2.	Gram Panchayat	Gram panchayat consists of 15-30 elected members. It covers a population of 5000 to 20000. It is chaired by the president, vice-president and a secretary. The gram is an executive organ of Gram Sabha and is responsible for overall planning and development of the villages. The panchayat secretary has been given powers to function for wide areas such as maintenance of sanitation and public health, socioeconomic development of the village. Gram Panchayat is involved in planning and organizing of various health activities in the villages. One of the panchayat members is given the responsibility for coordinating health activities.
3.	Nyaya Panchayat	Nyaya Panchayat is comprised of 5 members from the panchayat. It tries to solve the dispute between two parties/groups/ individuals over certain matters on mutual consent. Thus, saves the trouble of going to formal judicial system.

Panchayat Raj at Block Level

The Panchayat Raj institution at the Block level is known as **Panchayat Samiti.** The Panchayat Samiti includes following members, Sarpanches from all the Gram Panchayats in the Block: MLAs and MPs residing in the area; representative of women, schedule castes, schedule tribes and cooperative societies. The block development officer is the ex-officio secretary of the Panchayat Samiti. The Panchayat Samiti is responsible for Block development activities under the community development program.

Panchayat Raj at District Level

The Panchayat Raj institution at District level is known as Zila Parishad. The Zila Parishad includes the following members: the heads of the Gram Samities in the District; MLAs and MPs from the District, representatives of women, schedule castes, schedule tribes, two persons who have experience in administration, rural development, etc. the collector of the district is the non-voting member. The Zila Parishad is headed by the chairman also known as Adhikasha. The Zila Parishad in general supervise and coordinate development programs being carried by the Gram Samities in the Block of a District.

CONCLUSION

The villages have a sense of unity. Their customs, convention and culture are common. In a village, neighborhood is very important. In a village, each other and have good neighborly relationships. The people in the villages have great faith in religion. They lead a simple life. They are free from metal conflicts. They are sincere, honest and hardworking. India is a land of villages. The bulk of its population lives in villages. Till the middle of 19th century every village was self contained; isolated self sufficient unit. But changing political and economic conditions have changed these characteristics of the village. Indian villages are known for an atmosphere of peace and simplicity. Even there lot of change and the villages have become the most active centers of political life in the country. The villagers are strongly attached to old customs and traditions. Indian villages are known for their poverty and illiteracy. In ancient India villages enjoyed fair amount of autonomy of self government. British introduced highly centralized system of administration. Today we are again trying to review the old Panchayat Raj system. The villagers in India are today passing through a transitional period.

BIBLIOGRAPHY

1. Barnes. An Introduction to the History of Sociology. The University of Chicago Press.
2. K Davis. Human Society. Surjeet Publications, New Delhi, 1981.
3. Murphy G, Murphy LB. Experimental Social Psychology. Harper & Bos, New York, 1931.
4. Murray HA. Explorations in Personality. Oxford University Press, New York, 1938.
5. Newcomb TM. Personality and Social Change Attitude Formation in a Student Community, Dryden, New York, 1943.
6. NJ Smelser. Sociology. Prentice Hall, India Ltd., 1993.
7. Ogburn and Nimkoff. A Handbook of Sociology. Eurasia Publishing House, New Delhi.
8. P Gisbert. Fundamentals of Sociology. Orient Longman.
9. RN Sharma. Principles of Sociology, Rajahamsa Pakistani, Meerut.
10. Robert Bierstedt. The Social Order. Tata McGraw Hill, 1970.
11. Ronald Fletcher. The Making of Sociology, Vol 1 and 11. Rawat Publication.
12. Samuel Koening Barnes and Noble. An Introduction to the Science of Society, 1968.
13. Vilhelm Aubert Heineuann. Elements of Sociology, Educational Books Ltd. London, 1969.
14. Young and Mack. Systematic Sociology, East-West Press, New Delhi, 1972.

33 *Urban Community*

DEFINITIONS

1. **Urban:** An urban community is a group of people having a certain minimum population and possessing certain specialized economic, nomic, political, and social structure.
2. **City:** A city is a limited geographical area inhibited by a large and closely settled population having many common interests and institutions under local government authorities by the state.
3. **Urbanism:** Urbanism is a process of development. It refers to the movement of population from rural to urban areas. It is not merely shifting of people from village to city but also change of work pattern from agriculture to urban type of work like industry, trade, services, etc.
4. **Regional community:** Regional community defined as an area within which the people and the different constituent's communities are conspicuously more interdependent than they are with people of other areas.
5. **Regionalism:** The community feeling within a region is called regionalism. Regionalism gives man a feeling of oneness with his fellow and with the earth they share. It involves a cultural wholeness. The people of a region have attitude that look towards a large unit of stimulation, relationship and growth.
6. **Slum:** Slum is a building, group of buildings or area characterized by overcrowding with deterioration in civic amenities, unsanitary conditions or absence of facilities or amenities with endanger the health, safety, and morals of its inhabitants or the community.
7. **Metropolis:** The term metropolis means mother city. Such cities were dependent culturally, politically and economically on their mothers. In recent periods the term metropolis was used to such cities which grew in large propositions and gained super national importance. London was considered as a metropolis in 1820 itself because of the population exceeded 1 million.
8. **Tribes:** Group of families bearing a common name speaking a common dialect, occupying a common territory.
9. **Tribal welfare:** Central and State Governments have undertaken tribal welfare measures along with the help of voluntary agencies, to alleviate the tribal from ignorance, illiteracy and poverty with the following welfare programs.
10. **Tribal community:** Tribal is referred to as nomads, Girijans, original inhabitants of the country, adipraja, etc. Tribals live faraway from the so-called civilized people.

INTRODUCTION

The term urban is derived from the Latin word Urbanus. Urbanus means a city or a town. Towns and cities of India make up the urban communities with about 20% of the population. Compared with other countries India has a much higher rural population, but the urban population increasing rapidly. Town and cities are over-crowing and always expanding. In urban areas most of the people have to work in connection with industry, the manufacture, trade, transport of goods and materials. In urban social life relations are for short-time and impersonal. There is no feeling of oneness, and it is a case of each person for himself. There is keen competition. The basis of urban social life is class rather than caste, and social class depends on economic status, some people by working hard, or by other means, may get rich quickly, and move from lower to middle or even upper class.

Life is quite different in towns and cities than in villages. Traditions, customs, and mores do not have much influence over those living in urban areas. For those living in urban areas family life is less disciplined and there is no community support. There is much more mixing among people of very different background. This brings about changes in habits and attitudes. In India, cities exists from a long-time, cities like—Ayodhya, Pataliputra, Magadha, etc. are well-known ancient cities. Urban self-government was absent in ancient India. Because of urbanization the number of cities began to grow. Like in other parts of the world, in India too cities have increased by immigration of villagers.

DEFINITIONS OF URBAN COMMUNITY

1. Urban community is defined as a population aggregate whose occupations are non-agricultural and specialized activities—*James Quinn*.
2. An urban community possesses a high population density, predominance of nonagricultural occupations, complex division of labor, whose relations is characterized as secondary and depends upon formal social controls.
3. City is a state of mind, a body of customs and traditions and the organized attitudes and sentiments that are inherent in these customs. Thus, we find that city or the urban community has a limited area, a local government and certain striking traits quite different from the rural community—*Robert Park*.
4. A city is a limited geographical area inhabited by a large and closely settled population having many common interest and institutions under a local government authorized by the state—*Howard Woolston*.

URBANIZM

Urbanizm means a way of behavior and thinking. Urbanization refers to certain features like transiency, superficiality, anonymity, impersonal relations, highly mobile and dynamic. This kind of life pattern is extended to rural areas because of vast network of communications. Urbanization is a process of development. It refers to the movement of population from rural to urban areas. It is not merely shifting of people from village to city but also change of work pattern from agriculture to urban type of work like industry, trade, service, etc. According to Anderson, urbanization is a two way process. It involves not only the movement of people from villages to cities change of occupations but involves basic changes in thinking and behavior of people.

CLASSIFICATIONS OF CITIES

Cities may be classified in various ways. Gist and Halbert gave six-fold classifications basing it on the functional concepts:

1. Production centers, such as Jamshedpur for Iron and Steel, Ahmedabad for Textile, Danbury for Hats, Akron for Rubber.

2. Centers for trade and commerce, for example, New York, Hamburg, Amsterdam, Delhi, Ludhiana.
3. Political capitals for instance, New Delhi, Chandigarh, Washington, London.
4. Cultural centers like Oxford, Cambridge, Santiniketan, and Varanasi.
5. Resort cities like Monte Carlo, Padam Beach, Srinagar, and Shimla.
6. Diversified cities, which have a great many varied interests and not outstanding in any particular activity.

EE Muntz has suggested principle activity as the basis for classification of the cities:

Sl.No.	Types	Description
1.	Defense cities	Which were built for the purpose of defense with walls around them, for instance Quebec, Mexico, Manila.
2.	Commercial cities	London, New York, Mumbai.
3.	Manufacturing or industrial cities	Massachusetts, Jamshedpur, Manchester.
4.	Political cities	New Delhi, Chandigarh, Washington in which governmental activities are centered.
5.	Religious cities	Jerusalem, Vatican, Jeddah.
6.	Educational cities	Oxford, Cambridge, Santiniketan.
7.	Resort cities	Monte Carlo, Srinagar.

On the basis of size urban areas are classified as:

Sl.No.	Types	Description
1.	Town	Consists of 5000 to 50,000 population.
2.	City	Consists of 50,000 and above.
3.	Metropolis	Consists of 100,000 and above.

CHARACTERISTICS OF URBAN COMMUNITY

1. **Impersonality of social relations:** The most striking feature of the social aspect of urban life is its impersonality. The chief reason for this state of affairs is that people in cities do not regard affectionately other persons and do not have any respect for them. They love and respect goods and things in preference to human being. Every commodity and service in urban society is evaluated in terms of cash; therefore, everything in city is for sale and purchase. Nothing has intrinsic value in the urban context: All can be measured in terms of cash. Every service rendered by someone to someone has its price. Due to the overwhelming influence of materializm every kind of commodity and every kind of human relation has its price. The cash nexus completely dominates the urban life.
2. **Mechanical social life:** As a consequence of impersonality of relations, industrialization and the widespread use of modern sophisticated technical gadgetry the urban life has become mechanical. It has lost all creativity. In urban, the person meets numerous people daily. A city-dweller rarely forms close relationships with anyone, radio, television and newspaper encourage indirectness and formality of relationships because due to these one has not to depend on any one for news and information. Due to temporary, casual and calculated relations among

individuals, few permanent, stable and deep relationships develop in cities. Even when the relationship is durable and longstanding, it does not grow in depth and intimacy because of its utilization bias.

3. **Secondary control:** Due to impersonality of social relations and mechanical nature of the social life, primary controls are not effective in urban context. There is little control of family, caste and Biradari upon the conduct and behavior of the individual. An urban man is under the control of the law enforcing agencies of the government only. Therefore, in cities laws and police assumes great significance and very crucial role. Often the relations amongst the members of such societies because so intimate that the control exercised by them because the same as the primary control. Sometimes, clubs and societies in cities perform the functions of family, church and neighborhood.

4. **Ostentation and show:** In urban life there is too much emphasis on ostentation. Erich Fromm has elaborately depicted a forceful picture of this urban proclivity in his book 'The Sane Society'. The urban people are so addicted to ostention that the value a thing which impresses them rather they are impressed if it is decorative, out of way, unusual or rare. They want to be popular, to be respected in recognition of the pomp and show of their possessions. There is indeed so much emphasis on the outward show, the brightness and glamour of dress, perfumes and such things that it is doubtful if the urban man ever gets time to look into himself, to reflect and ponder.

5. **Fashion:** As consequences of the tendency towards ostentation and show off, the fashion flourishes and is the order of the day in cities. The trends in fashion are determined by popular leaders, film actors, and actress. The ladies fashion in hair dress, clothing, ornaments and mannerism follow the trends set by the film personalities. Similarly, young men follow very closely the fashions of their film heroes in matter of dress, speech and even smoking. The trend in fashion is usually set by leading metropolises. People in small town simply copy these. In India people of Mumbai and Delhi lead in fashion and others follow their suit.

6. **Dynamism:** Another feature of the social life in the urban society is that it is far more dynamic and mobile than the life in the village. The dynamicity and mobility of urban life is of many kinds. For example, we find frequent change of residence in cities. This keeps people moving the shifting. The change of residence in cities is due to the fact that majority of people in cities live in tenanted houses. Therefore, they always so manage their affairs so to be able to shift easily and at a short notice. The change of residence can be due to a number of factors: Transfer, quarrel between tenants and landlords; availability of better or cheaper accommodation, etc. The government servants are transferred periodically and they have to change their residence from time-to-time. The social mobility of urban life affects social relations. Generally an increase in the social mobility is accompanied by intensification of impersonality and unattachedness or social relations. It also leads to personal and social disorganization.

7. **Lack of neighborly feeling:** In cities we find lack of feelings of neighborliness. The social relations are motivated and calculated; these are totally devoid of love and sympathy. Generally, speaking the feeling of neighborliness is in inverse proportion to the size of the city and the density of its population. In cities the residential and industrial complexes are usually separated by great distances. Therefore, people leave their homes early in the morning and return fairly late in the evening utterly exhausted. Sunday and other holidays are spent in doing household chores. Thus, they get virtually no time to meet their neighbors and spend some time with them.

8. **Heightening of conflicts and competition:** In urban life we find a great deal of conflict and competition. With rise the mechanical nature of urban life and it is artificially the mental conflicts

are also on the rise. In the gaudy life of the cities a man is beset with so many desires some of which are so at variances that it is small wounder that neuroses are so common in the cities. As a consequence of conflicting desires the life is full of discontent and sorrow. Besides social and mental conflicts there is also competition in the economic life.

9. **Rapidly information of association:** Another special feature of city life is the abundance of voluntary associations and the speed with which these spring up. In cities we fine diversity of self interests, aptitudes, aspirations, aims and purposes in order to meet this diversity a large variety of associations are springing up, therefore, there is a plethora of voluntary associations in cities. Some of these associations have usurped the functions of family and neighborhood.

10. **Position of women:** As MacIver observes, the individualization of women has been fostered by urban life and the resulting free reciprocity of relationship between men and women a significant influence on whole structure of society. City women are working in workshop and factory, college and hospital.

11. **Economic status:** Cities provide opportunity for personal development such as modern business, employment opportunities, standard of living development, great achievement and better living in the urban with social relationship.

12. **Educational status:** The educational facilities in urban is improved. Elementary schools in a better equipped than in the rural. Most training schools, colleges and technical schools are urban. Many libraries are situated in urban.

URBAN COMMUNITY

1. **Namelessness:** The urban groups have, as Bogardus observes, a reputation for namelessness. By virtue of its size and population, the city cannot be primary group. The inhabitants of a city do not come into primary contact with each other. They meet and speak without knowing each other's name. A citizen may live for several years in a city and may not know the names of one-third of the people who live in the same city area. The urban world puts a premium on varied recognition. In short, urban contacts are segmental.

2. **Homelessness:** Homelessness is another disturbing feature of city community. The house problem in a big city is very acute. Many low class people pass their nights on pavement. The middle class people have but insufficient accommodation, a room or two and that also on the sixth or seventh floor.

3. **Class extremes:** Class extremes characterize urban community. In a city are found the richest as well as the poorest people, the people rolling in luxury and living in grand mansions as well as the people living on pavements and hardly getting two meals a day.

4. **Social heterogeneity:** The city is more heterogenous than the village. It has been the melting pot of races, peoples, and cultures and is a most favorable breeding ground of new biological and cultural hybrids. It has not only tolerated but rewarded individuals differences. It has brought together people from the ends of the earth because they are different and thus useful to one another rather than because they are homogeneous and like mind.

5. **Social distance:** Social distance is a product of anonymity and heterogeneity. The city dweller feels lonely. There is masking of one's true feelings. The routine social contracts are impersonal and segmented.

6. **Energy and speed:** Energy and speed are the final traits of a city. People with ambition work at a tremendous speed, day and night, which stimulate others also to work similarity. Stimulation and inter-stimulation are endless. Urban life produces greater emotional tension and insecurity

than does rural life. Cities may be called consumers of population. They are consumers of population in the sense also than due to congestion, insanitariness and unhealthiness they adversely affect health of the inhabitants.

REGIONAL COMMUNITY

Another important social unit is the regional area. A region is a large area where there are a good many resemblances among the inhabitants. A region may not coincide with state or national boundaries. It usually combines rural and urban communities into one unit. Regional community is marked because one may live his entire life with it or his social relationships may be found within it. But one cannot live a complete life say within a church or a business organization. But one can do it in a tribe or a city. The modern civilized communities are much less self-contained. We may live at the metropolis and be a member of a small community or we may live in a village and be a part of a larger community.

Definition

Regional community defined as an area within which the people and the different constituent communities are conspicuously more inter-dependent than they are with people of other areas—*Lundberg*.

Regionalism

The community feeling within a region is called regionalizm. There is a difference between regionalizm and sectionalizm. The former implies an integral relationship with a large whole, while the later suggests segregation, separation and isolation. Sectionalizm is a narrow loyalty to local interests and historic sentiments. Regionalizm gives man a feeling of oneness with his fellow and with the earth they share. It involves a cultural wholeness. The people of a region have attitude that look towards a large unit of stimulation, relationship and growth. It includes unity in economic and social functioning.

Special Feature of Regional Community

A regional community is that it must occupy a definite territory. A normad community like the gypsies has a local though a changing habitation. At a given time they occupy a definite locality. But most of the so called communities are settled.

Aims of Regionalism

A fundamental aim of regionalism is the development of an integrated large community within which city and country each has its place and makes its contribution. Each region is a locality having a specific geographic character, certain common properties of soil, climate, vegetation, agriculture and technical exploitation. This is the geographical requirement of a region. Besides, a religion in so far as it is an integrated area of social life exhibits a balance state of dynamic equilibrium, between its various parts. Region is a community large enough to encompass a variety of interests and activities, urban and rural, industrial and agricultural, to ensure balance. Region must be a balance and integrated community.

Types of Regions

Odum and Moore have distinguished between five kinds of regions.
1. A physical region is one which is demarcated by geographical factors. A large river valley surrounded by mountains is a well-known type of physical region.
2. A metropolitan region is a large city with its suburbs and all the surrounding area whose trading activities are carried on in the city.
3. A sectional region is one in which a particular set of folkways prevail.
4. An administrative region is governed by political boundaries determined by convenience or by accident or by political planning.
5. Then there is the group-of-states region which usually possesses physical similarity, homogeneity and cultural uniformities.

Regions in India

Under the States Reorganization Act, 1956, India was divided into four different zones.
1. Northern Zone including Jammu and Kahmir, Panjab, Rajasthan, Uttar Pradesh and Delhi.
2. Western Zone including Maharashtra and Gujarat.
3. Southern Zone including Chennai, Mysore and Kerala.
4. Eastern Zone including Assam, Bihar, Orissa and West Bengal.

Each state within a zone has its own language, its own traditions and its own special problems. In this country there are variations of geographic factors, industrial and agricultural techniques, consumption habits and standards and of nationality differences which are great difficulties in furthering the development of integrated regions which demand a more complete unification of interests.

CITIES AND THEIR GROWTH

An understanding of the origin of the cities is a simpler problem. Cities came into existence since many thousand years ago. Ancient cities arose in the Nile, Tigris-Euphrates and Indus river valleys. Great cities like Harappa, Mohanjodaro in India, Memphis and Thebes in Egypt, Rome in Italy and Athens in Greece are the ancient cities. During the medevil period, commercial activities and the political factors, religions were chiefly responsible for the growth of cities. Urbanization became a world wide phenomenon after the 18th century. Some of the factors that gave impetus to the development of cities are as follows:
1. Industrial revolution: The advent of mechanical power to textile and metal industries.
2. The new sources of power: Like steam, electricity and oil. Establishment of large factories.
3. The development of urban: Market, trade, and commerce.
4. Progress in science and technology: Countless invention and discoveries.
5. Development of modern means of transport and communication: Railways, automobiles, aeroplanes, telephone, telegraph, radio, TV and computer.
6. Migration of rural people in search of jobs to cities—due to increased birth rates a significant proportion of the population shifted to urban centers.
7. Education and recreation facilities.
8. Political centers or capital cities, military centers, industrial centers, religious centers (places like Haridwar, Tirupathi, and Varanasi) and educational centers have developed as cities.

The urban population gradually increased. The decline in percentage of rural population and the raise in urban population is indicating the growth of cities. In India, the urban population was 109.11 millions in 1971 which was increased to 160.1 million in 1991 and increased to 291 millions by 2001. In India, new towns came into existence and the old towns grew as cities and cities like Kolkata, Mumbai, Chennai, Delhi, Bangalore, Hyderabad developed as metropolitan cities with more than 50 lakh population.

Metropolis

The term metropolis means mother city. In ancient period the Greek established their colonies in foreign countries. Such cities were dependent culturally, politically and economically on their mothers. In recent periods the term metropolis was used to such cities which grew in large proportions, and gained super national importance. London was considered as a metropolis in 1820 itself because its population exceeded 1 million. A century later 50 cities has a population of more than 1 million. Such cities are called Giant city.

URBAN SOCIAL PROBLEMS

The rapid urbanization and industrialization processes are responsible for the certain social problems. It is said that city is a center of attraction and at the same time it is pathological.

The common social problems are:
1. Over crowding.
2. Road accidents.
3. Growth of slums.
4. Poverty.
5. Antisocial activities.
6. Political unrest.
7. Failure of people adjusts.
8. Prostitution.
9. Crime and delinquency.
10. Begging.
11. Mental illness/conflicts/disease.
12. Alcoholizm.
13. Drug additiction.
14. Gambling.
15. Smoking.

Common Problems in India

1. **Death and diseases:** In earlier days the cities suffered from different kinds of epidemics. Medical knowledge was meager and health care services were not developed. Hygienic measures were primitive and poor. Consequently, the death rates and incidence of diseases were higher in cities. In modern city now-a-days more and more hospitals have been established. Highly qualified and superspecialty doctors and well-trained paramedical health team involved in super specialized medical, surgical and rehabilitative care. Still occurrence of death and diseases are present due new existing social and man made troubles.

2. **Pollution:** Pollution occurs because of big factories, traffic congestion, smoke, excessive dirt, dust and other types of air contamination, many diseases like respiratory problems, asthma, TB, etc. will spread at a higher rate and there is higher mortality rate. Day-by-day pollutions are increasing at the same time controlling measures also carried out by the exports.

3. **Mental diseases:** City life is very busy, excessive noise, glaring, lights of automobiles, economic pressures, create stress and strain. All these create mental tensions and serious problems and leads to mental illness. Isolation is another cause of emotional disturbance such a situation in extreme cases of individuals, leads to suicide.

4. **Slums and housing problems:** Since the dawn of industrial revolution man has gravitated to cities in search of economic opportunities. In cities he can seek remunerative jobs. Cities made the greatest progress in education, trade, commerce. The new migrants may occupy an area near the place of their work and may construct temporary huts or sheds and began to live in such residential areas. The over crowding of such areas, without any basic amenities become slum.

5. **Transportation congestion:** Transport facility in big cities is a major problem. School children find it difficult to go to their schools because of rush. The increasing use of automobiles, make the traffic congestion. They pollute the environment with heavy smoke.

6. **Sanitation:** Cities and towns in India have failed to provide good sanitation facility. Municipalities or cooperation have failed to remove the garbage and clean the drains. The sweepers are not sincerely performing their duties. The spread of slum adds to the filth and uncleanliness. Because unhealthy sanitation, the diseases like diarrhea, diphtheria, malaria, etc. spread among citizens.

7. **Corruption:** Corruption is rampant in government offices and city corporations.

8. **Inadequate water supply and drainage system:** Water management is a serious problem in cities. Most of the cities face the problem of water supply. No city has the facility of supplying water for 24 hours. Many small towns are depending upon tube wells or tanks through the government's aim are to provide clean water supply to all the city dwellers, it has failed to formulate a national policy. Drainage system in cities is equally bad. Stagnant water can be seen in every city to lack of proper drainage and the over crowding of houses. Consequently the cities become the breeding places of mosquitoes and cause diseases like malaria, dengue fever, chickengunia, etc.

9. **Poverty:** Poverty is a major social problem in most of the underdeveloped and developing countries. Poverty is less purchasing capacity or poor economy. Poverty is the most important social as well as health problem. Some of the causes of poverty are personal, while others are geographical, economic and social. In capacity of the individual to earn due to faulty heredity, environment, unfavorable physical conditions such as poor natural resources and misdistribution of the available resources.

10. **Unemployment:** Unemployment in youth both educated and uneducated is a major social problem in India. Most of the unemployment are educated youth. The present system of education is responsible for unemployment.

11. **Crime:** Crime is an act forbidden by law and every crime has a penalty presented by law. Crime is always an Antisocial Act and thus a social problem. Some people commit crime out of frustration due to poverty, unemployment and coercion by superiors and powerful man but others do it because of a craving for the riches, fame and power like business men, professionals and politicians.

Measures to Solve the Urban Problems

In order to solve the problems of the city, effective measures must be taken. The following measures are suggested:

1. Prevention of migration.
2. To arrest the individual growth in a particular place. Decentralization of industries.
3. Systematic urban planning and development.
4. Effective and corrupt free local self governance.
5. To improve the infrastructure and to provide better healthy civic amenities.
6. Decentralized administration in which the local people must participate.
7. Organization of free health check-up camps and supply of free medicines to poor people.
8. Establishment of health centers in all thickly populated mohallas. Health education must be given about the use of drinking water, nutrition, community health services must be provided by trained health personnel's.

FACTORS INFLUENCES URBAN COMMUNITY

Social Effects of Urbanization

Urbanization and industrialization brought many changes in the society. The family structure, the status of man, caste and class, values of society, social relationships, etc.

1. **Urbanization and family:** Urbanization has affected the family structure, functions and relations. In India, the traditional joint family has been replaced by nuclear family. The trend today is towards a break in joint family. Urban family is based on equalitarian principles. Both husband and wife share their view in decision making. In cities most of the families both the partners are employed.
2. **Urbanization and castes:** Urbanization caused enormous change in caste and family. The three basic features of caste that are affected by urbanization and education are heredity, hierarchy and endogamy. The urbanites are educated and their relationships are not governed strictly by caste norms. We find change in commensality, material relations, social relations and occupational relations. Another important tendency, one can find is formation of caste associations and struggle for getting more and more governmental concessions in an organized manner.
3. **Urbanization and status of women:** The status of women in ancient India was high. But her position was declined during later periods, women was considered inferior, denied any right. She was suppressed and secluded, subjected to harassment. But after 19th century because of the efforts of reformist's new legislative measures, national movement, establishment of educational institutions, industrialization and urbanization led to the great emancipation of the Indian women.

SLUM

A slum is an over crowed locality with poor housing conditions, dirty and dark streets, unsanitary conditions, lack of civic amenities where poverty stricken, diseased, addicts, beggars, criminals, delinquents, prostitutes and other people dwell. These are generally called blighted areas. Even middle class people also are forced to live in such places.

The people living in the slum are poor wage earners, sweepers, casual laborers, hawkers, salesmen, beedi making laborers, handcart pullers, rickshaws, auto drivers, construction workers; homeless, habitual criminals reside in such substandard areas.

Feature of Slum

1. Overcrowding, poor environmental conditions.
2. Scarcity of health and family welfare services.
3. Absence of minimum level of residential accommodation.

COMMUNITY DEVELOPMENT PROJECT

The Planning Commission, Government of India has defined community development as an attempt to bring about a social and economical transformation of village life through the efforts of the people themselves. Community development was started for the development of rural community or urban community. The Community Development Program is aimed at a comprehensive and all round development of people.

Community Development Program was made in India in 1952 during the first-five-year plan to involve the rural population in the process of planning their own welfare measures. A program known as the Community Development Program was lunched on 2nd October 1952 for the all round development of the rural areas. This community development process designed to promote better living of the whole community with the active participation by the community itself along with governmental effort.

Activities of Community Development Program

1. Interpretation of the health needs of villages to the authorities responsible for planning and implementing the health program.
2. Improvement of agriculture.
3. Improvement of establishment of primary health centers and subcenters.
4. Improvement of housing through self help.
5. Social welfare and training in rural arts.
6. Crafts and industries to local people.

Levels of community program, development program implementation:

1. **At central level:** The program is under agriculture and irrigation ministry.
2. **At the state level:** There is a committee, with Chief Minister as Chairman and ministers of different departments as its members.
3. **As the district level:** The district board of planning has its elective members representing Members of Parliament, Members of Legislative Assembly and heads of the block level panchayat, headed by district collector.
4. **At the block level:** Block Developmental Officer and eight extension officer each from agriculture, animal husbandry, cottage industry, panchayats, cooperative society, social education, women and child welfare are appointed.
5. **At village level:** Panchayat assisted by gram sevaks (one each for 10 villages are appointed) and extension workers. There are female sevikas and dais to carry on women and children welfare activities.

Aims of community development project:

1. Integrated development of rural community covering, social, cultural and economic aspects of rural life.
2. Fullest development of available material and human resources.
3. Development of a sense of responsibility and awareness among the villagers.

4. Development of initiative among the villages.
5. Development of agriculture and allied matters like animal husbandry.
6. Development of social life by providing better communication.
7. Developing of cottage industries.
8. Providing more opportunities for employment.
9. Development of cooperative effort at rural level.
10. Women and child welfare.

Since this program is aimed for overall progress of the people; by the people and for the people, it is desired that all the people of community must be involved for obtain the target.

CONCLUSION

The city or the urban community came into being after the development of villages. There were cities in ancient times also, but most of them were of importance due to religion, policies or trade and commerce. The urban man is engaged in large number of diverse occupations such as industry, trade, commerce, education, government and recreation. Urban society show serious problems of social disorganization, urbanization and industrialization produce a changed physical environment and economic organization. Urbanization changes the social economic and political institutions.

BIBLIOGRAPHY

1. Alex Inkles. What is sociology? An Introduction to the Discipline and Profession, Prentice Hall, Mc, New Jersey, 1964.
2. Betty Yorburg. Introduction to Sociology, Harper and Row Pub Co., New York, 1982.
3. Elbert W Steward. Sociology: The Human Science, McGraw-Hill Book Co, New York, 1978.
4. Emile Durkheim. Suicide, John Spaulding and George Simpson (trans) Free Press, New York, 1966.
5. George Ritzer. Social Relations: Dynamic Perspectives, Allyn and Bacon Inc., Boston, 1974.
6. Harry M Johnson. Sociology: A Systematic Introduction, Allied Publishers Ltd, Mumbai.
7. Kingsley Davis. Human society, Macmillan Co, New York, 1949.
8. Max Weber, (HH Gerth and C Wright Mills (Ed and Translated). Essay in sociology, Oxford University Press, New York, 1958.
9. Morris Ginsberg. Sociology, Thorston and Butterworth London, 1934.
10. PA Sorokin. Society, culture and personality, Harpet and Bros, New York, 1947.
11. Samuel Koenig. Sociology: An introduction to the science of society, Barnest and noble, Mc. New York, 1968.

34 *Social Stratification*

DEFINITIONS

1. **Social stratification:** Social stratification is the division of society in permanent groups or categories linked with each other by relationships of superiority and subordination. Stratification is a horizontal division of society into higher and lowers social units.

2. **Social equilibrium:** Every society in order to have proper organization must have proper social equilibrium. It means that one proper group should not dominate over others. This cannot take place if the society is divided into various groups and people have different functions to discharge. Because of these functions they shall be mutually dependent and this mutual dependence shall be responsible for maintaining the social equilibrium.

3. **Caste stratification:** In this type of stratification the hierarchical order of different classes is determined on the basis of birth. Apart from it, the membership of groups is also determined on the basis of birth. Normally, in Hindu society there are four castes, viz. Brahmin, Kshatriya, Vaishya and Shudras. These castes have further been divided into sub-castes.

4. **Racial stratification:** This is another form of social stratification for which hierarchical order or the superiority of one class is relevance to the other is determined on the basis of the membership of a particular race. In such a type of stratification is not possible for people to leave one race and join the other.

5. **Class stratification:** This type of stratification is based on economic consideration and other personal and individual attainments. In such a society it is possible for the members of a particular class to move into another class, as also people are considered superior or inferior to one another.

6. **Open-class structure:** The open-class structure is based upon achieved criteria. There is complete freedom of association between the members of all strata, including intermarriage and equalitarian social relations. Vertical mobility is possible and probable from the bottom to the top. However, just as there has never been a pure caste society, there has never been a completely open-class structure.

7. **Caste society:** The caste society in its pure form is composed of strata based entirely upon ascribed criteria. There is very little association between members of the different strata, and the few relations permitted are severely limited and formally prescribed, e.g. master servant, professional-client relations. Marriage between castes is prohibited, and there is neither career nor generational mobility in the pure caste society. Each person is born into a caste, marries within his caste, and has children who stay in the caste. Although there has probably never

been a society which met all the criteria of caste organization, traditional India and the ancient India had caste like structures.

8. **Class system:** Class is a group of people having the same social status with respect to certain characteristics. These characteristics are not ascribed (given by birth) usually but are earned through individual efforts.

9. **Slavery:** Slavery is a form of social stratification involving great social inequality and the ownership of some persons by others. Slavery as an established institution existed in almost all the early civilization.

10. **Primitive communalizm:** Primitive communalizm is a form of stratification characterized by a high degree of sharing and minimal social inequality.

INTRODUCTION

Social stratification is a process by which individuals and groups are ranked in more or less enduring hierarchy of status. Every society is divided into higher and lower social units. Every society is divided into more or less distinct groups. Even most primitive societies had some form of social stratification. Some individuals and groups are rated higher than others on the basis of opportunities and privileges that they enjoy. For example, in India doctors or engineers are rated higher than teachers. As a class the formers have a higher social prestige. The prestige attached to different positions becomes a part of the social order and that is stratification.

Stratification tends to restrict interaction, so that there is more interaction of a given sort within strata than between strata. In a given stratification system, certain kinds of interaction may be more restricted than others. In seeking a marriage partner, in choosing a profession, in making friends there may exist more restrictions than in the flow of automobile traffic. Social stratification involves inequality, arising either from the actual functions performed by the persons involved or from the superior power and control of resources possessed by certain individuals or groups or both.

DEFINITIONS OF SOCIAL STRATIFICATION

1. Social stratification is an horizontal division of society into higher and lower social units—*Raymond W Murray.*
2. Social stratification means the differentiation of a given population into hierarchically superimposed classes—*Sorokin.*
3. Social stratification is the division of society into permanent groups or categories linked with each other by the relationship of superiority and subordination—*Gisbert.*
4. Social stratification defined as a pattern of superimposed status of a person or a group or persons in society with the result that there comes to exist people, high or low, superior or inferior—*John F Cuber and William F Kenkel.*
5. Social stratification is a system of differentiation which includes a hierarchy of social position whose occupants are treated as superior, equal or inferior relative to one another in socially important aspects—*Kurt B Mayer.*
6. A stratified society is one marked by inequality, by differences among people that are evaluated by them as being lower and higher—*Lundberg.*
7. Social stratification is the ranking of individuals on a scale of superiority-equality, according to some commonly accepted basis of valuation—*Williams.*
8. Stratification is a process by which the individuals and groups are ranked more or less enduring hierarchy of status—*Ogburn and Nimkoff.*

9. Social stratification is the division of society into permanent groups or categories linked with each other by the relationship of superiority and subordination—*Gilbert*.
10. Social stratification refers to arrangement of any social group or society into a hierarchy of positions that are unequal with regard to power, property, social evaluation and/or psychic gratification—*Melvin M Tumin*.

FUNCTIONS OF STRATIFICATION

1. Stratification provides a sense of competition and thus all try to go up and find a higher place in society.
2. Social stratification makes people responsible for the nature of work that they are doing.
3. Social stratification helps in deciding roles and functions of each category of people living in the society.
4. Stratification is also needed to give recognition to those who are able and capable, so that all are not clubbed together with the inefficient.
5. Stratification is also essential for locating status of a person in society. Without stratification it will be difficult to locate people and degree of their wisdom, initiative and knowledge.
6. Stratification provides for the placement and motivation of individuals to affect the performance of their necessary social duties.
7. It provides a system of reward and inducement to members for carrying out various duties associated with various positions.
8. The rewards, usually economic, prestige and leisure are built into social positions so that, being unequal; they result in inequality of positions.

CHARACTERISTICS OF STRATIFICATION

According to MM Tumin, the main attributes or characteristics of stratification are as follows:

Sl.No	Characteristics	Description
1	It is social	It does not represent biologically caused inequalities. It is true that such factors as strength, intelligence, age, and sex can often serve as the basis on which statuses or strata are distinguished. For example, the principle of a college attains a dominant position neither by his physical strength nor by his age but having the socially defined traits.
2	It is ancient	The stratification system is quite old. According to historical and archeological records, stratification was present even in the small wandering bands. Age and sex were the main criteria of stratification then. Difference between the rich and poor, powerful and humble, freemen and slaves was there in almost all the ancient civilization.
3	It is universal	The stratification system is a worldwide phenomenon. Difference between the rich and the poor or the haves and the have not is evident everywhere. Even in the nonliterate societies stratification is very much present. As Sorokin has said, all permanently organized groups are stratified.
4	It is in diverse forms	Stratification is not uniform in all societies. It is different from one society to another society. The ancient Greek society was divided into freeman and slaves and so on. Class and caste are general forms of

Contd...

Contd...

Sl.No	Characteristics	Description
		stratification to be found in modern world. It is a highly complex in modern civilized societies. Estate system existed during the Medieval period.
5.	It is consequential	The stratification system has its own consequences. The most important, most desired, and often the scarcest things in human life are distributed unequally because of stratification. The system leads to two main kinds of consequences: Life chances and lifestyles. Life chances refer to such things as infant, mortality, longevity, physical and mental illness, childlessness, marital conflict, separation and divorce. Life styles include such matter as the modes of housing, residential area, one's education, means of recreation, relationships between the parents and children, the kind of books and magazines and TV show to which one is exposed, one's mode of conveyance and so on. Life chances are more involuntary, while lifestyles reflect differences in preferences, tastes and values.

ORIGIN OF SOCIAL STRATIFICATION

There are two main theories concerning the origin of social stratification:
1. Theory of economic determination of Karl Marx—which is referred to as the conflict theory.
2. The functional theory.

Sl.No.	Types	Description
1.	Theory of economic determinism or the conflict theory	According to Karl Marx, economic factors are responsible for the emergence of different social strata or social classes. Therefore, social classes are defined by their relation to the means of production. Thus there are, in every society, two mutually conflicting classes—the class of the capitalists and the class of workers or the rich and the poor. Gumplowicz and Oppenheimer and others have argued that the origin of social stratification is to be found in the conquest of one group by another.
2.	Functionalist theory	Kingsley Davis, PA Sorokin, MacIver and other rejected the conflict theory of Marx. Sorokin maintained that conflict may facilitate stratification but has never originated it. He attributed social stratification mainly to inherited individual differences in environment conditions. Kingsley Davis has stated that the stratification system is universal. According to him, it has come into being due to the functional necessity of the social system. Functional theory emphasizes the integrating function of social stratification based upon individual merits and reward. Both have their own merits and demerits.

FORMS OF SOCIAL STRATIFICATION

Sl.No.	Types	Description
1.	Primitive communalism	Primitive communalism is a form of stratification characterized by a high degree of sharing and minimal social inequality. In societies practising primitive communalism, often some individuals achieve relatively high status as chief, respected leader, medicine man or shaman. But the rewards associated with the so-called high status are mainly harmony. Hence the level of the social inequality, in general, is very low. It is observed that primitive communalism is common in hunting and food gathering societies.
2.	Slavery	Slavery is a form of social stratification involving great social inequality and the ownership of some persons by others. Slavery as an established institution existed in almost all the early civilizations. It reached its peak in the early Roman Empire. Slavery is common to early agararian societies. It is frequently the result of a war in which the vanquished with their women and children became utterly dependent on their conquerors.
3.	Estates system	The system emerged in the ancient Roman Empire and existed in Europe until very recent times. The estate system consisted three main divisions— the clergy, the nobility and the commoners or the ordinary people.
4.	Caste system	The caste system as a form of social stratification is peculiar to India. Caste is a hereditary type of social group. The Hindu social order is based on the caste system. The group or caste has a common name and a traditional occupation. The membership is by birth; the members have many castes within their own groups (sub-castes) or else be treated as outcastes.
5.	Class system	Class is a group of people having the same social status with respect to certain characteristics. These characteristics are not ascribed (given by birth) usually, but are earned through individual efforts.

BIBLIOGRAPHY

1. A Cartwright. Patients and their Doctors, Routledge and Kegan Paul, London, 1967.
2. Betty Yorburg. Introduction to Sociology, Harper and Row Pub Co., New York, 1982.
3. EC Hughes et al. Twenty thousand nurses tell their story, JB Lippincott, Philadelphia, 1958.
4. F Davis (Ed). The Nursing Profession, John Wiley, New York, 1966.
5. IEB Menzies. The Functioning of Social Systems as a Defence against Anxieties Tauistocic Pamphlet No. 3, London, 1961.
6. J Klein. The Study of Groups, Routledge and Kegan Paul, London, 1967.
7. J Macquire. Threshold to Nursing, (Occasional) Papers on Social-Administration, Bell London, 30, 1969.
8. Jack Nobbs. Sociology in Context, Macmillan Education, London, 1983.
9. Leo W Simmons, Harold G Wolff. Social Science in Medicine Little Brow, Boston, 1954.
10. P Kelvin. The Basis of Social Behavior, Holt, Rinehart and Winston, London, 1970.
11. Smith Abel B. A History of the Nursing Profession, Heinemann, London, 1960.
12. William J Goode. Principles of Sociology, Tata McGrow-Hill Pub. Co., New Delhi, 1979.

Caste System

35

DEFINITIONS

1. **Caste:** Caste as a collection of families-bearing a common name claiming a common descent from a mythical ancestor, professing to follow the same hereditary calling, forming a single homogenous community. Caste as "a hereditary endogamous group having a traditional occupation".

2. **Varna:** Hindu Social Organization is broadly classified into four divisions. These are called Chathur Varna system. The four Varna are Brahmin, Kshatriya, Vaishya, and Shudra. Varna means color and applicable to the Arya and Dasa Varna.

3. **Racial purity:** It has preserved the racial purity of higher caste by forbidding indiscriminate intermarriages and has greatly fostered the habits of cleaning by insisting on ritual purity.

4. **Cultural diffusion:** Cultural diffusion helps in caste customs, beliefs, skill, behavior, the trade secrets are passed on from generation to generation. Culture thus carried from one age to another.

5. **Untouchablity:** Untouchablity is a hatefullest expression of caste. Large section of people is reduced to the state of virtual slavery. In addition, it has also carried many other social evils like child marriage, dowry system, purda system and casteism.

6. **Undemocratic:** The caste system is undemocratic because in denies equal rights to all irrespective of their castes, creed or color. Social barriers are erected specially in the way of lower class individuals who are not given freedom for the mental and physical development and are not provided with opportunities for that.

7. **Brahmins:** In caste system the Brahmins play in higher level role in the society. The primary function of the Brahmin caste is to perform various religious and ceremonial rituals.

8. **Gadaria:** The gadaria or shepherds are the herdsmen who keep sheep, goats, cows and buffaloes. They sell milk and get cash payment. After harvesting they take their animals to the fields. The gadarias also cultivate the land.

9. **Jajmani system:** Jajmani system is hereditary. The jajmani rights are property rights and hence are inherited according to the law of inheritance.

10. **Barter system:** The exchange of services is not based on money system but on barter system. The serving family gets things in exchange for the services rendered bi it; though in some cases it may also get money.

11. **Caste endogamy:** Caste endogamy may greatly affect the quality of the newborn children, resulting in physiological and psychological imbalances.

12. **Religious conversions:** The lower caste people and the untouchables are getting themselves converted to Islam and Christianity, due to the brutality of the upper class.
13. **Sanskitization:** It is the process in which the lower castes try to initiate the lifestyles of upper castes in their attempt to raise their social status. It is a process of upward mobility.
14. **Westernization:** Westernization refers to the change brought about in Indian society and culture as a result over 150 years of British rule and the term includes changes occurring at different levels—technology, institutions, ideology and values.

INTRODUCTION

The word caste is used in everyday life and we use it to distinguish one person from another. We say that such and such person belongs to a particular caste. In saying it we generally mean to convey that he is born of parents or is a member of the family said to belong to a particular caste. The word caste is derived from the Spanish word casta which means breed. Caste is a unique social institution of Indian society, originated from Varna system, described in the Vedas.

Caste system has been the predominant form of social stratification in India, and even today, it exerts considerable influence on our lives and social interaction. Caste is social phenomena found in almost all human societies but at nowhere it took such a well-defined and rigid form as it did it India. Caste is an institution most highly developed in India and it has profoundly influenced the life of the Hindus. Place of residence, mode of life, personal association, the type of food which one can eat and from whom one can accept food and water, occupation and the group in which he has to find his mate, are determined by his birth.

Social interaction between castes is very strictly limited and intercaste marriages are strictly prohibited. The caste system is always safeguard by social laws and sanctified by religion. The caste system is very conservative and lends great stability to society. It serves to hand over from one generation to another generation skills and secrets of craftsmanship, but it also acts as deterrent to the introduction of new and improved methods of production in industry and agriculture and results in an economy dependent on the interplay of a large number of segregated and sometimes conflicting interests.

DEFINITIONS OF CASTE SYSTEM

1. When status is wholly predetermined, so that men are born to their lot in life without any hope of changing it, then class takes the form of caste—*MacIver and Page*.
2. A caste is a social group having two characteristics: (1) membership is confined to those who are born of members, and include all people born, (2) the members are forbidden by an inexorable social law to marry outside the group—*Ketkar*.
3. Caste is a collection of families, bearing a common name, claiming a common descent, from a mythical ancestor, human and divine, professing to follow the same hereditary calling and regarded by those who are competent to give an opinion as forming a single homogeneous community—*Sir Herbert Risely*.
4. Caste is an endogamous group or collection of such groups bearing a common name, having the same traditional occupation claiming descent from the same source and commonly regarded as forming a single homogeneous community—*RA Gait*.
5. Caste is a system in which an individual's rank and its accompanying rights and obligations is ascribed on the basis of birth into a particular group—*Williams*.

6. Caste started as natural division of occupational classes and eventually upon receiving the religious sanction, became solidified into the existing caste system. The caste system comes into being when it becomes an integral part of religious dogma which divides the people into superior and inferior groups with different responsibilities, functions and standards of living—*Henry Maine*.
7. Caste is a system of stratification in which mobility up and down the status ladder, at least ideally may not occur—*AW Green*.
8. Caste is that extreme form of social class organization in which the position of individuals in the status hierarchy is determined by descent and birth—*Anderson and Parker*.
9. Caste as a collection of families or groups of families bearing a common name, claiming a decent from a mythical ancestor, human or divine, professing of follow the same hereditary calling and regarded by those who are competent to give an opinion as forming a single homogenous community—*Herbert Risley*.
10. A caste is an aggregate of persons whose share of obligations and privileges is fixed by birth sanctioned and supported by religion and magic—*Matindale and Monachesi*.

FEATURES OF CASTE SYSTEM

Kingsley Davis has mentioned certain common feature or tendencies which together distinguish Indian caste from other types of groups as follows.
1. The membership in the caste is hereditary.
2. This inherited membership is fixed for life.
3. Choice of marriage partner is strictly endogamous, for it must take place within the caste group.
4. Contact with other groups is further limited by restrictions on touching, associating with, dining with, eating food cooked by outsiders.
5. Consciousness of caste membership is further emphasized by the caste name.
6. The caste is united by a common traditional occupation.
7. The relative prestige of the different castes in any locality is well-established and jealously guarded.

DIFFERENCE BETWEEN CASTE AND CLASS

Sl.No.	Caste	Class
1.	Determined by birth	Determined by economic status.
2.	Untouchable	Changeable.
3.	Closed system	Open system.
4.	Restrictions on food and social intercourse	No restrictions on food or social intercourse.
5.	There is social distance between castes	There is no social distance between classes.
6.	Hereditary occupation—occupation restriction	Classes do not have hereditary occupation.
7.	There is endogamy	There is no endogamy.
8.	There is definite intercaste relationship. Example, Jajmani	There is no inter-class relationship.

Contd...

Contd...

Sl.No.	Caste	Class
9.	Status is ascribed	Status is achieved.
10.	Social distance between castes is more	Social distance is very less.
11.	In caste there is no caste consciousness	In class there is class consciousness
12.	Caste is based on inequalities and so not in favor of democratic values	Caste believes in equalities and favor of democracy.
13.	In caste system there are comparatively more strict restrictions in marriage	An individual has comparatively greater freedom in a class.
14.	Caste system does hinder democracy	Class system does not hinder democracy.

CHARACTERISTICS OF CASTE SYSTEM

1. **Caste is innate:** The membership of caste is determined by birth. A person remains the member of the caste into which he is born and his membership does not undergo any change even if change in his status, occupation, education, wealth, etc. takes place.
2. **There are laws concerning food in the caste:** Each individual caste has its own laws which govern the food habits of its members. Generally there are no restrictions against fruits, milk, butter, dry fruits, etc.
3. **Occupations of most castes are determined:** In Hindu religious tests the occupations of all Varnas were determined. According to manu the functions of Brahmin, Kahatriya, Vaishya and the Shudra were definite. In Hindu society even today in most cases the son of the blacksmith pursues the occupation of his father; the son of a carpenter becomes a carpenter while the son of a shoemaker becomes a shoemaker.
4. **Caste is endogamous:** The members of each of the many castes marry only within their own caste. Brahmin, Kshatiya, Vaishya and Shudra all marry within their respective castes. Westermark considers this to be chief characteristics of the caste. Hindu society does not sanctify intercaste marriage even now.
5. **Caste has laws concerning position and touchability:** The various castes in the Hindu social organization are divided into a hierarchy of ascent and descent one above the order. In this hierarchy the Brahmins have the highest and the untouchables the lowest position. In kerala a Namboodari Brahmin is defiled by the touch of a Nayar, but in the case of a member of Thiya caste a distance of 36 feet must be kept to avoid being defiled and in the case of members of the Pulayan caste the distance must be ninety-six feet. The stringent observation of the system of untouchability has resulted in some low caste of Hindu society being called untouchables who were consequently forbidden to make use of places of worship, cremation grounds, colleges, public roads and hostels, etc. and well-disallowed from living.

CONDITIONS FAVORING THE CASTE SYSTEM

1. **Geographic isolation:** Geographic isolation has a large part to play in rendering a society static and powerless. The absence of adequate means of transport leads to the geographical isolation, from others, of people who inhabit distantly situated areas and this foster old customs, mores, traditions and superstitions, all of which encourage the caste system.

2. **Static society:** Hindu society is a static society. There has never been any stupendous variation in its political situation and economic conditions. Its social mores, customs and traditions have failed to change over the ages as times have marched along. But this does not mean that Hindu society does not change at all.

3. **Foreign aggression:** A further contribution to the desirability and utility of the caste system was made by foreign aggression. Many scholars hold that the caste system started in India when the Aryans invaded the country. The Aryans were fair skinned and victors. The natives of India were black-skinned and the victims.

4. **Rural social structure:** The rural social structure is usually unchanged and static. Ancient traditions were better respected in it. As the rural structure weakens, or in other words, as urbanization in the country increases, the caste also becomes progressively weaker.

5. **Influence of religion:** The influence of religion is the most important factor contributing to the continuation of the caste system. The Hindu system is looked upon as a divine institution. People who violate it are considered sinners and it is believed that God will punish them. Due to this reason people do not have the courage to violate the laws of the caste system.

6. **Difference of race:** The existence of many races in the country led to formation of many strict laws concerning discrimination since each race endeavored to maintain its purity. In the mediaeval period of Indian history stringent laws concerning caste were laid to protect Hindu society form Muslims.

7. **Lack of education:** Lack of education occupies an important position among the factors which have encouraged the existence of caste system in Hindu society. An uneducated society is static and motionless.

CONDITIONS UNFAVORABLE TO CASTE

1. **Modern education:** The major part in weakening caste system is played by the existing education. Modern education is negative as regards religion. It emphasizes democratic values such as liberty, equality and fraternity. Modern education bears the stamp of scientific and independent thinking in the west. Education has encouraged inter caste marriage. The feeling of superiority and untouchability are being gradually eliminated from the minds of children of all castes studying in the same school.

2. **Industrialization:** Industrialization also led to decrease in the intensity of caste favor because persons from all castes sought and obtained employment in factories. As a result of industrialization individuals of all castes came into mutual contact in factories, hotels, markets, trains, trams and buses, etc. and the observance of laws concerning touchability became impossible.

3. **Increase in the importance of Wealth:** In the modern age, wealth is replacing caste as the basis of social prestige. Now days a person adopts the occupation which appear to him to be the most profitable. The consideration in the choice of a profession is no longer caste but individual capacity and facility in earning wealth.

4. **Movement of social emancipation:** As a result of the influence of modern education there has been a veritable flood of movements for social emancipation.

5. **Means of communication:** Means of communication developed along with the progress of industrialization. This put an end to geographical isolation and the thoughts, customs, etc. of various places influenced each other. It become difficult to maintain the rigidity of caste in the whirlwind of communication set into motion by industrialization through such means as buses, train, trams, cars, etc.

6. **Political agitation:** To end the discriminatory practices on the basis of the caste system was a part of the aim of the national agitation for a political awakening of people in India. The objective of this national movement was established of a democratic pattern of society in India.

7. **New legal machinery:** In the new legal machinery of the British government all castes were similarly punished for the same offences. The establishment of judicial courts deprived the caste panchayats of their power and they no longer retained the authority of punishing criminals. In the way the restrictions upon the opponents of the caste system were removed and gradually its laws also lost their meaning and significance.

8. **Appearance of new social classes:** The classes are appearing in the society. These social classes are replacing the caste. The organization of castes was vertical, that of classes is horizontal. As the class consciousness is increasing, caste consciousness is decreasing.

9. **Independence of India:** The most severe shock to the caste system was the country's gaining independence. Para 1 (2) of the constitution of independent India declared citizen equal. The fortress of the caste system collapsed and all foreign rules came to an end. According to untouchability Crime Act of 1955 it is a crime to prevent any one from using a public place.

TRENDS IN CASTE SYSTEM

From the beginning the caste system was opposed by Buddhism, Jainism, Sikhism, and later by Islam and Christianity. Various social and religious movements in medieval period, such as Bhakti Movement, veerahivism also condemned the rigidities of caste system, the supremacy of high castes and the principles of ritual purity and impurity. Several reformers like Yogi Veerabhmam in Andrapradesh, Basvanna and Kanakadasa in Karnataka, Narayana Guru in Kerala, Kabir Panth in North India, modern elites taking from Rajaram Mohan Roy to Mahatma Gandhiji and Ambaeskar tried to abolish the evils of caste system and particularly untouchability in India. But their efforts also failed. According GS Ghurye there is no fear of extinction of the caste-system in the near future due to the following two conditions.

1. **Election:** Due to establishment of democracy in India the legislative machinery is operated by representative elected by the people. The method of election has done much to encourage the caste system because the candidates want to achieve their end by drumming the cause of casteism among the votes. In this way people are asked to vote their caste candidate and the castism is maintained by the elected leaders after the elections are over. Political parties sponsor only that candidate for election in a particular area whose caste is the most numerous in the area.

2. **Protection of backward classes:** Indian constitution has provided for the protection of the backward and scheduled castes. Some posts are retained for them in government service. Some seats are also retained for them in the legislative assemblies. They are given all types of facilities and special scholarship for education. All these special rights have encouraged casteism very much in the backward caste since the caste is providing beneficial to them because of these prerogatives.

Modern Trends of Caste System

Sl. No.	Trends	Description
1.	Progress of class-consciousness	In India, on the one hand, the caste is becoming weaker due to the influence of such factors as industrialization, urbanization, increase in the means of transportation, popularity of English education, political and social awakening, democratic government and laws obsolishing untouchability, etc. and on the other such new organizations as labors unions, etc. on the basis of occupation, post, etc. are being established.
2.	Casteism	All these changes led people to believe that the caste system will generally take on the form of a class system. But while on the one hand class consciousness seems to be progressing, on the other one can see progress in casteism as, well. Most commonly, in the biggest business institutions and sometimes even in educational institutions what happens is that the people who are employed in various posts belong to the castes of the proprieties, organizers and senior officials. Casteism of a similar type prevails also in government services and senior officials. Casteism of a similar type prevails also in government services and political elections.

CASTE IN MODERN INDIA

The political independence of the country, besides the progress of industrialization, urbanization, secularization, etc. brought in a series of changes in the caste system.

Changes in the Traditional Features of Caste

1. **The religious basis of the caste has been attacked:** Caste is no more believed to be divinely ordained. It is being given more a social and secular meaning than a religious interpretation.
2. **Restrictions on food habits have been relaxed:** Distinction between pakka food and kachcha food has almost vanished. Food habits have become more a matter a personal choice than a caste rule. Still commensal taboos are not completely ignored especially in the rural areas.
3. **Caste is not very much associated with hereditary occupations:** Caste no longer determines the occupational carrier of an individual even Brahmins are found driving taxis, dealing with foot-wears and running non-vegetarian hotels and bars and so on.
4. **Endogamy, which is often called the very essence of the caste system, still prevails:** Inter-caste marriages though legally permitted, have not become the order of the day. Most of the legal, political, educational economic and other disabilities from which the lowest caste people had suffered, have been removed by the constitutional provisions.
5. **Caste continuous to be a segmental division of Hindu society:** Caste with its hierarchical system continuous to ascribe statuses to the individual. But the twin processes of sanskritization and westernization have made possible mobility both within and outside the framework of caste.
6. Caste panchayats, which used to control the behavior of caste members have either become very weak or disappeared.
7. **Restrictions imposed by the castes on social intercourse are very much relaxed:** Distinction between touchables and untouchables is not much felt especially in the community of literature people. However, instances of untouchability are heard is the rural areas.
8. The Jajmani system which used to govern the inter-caste relations especially in the villages has become very weak. In many places it has vanished. In places of intercaste dependence, intercaste strifes are found.

9. Caste today does not dictate individual's life nor does it restrict newly valued individuals freedom. Hence, it no longer acts as a barrier to the progress of an individual.

Changes in the Role of Caste

1. **Increase in the organizational power of caste:** Education makes people liberal, broad-minded, rational and democratic. Educated people are believed to be less conservative and superstitions. Hence, it was expected that with the growth of literacy in India, caste-mindedness and castesim would come down. On the country, caste-consciousness of the members has been increasing. Every caste wants to safeguard its interests. For fulfilling this purpose castes are getting themselves organized on the model of labor union.
2. **Political role of caste:** Caste and politics have come to affect each other now. Caste has become an inseparable aspect of our politics. In fact, it is tightening its hold on politics. Elections are fought more often on the basis of caste. Selection of candidates, voting analysis, selection of legislative party leaders, distribution of ministerial portfolios, etc. is very much based on caste.
3. **Protection for scheduled caste and other backward classes:** The constitution of India has made enough provision to protect the interest of scheduled castes and tribes. They are offered more political, educational and service opportunities through the reservation policy. Seats are reserved for them from Mandal panchayat to parliament and in all government departments. Though the reservation policy is against the declared goal of establishment of a casteless society, all political parties have supported it mostly, for political purposes.
4. **Sanskritization and westernization:** As MN Srinivas has pointed out, two important trends are witnessed in caste—the process of sanaskritization and that of westernization. The former refers to a process in which the lower castes tend to imitate the values, practices and other life-styles of some dominant upper castes. The latter denotes a process in which the upper-caste people tend to mould their life-styles on the models of westerners.
5. **Backward classes movement:** The non-Brahmin castes today are getting themselves more organized to challenge the supremacy of the Brahmins and to assert their rights. The movement against the Brahmin supremacy by the lower castes came to be known as backward class's movement. The backward class's movements have become vital political forces today. Its influence has changed the political scenario of the country. This movement has made the Brahmins politically weak and insignificant especially in Kerala and Tamilnadu.
6. **Competitive role of castes:** Mutual interdependence of castes which existed for centuries and was reinforced by the institutional system of Jajmani, is not found today. Live and let live policy which was once associated with the caste makes no sense today. On the country, each caste looks at the other with suspicion, contempt, and jealousy and finds in it a challenger, a competitor. Excessive caste-mindedness and caste-patriotism have added to this competition. This competitive spirit further strengthens caste-mindedness.

ORIGIN OF CASTE

The caste system of Indian society is considered as an offshoot of these four fold divisions of society. But when we examine the scriptural, historical, and ethnographic explanations we fine multifarious factors influencing the genesis and development of caste in India. The different views of the thinkers have led to the following theories regarding the origin of caste system.

Sl. No.	Origin	Description
1.	Traditional theory	It is based on the ancient literature of Hindu tradition. Purusha sukta of Rigveda explains that the four varnas Brahmin, Kshatriya, Vaishya and Sudra came into existence respectively from the mouth, arms, thighs and feet of the Bramhan. These four divisions are assigned different duties. The traditional theory explains the functions of the four varnas.
2.	Political theory	The emergence of Aryans on the land of India, their concern to maintain purity and the rising power of Brahmins are some of the factors that have generally crystallized into the formation of castes. Bramhins as a priestly class exercised authority over other classes. They imposed restrictions on food, drink, and marriage. They enjoyed special privileges, position and high ritual status.
3.	Occupational theory	Nesfiled held that caste is mainly occupational in origin. He maintains that the technical skills, particularly various artisan and craftsmen skills were passed on from generation to generation hereditarily. The occupations were practiced for a long period and inherited. So each occupational group came to be known as castes. These occupations have been socially graded on the basis of superiority and inferiority or clean and unclean occupations.
4.	Racial theory	Herbert risely is the chief protagonist of racial theory of caste origin. He showed that caste and race are inseparable, his books, the people of India, Tribes and castes of Bengal prove that physical aspects are related with social aspects. Human being can be classified into several racial groups on the basis of biological triads. The biological traits can be measured by anthropometric methods. Aryans were considered as belonging to superior race and the Dravidians as belonging to inferior.
5.	The theory of mana	Hutton has analyzed that the caste system in India came into existence because of primitive conception of Mana. Mana is a kind of secret mysterious power found in individuals, objects or places. Mana has powers to harm people. Therefore, people avoid all those individuals or objects in which the mana exists, as a protective measure. This is called the practice of Taboo.
6.	Religious theory	Some thinkers explained that, the belief in Dharma, Karma, Varna, Dharma and other Hindu religious factors are considered as bases of caste system.
7.	Evolution theory	According to evolution theory, the Indian caste system evolved gradually because of multifarious factors, like the varna system, racial factors of Aryans, and non-Aryans the belief in doctrine of karma, the occupational divisions of society, the selfish and clever devise of Bramhins. The rules and regulations introduced by different kings. Geographical and economic conditions and other factors are all contributed for the evolution of the caste system.

JAJMANI SYSTEM

The Jajmani system governed by relationship based on reciprocity in inter-caste relations in villages. The functional inter-dependence of castes is a marked feature of the Indian caste system in the villages. The Jajmani system as inter-family, inter-relationship pertaining to the patterning of superordinate-subordinate relations between patrons and suppliers of service. Jajmani relations entail ritual matters and social support as well as economic exchanges. The servicing castes perform the ritual and ceremonial duties at the Jajman's houses on occasions like birth, marriage and death. Jajmani originally referred to the client for whom a Brahmin priest perform rituals, but later on it came to be referred to the patron or recipient of specialized services.

Meaning of Jajmani System

Jajmani system refers to distribution whereby high caste land owing families (called Jajmans) are provided survives and products by various lower castes such as carpenter (Badagi), barbar (Nat), potters (Kumbars), blacksmith (Kummars), washerman (Dhobis), etc. they serving people called Kamina are paid in cash or in kind (grains, fodder, cloths, animal products like milk, butter, etc).

Features of Jajmani System

1. Jajmani system is hereditary.
2. The Jajmani rights rights are property rights and hence are inherited according to the law of inheritance.
3. Jajmani relations are permanent
4. The Jajmani links are between family rather than castes. Thus a family of Rajputs gets it metal tools from a particular family of the Lohar (blacksmith) caste and not from all Lohar castes in the village.
5. Jajmani system once useful in Indian society has gradually been reduced into exploitation of the lower castes. The higher castes exploit the lower caste people who find themselves helpless before the money power of their patrons.

Advantages of Jajmani System

1. It provides security of occupation, the occupation being hereditary.
2. It provides economic security as the Jajman looks after all the needs of the serving family.
3. It reinforces the relations between the Jajman and his parjan which are more personal then economic.

ADVANTAGES OF CASTE SYSTEM

1. Caste system helps in maintaining purity of blood, each caste people married within their own caste and such purity of blood was maintained.
2. Each caste took pride in its customs, rituals, traditions and ceremonies, etc. it has rightly been said that if today India has been in a position to preserve its ancient culture that is primarily due to caste system.
3. Caste system also helped in maintaining social and professional discipline.
4. Caste system has preserved our society from infiltration of all outside cultures.
5. Caste system developed a sense and spirit of cooperation in the society.

DEMERITS OF CASTE SYSTEM

1. The whole caste system is against national unity. It does not make the people feel that they are one.
2. The caste system is against democratic spirit. Democracy believes in human equality. But the caste system believes in inequality.
3. The caste system creates a false sense of prestige among higher castes. They felt that all other castes should work according to their advice.

Social Class System

36

DEFINITIONS

1. **Social class:** Social class is defined as the aggregate of persons having essentially the same social status in a given society. Social classes are aggregates of individuals who have the same opportunities of acquiring goods and the same exhibited standards of living.
2. **Social stratification:** Social stratification is a horizontal division of society into higher and lowers social units. Every society is divided into more or less distinct groups.
3. **Class:** Class is a group of individuals who through common descent.
4. **Middle class:** The middle class is a heterogenous group consisting not only of tradesmen but also of doctors, lawyers, engineers, teachers, architects and many other white-collar workers. The middle class, as its very name signifies, stands below the capitalist and above the proletariat class. It is inferior to the former but superior to the latter in social status.
5. **Open system:** Class is an open system, because, a person can change his status by his efforts.
6. **Opportunities:** Class system opens fresh opportunities to rise in life.
7. **Class consciousness:** The feeling of class consciousness is necessary to constitute a class but there is no need for any subject consciousness in the members of caste.
8. **Backward class:** The backward classes from an important category in Indian population. They are officially lighted and given special recognition in variety of contexts.
9. **Achieved status:** Status is achieved by the individual. There is scope for achievement. Hence status can be changed or improved.
10. **Tribe:** Tribe is a collection of families or group of families bearing a common name, members of which occupy the same territory, speak same language and observe certain taboos regarding marriage, profession or occupation and have developed a well-assessed system of reciprocity and mutuality of obligations.

The word `class' is by no means an unusual world. It is said that classism is increasing or that new classes are coming into being in India. The word class lends itself to a variety of uses, in the form of the landlord class and business class at one end and the Brahmin class and capitalist class at the other. Every society has many classes, the individual interests of all of which do not coincide. Each social class has its status in society in accordance with which it receives prestige in the society.

DEFINITIONS OF SOCIAL CLASS SYSTEM

1. Social class is defined as the aggregate of persons having essentially the same social status in a given society—*Ogburn and Nimkoff*.
2. A social class is a culturally defined group that is accorded a particular position or status within the population as a whole—*Lapiere*.
3. A social class is a portion of community marked off from the rest by social status—*MacIver*.
4. Social class is a category or group of persons having a definite status in society which permanently determines their relation to other groups—*P Gisbert*.
5. Social classes are aggregates of individuals who have the same opportunities of acquiring goods and the same exhibited standards of living—*Max Weber*.

DIFFERENT BASES OF SOCIAL CLASS

1. **Occupational basis:** Occupation is considered to be the basis of class division. According to this, individuals in superior occupations are treated as superior while those in inferior occupations are treated as inferior.
2. **Basis of manual labor:** Verblen looks upon manual labor as the basis of class-consciousness. People including in manual labor are looked upon as belonging to an inferior class while those in superior classes are engaged in administration, sport, war, religion and other activities.
3. **Various factors:** Cattel believes class consciousness to be the sum total of five factors, viz. prestige, mean IQ, average income, education of some years and the amount of birth restrictions. But class-consciousness is not based on these five factors only. It continually changes according to circumstances.

PRINCIPLES OF CLASS SYSTEM

1. The class of an individual is determined by his occupation, power and wealth. One caste escapes from a class or falls into it.
2. The class of an individual is based on his accomplishments. In other words the amount of award that an individual gets for his social labor determine his class.
3. In the class system, there is no restriction on marriage outside one's own class.

CHARACTERISTICS OF SOCIAL CLASS

1. **Class—A status group:** A social class is essentially a status group. Class is related to status. Different statuses arise in a society as people do different things, engage in different activities and pursue different vocations. The consideration of the class as a status group makes it possible to apply it to any society which has many strata.
2. **Universal:** Class system is almost a universal phenomenon. The class system appears in all the modern complex societies of the world.
3. **Social class—An open group:** Social classes are open groups. They represent an open social system. This means there are no restrictions, or at the most only very mild restrictions are imposed on the upward and downward movement of individuals in the social hierarchy.
4. **Class consciousness:** Class consciousness is the statement that characterizes the relations of men towards the members of their own and other classes.

5. **Mode of feeling:** In a class system we may observe three modes of feeling: (a) There is a feeling of equality in relation to the members of one's own class. (b) There is a feeling of inferiority in relation to those who occupy the higher status in the socioeconomic hierarchy. (c) There is a feeling of superiority in relation to those who occupy the lower status in the hierarchy.

6. **Element of prestige:** Each social class has its own status in society. Status is associated with prestige. The relative position of the class in the social set-up arises from the degree of prestige attached to the status. Thus, the status and prestige enjoyed by the running classes or rich classes in every society is superior to that of the class of commoners or the poor people.

7. **Social class—An economic group:** The basis of social classes is mostly economic, but they are not mere economic group or divisions. Subjective criteria such as class-consciousness, class-solidarity and class identification on the one hand, and the objective criteria such as wealth, property, income, education, occupation, etc. on the other are equally important in the class system.

8. **Achieved status and not ascribed status:** Status in the case of class system is achieved and not ascribed. Birth is not the criterion of status. Achievements of an individual mostly decide his status. Factors like income, occupations, wealth, education, lifestyles, etc. decide the status of an individual.

9. **Mode of living:** Lifestyles or the modes of living include such matters as the modes of dress, the kind of house and neighborhood one lives in, the means of recreation one resorts to, the cultural products one is able to enjoy, the relationship between parents and children, the kinds of books, magazines and TV show to which one is exposed, one's friend, one's mode of conveyance and communication, one's way of spending money and so on.

10. **Element of stability:** A social class is relatively a stable group. It is neither transitory nor unstable like a crowd or a mob.

CONCLUSION

Social interaction is governed by social stratification. Social stratification occurs when people accept the fact that families or individuals do not have equal access to the same privileges, power, prestige, occupation, or wealth. Human society is stratified and ranked in categories according to the distribution of privileges, power and prestige or on the basis of status. A caste system refers to a level or strata of people whose statuses are fixed for their lifetimes (ascribed status). Status is determined by birth. Mobility is not allowed in the caste system. A class system allows social mobility between the various classes. A social class is defined as the aggregate of persons having essentially the same social status in a given society.

37

Social Mobility

DEFINITIONS

1. **Social mobility:** Social mobility is the movement of a person or persons from one social status to another. Social mobility is the movement of individuals, families, groups, from one social position to another. The movement may either upward or downward, between higher and lower social classes more precisely, movement between one relatively full time, functionally significant social role and another that is evaluated as either higher or lower.

2. **Vertical mobility:** Vertical mobility refers to movement of people from one social status to another. Vertical mobility may be upward or downward. It also refers to movement in any or all of the three areas of living: Class, occupation and power.

3. **Horizontal mobility:** It refers to change of residence or job without status change, such as a teacher's leaving one school to work in another or even in a factory as a welfare officer.

4. **Social prestige:** Social prestige is ultimately depends upon the accepted values system. If certain qualities of achievements are socially valued, some people will strive from them.

5. **Industrialization:** Industrialization leads high degree of upward mobility. Industrialization creates a variety of new job opportunities. The chances for vertical mobility are unlimited contrary to it in the agricultural society the opportunities are very limited.

6. **Urbanization:** Urban society is characterized by a widely differentiated and open system of ranking. This led to a two dimensional mobility. First, the high degree of vertical mobility within the urban society. Secondly, the migration of population from rural areas to urban which effects the mobility pattern of the society.

7. **Mechanization:** Mechanization has affected the social mobility vertically in two ways. It has replaced the use of manpower at various occasions and created various job opportunities for semi-skilled labors.

8. **Social justice:** Social mobility providing equal chances or opportunities for social mobility for all social classes is a democratic commitment.

9. **Modernization:** Modernization is a process by which modern scientific knowledge is introduced in the society with the ultimate purpose of achieving a better and a more satisfactory life in the broadest sense of the term as accepted by the society concerned.

10. **Open versus closed:** A class system is an open system or raising levels. If a hierarchy becomes closed against vertical mobility, it ceases to be a class system and become a caste system. The class system is an open and flexible system while caste system is a closed and rigid system.

Social mobility is an act of moving from one social status to another. People in society continue to move up and down the status scale. This is called social mobility. Mobility may be for groups as well as individuals. In an open class, every individual's struggles to get into higher rank. But it depends on the background of his ascribed status and the available opportunities in the social set-up. Individuals are normally recognized in society through the statuses they occupy and the roles they enact. Not only the society is dynamic but also the individuals are dynamic.

Men are normally engaged in endless endeavor to enhance their statuses in society, move from lower position to higher position, secure superior job from an inferior one. For various reasons people of higher status and position may also be forced to come down to a lower status and position. A doctor or engineer enjoys greater prestige than a priest. Likewise, if a person becomes a minister from an ordinary shopkeeper, his status comes to his old shop, the status enjoyed by him as a minister is lost. Thus it is seen that people in society continue to move up and down the status scale. This movement is called social mobility. Mobility is to be distinguished from migration which is a movement in geographical space.

DEFINITIONS OF SOCIAL MOBILITY

1. Social mobility is the movement of a person or persons from one social status to another—*Wallace and Wallace.*
2. Social mobility refers to the movement of an individual or group from one social class or social stratum to another—*Dictionary of Sociology.*
3. Social mobility refers to the movement of individuals between different levels of social hierarchy, usually defined occupationally—*N Abercrombie.*
4. Mobility refers to any transition of an individual or social object or value; anything that has been created or modified by human activity–from one social position to another—*Sorokin.*
5. The term social mobility refers to the processes by which individuals move from one position to another in society positions which, by general consent, have been given specific hierarchical values—*Lipset and Bendix* (1960).
6. Social mobility is the movement of individuals, families, groups from one social position to another….. the changes in social position that interest the theory of social mobility are primarily variations in occupations, prestige, income, wealth, power and social status—*Goldhamer* (1968).
7. Social mobility is the movement either upward or downward, between higher and lower social classes or more precisely, movement between one relatively full time, functionally significant social role and another that is evaluated as either higher or lower. This movement is to be considered as a process occurring overtime, with individuals (and their family units) moving from one role and social class position to another—*Barber* (1957).

CLASSIFICATIONS / TYPES OF SOCIAL MOBILITY

1. **Horizontal mobility:** It refers to change of residence or job without status change, such as a teacher's leaving one school to work in another or even in a factory as a welfare officer.
2. **Vertical mobility:** It refers to movement of people from one social status to another. Vertical mobility may be upward or downward. It also refers to movement in any or all of the three areas of living: class, occupation and power.
3. **Open system mobility:** It refers to the free movement in status change. It neither does nor recognizes the formal fixation of status. In such a system, status can be achieved, mobility is motivated and encouraged. An individual is at liberty to improve his status and position.

4. **Closed system mobility:** It refers to status is based on birth or caste. It is impossible to change one's caste. The Indian society furnishes the example of closed model of mobility whereas the American society is an open model of mobility.
5. **Inter-general mobility:** It refers to mobility between generations, example movement between a father's generation and a son's generation. Today we find significant changes between the occupational structures of two generations. The present day industrial society is marked by inter-generational mobility.

FACTORS INFLUENCE SOCIAL MOBILITY

According to Henry M Johnson

1. **Social prestige:** It ultimately depends upon the accepted value system. If certain qualities of achievements are socially valued, some people will strive for them.
2. There is no content tendency for intelligence and other kinds of native capacity to be confined to upper classes. It has not been uncommon for the sons of farmers and laborers to rise to the highest position in society.
3. At varying rates of speed, changes are always occurring in the demand for different kinds of skill.
4. The birth rate of each class never exactly fills all the positions in the class.
5. Birth in upper classes sometimes fosters complacency in many persons.

Other Factors

1. **Social change:** In general the principal condition that favors or prevents mobility is the rate of social change. It may be noted that political, economic, religious or other revolutions may produce rapid social mobility so as to reduce the upper classes to the bottom of social scale and to elevate to the top, classes formerly at the bottom.
2. **Communication:** Any system that limits communication between classes and restricts knowledge of the conditions of life to one's own class will also tend to discourage social mobility.
3. **Division of labor:** The amount of social mobility is influenced by the degree of division of labor that exists in a society. If the division of labor is very highly developed and if the degree of specialization and skilled training is very high, it is correspondingly difficult for a person from one class to pass readily into other classes.
4. **Economic development:** Economic progress is the most important factor in determining the rate of mobility in any country. Economic progress is associated with industrialization and industrialization is associated with a higher rate of mobility.

DIMENSIONS OF SOCIAL MOBILITY

1. **Direction of social mobility:** Any movement in the social stratification may have three possible directions, for example, higher, lower or at the same level of the social rank held by the moving individuals or group. These movements have been respectively termed as upward, downward and horizontal mobility.
2. **Dimension of time:** From the perspective of the duration of time, social mobility has been classified into two categories, for example, intragenerational and interagenerational social mobility. Intergeneration mobility compares the social positions of parents and offsprings while intragenerational mobility compares the social positions of the same individual at different times.

3. **Unit of mobility:** The unit in social mobility may be an individual, family, or group. Individual mobility is the movement of individual alone which sometimes even dissociates him from his membership group. The group mobility demands homogeneity and the united efforts of all the members of the group. However, both individual and group are equally important units of social mobility.

4. **Context of social mobility:** Sorokin (1959) explained that no specific trend can be observed regarding the nature, amount and frequency of the mobility, thus social mobility can be understood only in the context of the particular ranking structure of the society.

5. **Amount of social mobility:** This dimension is concerned with the amount of social mobility in a society and its measurement. The amount of mobility varies from society to society influenced by various factors.

DETERMINANTS OF SOCIAL MOBILTY

Social mobility is multidimensional phenomenon. Directly or indirectly, to a greater or lesser extent various factors contribute into the social mobility in a society.

1. **Pattern of stratification:** Two contrary systems have been identified in the pattern of stratification, for example, the closed and the open system of stratification. Caste system of India is the best example of the closed stratification system. Contrary to it, class system of the western societies is the example of open ranking system.

2. **Industrialization:** It has been widely accepted that the industrialization, particularly at the initial stages, leads to a high degree of upward mobility. Industrialization creates a variety of new job opportunities. The chances for vertical mobility are unlimited, contrary to it in the agricultural society the opportunities are very limited.

3. **Urbanization:** Urban society is characterized by a widely differentiated and open system of ranking. This led to a two dimensional mobility. First, the high degree of vertical mobility within the urban society. Secondly, the migration of population from rural areas to urban which affects the mobility pattern of the society in various ways.

4. **Development of the means of transportation and mass communication:** This reduces the distance of space as well as time thus increasing the opportunities for social mobility. An individual can know about opportunity at a place far away from his residence. The scope of job opportunities has widened to a great extent with the means of transportation and communication and thus causing high rate of social mobility.

5. **Demographic variables:** Migration of population from one place to another within the country also generates social mobility. For example, migration of population from rural to urban areas, from cities to metropolitan cities, widens the scope of job opportunities and results in the high degree of social mobility.

6. **Opportunity structure of the society:** Opportunity structure of the society to a great extent determines the extent and nature of mobility. The role structure of the developed societies is highly differentiated and gives multiple opportunities to an individual for upward mobility.

7. **Motivational factor:** It is the aspiration for a high status in the individual and the group which leads to upwards social mobility.

8. **Mechanization:** Mechanization has affected the social mobility vertically in two ways. It has replaced the use of manpower at various occasions and created various job opportunities for semi-skilled laborers.

9. **Consumption pattern:** The consumption pattern of the society also influences the degree of social mobility. If the consumption pattern is clearly visible for different ranks, the degree of upward mobility will be higher.
10. **System of transfers and promotions:** The system of transfers and promotions in both private and government bureaucratic organizations also influence the social mobility.
11. **Governmental policies:** The governmental policies of every country directly, or indirectly, determine the pattern of social mobility.
12. **Leaders:** Mobility leader have also been found motivating their kinsmen to join them. For example the migrated people of Punjab motivated and helped their native persons to move out and achieve a better job opportunity.
13. Western impact and the western system of education and the equality of educational opportunities have greatly contributed to both horizontal and vertical mobility. Education helps in achieving better occupations particularly professional jobs like engineer, doctors, manager, etc. it helps in achieving high economic status and social prestige.

IMPORTANCE OF SOCIAL MOBILITY

1. Social mobility provides opportunity for the expression of individual talents. Social mobility becomes inevitable if the most important functions of the society are to be performed by the most capable persons.
2. **Social justice:** Social mobility providing equal chances or opportunities for social mobility for all social classes is a democratic commitment.
3. **Job satisfactions:** Social mobility is inclusive of occupational mobility also. In the traditional societies occupations are normally hereditary in character and hence children are obliged to follow the occupations of their parents whether they have a liking for it or not. Now in the modern industrial society things are different. People need not stick onto their parental occupations.
4. **Acts as a safety-valve:** Social mobility providing opportunity virtually means creating a safety-valve to escape from the danger. Since the lower classes are provided with an open chance to enhance their social status or to enter into the status-position of other upper class people by means of their performances; they do not normally organize themselves to dislodge the upper-class people of their status.
5. **Opportunity for competition:** Social mobility is of great importance in helping individuals to improve their capacity and work efficiency. It provides motivation for progress and higher attainments.
6. Education is often considered to be a potential means of social mobility. It provides advantages by increasing the individual's ability. The levels of education indicate differences in status. Social ability depends on the nature and contents of education.
7. Property is an important concept to indicate the social levels of individuals and group. In some families, property is inherited and in some others it is acquired.

CONCLUSION

Social mobility is the manifestation of the dynamic nature of society. Societies are not static but changeable. Individuals who constitute the basic social units of society are also moving up and down in the status hierarchy. They also move from one place to another and from one occupation to another. Not only the individuals are mobile even the groups are subjected to mobility. Thus it is clear social mobility may be understood as the movement of an individual or group from one status or position to that of another.

Race

38

DEFINITIONS

1. **Race:** Race is a large, biological human grouping with number of distinctive inherited characteristics which vary with certain range. A race is a valid biological concept. It is a group united by heredity, a breed or genetic strain or subspecies.

2. **Prejudice:** Prejudice is an attitude that predisposes a person to think, perceive, feel and act in favorable or unfavorable ways toward a group or its individual members.

3. **Ethnic:** Ethnic group defined as a social division whose members share a distinctive social and cultural tradition, maintained within the group from generation-to-generation.

4. **Ethnocentrism:** Ethnocentrism is the belief that the values and norms of one's own group are superior to the other. Ethnocentrism is one's own emotional reaction or moral adjustments towards other culture.

5. **Minorities:** Minorities defined as a group of people because of their physical or cultural characteristics are signed out from the others in the society, and are subjected to social difference and unequal treatment and collective discrimination.

6. **Caucasians:** Caucasians are generally called white race and confined to different parts of Europe and Asia. They are white skinned, narrow nose, wavy hair, stature varies from tall to medium and lips are thin.

7. **Negroes:** Negroes are generally called black race. They are confined to Africa and Oceania. Their physical traits are black skin color , broad nose, woolly hair, broad head, and thick lips, tall to short stature.

8. **Mongolians:** Mongolians are generally called yellow race. They are confined to Mongolia, china, Japan, Indonesia, Burma, Tibet, Himalayan region, etc. Their physical traits are yellow skin, strait black hair, medium stature, closed eyes.

9. **Parsees:** The Parsees are an ethno-religious minority in India. Their population is small in number, less than one lakh. They are concentrated in Mumbai and Gujarat. But their role in economic social and political fields is significant.

10. **Linguistic minorities:** India is a land of multilinguistic group. The different states of India have been reorganized on the basis of languages. In all states adequate facilities have been provided for instruction in the regional language or state language at the primary stage of education.

INTRODUCTION

A race is a socially constructed category composed of people who share biologically transmitted traits that members of a society consider important. People may classify each other racially based on physical characteristics such as skin color, facial features, hair textures and body shape. Race is a group which shares in common a certain set of innate physical characters and a geographical origin within certain area. In this way, a race lives in a definite geographical area and has some definite innate characteristics. The biological concept of race arises as result of failure to realize that race is not a sociological term but is distinctly a biological and anthropological concept.

If we go through the history of mankind, we find man in the earliest periods lived in small homogeneous society. After few thousands years as a result of migration, conquest continued and extensive contact between different members of society and inter-mixture of people resulted in the creation of different social categories. Social differences occur on the basis of race, language, religion, culture, ativism, etc. Based on such criteria people developed differential attitude and unequal treatment.

DEFINITIONS OF THE RACE

1. A race is a large, biological, human grouping with a number of distinctive inherited characteristics which vary within a certain range—*AW Green*.
2. A race is a large group of people distinguished by inherited physical differences—*J Biesanz* and *M Biesanz*.
3. A race is a biologically inherited group possessing a distinctive combination of physical traits that tend to breed true from generation to generation—*Hoebel*.
4. A race, in short, is a group of related intermarrying individuals, that is, a population which differs from other population in the relative common-ness of certain hereditary traits—*LC Dunn*.
5. A race is a valid biological concept. It is a group united by heredity, a breed or genetic strain or subspecies—*AL Krober*.
6. A race is a large division of human being distinguished from other by relatively obvious physical characteristics presumed to be biologically inherited and remaining relatively constant through numerous generations—*Paul AF Walter*.

KINDS OF RACE

Physical anthropology is chiefly concerned with the classification of men into race. On the basis of different physical traits, numbers of classifications have been formulated. The Races of the world are primarily divided into three kinds. They are Caucasians (white race), Negroes (Black race) and Mongolian race (yellow race).

Sl.No.	Kinds	Description
1.	Caucasians(White Race)	They are generally called white race and confined to different parts of Europe and Asia. They have white skinned, narrow nose, wavy hair, stature veries from tall to medium and lips are thin. The sub-race of Caucasians are Nordic, Alpine, Mediterranean, Ainu, Indodravidian, etc.
2.	Negroes (Black Race)	They are generally called black race. They are confined to Asia, Africa, and Oceania. Their physical traits are black skin color, broad nose, wooly hair, broad head, and thick lips, tall to short stature. The sub-races are African negroes, Melenasian, Negritos, Nilotic Negroes, Bushman Hottentot and Pygmy.

Contd...

Contd...

Sl.No.	Kinds	Description
3.	Mongolians (Yellow Race)	They are generally called yellow race. They are confined to Magnolia, China, Japan, Burma, Tibet, Himalayan region, etc. Their physical traits are yellow skin, strait black hair, medium stature, closed eyes. The sub-races of Mongolians are: Classic Mongoloid, Eskimos, Indonesians and American Indians.
4.	Australoid	Australoid is one of the major races. They are found in Australia. Their physical traits are, low forehead, broad nose, medium lips, wavy hair, narrowhead, skin color dark brown, medium stature.

RACE AS A BIOLOGICAL CONCEPT

Racial groups are no doubt refer to biological categories that represent common observable hereditary traits. Race is a group which shares in common a certain set of intimate physical characteristics and geographical origin within a certain area. Historically, three diagnostics traits have been used to divide the human species into races: Skin color, hair, form and various combination of nose, face and lip shapes. The discoveries of fossil man in different parts of the world reveal that man is biologically related to prehistoric men like java man, Neanderthal man and Cro-magnon man. Thus finally anthropologists have come to the conclusion that living men are evolved from a single species namely Homosapiens. Though man evolved from single species biological differences occurred. Such kind of differentiation is due to hereditary processes, mutation (variation in genes), natural selection, isolation, in breeding and interbreeding process.

General Views of Race as a Biological Concept

1. Sutherland and Woodword described, race is a broad association of persons of familiar biological heritage, who are united in sentiment by common cultural traditions and who in time of conflict seek to claim rights to better social position on the basis of an inherited quality.
2. Scientifically speaking the term race is a biological concept. Race means a sub-division of human species that possess common biological trait. According to AL Kroeber, a race is a valid biological concept. It is a group united by heredity, a breed or genetic stain.
3. Linton has defined that race consists of a number of breeds which share certain physical traits.
4. Charles Darwin expounded the theory of biological evolution and explained that all species have evolved from simple to complex form. He rejected all the old beliefs with regard to creation. Man is the product of evolution like other species. He is classified under mammals; especially he is closely related to primates.
5. According to Penniman, race is a genetic class in which there are many indefinite and mutually related genetic characteristics, by means of which it can be distinguished from other classes and on the basis of which the conditions of contributions, separation among offsprings and future generation can be distinguished.
6. According to Professor Dunn, races are biological sub-groups within a single species. Homo sapiens, in which the similar heredity which the whole species has in common far outweighs the relative and minor ways in which the sub-groups are different.

Biological Determinants of Race

Color and distribution of the hair on the head, the face and the body, hair forms are grouped as:
- Soft straight hair as the Mongols and Chinese's (Leiotrichy).
- Smooth curly hair of India, Western Europe, Australia and South Africa (Cymotrichy).
- Thick curly hair as of the Negroes (Ulotrichy).

RACES IN INDIA

According to Sir Herbert Risley, India has seven racial types:

Sl.No.	Kinds	Location
1.	Pre-Dravidian	Surviving among primitive tribes to the hills and jungles, such as Bhils.
2.	The Dravidian	Living in southern peninsula up to the Gangetic valley.
3.	Indo-Aryan	Kashmir, Punjab, and Rajputana.
4.	Aryo-Dravidian	Gangetic valley.
5.	Cytho-Dravidian	Running east of Indus.
6.	Mongoloid	Found in Assam, and the foothills of the eastern Himalayas.
7.	Mangola-Dravidian	

UNESCO CONCEPTION OF RACE

UNESCO arranged a conference of all prominent sociologists, anthropologists and psychologists in order to determine a single conception of race. The conference gave the following judgements concerning race:

1. Fundamentally, the entire human species has one origin and all men are homosapiens.
2. National groups, religious groups, geographical groups, cultural groups, linguistic groups, etc. are all entirely unconnected with and unrelated to race.
3. Some races make claims of purity but this is not true. Today pure races cannot be found anywhere in the world. The process of mixing of races originated long back.
4. The differences found to exist between the physical characteristics of men are due both to heredity arise due to the process known as mutation and in-breeding.
5. Human races can be classified but these classifications are based on physical traits. They have no relation of any kind of mental or intellectual superiority or inferiority.
6. The inner capacity for the development of mind and culture is found equally in every race. Hence distinction between races cannot be based on cultural differences or levels of intelligence. Intelligent people are to be found in all races.
7. It is possible that in one nation the degree of racial differences may be greater while in another nation it may be of greater or a lesser degree.
8. Evidence in support of the fact that the race has no important effects in the social and cultural differences between various human groups has been found in historical and sociological studies.
9. That from biological point of view, mixing of races is deleterious, is an essentially incorrect and invalid belief.

CHARACTERISTICS OF RACE

1. Race is a group of intermarrying people who are born of common ancestors, possess similar physical traits and have feeling.
2. Inbreeding renders permanent physical characteristics of the race and due to them one race can be distinguished from another. One major cause in inbreeding is geographical isolation.
3. Racial traits are determined by hereditary, for example, skin, color, stature, hair, eyes, etc. on the basis of those traits we may identify an individual as a member of a particular race.
4. Racial hereditary includes the traits which are relatively constant in spite of environmental effects. They transmit from one generation to another.

Indefinite Physical Traits

1. **Color of the skin:** Usually, on the basis of color of the skin people differentiated between the white, yellow, and black races, etc. The color of the skin distinctions are made as leucoderm-Caucasian, xanthoderm-Mongolian, Melanoderm-Negro.
2. **Texture and color of the hair:** The texture and color of hair is another indefinite physical trait of race. There are the three following distinctions of hair on the basis of texture–Leiotrichy (soft straight hair) as on the Mongols and Chinese. Cymotrichy (smooth curly hair) as of the inhabitants of India, western Europe, Australia and north-east Africa, Ulotrichy (thick curly hair) as of Negros.
3. **Structure and color of eyes:** There are three distinctions of the color of the eyes—white, grey and yellow. The structure of the orifice of the eye is usually horizontal but at same places diagonal eyes are found as in southern Europe and north Africa.

Definite Physical Traits

1. **Stature:** Definite races are distinguished on the basis of differences in stature. Topinard has classified height in the following manner:

Sl.No.	Kinds	Measurements
1.	Tall stature	170 cms (5 feet 8 inches to 10 inches)
2.	Above average stature	165 cms (5 feet 5 inches to 7 inches)
3.	Short stature	160 cms (below 5 feet 5 inches)

2. **Structure of the head:** Heads are classified in three classes according to the ratio of length and width. The structure of the head can be known by the ratio of its length to its breath. The cephalic index can be calculated by multiplying the width of the head by 100 and by dividing the product by its length.

Sl.No.	Kinds	Dividing with
1.	Dolicocephalic	75
2.	Mesocephalic	75 to 80
3.	Brachycaphalic	80

3. **Structure of Nose:** Taking the length of the nose as 100, the percentage of its width is calculated. The resultant figure is calculated nasal index. It is this which helps to determine the

structure of the nose. According to the nasal index the nasal structure is also classified in three classes:

Sl.No.	Kinds	Location
1.	Leptorrhine (thin)	70%—typical of Punjab.
2.	Mesorrhine (medium)	Above 76%—this type found in the people of Uttar Pradesh.
3.	Platrrhine	Above 85%—nasal index of this type found in Chennai, Madhya Pradesh, Nagpur areas of India.

4. **Blood group:** The blood group is one such racial trait which remains unaffected by changes in the environment. There are four groups of blood groups: A, B, AB and O. In every race, people who have these blood groups are to be found.
5. **Length of hands and feet:** Among different races the lengths of the hands and feet do not coincide.
6. **Perimeter of chest:** Differences in the chest measurements between people of different races are to be found.

ETHNICITY

Ethnicity is a shared cultural heritage. People define themselves or others as members of an ethnic category based on having common ancestors, language or religion that confers a distinctive social identity. Like race, ethnicity is socially constructed on an individual level, people play up or play down cultural traits so that they fit in or stand apart from the surrounding society.

Definition

Ethnic group defined as a social division whose members share a distinctive social and cultural tradition, maintained within the group from generation to generation—*MacIver and Page.*

Meaning of Ethnicity

Ethnicity refers to a shared identity related to social and cultural heritage such as values, languages, geographical space, and racial characteristics. Members of an ethnic group feel a common sense of identity. Individuals may declare their ethnic identity. Therefore, cultural background is a fundamental component of one's ethnic background or ethnicity, a group within the social system that claims to possess variable traits such as a common religion or language.

Ethnocentrism

Ethnocentrism is the belief that the values and norms of one's own group are superior to the other. Ethnocentrism is one's own emotional reactions or moral adjustments towards other cultures. It is loyalty to one's own group. But in reality the values and norms of the other groups are as important as our own.

MINORITIES

A minority is any category of people distinguished by physical or cultural diffe_ence that a society sets apart and subordinates. Both race and ethnicity are the basis for minority standing. Man separated from man not only on the basis of race but also socially distinguished on the basis of national, religious, linguistic and other group traditions. Such social divisions are called ethnic groups and minorities.

Definitions

1. Minority is defined as a group of people because of their physical or cultural characteristics are singled out from the others in the society, and are subjected to social difference and unequal treatment and collective discrimination—*Louis*.
2. Minority is defined as a group of people living on a soil which they have occupied from times immemorial but who through change of boundaries have politically subordinated—*Europe Minority Association*.
3. Minorities are those non-dominant groups in a population who wish to preserve stable ethic, religious or linguistic traditions or characteristics markedly different from the rest of the population—*United Nations sub-Commission*.

Characteristics of Minority

1. They share a distinctive identity, which may be based on physical or cultural traits.
2. Minority has subordinated status.
3. In the dominant majority group relations, there exists conflicting situations.
4. Minorities are self-conscious unit.
5. Membership in a minority is transmitted by birth and they are endogamous.
6. They are collectively exploited by the majority groups.
7. The members of the minority groups are held in low esteem and they are segregated and isolated and subject to ridicule.
8. They are deprived of educational, political occupational and other opportunities.

Minority Groups in India

Indian constitutional experts have identified the different elements of the minority problems in India. Articles 29 and 30 of the Indian Constitution guarantee the protection and interests of minorities in India. Article 29 envisages that any section of citizen having distinct language script or culture of its own shall have the right to conserve the same. Article 30 protects the interests of minorities based on religion or language to establish and administer educational institutions. The minorities in India are generally classified into two groups mainly of religious minorities and linguistic minorities.

Religious Minorities

Sl.No.	Minority group	Description
1.	Muslims	Muslims are the largest religious minorities in India. They are belonging to Islamic religion, who constitute 12.12% as per 1995 censes report. Islam as a religion began to flourish during the time of Qutubdin. It was during the rule of Moghuls, larger number of Hindus was converted to Islam and Mosques were constructed all over India. During the national struggle for independence different sections of Muslim had different view and particularly Muslim league favored the partition. As a result India was divided into Pakistan and India in 1947. The division of the country has led to displacement of Hindus, Muslims and Sikhs.

Contd...

Sl.No.	Minority group	Description
2.	Christians	The Christians constitute the 2.60% of the total population. It is the second largest religious minority in India. Christianity as a religion began to spread after the advent of Europeans. After the consolidation of the British administration, the Christian missionaries were very active in the field of education and in spread of their religion. The new religion accepted by many Hindus, particularly, the low caste people and tribal people. Christian missionaries started many schools, colleges and hospitals. They made a remarkable contribution in the field of education and health.
3.	Sikhs	Sikhs constitute the third largest religious minority. They constitute less than 2% of India's population. They are concentrated in Punjab and spread in different states in India and abroad. They are the followers of Sikhism. Sikhism was started as a reform movement against the dogmas of Hinduism. Guru Nanak was the founder of this religion. Sikh shrines are called Gurudwaras. The Golden temple of Amritsar is the sacred shrine in Punjab. The contribution of Sikhs to the development of industries is unique, they are patriotic citizens of India.
4.	Parsees	The parsees are an ethno-religious minority in India. Their population is small in number, less than one lakh. They are concentrated in Mumbai and in Gujarat. But their role in economic social and political fields is significant. They migrated from their homeland Persia in 7th century AD, when Muslim invaded their country. They are the smallest minorities and strictly loyal to the nation. Thus the contribution of parsess to political, economic and industrial development is great. Their relationships with Indians are bound in brotherly relations and affection to all the children of the soil.
5.	Anglo-Indians	Anglo-Indians are a microscopic minority in India and their population is 3 lakh. It is a racial, religious and linguistic minority group. Anglo-Indian is an ethnic group came into existence due to the inter-mixture of Britishers and Indians. The community is 100% literate and urbanized. The Government of India has safe guarded its interest through Constitutional measures. This community is provided two seats in Parliament through nomination by the President of India.

Linguistic Minorities

India is a land of multi-linguistic groups. The different states of India have been re-organized on the basis of languages. In all states adequate facilities have been provided for instruction in the regional language or state language at the primary stage of education.

CONCLUSION

Race is one of those terms used with a variety of meaning. The Greek classified all mankind as either Greek or barbarian yet one of these is a racial group. The term race is sometimes used as synonymous with nationality. Thus French, Chinese and German are spoken of as races. The German and French are nations. A nation does not necessarily consist of individuals with uniform physical characteristics. Sometimes it has been frequently confused with language, as well as with religion. The word race has been sometimes used in a very wide sense and we speak of human race thus including all the human beings.

39

Social System

DEFINITIONS

1. **Social system:** Social system is a system of interdependent interactive processes. In other words, a social system refers to individual actors interacting with each other in accordance with shared cultural norms and values. A social system consists in plurality of individual actors, interacting with each other in a situation or environment.
2. **Status:** Status is a term used to denote comparative amounts of prestige, difference or respect accorded to persons who play different roles in a group. Status refers to an individual's total standing in society.
3. **Achieved status:** Achievement of status refers to individual accomplishments and individual failure. A person by his own effort, in spite of many obstacles can change his status.
4. **Social role:** Social role as the culturally defined pattern of behavior expected or required of persons in a specific social position.
5. **Ascribed status:** It is a social position, a person receives at birth or assumes involuntarily later life. This status is not based on individual ability, skill effort or accomplishment. This status is obtained on inheritance in the society.
6. **Norms:** Norms are standards of group behavior. When a number of individual does interact, a set of standards develop that regulate their relationship and modes of behavior. These standards of group behavior are called social norms.
7. **Folkways:** Folkways are unconscious spontaneous and uncoordinated adjustments of individual to his environment.
8. **Role:** A role is a set of socially expected and approved behavior pattern, consisting of both duties and privileges, associated with a particular position in a group.
9. **Individual achievements:** Individual achievements are very significant in determining social status. This may be in the field of education, occupation, sports, literature, art, science or any other field.
10. **Social act:** Social act or action is a process in the social system that motivates the individual or individuals in the case of group. The action is not an unexpected response to a particular situation or stimuli. It indicates that the actor has a system of expectations relative to his own need arrangements.

INTRODUCTION

Society is a web of social organizations. In this way, social organization is a system of social relationships. Social relationships are complex. They are composed into numerous small groups.

In these groups are individuals. Social system refers to individual actors interacting with each other in accordance with standard cultural norms. The individual who participates in interactive relationships influences the other individuals and groups. Interactions and inter-relationships between different individuals and social groups create a system called social system.

DEFINITIONS OF SOCIAL SYSTEM

1. A social system basically consists of two or more individuals interacting directly or indirectly in a bounded situation—*Mitchell Duncan*.
2. A social system is defined in terms of two or more social actors engaged in more or less stable interaction within a bounded environment—*A Dictionary of Sociology*.
3. A social system is a set of persons or groups who interact with one another, the set is conceived of as a social unit distinct from the particular persons who composes it—*David Popenoe*.
4. A social system consists in a plurality of individual actors, interacting with each other in a situation of environment ......who have motives to the optimization of gratification and whose relation to their situation is defined and meditated in terms of a system of culturally structured and shared symbols.

CHARACTERISTICS OF SOCIAL SYSTEM

Sl.No.	Characteristics	Description
1.	Inter-related acts	Social system composed of inter-related acts, because it produces social relationship.
2.	Give rise to higher order	Participation of actors in their positional aspect and processual aspect give rise to higher order unit namely statuses and roles.
3.	Based on regulative norms	Statuses and roles are determined by norms like beliefs, traditions, customs, mores, laws, institutions, etc.
4.	It has a structure	Social system has a structure. It includes various types of subgroups and roles.
5.	Related to cultural values	The cultural value motivates to maintain equilibrium between different parts.
6.	Social system is inter-connected	The parts or elements of social system are inter-connected and assigned with certain functions.
7.	Social system is dynamic	Social system changes from time to time, in spite of changes, continues to exist by solving the social needs. The social needs of the social system are adaptation, goal attainment, integration, and pattern maintence and tension management.
8.	Efficiency	Social relationships with respect to the appropriate ways of behavior, the norm of efficiency, is of great importance in the social system.

STATUS

Status is a term used to designate the comparative amounts of prestige, difference or respect accorded to persons who have been assigned different roles in a group or community. The status of a person is high if the role, he is playing, is considered important by the group. If the role is regarded less high, its performer may be accorded lower status. Thus the status of a person is based on social evaluations.

Definitions

1. Status is the worth of a person as estimated by a group or a class of persons—*Secord and Bukman.*
2. Status is the rank-order position assigned by a group to a role or to a set of roles—*Ogburn and Nimkoff.*
3. Status is the social position that determines for its possessor, apart from his personal attributes or social services, a degree of respect, prestige and influence—*MacIver.*
4. Status is a position in the general institutional system, recognized and supported by the entire society spontaneously evolved rather than deliberately created, rooted in the folkways and mores—*Davis.*
5. Status defined as a position in social aggregate identified with a pattern of prestige symbols and actions—*Martindale and Menachesi.*
6. A status is a position in a social group or grouping, in relation to other positions held by other individuals in the group or grouping—*Green.*
7. Status means the location of the individual within the group, his place in the social network of reciprocal obligations and privileges, rights and duties—*Mazumdar.*
8. Status is the social position that determines for its possessor, apart from his personal attribute or social service, a degree of respect, prestige and influence—*MacIver and Page.*
9. A status is a position in a social group or grouping, a relation to other position held by other individuals in the group or grouping—*Morris Ginsberg.*
10. Status is the place in a particular system, which certain individuals occupy at a particular time—*Ralph Linton.*
11. Status refers to an individual's total standing in society—*Johnson.*

Nature of Status

The word status is used to refer to an individual's total standing in society. In that sense, it embraces all his particular statuses and roles especially in so far as they bear upon general social standing. As we know each person occupies many different roles. He is a father, a doctor, the president of rotary club, and a player of tennis. As a father he is neglectful of his children and does not carry out the requirements of his position, but as a doctor he gives most of his time to his profession and does well. He is a good player but a poor president. In such a case we will have to qualify our statement when we make his status evaluation.

Characteristics of Status

1. **Ascribed status:** This is a social position a person receives at birth or assumes involuntarily later in life. This status is not based on individual ability, skill effort or accomplishment. This status is obtained on inheritance in the society. Sex and age statuses are the most obvious and universal. Example of ascribed status includes being a daughter, a Cuban, a teenager, or a widower.

Sl.No.	Characteristics	Description
1.	Sex	Sex difference is one of the bases of the ascription of life time statuses. Because it is visible biological fact that appears at birth.
2.	Age	Age is another criterion which is visible physiological fact in determining the status. Age is steadily changing and the ascription of status will be determined on the basis of age relationship. For example, between parent and child, elder brother and younger brother.
3.	Kinship	Kinship is another factor that determines the status of a person. An infant's status is identified in relation to the parents and siblings. Kinship connections determine the individual status.
4.	Wealth	Wealth is another criteria of social status. The source of wealth is socially significant. Wealth may be inherited; the inherited wealth or property enhances the prestige of persons.
5.	Race and caste	In multi-raced societies like America, it is the racial group which determines social status. The white race has always superior status as compared to other races like Negro or Mongoloid.

2. **Achieved status:** It is a status achieved by an individual through his own efforts with competitive spirit and showing special abilities, knowledge and skill. It also refers to a social position a person assumes voluntarily that reflects personal ability and effort. For example, many occupational statuses are considered to be achieved status as advocate, doctor, professor, author, etc.

Sl.No.	Characteristics	Description
1.	Occupation	Occupation is also a significant determinant of social status. Certain occupations like national or provincial services, doctors and engineers are more reputed in the society as compared with several others.
2.	Education	The level of education also is important in the determination of social status. A highly educated or technically qualified and trained person has greater respect and honor in the society.
3.	Political authority	In the modern world, persons well-planned in political life, especially those who hold positions in the government, have very high status.
4.	Marriage	Marriage automatically gives the status of a husband or wife and further that of a daughter-in-law, son-in-law, brother-in-law, sister-in-law and several other related statuses.
5.	Individual achievements	In contemporary society, individual achievements are significant in determining social status,. This may be in the field of education, occupation, sports, literature, art, science or any other field.

3. **Master status:** It is a status that a society defines as having special importance for social identity, often shaping a person's entire life. For most people, one's occupation is a master status because it conveys a great deal about social background, education and income.

IMPORTANCE OF SOCIAL STATUS

1. The social status is of great importance both for the individual and society. An individual wins respect in society by virtue of his status. An increase in the individual's status entitles him to more respect than before.
2. Marriages in almost every society are contracted on basis of social status. It is common knowledge and an everyday occurrence that many marriages are not contracted simply because of differences in the social status or in the financial condition of the parents of the boy and the girl. Everyone wants to marry his son and daughter into a family of an equal or better footing in society. An individual wins respect in society by virtue of his social status.
3. Every social status is recognizable from some symbols of respect. These symbols of respect change along with changes in social status. An increase in the individual's social status entitles him to more respect than before irrespective of whether this increase or improvement is due to marriage or the acquisition of skill in some art or knowledge or due to his having moved into some higher office.
4. The roles of an individual also changes along with his social status. Different roles are conjoined to different social positions. Actually the very object in having difference in the statuses within society is to facilitate the division of work among people according to their ability.
5. Status system is a universal characteristic of human society. It constitutes the basic organization of group life and determines who is to carry what. Status system is necessary in the specialization of functions, and in the coordination of the specialized functions of a community. It is important for affording incentives for effort and in promoting the sense of responsibility, dependability and stability so necessary for cooperative living.

ELEMENTS OF SOCIAL SYSTEM

The social system is constituted by the actions of individuals. It involves participation of an actor in a progress of interactive relationship. This participation has two main aspects: The positional aspect and the processional aspect.

Sl.No.	Elements	Description
1.	The act	Social act or action is a process in the social system that motivates the individual or individuals in the case of group. The action is not an unexpected response to a particular situation or stimuli. It indicates that the actor has a system of expectations relative to his own need-arrangements.
2.	The actor	The actor is also a significant unit of social system. It is he who holds a status and performs a role. A social system must have a sufficient proportion of its actors. These actors must be sufficiently motivated to act according to the requirements of its role system. The social system must also be adapted to the minimum needs of the individual actor.

Contd...

Contd...

| 3 | The role and status | The social system involves the participation of actor in a process of interactive relationship. The participation has two aspects—the role aspect and the status aspect. Role denotes the functional significance of the actor for the social system. Status denotes the place of the actor in the social system. |

CLASSIFICATIONS OF SOCIAL SYSTEM

Sl.No.	Classification	Description
1.	Classification by Morgan and other Evolutionist	Classifications based on evolution: 1. Savagery social system 2. Barbarian social system 3. Civilized social system Classification based on livelihood: 1. Hunting social system 2. Pastoral social system 3. Agricultural social system 4. Industrial social system
2.	Durkheim's classification	Described as two kinds of social system: 1. Mechanical social system 2. Organic social system
3.	Sorokin's classification	Classifications based on cultural system: 1. Sensate 2. Ideational 3. Idealistic

STATUS AND OFFICE

There is a close inter-dependence between the office and status. Occupational position is often a status and office both. Office designates the position of occupation by a person in a social organization governed by specific and definite rules, more generally achieved than ascribed. The examples are the office of a principal, the editor, the manager, the director, professional organizational counselor, etc. It is clear that holding an office may give a status. The kind of status, it gives, depends upon the importance, scope and function of the office. There are two ways of attaching status to an office. Firstly, we attach an invidious value to an office as such independently of who occupies it or how its requirements are carried out. Secondly, we attach value to the individual according to how well or ill he carries out the obligations of that office. The first kind of invidious value or evaluation is called prestige. The second one is called esteem. People attach high value to particular job irrespective of the individuals who hold it.

STATUS COMPARISION

Persons generally compare themselves and others with respect to status. The people with whom a person compares himself and the degree to which he makes the comparison are determined by principles of distributive justice, the person's perception of his power and the conditions allowing ease for comparison. The following are the conditions under which status comparisons are made:

1. Each person must be able to observe the rewards, costs and investments of others so that he can compare them with his own.
2. Each person must have approximately the same power to obtain rewards or avoids costs.
3. A person will compare himself only with those whose rewards and costs are not too different from his own.
4. Comparisons are likely to be made with persons having similar investments because they should experience similar rewards and costs.

ROLE

The word role means the roll on which an actor, part was written. The social system is based on a division of labor in which every person is assigned a specific task. The task performed by an individual makes up the role he is expected to play in the life and community. Since the role is a set of expectations, it, therefore, implies that one role cannot be defined without referring to another. There cannot be a parent without a child, or an employer without an employee. In this sense, roles are but a series of rights and duties that is they represent reciprocal relations among individuals. Holding the status of student, for example, means one will attend classes, complete assignments and more broadly, devote a lot of time to personal enrichment through academic study.

Definitions

1. A role is the function of a status—*Young and Mack.*
2. Role is a pattern of behavior expected of an individual in a certain group or situation—*Lundberg.*
3. A role is a set of socially expected and approved behavior patterns, consisting of both duties and privileges, associated with a particular position of a group—*Ogburn and Nimkoff.*
4. Role is the dynamic or the behavior aspect of status.... A role is what an individual does in the status he occupies—*Robert Bierstedt.*
5. A social role is the expected behavior associated with a social position—*Duncan Mitchell.*
6. Role is defined as behavior expected of someone who holds a particular status—*Liton.*

Role Set

Robert Merton (1968) introduced the term role set to identify a number of roles attached to a single status. For example four statuses of one individual, each status linked to a different role set.

1. As a professor, this person interacts with students (teacher role) and with academics (the colleague role).
2. As a researcher, gathers and analyzes data (the laboratory role).
3. The man occupies the status of husband with conjugal role (such as confidante and sexual partner) towards his wife, with whom he shares a domestic role towards the household.
4. He holds the status of father, with routine responsibilities of his children (protective role), as well as towards their school and other organizations in his community (the civic role).

Role Conflict and Role Stain

A social group, as already observed, carries on its life smoothly and harmoniously to the extent that roles are clearly assigned and each member accepts and fulfills the assigned role according to expectations. Each person participates in a number of groups or sub-groups in different capacities. So one individual is required to play a number of different roles. An individual, in his total personality structure, has to play many roles according to social expectations. This has resulted in adjustments of difficulty and creates confusion. Incompatibility between two roles called role conflict. Such role conflicts result in departure from the conformity to some of the expectations or may result in deviation.

Causes of Role Conflict

1. Culture heterogeneity and complexity of the social system.
2. Different roles of an individual in different groups.
3. The possibility of confusion over the appropriateness of a case.
4. When two or more persons are authorized to perform some functions.
5. When the functions are below the status of the individual.
6. Differences in the expected behavior from the person assigned a role.
7. Differences in the perception of one's duties and responsibilities.

Roles in modern society are numerous, complex, highly diversified and sometimes in conflict. In periods of rapid social change, the nervous strain of conflicting roles is greater because the requirements of each role and the expectations of the community regarding them are uncertain. To the extent the different roles are clearly allocated and to the extent the rights and duties inherent in each role clearly understood and to the extent everyone behaves in his role as expected, the social system will run smoothly and with a minimum of strain on the individual personality.

CONCLUSION

Status and role are important element of any society. In fact, Talcott Parsons, a prominent sociologist has held that sociology itself is a collection of status and roles of people. Social organization and disorganization are based on status and role. Social change also is on the basis of change of status and role. Social system is an orderly and systematic arrangement of social interactions. It is a network of interactive relationship. It may be defined as a plurality of individuals interacting with each other according to shared cultural norms and meaning. The constituents parts of social system are individuals. Each individual has a role to play.

40 *Social Organization*

DEFINITIONS

1. **Social organization:** Social organization is the organization of the society and it is a system of social relationships. Social organization is a result of the interaction of forces (integration and differentiation) within the social groups. The groups are part of social organization.
2. **Accommodation:** Accommodation denotes acquired changes in the behavior of individuals which help them to adjust to their environment.
3. **Assimilation:** Assimilation is the process, whereby individuals or groups once dissimilar become similar and identified in their interest and outlook.
4. **Association:** An association is a group of people organized for a particular purpose or a limited number of purposes. An association is not a community but a group within a community. Membership of an association is voluntary but the membership of community is compulsory.
5. **UNICEF:** It is a specialized agency to deal with welfare and rehabilitation of children. It gives assistance to underdeveloped countries for maternal and child health, nutrition, environmental sanitation, provision of safe drinking water, health centers, health education and other programs which would benefit children directly or indirectly.
6. **UNDP:** United Nations development program provides funds to help poor nations to develop their human and natural resources more fully. Assistance is given for different projects connected with agriculture, industry, education, science, social welfare and health.
7. **FAO:** Food and agriculture organization (FAO) aims to help the nations to raise their standards of living to improve the nutrition, to increase efficiency in farming, forestry, and fisheries, to improve the conditions of rural people.
8. **Red Cross Society:** It is a non-political international humanitarian organization devoted to the services of humanity in times of war and peace. Indian red cross is primarily concerned with providing various amenities to military hospitals, for disabled people and disaster services.
9. **Central Social Service Welfare Board:** It is a semi-government organization. Its functions are surveying the needs of voluntary welfare organizations, promoting and initiating voluntary organizations and rendering financial aid to deserving organizations and services.
10. **UNFPA:** United nations fund for population activities (UNFPA) has been helping India since 1974 to develop the capacity for manufacture of contraceptives, population education programs, new techniques in maternal and child health care and also training of grassroot level health worker.

INTRODUCTION

Social organization is the organization of society. Society is a web of social relationships. In this way, social organization is a system of social relationship. Social relationships are complex. They are composed into numerous small groups. In these groups of individuals. The mutual relationships between individuals are controlled and regulated by institutions and associations. Social organization includes and comprehends the cultural institutions and their inter-relationships in addition to the unorganized activities of the group.

DEFINITIONS OF SOCIAL ORGANIZATION

1. Social organization is meant the totality of cultural institutions and their inter-relationship together with the body of the unorganized activities characteristic of the group—*Reuter and Hart.*
2. Social organization is a state of being, a condition in which the various institutions in a society are functioning in accordance with their recognized or implied purpose—*Elliott and Merrill.*
3. Social organization in a whole composed of cooperating specialized parts—*Lumley.*
4. Social organization is a system by which the parts of society are related to each other and to the whole society in a meaningful way—*ME Jones.*
5. The most important bases of social organization are sex, age, kinship, locality, social status, political power, occupation, religion and magic, totemism and voluntary associations—*Ralph Piddington.*

CHARACTERISTICS OF SOCIAL ORGANIZATION

1. The organization of this system is the inter-relationship of its constituents. The constituents of society are institutions, associations and groups.
2. A society can be described as organized only when all these various organs function smoothly and without friction, and adequately perform their functions.
3. Social organization is the system by which the parts of sociology are related to each other and to the whole society in a meaningful way.
4. Social organization that maintains an active synthesis between the mutual activities of various units of society. Society has some implicit and explicit objectives for the attainment of which its parts work.

SOCIAL ORGANIZATION AND SOCIAL GROUP

The group is a part of the social organization. The processes of integration and differentiation always continue actively as a result of which large group are constantly being disintegrated or divided into smaller ones while the smaller ones are integrated into big groups. These are the processes of social organization. Social organization is the net result of the interaction of these two forces within social groups. In this way social organization is based on social groups.

According to George Peter Murdock, social organization is the organization in small groups, particularly in those groups which are based on age, blood relationships, occupation, habitation, ownership of property and status. Actually social organization can be said to be the pattern of inter-group relationships. What are the natural relations of various groups in any society; this depends upon its social organization. In this way there is a very intimate relation between social group and social organization.

FEATURES OF SOCIAL ORGANIZATION

1. **Unanimity among the members of society:** The existence of unanimity among the members of the society is a feature of social organization. In its absence, conflict will arise between them and social disorganization will set in. For example, in ancient India the difference between the status of Brahmins, Kahatriyas, and Vaishyas, and the Shudras was very great. The activities of these groups also different and the ones undertaken by the Shudras were worse than those of other castes.

2. **Promptness in accepting status and roles:** Unanimity among members of a society can be maintained only so long as people are prompt and ready to accept their status and respective roles within the social organization. In society it is not possible to apportion roles to all individuals in such a way that everyone gets same and equal work. Just as every tool and parts has its own position and function in a machine, so are the functions of people in society divided. A body can function only as long as all its various organs perform their respective functions. Much the same can be said of society. In society one comes across differences in the social status of different individual who differ in respect of their sex, age, status, physical capability, skill and duties. The role of individuals is determined on the basis of the social status.

3. **Control of society on the activities of the individuals:** The members of society will be prompt in accepting their status and role only when society will be prompt in accepting their status and role only when society has control over them. Society exercises this control through the media of habits, customs, traditions, mores, rituals and institutions. It is this which creates unanimity is society. Social disorganization starts the moment this control of society is lifted from upon the members.

TYPES OF SOCIAL ORGANIZATION

Sl.No	Types	Description
1.	Family	The family is the basic unit in all societies. It is a group of biologically related individual living together and eating from a common kitchen.
2.	Religion and caste	The caste system in India is an example of a closed class, i.e. there is no mobility or shifting from one class to another and the members remain throughout life time wherein they are born. Each caste is governed by certain rules and sanctions relating to endogamy. Food taboos, ritual purity, etc. each caste group within a village is expected to give certain standardized services to the families of other castes.
3.	Temporary social groups	1. **Crowd:** When a group of people some together temporarily for a short period, motivated by a common interest or curiosity is known as crowd. 2. **The mob:** The mob essentially a crowd, but has a leader who forces the members into action. There may be a symbol in the shape of a flag or slogan. The mob is more emotional than a crowd. 3. **The herd:** This is also a crowd with a leader. Here the members of the group have to follow the orders of the leader without question, e.g., tourist group under a guide.
4.	Permanent spatial groups	1. **The band:** It is the most elementary community of a few families living together. Here the group has organized itself and follows a pattern of life, e.g. gypsies in India.

Contd...

Contd...

Sl.No	Types	Description
		2. **Village:** The village is a small collection of people permanently settled down in a locality with their homes and cultural equipments.
		3. **Towns and cities:** From a sociological point of view, a city or town may be defined as a relatively large, dense and permanent settlement of socially heterogeneous individuals. The community is sub-divided into smaller groups on the basis of wealth and social class.
5.	Government and political organization	Government is an association of which law is the institutional activity. There is no society which lacks government. It is the supreme agent authorized to regulate the balanced social life in the interests of the public.

FORMAL ORGANIZATIONS

A century ago, most people lived in small groups of family, friends, and neighbors. Today, our lives revolve more and more around formal organizations, large secondary groups organized to achieve their goals efficiently. Formal organizations such as business corporations and government agencies differ from families and neighborhoods in an important way: Their greater size makes social relations less personal and fosters a formal, planned atmosphere. In other words, formal organizations operate in a deliberate way, not to meet personal needs but to accomplish complex jobs.

Types of Formal Organizations

Amitai Etzioi (1975) identified three types of formal organizations, distinguish by the reason people participate: utilitarian organizations, normative organizations and coercive organizations.
1. **Utilitarian organizations**: Just about every one works for income belongs to a utilitarian organization, one that pays people for their efforts. Large business, for example, generates profits for their owner and income for their employees.
2. **Normative organizations:** People join normative organizations not for income but to pursue some goal they think is morally worthwhile. Sometimes called voluntary associations, these include community service groups (such as the PTA, the Lions Club, the League of Women Voter and Red Cross), as well as political parties and religious organizations.
3. **Coercive organizations:** Coercive organizations have an involuntary membership. That is, people are forced to join these organizations as a form of punishment (prisons) or treatment (some psychiatric hospitals). Coercive organization has special physical features, such as locked doors and barred windows, and is supervised by security personnel.

VOLUNTARY SOCIAL HEALTH AGENCIES

Sl.No.	Organization	Description
1.	WHO (World Health Organization)	The WHO is a branch of the UNO and it started functioning in 1948, and has its headquarters in Geneva, Switzerland. The main objective of the WHO is the attainment of all people of the world the highest level of health. The current objective is health for all by 2010. It renders valuable services in the prevention and control of specific diseases like AIDS. It tries best to prevent the spread of the disease.
2.	UNICEF (United Nations International Children's Emergency Fund)	This is a specialized agency to deal with welfare and rehabilitation of children. It gives much assistance to underdeveloped countries for maternal child health, nutrition, environment sanitation, and

Contd...

Contd...

Sl.No.	Organization	Description
		provision of safe drinking water, health centers, health education and other program which would benefit children directly or indirectly. It gives substantial aid to nations for the production of vaccines.
3.	United Nations Development Program (UNDP)	This provides funds to help the poor nations to develop their human and natural resources more fully. Assistance is given for different projects connected with agriculture, industry, education, science, social welfare and health.
4.	United Nations Fund for Population Activities (UNFPAA)	It has been helping India since 1974 to develop the capacity for manufacture of contraceptives, population education program, new techniques in maternal and child health care and also training of grass root level health worker.
5.	Food and Agriculture Organization of the UNO (FAO)	The FAO aims to help the nations to raise their standards of living to improve the nutrition, to increase efficiency in farming, forestry and fisheries, to improve the conditions of rural people. Its primary concern is to increase food production to meet the needs of the increasing population.
6.	Red Cross Society	The Red Cross Society is a non-political International Humanitarian organization devoted to the service of humanity in times of war and peace. The Indian red cross is primarily concerned with providing various amenities to military hospitals, for disabled people, and disaster services.
7.	Indian Council of Child Welfare (ICCW)	It was established in 1952. It is associated with the International Union of Child Welfare. It strives hard to provide opportunities and facilities by law and other means to every child to develop physically, mentally, morally, spiritually and socially under healthy and normal conditions.
8.	Central Social Welfare	This is semi-government organization. It was set-up by the board. Government of India in August 1953. Their functions are surveying the needs of voluntary welfare organizations, promoting and initiating voluntary organizations and rendering financial aid to deserving organizations and services.
9.	Hind Kusht Nivaran Sangh	It was founded in 1950 with its headquarters in New Delhi. Its precursor was the Indian Council of the British Empire Leprosy Relief Association, which was dissolved in 1950. The program of work of the sangh includes rendering of financial assistance to various leprosy homes and clinics, health education through publications and posters, training of medical workers and physiotherapists, conducting research and field investigations, etc.
10.	Tuberculosis Association of India	The Tuberculosis Association of India was formed in 1939. It has branches in all the states in India. The activities of this association comprise organizing a TB Seal campaign every year to raise funds, training of doctors, health visitors and social worker in antituberculosis work, promotion of health education and promotion of consultations and conferences.

Contd...

Contd...

Sl.No.	Organization	Description
11.	Bharat Sevak Samaj	It is a non-political and non-official organization was formed in 1952. one of the prime objectives is to help people to achieve health by their own efforts. The important activity is improvement of sanitation.
12.	The Kasturba Memorial Fund	The Kasturaba memorial fund was established in the memory of Kasturaba Gandhi in 1944. The main objective of the trust is to improve the condition of Indian rural women. It has several institutions and does valuable services in educating rural girls and also social education and uplifting of villages.
13.	Family Planning Association of India	It was established in 1949 and has done pioneering work in the area of family planning. Its headquarters are in Mumbai and it has branches in several cities. The association also trains doctors and health workers in family planning techniques. The association also answers family planning quires.
14.	All India Women's Conference	It is a women's voluntary welfare organization established in 1926. They run maternal child welfare clinics, medical centers, adult education centers, family planning clinics, milk centers and cooperatives.
15.	Professional bodies	The Indian medical association, the trained nurses association of India, Indian dental association, Indian pharmacological association, these professional bodies conduct annual conferences, publish journals, arrange scientific sessions and exhibitions to set-up standards of professional education.
16.	All India Blind Relief Society	It was established in 1946, with an objective of coordinating different institutions working for the blind. It organizes eye camps and lot of other relief work for the welfare of the blind.
17.	Christian Churches and Institutions	Christian medical association of India, Catholic medical association of India, young men Christian association, young women Christian association are doing much work in the forms of relief in disaster like floods, earthquakes and famines, education and welfare for women and children. The Christian churches in India are running large number of schools, colleges, hostels, orphanages, training centers hospitals and welfare centers.
18.	Other organizations	The Ramakrishna mission, Aryasamaj rotary international, lions international, Rockefeller foundation, ford foundation, cooperative for American relief everywhere (CARE) and many other national and international organizations have played and are playing a significant role in solving a large number of socioeconomic problems in India.

CONCLUSION

Social organization is the organization of society. Society is a web of social relationships. In this way, social organization is the system of social relationships. Social relationships are complex. They are composed into numerous small groups. In these groups are individuals. The mutual relationship between individuals are controlled and regulated by institutions and associations. Hence, institutions and associations along with individuals and groups form a part of the social organization. Hence, it is social organization that maintains an active synthesis between the mutual activities of various units of society.

41 Social Disorganization

DEFINITIONS

1. **Social disorganization:** Social disorganization is a state of disequilibrium and a lack of social solidarity or consensus among the members of a society.
2. **Cultural lag:** Cultural lag is the imbalance in the rate and speed of change between the material culture and non-material culture. Social change that disorganization is caused primarily by the unequal rates of change in the different parts of culture, resulting in conflict between them.
3. **Natural catastrophes:** A maladjustment or conflict between man and his natural environment, especially under circumstances of radical change such as epidemics, floods. Famines, wars, etc. Natural catastrophes can cause social disorganization; the sudden death of a leader may create a crisis and throw the society out of gear.
4. **Social pathology:** Social pathology is the process and results of the process whereby in any given society, some people are socialized in such a way as to develop thought and/or behavior patterns that are defined as disapproved deviations.
5. **Deviant behavior:** Deviant behavior is conduct that the people of a society generally regard as aberrant, disturbing, improper, immoral and for which specific social control effects are likely to be found.
6. **Social problem:** Social problem is a way of behavior that is regarded as violation of one or more generally accepted or approved norms. Social problems are behavior patterns or conditions that are considered objectionable or undesirable by many members of a society.
7. **Individual disorganization:** Individual or personal disorganization they included juvenile delinquency, various types of crime, insanity, drunkenness and suicide.
8. **Family social disorganization:** Family social disorganization symptoms include divorce, illegitimate births, desertion and venereal diseases.
9. **Community social disorganization:** It may include poverty, unemployment, crime and political corruption.

INTRODUCTION

Society is a web of social relationships. In an organized society these relationships remain organized. In a disorganized society these relationships remain organized. The process whereby social relations become disorganized is known as social disorganization. Social organization inclusive of habits, institutions, associations, etc. in the process of disorganization all these become disorganized. Social disorganization is the process opposed to social organization. Social disorganization refers to serious maladjustments rather than maladjustments in society so that they fail to satisfy the needs of the individuals satisfactorily.

Social disorganization, as the process by which the relationship between members of a group are broken or dissolved. Social disorganization occurs when there is a change in the equilibrium of force, a breakdown of the social structure; so that former patterns no longer apply and accepted forms of social control no longer function effectively. Social organization and social disorganization are relative terms. Social disorganization occurs when there is a change in the equilibrium of forces, so that many former expectations no longer apply and many forms of social controls no longer function effectively.

DEFINITIONS OF SOCIAL DISORGANIZATION

1. Social disorganization is the process. Social pertains to society or social relationships while the word disorganization is indicative of breaking or disruption or disintegration which speaks of the annihilation, destruction, or breaking of social relations between the members—*Elliott and Merrill*.
2. Social disorganization is a disturbance in the patterns and mechanism of human relations—*RFL Faris*.
3. Social disorganization is decrease of the influence of existing social rules of behavior upon the individual member of the group—*Thomas and Znaniecki*.
4. Social disorganization as a state of disequilibrium and a lack of social solidarity or consensus among the members of a society—*Emile Durkheim*.
5. Social disorganization is the process by which the relationships between members of a group are shaken—*Mowerer*.

CAUSES OF SOCIAL DISORGANIZATION

Social organization is a complex process and to attribute it to one cause is to commit a fallacy. Social disorganization is created due to scientific and technological inventions on the one hand and clashing interests of economic, social, and political classes on the other.

1. **Social change:** Social structure is dynamic. Its various element modes, mores, institutions, associations, etc. are constantly changing. In it the old mores come into conflict with novel patterns and old institutions enter into strife with newer institutions, the result of which is the unanimity of society destroyed.
2. **Division of labor:** According to Emile Durkheim, extreme division of labor is the cause of social disorganization. Division of labor is generally productive of social solidarity; but which it becomes excessive and complex then solidarity diminishes or disappears and social equilibrium is disturbed. Extreme division of labor gives raise to economic crises of all kinds, class struggle and industrial strife, and leads to demoralization of individuals, the family and community.
3. **Violation of social rules:** According to WI Thomas and Znaniecki, when the rules and regulations of society fail to keep individuals under control, social disorganization sets in. In society there are always individuals who violate social rules. This has a disorganizing effect upon social institutions, and unless the violations are cheeked, they may eventually lead to the death of institutions.
4. **Cultural lag:** Cultural lag is also one cause of social disorganization. Cultural lag is the name given to the phenomenon wherein an element of a culture fails to keep up with the others in the process of change. This creates confusion in society and social disorganization sets in. Non-physical elements change at a slow rate and their change lags behind the change in the physical elements. Beliefs and thoughts change with great difficulty but not much time is needed for the adaptation of material things.

5. **Industrialization:** Economic system had led to capitalism, exploitation and class conflicts. It has also contributed to unemployment, crime, immobility, family disorganization, urbanization and its evils.

6. **Change in social values:** Social organization derives its strength from social values. This organization is destroyed when some injury is inflicted upon them and the process of disorganization sets in. Elliott and Merrill has written without social values neither social organization nor social disorganization would exist. Changes in the social values necessitate new social institutions and associations. These come into conflict with the existing order, institutions and association this creates disorder in society. The status and roles of people change in accordance with the change in social values.

7. **War:** War also is one cause of social disorganization because it introduces confusion and disorder in society. The young men community is consumed in a way, young women are widows, and soldiers have to be far way from their families. Social values are also injured by war. The value of human life is reduced. Murders, arson and rape increase.

8. **Crisis:** Thomas writes crisis is any occurrence which interrupts smoothly running habits by focusing attention upon a conflict situation.
   a. *Precipitate:* Precipitate crisis is that which is so sudden so to deprive people of their senses such as the death of a great leader, a terrible accident, famine, catastrophe, etc. These crises change the situations and functions of many million individuals.
   b. *Cumulative:* A cumulative crisis, as the name is indicative of its nature, is not manifested instantaneously but gradually takes root and develops as a result of many successive incidents. In Indian union, and the consequent creation of Pakistan was just such a cumulative crisis.

9. **Technological interventions:** Industrial revolution was essentially a technological change, but it ushered in a serious modification in social interactions. Modern means of communication, scientific inventions altered the economic and social structure.

10. **Natural catastrophies:** A maladjustment or conflict between man and his natural environment, especially under circumstances of radical change such as epidemic, floods, famines, wars, etc. such conditions significantly disrupt the normal functioning, not only of certain units of society, but of the entire society.

11. **Conflict of norms:** The norms within society may conflict with changes in patterns of economic or other aspect of life and may lead to disorganization. When ethnic and religious groups with differing norms cone into contact, there arises a conflict of norms. The changing society there may occur conflicts of norms between older and younger generations.

Causes Pointed out by Sociologist

Sl.No.	Sociologist view	Classification
1.	Eilliot and Merril	1. The social process namely cultural, political, and economic. 2. Cultural lag. 3. Conflicting attitudes and values. 4. Social crisis.
2.	Karl Manheim	1. Geographical factors. 2. The biological factors. 3. Cultural factors. 4. The technological factors. 5. Psychological factors.

Difference between Social Organization and Disorganization

Sl.No.	Social organization	Social disorganization
1.	Unanimity	Multiplicity of opinions.
2.	Homogeneity	Heterogeneity of population.
3.	Mutual faith	Mutual distrust.
4.	Similarity in interest and attitudes	Individuality and variety in interest and attitudes.
5.	Intelligent behavior	Hedonistic behavior.
6.	Emphasis on duties	Emphasis on rights.
7.	Protection of sacred elements	Degeneration of sacred elements.
8.	Sincerity	Ostentation.
9.	Peace and happiness	Disturbance and pain.
10.	Synthesis between status and functions	Contradiction between status and functions.
11.	Clarity of situation and activities	Lack of clarity of situation and activities.
12.	Synthesis of mores	Conflict of mores.
13.	Synthesis between institutions	Conflict between institutions.
14.	System in the symbols and tools of relationships	Disorder in tools and symbols.
15.	Strong social control	Absence of social control.
16.	Adjustment between society and individual	Conflicts between society and individual.
17.	Respect of social laws	Disregard of social laws.
18.	Adjustment between the various parts of society	Conflict between the various parts of society.

In this way, the process of social disorganization is completely opposed to the progress of social organization is a tool. Social disorganization is the disintegration of this tool.

CHARACTERISTICS OF SOCIAL DISORGANIZATION

1. **Conflict of mores and of institutions:** In every society, there are some mores and institutions on the basis of which the life of the members proceeds smoothly and in an organized manner. With the passage of time these mores and institutions becomes obsolete and antiquated and fail to satisfy the needs of the members of society. Ever new ideals arise and new institutions are formed out of difference of opinion and of ideals. In this way society is broken up into numerous groups.
2. **Transfer of functions from one group to another:** The functions of every group are determined in an organized society. But society is always dynamic and these functions of the groups cannot remain the same for a long time. As time, passes the functions of one group are transferred to another. This is not conductive to any precise definition of the functions of the various groups and they tend to become disorganized.
3. **Personal individualization:** In an organized society the functions of an individual are determined on the basis of the social organization. From the social viewpoint, marriage, family, occupation, etc. were based on some definite patterns ancient India. But the modern age of individualism every person thinks upon all the important matters of life from his own individual view point.

4. **Changes in social structure:** A change in the social structure means change in the role or function of status of its members. In an organized society, the status and functions of each individual are defined any everyone works accordingly. This maintains the society in an organized condition. But as the time passes, changes in social values and thinking are accompanied by changes in these status and functions. This change takes away the precise definition of an individual's status and function and they please. Due to this, social disorganization sets in.

SYMPTOMS OF SOCIAL DISORGANIZATION

Social disorganization is an indication of the existence of diseased or disruptive elements in society. Mabel A Elliot and Francis E Merrill have pointed out that social disorganization may be of three types.

Sl.No.	Types	Symptoms of disorganization
1.	Individual social disorganization	Individual or personal disorganization they included juvenile delinquency, various types of crime, insanity, drunkenness, suicide.
2.	Family social disorganization	Symptoms of family disorganization they included divorce, illegitimate births, desertion and venereal diseases.
3.	Community social disorganization	It may included poverty, unemployment, crime and political corruption.

Calvin F Suhmid listed the following symptoms of disorganized communities: High rate of population mobility, high rates of divorce, desertion, illegitimacy, dependency, delinquency and criminality, a disproportionately high rate of males, a low rate of home ownership, high rate of suicides, commercialized vice and death from disease and alcoholism.

Herbert A Bloch divided the symptoms of social disorganization into two categories: The sociological and the literary-ideological.

Sl.No.	Types	Symptoms of disorganization
1.	Sociological	Sociological symptoms into three classes: Individual, family and community.
2.	Literary-ideological	He meant certain tendencies appearing in literary and artistic works which indicate tendencies appearing in literary and artistic works which indicate a disturbed state of mind.

Faris has enumerated the following symptoms of social disorganization:
1. Formalism.
2. The decline of sacred elements.
3. Individuality of interests and tastes.
4. Emphasis of personal freedom and individual rights.
5. Hedonistic behavior.
6. Population heterogeneity.
7. Mutual distrust.
8. Unrest phenomena.

CONCLUSION

Social disorganization, therefore, is to be considered in terms of functional disequilibrium. It is disequilibrium within customs, institutions, groups, communities and societies. Comparing social disorganization with social organization. Queen and Haper writes, if social organization means the development of relationships which persons and groups find mutually satisfactory, then disorganization means their replacement by relationships which bring disappointment, thwarted wishes, irritation and unhappiness.

Social Problems

DEFINITIONS

1. **Prostitute:** A prostitute may be defined as "An individual (male or female) who for some kind of reward (Monetary or otherwise) or for some other form of personal satisfaction and as a part or full time profession, engages in normal or abnormal sexual intercourse with various persons who may be of the same sex as or the opposite sex to the prostitute.

2. **Dowry:** Dowry is the property which a women bring with her or is given to her at the marriage.

3. **Juvenile delinquency:** Juvenile delinquency involves wrong-doing by a child or young person who is under an age specified by the law of the place considered.

4. **Poverty:** Poverty as "that condition in which a person either because of inadequate income or unwise expenditure does not maintain a scale of living high among to provide for his physical and mental efficiency and to enable him and his natural dependents of function usefully according to the standards of the society of which he is a member."

5. **Unemployment:** Unemployment is a condition of the labor market in which the supply of labor is greater than the number of available openings.

6. **Crime:** Crime is a antisocial behavior that has violated public sentiment to such an extent as to be forbidden by statute.

7. **Alcoholism:** Addition to alcoholism and excessive drinking has disastrous physiological, psychological and sociomoral effects. Alcoholic means a drinker, who is an excessive drinker, with out which he cannot live. Such persons are called drunkards, who are mentally disturbed, physiologically affected. Demoralized and socially and economically maladjusted.

8. **Drug abuse:** Drug abuse is a serious social problem that confronts youth of India. The problems arise mainly due to failure to internalize norms, through frustration and habit formation. The message from the narcotic control bureau and other agencies is drug abuse is life abuse.

9. **Women abuse:** Women abuse is a serious and widespread societal problem. Women from all ages, racial and ethic background, sexual orientations, socioeconomic classes, religious, ability levels and professionals can experience abuse.

10. **Child abuse:** Child abuse is the term referred to children who have received serious physical injury causes willfully. Child abuse is harm to, or neglect of, a child by another person, whether adult or child.

INTRODUCTION

Sociology is primarily concerned with the study of social disorganization and social problems. Social problems show abnormal or pathological signs in social relationships. They are the conditions that threaten the well-being of society. Every social problem implies three things, firstly—that something should be done to change the situation which constitutes a problem, secondly—that the existing social order will have to be changed to solve the problem, thirdly—that situation regarded a problem is undesirable but not inevitable. The people deplore the situation because they think that it can be reformed or eliminated. It may also be noted that a situation becomes a problem only after the people become aware that certain cherished valuations are threatened by conditions which have become acute. Without such awareness no situation can be identified as a problem.

DEFINITIONS OF SOCIAL PROBLEMS

1. Social problem defined as any difficulty or misbehavior of a fairly large number of persons which we wish to remove or correct—*Lawrence K Frank*.
2. Social problem defined as a condition affecting a significant number of people in ways considered undesirable, and about which it is felt something can be done through collective social action—*Paul B Harton and Gerald R Leslie*.
3. A social problem as a condition which is defined by a considerable number of persons as deviated from social norm which they cherish—*Richard C Fuller and Richard R Meyers*.
4. A social problem is any deviant behavior in a disapproved direction of such a degree that it exceeds the tolerance limit of community—*Lundberg*.
5. A social problem is a set of conditions which are defined as morally wrong by the majority or substantial minority within a society—*Green*.
6. Social problems as a way of behavior that is regarded as violation of one or more generally accepted or approved norms—*Robert Nisbet*.
7. Social problems are behavior patterns or conditions that are considered objectionable or undesirable by many members of a society—*Madan*.
8. Social pathology as the process and the results of the process whereby in any given society, some people are socialized in such a way as to develop thought and/or behavior patterns that are defined as disapproved deviations, such as deviations, such deviations assuming a verity of forms, e.g. mental illness, prostitution, alcoholism, drug addition, crime, juvenile delinquency, sometimes used synonymously with social problems and with social disorganization—*Thomas Ford Hoult in the Dictionary of Modern Sociology (1969)*.
9. A social problem is any deviant behavior in a disapproved direction of such a degree that it exceeds the tolerance limit of the community—*Lundberg*.

FEATURES OF SOCIAL PROBLEMS

1. Social problems are deviations from the general norms (rules) of the society by a large number of members. This is called anomie, it means normallessness.
2. Social problems are common to all societies, but they are vary from society-to-society.
3. All social problems are interconnected.
4. Social problems are harmful to society. They threaten the well-being of the society and disrupt the social equilibrium.
5. Social problems require collective effort for their solution.
6. Social problems arise due to social maladjustments. They are the pathological conditions of society.

CLASSIFICATION OF SOCIAL PROBLEMS

Some sociologists have made an attempt to classify social problems. Harold A Phelps classified them under four categories corresponding to the four major sources.

Sl.No.	Type	Description
1.	Economic	Poverty, unemployment, dependency, etc.
2.	Biological	Physical diseases and defects.
3.	Biopsychological	Neurosis, psychosis, epilepsy, feeble mindedness, suicide, and alcoholism.
4.	Cultural	Problems of old age, the homeless and the widowed, illegitimacy, crime and juvenile delinquency.

In America the Report of the President's Committee on Recent Social Trends Attributed social problems to inadequacies in physical heritage, biological heritage, and social policy.

Sl.No.	Type	Description
1.	Physical heritage	It includes problems like depletion and conservation of natural resources.
2.	Biological heritage	It includes problems of population quantity, quality, growth, decline and flexibility, as well as problems of eugenics and birth control.
3.	Social heritage	It includes problems involving technological changes, unemployment, business, cycles and depression, education, politics, religion, public health, law of enforcement and minority groups.

CAUSES OF SOCIAL PROBLEMS

Merton analysis that social problems generally occur due to disorganization and deviant behavior or individual disorganization. These two concepts are closely related to social problems. Social problems exist in all societies. They arise out of pathological social conditions. There are multiple causes of social problems. The causes of social problems are the same as that of social disorganization. Social disorganization creates many social problems and social problems lead to social disorganization. These are inter-related and interdependent.

1. Maladjustments among the individuals, due to different social, cultural, and economical settings.
2. Ineffective means of social control.
3. Conflict of values and degeneration of values.
4. Malfunctioning of social, economic, political and religious systems.
5. Incompatible rates of social change cause social problems.

Elements to Identify Social Problems

Three elements must be identified in social problems:
1. A large of people are involved in the problem or affected.
2. The problem is considered as undesirable by society.
3. Something can be done to rectify the problem.

Conclusion

Sociology primarily concerned with the study of social disorganization and social problems. Social problems show abnormal or pathological sign in social relations. They are the conditions that threaten the well-being of society. The origin of social problems lies not in a single cause but in many causes which cannot be put under a single theory. A problem may be due to a combination of physical, biological, mental, and cultural factors or any one of them. No hard and fast rule can be laid down about the cause of social problems.

POVERTY

Introduction

Poverty is socioeconomic problem of the developing and underdeveloped countries. Poverty means inability to secure the minimum consumption requirements for life, health and efficiency. Poverty is a condition of an acute lack of basic needs for livelihood. A poor man is one who is unable to get a square meal a day. Economist and planners are of the opinion that lack of financial resources required by a person to subsist and the life below a minimum subsistence level is called poverty.

Definitions

1. Poverty is the insufficient supply of those things which are requisite for an individual to maintain himself and those dependent upon him in health and vigor—*Goddard*.
2. Poverty is defined as that condition in which a person either because of inadequate income or unwise expenditure, does not maintain a scale of living high enough to provide for his physical and mental efficiency and to enable him and his natural dependents to function usually according to the standards of society of which he is a member—*John L Gillin*.
3. Poverty is the deprivation of something necessary for subsistence and physical efficiency—*EJ Ross*.
4. Poverty is deprivation of those minimal levels of food, health, housing, education and recreation in a society—*Harrington*.
5. Poverty is insufficient supply of those things which are requisite for an individual to maintain himself and those dependent upon him in health and vigor—*TG Goddard*.

Influences of Poverty on Health

The health consequences of poverty are severe. The poor die younger and suffer more from disability. They are exposed to greater risk from unhealthy conditions at home and at work. Malnutrition and the legacy of past illness mean that they are more likely to fall ill and slower to recover, especially if they have little access to health care. When a family's bread winner becomes ill, other members of the household may at first cope by working harder themselves and by reducing consumption, even of food.

Poverty wields its destructive influence at every stage of human life from the movement of conception to the grave. Poverty is the main reasons why babies are not vaccinated, clean water and sanitation are not provided, and curative drug and other treatments are unavailable. It is the main cause of low life expectancy, low birth weight babies, higher maternal mortality, handicap and disability, mental illness, stress, suicide, family disintegrity and substance abuse.

Factors Responsible for Poverty

1. Incapacity of the individual, which may be due to a faulty heredity or to the environment.
2. Unfavorable physical conditions, such as poor natural resources, bad climate and weather and epidemics.
3. Misdistribution of wealth and of income and the imperfect functioning of our economic institutions.

Causes of Poverty

1. Irregular, insufficient and poorly paid employment is, perhaps, the greatest cause of poverty. Unprovided old age, death or the disability of the wage earner, unprovided widowhood, orphanhood and the like also frequently result in poverty.
2. Poverty can also be caused by environmental factors- outcome of insufficient natural resources in one such factor.
3. Poverty may be due to lack of education and important legislation such as an inadequate punitive system.
4. The subjective causes of poverty include individual circumstances and inequalities, character defects and moral handicaps risk high among personal causes of poverty.
5. Idleness, laziness, poor health, extravagance, wastage, poor judgment, ignorance, vanity, incompetency, unemployment, etc. are frequent causes of poverty.
6. Bad habits, immorality, dishonesty, betting, gambling, alcoholism, drug addition, etc. may lead to poverty.

ML Jhingan listed the following as the principal causes of poverty.

1. Underdeveloped country.
2. Inequality of income and wealth.
3. Low per capita income.
4. Inadequate growth rate.
5. High growth of population.
6. Unemployment.
7. Low consumption.
8. Regional disparities.
9. Low availability of essentials.
10. Inflation.
11. Outdated technology.
12. Capital deficiency.
13. Social factors.

Poverty in India

In India, poverty is the most important problem. Each year more than 5 million people are added to the growing multitude of the poor. The main cause of poverty is the personal ownership and monopoly of the individual on the land. In cities where land is valuable we find extremes of poverty and richness. Some of the causes of poverty are personal while others are geographical, economic and social incapacity of the individual due to faulty heredity or to the environment, unfavorable physical conditions such as poor natural resources and misdistribution of the available resources are the main causes of poverty.

In India, there are caught in various circle of poverty due to the prevalent sociocultural institutions. In order to fulfill social obligations and observe religious ceremonies people spend extravagantly. With already low income levels and negligible saving the chances of borrowing are great. The level of indebtedness is both the cause and effort of poverty. Poverty is the most obvious problem in India. According to 2003 estimated about 28.6% (308.59 million) population of the country is living below the poverty line.

Effects of Poverty

Poverty and its vicious circle always undermine physical and mental ability. The moral effects of poverty are also being noted. Bad housing and living conditions, overcrowded rooms and squalor, worry and malnutrition, all lead to ill health, and the moral effects of poverty are sometimes so grave to result in lack of self confidence and initiative, so essential to lead a prosperous life.

Remedial Measures

Since poverty and inequality are inseparable in the case of India, the policy measures for reducing inequalities in income and wealth are equally applicable for the removal of poverty.

1. **Spread of education:** Education should be made compulsory at least up to high school standard. This will broaden the total outlook of the people and adopt better ways of life.
2. **Development of supporting occupations:** There must be massive employment generation will sustain and will be sustained by great availability of wages goods. There should facilities for supplementary employment such as handicrafts, weaving, and pottery may be helpful.
3. **Family welfare programs:** These should be intensified at the village level, so that all unwanted births are avoided and the burden of over-population is reduced.
4. **Fixing minimum wages:** Just as in the factory, minimum wages should be fixed for the labors also, and it should be actually implemented.
5. **The institutional** reform and the fiscal policy must be oriented to reduce inequality alongside increased productivity.
6. **The backward regions** and classes have a high incidence of poverty. Their development must receive high priority.

Conclusion

Poverty is that condition in which a person, either because of inadequate income or unwise expenditure, does not maintain a scale of living high enough to provide for his physical and mental efficiency and to enable him and his natural dependent to function usually according to the standards of society of which he is a member. The Government of India has lunched 20 pointed programs to remove poverty from the land through various measures and we may hope that a day will come when all the people and we may hope that a day will come when all the people will be least assured of the basic necessities of life.

ILLITERACY

Introduction

Illiteracy is a great curse both to the life of the individual and the life of the nation. Education and self realized people are the assets of a nation; the strength of a nation is the seen total of the strengths of the people inhabiting its territories. The illiterate, poor and backward people are liabilities rather than assests to the nation. The 1948, the declaration of Human Rights started that everyone has a right to education. Yet even today, this right is being denied to millions of children. Education is a crucial element; development can either be broad based or sustained. The benefits that accrue to a country by having a literate population are multidimensional. Spread of literacy is generally associated with modernization, urbanization, industrialization, communication, and commerce.

Importance of Illiteracy in India

Education forms an important input in the overall development of individuals enabling them to comprehend their social, political, and cultural environment better, and respond to its appropriately. Higher levels of education and literacy lead to a greater awareness and also contribute to improvement of economic conditions, and is prerequisite for acquiring various skills and better use of health care facilities.

Statistics of Illiteracy in India

It was decided in 1991 census to use the term literacy rate for the population relating to seven years age and above. A person is deemed as literature if he or she can read and write with understanding in any language. A person who can merely read but cannot write is not considered literate. The same concept has been continued in census 2001 also. The literacy rate taking in account the total population in the denominator has now been termed as crude literacy rate. The significant millstone reached in census 2001 is that the total number of illiterate has come down from 328.1 million in 1991 to 296.2 million. Thus, for the independence, there is a decline in the absolute number of illiterates in the country. This is a major shift in improving the literacy status of India.

India claims the dubious distinction of leading the world in the number of illiterates. It also has a vast and rich experience in illiterates. It also has a vast and rich experience in literacy work on which to draw. The national literacy movement (NLM) provides technical support and leadership in targeting the estimated 121 million illiterates in the 15-35 age groups. The total literacy campaigns (TLC's) which grew out of the successful mass literacy movement in Kerala, have spread 212 districts of India.

Remedial Measures

Government of India has made education compulsory up to the age of 14 years in the country. Though considerable progress has been in expanding primary education, a major concern is high drop out rates in the first few years of schooling. In India, National Adult Education Program was inaugurated 2nd October 1978, but its actual implementation in all seriousness began from 1st January, 1980 where adult education projects were stared all over the country. Though it is a national program and financed by the Central Government, it is implemented by the State Government.

Problems of Illiteracy

India is one of the poorest countries of the world due to glaring fact of stark illiterate in the country. India is the only country which has suffered for more than seven countries of servitude. Ignorance and poverty go hand in hand with illiteracy. Illiteracy also causes them to dwell in dirt and filths and does not give them opportunity to become cultured. Being illiterate the villagers cannot become acquainted with the latest developments in modern science, and consequently agriculture and cottage industries are deprived of the degree of progress. It is due to illiteracy, that the rural people are ignored of the basic principles of health which makes them easy prey to sickness.

Conclusion

A literate and educated man can get some benefits from the experience of others but not forth illiterate person. For an illiterate person the whole world looks dark. Man is not simply body but is also spirit, mind, and intellect; while his physical development takes place by taking good food his mental and intellectual development takes place through education. Literacy is not the education but it is certainly the gate through which education passes to the castle of human kind.

FOOD SUPPLIES

Introduction

Food is the prime necessity of life. The discoveries of last fifty years have proved that nutritious food is necessary for good health and body movements of man. Apart from national agencies, international agencies like FAO, WHO, and UNICEF have spend money to evoke interest in people about their food and health and efforts have been made to activities various human resources in the direction. The regular surveys are conducted all over the world to calculate the amount of food needed for different working conditions. The survey conducted by different agencies show that the different diet of vulnerable groups like infants, pregnant women, and lactating women are deficient in protein, calcium, vitamin A, and B complex.

Definitions

1. Food is defined as anything solid, liquid, or semisolid which, when ingested putting into the mouth, digested and assimilated, and nourishes the body—*Rajammal P Devadas*.
2. Nutrition is that condition which permits the development and maintenance of the highest state of fitness—*Rajammal P Devadas*.

Problems of Food Supply in India

Since independence India has been facing serious shortage of food problems. We had to depend on food imports even for our survival but now the situation has considerably improved. The nation has crossed many hurdles and is on the path of self-reliance. Now we are not to depend on other nations. Sometimes, agriculturist is forced to borrow funds from moneylender at very high rate of interest and so generally he is forced to sell his produce to pay off his debts. He is sometimes not able to purchase fertilizer, good seeds, etc. due to in adequacy of funds. The technical reasons responsible for the low yields are:
1. Defective soil and soil erosion.
2. Crop diseases and posts.
3. Irregular and uncertain rains and lack of irrigation.
4. Ignorance and weakness of the cultivator.
5. Old and outmoded agricultural implements.
6. Lack of good seeds.
7. Lack of manures.
8. Inferior breed of castle.
9. Defective methods of cultivation and cropping.

   Government of India has launched several nutritional program to tackle major problems of malnutrition prevailing in India.
1. Applied Nutrition Program.
2. Mid-day School Meal Program.
3. National Goiter Control Program.

4. Supplementary Feeding Program.
5. Prophylaxis Against Anemia.
6. Vitamin A Prophylaxis for the Prevention of Blindness.

Food and Agriculture Organization (FAO)

The food and agriculture organization (FAO) was formed in 1945 with headquarters in Rome. It was the first United Nations Organization specialized agency created to look after several areas of world cooperation. The chief aims of food and agriculture organization are:
1. To help nations raising living standards.
2. To improve nutrition of the people of all countries.
3. To increase the efficiency of farming, forestry and fisheries.
4. To the better condition of rural people and through all these means, to widen the opportunity of all people for productive work.

The FAO's primary concern is the increased production of food to keep pace with the ever-growing world population. The most important aspect of FAO's work is towards ensuring that the food is consumed by the people, who need it, in sufficient quantities and in right proportions, to develop and maintain a better state of nutrition throughout the world. The FAO is also collaborating with other international agencies in the applied nutrition program. The joint WHO / FAO expert committees have provided the basis for many cooperative activities such as nutritional surveys, training courses, seminars and coordination of research program.

Conclusion

Agriculture is sometimes a gamble. The farmer may not get in when he needs it the most. Of there may be excessive rain causing floods. Perhaps the harvest may be a failure and that may reduce him to poverty. The factors responsible for creating food problems can conveniently be grouped under categories of factors affecting the demand and those affecting supply of gain. The growing population will have to be fed.

HOUSING PROBLEMS

Introduction

Housing is the modern concept includes not only the physical structure providing shelter, but also the immediate surroundings, and the related community services and facilities. The WHO prefers to use term residential environment which is defined as the physical structure than man uses and environs of the structure including all necessary services, facilities equipment and devices needed or described for the physical and mental health and the social well-being of the family and the individual.

Criteria for Healthful Housing

An expert committee of the WHO recommended the following criteria for healthful housing similar to the basic principles of healthful housing published by American Public Health Association.
1. Healthful housing provides physical protection and shelter.
2. Provides adequately for cooking, eating, washing and excretory functions.
3. It is designed, constructed, maintained and used in a manner such as to prevent the spread of communicable diseases.
4. It provides for protection for hazards of exposure to noise and pollution.

5. Is free from unsafe physical arrangements due to construction or maintenance and from toxic or harmful materials.
6. Encourage personal and community development, promotes social relationships, reflects a regard for ecological principles, and by these means promotes mental health.

Housing and Health

Housing is part of the total environment of man and being a part, it is to some extent responsible for the status of man's health and well-being. It is difficult, however, to demonstrate the specific cause and effect relationship because housing embraces so many facets of environment.

Sl.No.	Problems	Diseases
1.	Respiratory infection	Common cold, tuberculosis, influenza, diphtheria, bronchitis, measles, whooping cough, etc.
2.	Skin infections	Scabies, ringworm, impetigo, leprosy.
3.	Rat infestation	Plague.
4.	Arthropods	Houseflies, mosquitoes, fleas and bugs.
5.	Morbidity and mortality	High morbidity and mortality rates are observed where housing conditions are substandards.

Housing and Amenities

Social houses and basic amenities such as soundings safe drinking water facilities, safe disposal of waste, better sanitary facilities, etc. are conducive to good health. A house with adequate space, good cross-ventilation and a pleasant view from every window, with adequate space for children to play at home and neighborhood with adequate privacy and separate room for sick persons, all provide a congenial environment for a happy life and better health for the inmates.

Rao (1982) states in third world countries 80% of all sickness and disease is attributable to inadequate water sanitation, which include the efforts of drinking contaminated water, and water acting as breeding ground for vectors and diseases. He also identified a combination of factors such as scarcity of water supply, poor housing conditions, substandard drainage, overcrowding and conditions conducive to insect breeding as increasing the risk of infant mortality (SVR Rao, A review of water sanitation and health for all. Indian Journal of Public Health Vol. XXVI, No.1, Jan-March 1983).

Ashraf (1990) observed a common trend of high infant mortality rate (IMR) in populations with poor housing and lack of basic amenities residing in rural and hilly region of Uttar Pradesh. **According to his study IMR of families were.**

Sl.No.	Areas	Rural	Hilly
1.	Residing in kutcha houses	220.8	302.9
2.	With insufficient ventilation	232.0	191.0
3.	With severe smoke inside their dwelling	285.7	220.1
4.	Open latrine	220.5	141.8
5.	With place of garbage disposal near their houses	228.4	147.1

(Ashraf MS, Infant Mortality in Rural India, A diagnostic study, Print House, Lacknow, India, 1990)

Dr Radhakamal Mukherjee in his famous study Indian working class has pointed out that infant mortality is high in one roomed tenements. An over crowded room, which lacks ventilation, with its floor wet almost all the time, leads to the development of respiratory diseases and also enhances spreading of infections diseases.

PROSTITUTION

Introduction

Prostration is one of the social vices, which prevailed from times immemorial. Generally, prostration means illicit sex union for mercenary induced or something else she needs. Prostitution the performance of sexual acts solely for the purposes of material gain. Persons prostitute themselves when they grant sexual favors to other in exchange for money, gifts, or other payment and in so doing use their bodies as commodities. Prostitution is described as a figure which is certainly the more mournful and awful upon which the eye of the immoralist can dwell. Prostitution is not to be confused with the illicit sex union of lover. In prostitution there is no affection. Sex favors are not granted on an affection basis, rather money.

Definitions

1. Prostitution which involves illicit sex union on a promiscuous and mercenary basis with accompanying emotional difference—*Elloit and Merill.*
2. Prostitution may be defined as the practice of habitual or intermittent sexual union more or less promiscuous, for mercenary inducement. It is thus characterized by three elements payment, usually involving the passing of money, although gifts or pleasure may constitute equivalent consideration; promiscuity, with the possible of choice; the emotional indifference, which may be inferred from payment and promiscuity—*Encyclopedia of the Social Sciences.*
3. Prostitution defined as women who offer her body to indiscriminate sexual intercourse's for hire—*The Oxford English Dictionary.*
4. Prostitution defined as the practice of habitual or intermittent sexual union, more or less promiscuous (indiscriminate), for mercenary inducement with accompanying emotional differences—*Goeffrey.*

Elements of Prostitution

1. Illicit and promiscuous sexual intercourse.
2. Hiring sex for money or unkind.
3. Lack of affection or personal interest.

Various Terms used in Prostitution

1. **Procurers:** Procurer is a person who procurers the girls and supply them to the sex market. There is always demand for freshness in the sex market, so those who loose their charm, who becomes diseased, will be replaced by new victims.
2. **Pimps:** A pimp is one who makes business contracts for the prostitute. He finds the customers and brings them to the brothel houses or lodges.
3. **Brothel keeper:** A brothel keeper is one who provides accommodation for new comers and encourages them in the profession. She takes fifty percentage of their earning. Generally, ex-prostitutes run brothels.

Causes of Prostitution

The main cause is biological in nature. The sex urge in human being though controlled by sex norms and the institution of marriage, it is impossible to control in all cases. Among males, the unmarried, the married and widowers, all the three categories indulge in the fulfillment of sexual urges.

Sl.No.	Causes	Description
1.	Poverty	The primary cause of prostitution is hunger. Prostitutes enter into this profession out of sheer economic necessity.
2.	Child widows	Child marriage was widely practiced and child widows were abundant in number. Once widowed, they were neglected, ill-treated or even abandoned. Most of these young widows often become prostitutes.
3.	Broken home and neglect of girls	In many broken homes, children are abandoned by father or mother. Without proper care and guidance, many of them turn to evil ways like prostitution.
4.	Growth of modern cities	Modern and urban centers facilitate prostitution in many ways. All the cities have large number of unmatched men. The anonymity existing in cities facilities the prostitutes to operate in an unobtrusive way.
5.	Unsatisfactory and marital life	Dissatisfaction in sexual life may especially be one reason which pushes women into prostitution.
6	Desire for luxury	Many young women are turned towards prostitution today just to lead a life of affluence. The meager salary or income of their parents or husbands cannot buy the luxuries they desire and often take up prostitution as a part time activity.

Factors Influences Prostitution

1. Dr Puneher and Ms Rao Poverty, inadequate housing conditions and other economic factors. Death of parents or husband, domestic causes like treatment or neglect or parents, husband or relations.
2. Kidnapping, bad influences, illegitimate pregnancy, etc. Desire for easy life low moral values are the main causes of prostitution.
3. Restriction on widow remarriage and the practice of socioreligious custom of dedicating the girls to goddess, Devadasi system. This system prevalent in North Karnataka and Maharashtra.
4. Urbanization and industrialization are also simulative factors in causing prostitution. In city environment the free movement of men and women, the unwhole some recreational centers, like cinema, bars, clubs, dancing halls, cabretts, lodges, brothel houses, have led to the trade in sex and exploitation of women.

Evil Effects of Prostitution

1	Prostitution and personal disorganization	The person who indulges in prostitution receives condemnation by the public. Due to double standards values the women suffer great personal deterioration. Sexual vices results in personal demoralization, loss of status. The prostitute loses all self-respect, and acts merely as a machine.

Contd...

Contd...

Sl.No.	Evil effects	Description
		She lacks of normal emotions and moral values. She often becomes vindictive and tries to bring more men to downfall. Even in the males, it causes a lot of disorganization.
2.	Prostitution and family disorganization	Prostitution affects not only the individuals but also family. Promiscuous sex relationships cause's sexually transmitted diseases like gonorrhea, syphilis, AIDS and other diseases. Illegitimate sex relations develops family friction and ultimately results in family disorganization. The person who habitually visits a prostitute loses any interest in his own family. Harmonious relationship within his family is affected. Husband-wife relationship is shattered. Even if a married woman goes into prostitution, with the consent of her husband, frictions, tensions and conflicts are unavoidable.
3.	Prostitution and community disorganization	Prostitution leads to widespread community disorganization. Prostitution leads to commercial exploitation. It has created various brothers, call flats, disorderly hotels to carry on the business secretly. Such places are the breeding centers of venereal diseases and other health hazards in the community. It has been reported that more than 30% of female sex workers are infected with HIV.
4.	Prostitution and economic problems	Any man who goes to prostitute regularly loses a lot of money in the manner. His economic condition is adversely affected and his family also suffers due to his delinquency.
5.	Prostitution and health hazards	Prostitution affects both the prostitute and the customers are in danger of serious health problems. Venereal diseases like gonorrhea and syphilis are transmitted through sexual contacts. The AIDS is mainly transmitted through sexual contact.
6.	Prostitution and moral degeneration	Prostitution defines results in moral degradation of the entire society. When a large number of women are engaged in such a profession and when large number of men indulges in illicit sex, moral standards of the society cannot be upheld.
7.	Prostitution and women degradation	With increasing trends of prostitution, women are losing respect in the society. Women are more and more looked upon sex symbols and the high ideals of womanhood cherished in our tradition are in peril. The unhealthy physical and social environment under which the prostitutes lived are shocking and absolutely demoralizing.

Prevention and Control of Prostitution

Legislative Measures

During the British rule various provisions were made in the ICP to control the sexual offences. The code provided an imprisonment up to one year or fine or both for insulting the modesty of any women. No one should compel her to marry or she may be forced to illicit intercourse. Sexual intercourse with women under 16 years of age is considered as rape.

In 1923, the Bombay Prevention of Prostitution Act was passed. According to this act making a living on the earnings of prostitution, soliciting in a public places, procuring, keeping a brothel and prostitution in prohibited areas were considered offences.

In 1956, Suppression of Immoral Traffic Act was passed by the Parliament. This is generally called SITA which gives wider power to the states to deal with the problem of prostitutes. This act has made provision to punish the person who keeps or manage a brothel. Any person indulged in procuring women for the purpose of earning money is to be severely punished, i.e. rigorous imprisonment between 1 to 3 years and fine of Rs. 2000, special police officers deal with the offences.

Preventive Measures

1. Facilities for vocational and moral training for women for lower economic stratum should be provided.
2. Rescue homes, shelter home and other facilities should be provided for the poor and destitute women. Girls who are in moral danger should be put in reformatories or institutions where they can be kept safe from the clutches of antisocial elements. In these institutions facilitates for vocational training should be provided, so that girls will be economically independent.
3. Men and women should be educated about the health practices to be followed with regard to sex. So sex education is very essential. There should be sex education at school and college levels. Girls should be taught the danger of sex exploitation by males.
4. Social education and propaganda also are important measures to fight this evil. A healthy public opinion should be created against illicit sex relations.
5. Health worker and social worker should take the task of publicity and propaganda through educative literature, TV program, films, etc.

Prohibitory Measures

1. Medical examination of all prostitutes should be conducted frequently. Any women who is found be infected should be segregated immediately, and should not be allowed to receive customers till she is cured.
2. Licensing system of prostitutes will be helpful if it is permitted by law. This will facilitate to have constant check over them.
3. Medical personnel dealing with prostitute should be specially trained. Sympathetic, efficient, and free care should be provided to prostitutes because many of them are very poor and helpless.

Prophylaxis

1. The prophylactic measures include prevention of communicable diseases and improvement of hygienic conditions.
2. The prostitutes and the customers should be instructed to use protective measures. Condoms may be used by males and females can use chemical disinfectives after the exposure.
3. Young men should be educated to practice continence and develop healthy habits of recreation.

Conclusion

Prostitution represents an extreme case of sexual stratification in which the commoditization of female sexuality contributes to women's devaluation and objectification. Ownership and exchange of female sexuality serves as the core element of our entire gender system. Prostitution today is the result of only disappointment and unsatisfied longings of young men and young women who find it convenient to enter in to this relationship for a money consideration. Prostitution is its connection results with serious diseases. The studies made on this matter in different parts of the country indicate a very high percentage of venereal diseases among prostitutes.

RIGHTS OF WOMEN AND CHILDREN

Rights of Women

Introduction

Womens are vital element of society. A society's progress largely depends on women, and therefore, they need to be considered as important pillar not only a domestic life but also in social life. In India, the status of women is based on religious and political factors. Sociological explanations about women are rooted in the ancient scriptures, during Vedic period women enjoyed high status in society. Women were the central figure in the family life. She had educational status and free to take decisions.

Status of Women in India

Sl.No.	Period	Status of women
1.	Vedic period	Women enjoyed high status in society. A woman was the central figure in the family life. She could participate in religious and public functions. She had educational status and free to take decisions. She was the guide and companion of man.
2.	Post-Vedic and later	The status of women gradually decline. The women was treated as a subordinate and inferior to man.
3.	During Medieval period	Particularly during Muslim rule the gender discrimination, exploitation and cruelty towards women increased to such extent, that she lost her individuality and freedom. Strict controls were imposed, education was denied, no property rights and lost her freedom. She must be subordinate to her husband; she had to follow the ideal of *pativrathya*. The inhuman practices like female infanticide, child marriage, harassment of widow, sati system, the dowry, parda system and other ill treatment hindered the growth of women independently.
4.	During British period	During the British rule the Indians were very much influenced by the western culture. Britishers established courts, introduced schools, and colleges and encouraged education of girls. The ideals of liberty and equality rational thinking opened the gateways of western culture. The social reformers and elites like Raja Ram Mohan Roy, Dayananda Saraswati, Swamy Vivekananda, Malabari, Eswarachandra Vidya Sagar, Ranade, Gokhale, Gandhiji, Ambedkar and others persuaded the British ruler to enact progressive legislations like abolition of sati, enhancement of age at marriage, widow-remarriage, divorce act, dowry prohibition act, start separate schools and colleges for girls and provide employment opportunities.
5.	After independence	Various Women Welfare Program have been implemented. The National Women Commission, Women Development Corporations, NGO's has initiated several programs for the empowerment of women. No doubt such effort have not only improved the socioeconomic status of women but also awakened the women folk to realize their rights.

Violence Against Women

The alarming social reality about women is that the violence against women is increasing. The following records of the Parliament, as reported in a newspaper are an illustration to show women is not safe in streets as well as in house. At the last session of the Parliament by the end of 2005, the facts and figures shown:

1. In every 26 minutes, a woman is molested.
2. In every 34 minutes a rape takes place.
3. In every 42 minutes a sexual harassment occurs.
4. In every 93 minutes a woman is burnt to death over dowry.

Further statistic (Viyaya Times 15.1.2006) revealed that:

1. 45% of the women are slapped, kicked or beaten by their husbands.
2. 75% of battered women contemplate suicide.
3. 5 crore women in India suffer from violence in their homes.
4. Only 1% of them have the courage to report the abuse.

The classifications of violence against women:

1. Kidnapping, torture, rape, abduction, murder.
2. Dowry deaths, burning, hanging, poisoning, etc. Ill-treatment of widows and elderly women.
3. Molestation, eve-teasing, immoral traffic, sexual harassment, wife-battering, kicking, snapping, verbal abuse, harassment of women at work place.

Commonly seen Indian society violence:

1. **Rape:** In India, the number of rape cases is said to be 30 per day according to statistics between 1990-1994. The victims of rape are highest in the age group of 16-30 years. Though rape is a Criminal Act, not all cases are reported and punished.
2. **Harassment of women at work places:** The poor girls and employees belonging to middle class are sexually humiliated by the employers, maid servants by their masters, dailywage earners by contractors and middlemen.
3. **Dowry:** Though the Dowry Prohibition Act 1961 has banned the practice of dowry, in reality it exists. The demands of dowry have increased. The dowry deaths also increased every year. In 1994, the cruelty by husband and in-law was reported to be 25946. Thousands of girls have been burnt by in-laws for sake of dowry.
4. **Wife-battering:** Wife-battering is also a serious violence against women which range from slaps, kicks to broken bones, torture and even attempt to murder. The empirical studies made by Prof Ram Ahuja have revealed that the causes of wife-battering are sexual maladjustment, emotional disturbances, alcoholism, jealousy and illiteracy of wives.

The UN Special Rapporteur—Violent against Women

1. Unequal power relations between men and women.
2. Denial of economic power and economic independence to women, economically disadvantaged women are more vulnerable to sexual harassment, trafficking and sexual slavery.
3. Family (despite being a source of human values) is the violence against women and a socialization process which may result in justifying and a socialization process which may result in justifying violence against women.
4. Modern technology especially reproductive technology that facilitates preselection of sex of the child has resulted in killing of female fetuses and selective abortion.
5. Sexuality, violence is often used as an instrument to control femal sexual behavior, rape, sexual harassment, trafficking, female genital mutilation; all involves forms of violence which are an assault on female sexuality.

6. Ideologies which justify the subordinate position of women are another cause of violence against women. Custom, tradition, and religion are frequently invoked to justify the use of violence against women.

7. Doctrines of privacy and the concept of the sanctity of the family are other causes of violence against women.

8. Patterns of conflict resolution process in a given society are also linked to violence against women. Violence against women is likely to be more in societies where violence is an important part of the conflict resolution process.

9. Militarization leads to greater abuse with regard to women. Rapes as an instrument of war are perhaps the greatest manifestation of this phenomenon.

10. The great cause of violence against women is government inaction with regard to crimes of violence against women.

Organizational Norms of Womens Right

1. **International norms:** The committee established under the convention on the elimination of all forms of discrimination against women (CEDAW) in its general recommendation 19 dealt entirely with the question of violence against women. The committee stated that, gender-based violence is a form of discrimination that seriously inhibits women's ability to enjoy rights and freedoms on the basis of equality with men.

2. **Women and human rights:** As early in 1946, the commission on the status of women was established to deal with women's issues. The universal declaration of human rights had affirmed the principle of the inadmissibility of discrimination and proclaimed that all human being are born free equal in dignity and rights and that everyone is entitled to all the rights and freedom set forth therein, without distinction of any kind, including distinction based on sex.

3. **Fundamental rights:** All the fundamental rights contained in par-III, article 12 to 35 are applicable to all citizens irrespective of sex, certain fundamental rights contain specific and positive to protect the rights of women. Article 15(3) the constitution specifically on grounds of religion, race, caste, sex, place of birth as contained in article 15, shall not prevent the state from making any special provision for women and children. Clause (3) of article 15, which permits special provision for women and children, has been widely resorted to, by the state and the courts have always upheld the validity of special measures in legislation or executive orders favoring women.

4. **Beijing conference (1995):** The fourth world conference of women, held 1995 (4-15 September, 1995) in Beijing, commonly called Beijing conference stated that women's rights are human rights. The conference called for the integration of women's human rights in the work of the different human rights bodies of the United Nations.

5. **Asian women's movement:** Women's movements are now active in all Asian countries, extending into all classes, active in social and political agitation and aiming to make all women conscious of their subordination. These growing movements have taken up many issues that affects women dowry deaths, rape, abortion, prostitution and against economic exploitation and political margination.

6. **Rights of women to economic development:** Recently the Supreme Court has highlighted the rights of the women in India to eliminate gender-based discrimination particularly in respect of property so as to attain economic empowerment. The court while referring to the Vienna declaration on the CEDAW which was rectified by the United National Organization on 18.12.1979 and by the Government of India on 8.8.1993 elaborately discussed the principles of equality of rights and respect of women dignity.

Women Abuse

Women abuse is the actual or threatened physical, psychological, sexual, financial, verbal, or spiritual abuse of a women by someone with whom she, has or had an intimate, familial or romantic relationship. Women abuse is a serious and widespread societal problem. Women from all ages, racial and ethic background, sexual orientations, socio-economic classes, religious, ability levels, and professions can experience abuse.

Types of abuse
1. **Psychological abuse:** Threats, insults, and put-down can be just as damaging as physical abuse because they endanger women's feelings of self-worth and her ability to control her own life.
2. **Financial abuse:** A woman who is prevented from finding a job, or who is not allowed to have a bank account or keep any income is an example of financial abuse.
3. **Social abuse:** When a woman is kept totally dependent on her partner and isolated from the support of her peers, friends and family.
4. **Sexual abuse:** Being forced as women to do or watch something sexual without our consent, or to have pain inflicted on you during sexual intercourse.
5. **Physical abuse:** Hitting, punching, slapping, biting, kicking, bruising, pinching, breaking bones, using weapons are obvious examples.
6. **Domestic violence:** Domestic violence occurs when you are in a relationship where your partner controls and dominates you, usually through violence, threat of violence, or by controlling your social life and finance.

Cycle of abuse
The cycle of relationship violence shows how abuse becomes a vicious pattern made up of the following stages:
1. The build-up phase—tension rise.
2. Stand over phase—partner becomes threatening, angry, insulting, verbally abusive.
3. The explosion phase—the violence occurs.
4. The remorse phase—partner is apologetic and promises never to do it again.
5. The pursuit phase—partner attempts to win-up back by promising to change.
6. The honeymoon phase—things are calm and perhaps even loving.
7. The build-up phase—tension being rise again.

Prevention of women's abuse
There are two methods which can be prevented the violence against women.
1. **Legislative method:** Various social legislations like Indian Penal Code, Anti-Dowry Act, 1961 and subsequent amendment, Widows Remarriage Act, Women's Property Act, Divorce Act, etc. but problems of women cannot be solved by legislative measures. Because many cases of women abuse will not come before the police or court of law. Moreover women are reluctant to approach the law courts. They silently suffer.
2. **Social measures:** The other measures that can prevent the abuse of women and their harassment is through social measures. The improvement of the status of women in society through education, employment opportunities, economic status and development of awareness among women. These measures no doubt reduce the exploitation of women to a certain extent. The women organization should function effectively to protect the helpless women, the victims of rape, dowry, harassment, and other must be provided short-term accommodation and should create awakening in the society, by asserting their rights.

Unmarried Mother

The important function of family is the task of procreation and child rearing. Marriage is an institutional arrangement found in all societies, which controls the desire for varied sexual experience. No doubt the marital relations control the sexual needs of the male and female. An unmarried mother is socially stigmatized and the birth of a child before marriage is considered as illegitimate birth. The problem of unmarried mothers is a social problem, which exists in all societies, but will not be publicized with the facts.

Causes of unmarried mother

The causes of unmarried mother are instability of modern family, divorce and separation, suppression of the expression of sex desire, young women who are lured into romanticism and include in sexual activity before marriage and become pregnant. In olden days the girls use to be married in their early age. But in modern societies, late marriages are preferred; many parents are unable to find the suitable bridegroom because of their economic insatiability to pay the dowry.

Problems of unmarried mother

Young men and women work together in offices, factories, and other public places. This has increased the social contacts between the opposite sex. Consequently, premarital and extramarital relations resulted in the higher proportion of illegitimate births and unmarried mother. The parents to avoid embarrassment resort to abortion or they may even kill the illegitimate children. A large number of pregnant girls before marriage may commit suicide. The new born children of unwed mothers are also ill-treated and are called bastard children. Thus, unwed mothers are socially dishonored.

Remedial measures

Society has to develop a humanitarian and sympathetic attitude. The women welfare organizations and the other authorities must find out the causes of their problems and must think of solving their problems. More and more orphanages have to be started to help the children. State should extent it's helping hand by providing training and employment opportunities to unwed mother to lead a dignified life.

Right of Children

The concept of the right of the child is of relatively recent origin. The changes in the social attitudes regarding children brought about transformation in their legal status also, for example, before the nineteenth century; the predominant notion in the west was that of child as property. The social legislation that accompanied the industrial revolution and the change in the legal status of child. The beginning of the twentieth century witnessed tremendous changes in the recognition of the child as an independent entity. In addition, there was also, a growing recognition that children should be provided special care. This was reflected in the declaration adopted by the League of Nations in 1924 that stressed protection of children from hunger and other material needs.

Fundamental Principles of the Convention

1. **Respect for the child's opinion:** The corollary to children as subjects of rights is the principle that their opinion should be respected. It means that child has the right to freedom of expression, freedom of thought, freedom of conscience and freedom of assembly.
2. **Each child has rights:** The recognition that children have equal value as an adult implies that all children should enjoy rights is fundamental to the convention. The principle is based on the notion that children are subjects and not objects of the rights.

3. **Equal value as human rights:** An underlying principle of the convention is that of according children the same values as adults. The principle stressed that childhood has value in itself.
4. **Best interests of the child:** While children have equal values as grownups they also need the protection and support from the society for enjoying their childhood. The principle of best interests of the child balances the need for providing protection to children while respecting.

Indian Constitution of Child Right

1. Article 15-3 nothing in this article shall prevent the state from making any special provision for women and children.
2. Article 24 prohibition of employment of children in factories, etc.
3. No child below the age of 14 years shall be employed to work in any factory or mine or engaged in any other hazardous employment.
4. The Supreme Court of India 1990, SC 292 (Justice Rangnath Misra, Justice MN Venkatachaliah and Justice PB Sawant) held that segregating prostitutes, children by locating separate schools and providing separate hostels, would not be in the interest of such children. Once children are born to prostitutes, it is in the interest of such children of the society at large, that the children of the society at large, that the children of prostitutes should be segregated from their mother and be allowed to mingle with others and become part of the society.
5. Age of a child under Act has been prescribed 14 years. The employment of children (amendment) Act, 1978 prohibits employment below the age of 15 years in railways premises.
6. The Apprentices Act, 1961 prohibits a person under age of 14 years. The Motor Transport Act, 1961 prohibits the employment of children under 15 years of age.
7. The Factories Act, 1948 prescribes minimum age of employment in factories to 14 years.
8. The Merchant Shipping Act, 1958 prohibits children 15 years to be engaged to work in any capacity in any ship.
9. The Employment of Children (amendment) Act, 1951 prohibits the employment of children between the age of 15 and 17 years.
10. The Factories (amendment) Act, 1954 prohibits employment at night under 17 years of age.
11. The Mines Act, 1952 prohibits the employment under 15 years.

Rights of the Child

1. Right to life (article 6. para 1).
2. Right to acquire nationality (article 7).
3. Right to freedom of expression (article 13, para 1).
4. Right of freedom of thought, conscience and religion (article 14, para-1).
5. Right of freedom of association and to freedom peaceful assembly (article 15, para-1).
6. Right to education (article 28, para-1).
7. Right to benefit from social security (article 26, para-1).
8. Right to standard of living adequate for child's physical, mental, spiritual and social development (article 27, para-1).
9. Right to the enjoyment of the highest attainable standard of health and the facilities for the treatment of illness and rehabilitation of health (article 24, para-1).
10. Right the protection of the law against arbitrary or unlawful interference with his or her privacy, family, home, or correspondence (article 16, para-1).

International Covenant

Article 24 of the International Covenant on Civil and Political Rights, 1966 spells out,

1. Every child shall have, without an discrimination as to race, color, sex, language, religion, national and social origin, property of birth, the right to such measures of protection as are required by his status as a minor, on the part of his family, society and the state.
2. Every child shall be registered immediately after and shall have a name.
3. Every child as the right to acquire a nationality.
4. Article 10 (3) of the international covenant on economic, social and cultural rights, 1966, lay down, special measures of protection and assistance should be taken on behalf of children and young persons without any discrimination for reasons of parentage or other conditions.

Important Laws Affecting Children in India

India is a secular country having multicultural dimensions, multiliguistics and various religions so the children protected is to be viewed from various angles in this regards.

1. The Child Marriage Restraint Act, 1929.
2. A Guardian and Wards Act, 1890.
3. The Hindu Adoption and Maintenance Act, 1956.
4. The Hindu Minority and Guardianship Act, 1956.
5. The Hindu Succession Act, 1956.

Conclusion

National Policy for Children, 1974 envisages the scheme of integrated child development services with 33 integrated children developed schemes in blocks/project. The scheme provides for an integrated package of services comprising supplementary nutrition, immunization, health checkup, referral services, preschool nonformal education and health and nutritional education for mother. These programs are being implemented and looked after with the help of cooperative for American relief everywhere care and World Food Program and UNICEF.

VULNERABLE GROUPS: ELDERLY AND HANDICAPPED

Elderly

Introduction

Aging is a natural phenomenon which has not only profound personal implications for the individuals but also implication for the society. Man has throughout the ages reflected upon changes occurring in behavior and implement with advancing ages. Aging begins with conception and terminates with death. Difference countries have laws setting out and age, which one is called an elderly people. There are many variations in defining aging. Some consider aging relative, asserting that chronological age is not a good predictor of any things because of the great individual differences found in the aging population.

Aged and Society

The old civilized societies the elderly people generally enjoyed a high status. The status was assumed because of the experience and knowledge of the age that helped the family and society.

Categorizing the Aging Population

1. Young old: 65 to 75 years.
2. Old: 75 to 85 years.
3. Old-old: 85 to 100 years.
4. Elite old: over 100 years.

Types of Age

1. **Chronological age:** Chronological age markers may associate with specific events. They have broad social and personal significance in most of the societies in all stages of the life cycle. They also provide social regulation of the aging process. Chronological age is a poor index of aging since it does not take into account the range of individual difference among people.
2. **Biological age:** The biological age of an individual can be defined as an estimate of the span. The measurement of biological age would encompass measurements of the functional capacities of the vital life limiting organ systems.
3. **Psychological age:** Psychological age is released through the adaptive capacity of an individual to changing environmental demands the ability to adjust with time and situation. The study of psychological age involves the study of memory, learning, intelligence, skills, feeling, motivation and emotions.
4. **Social age:** Change in the social age of the individual is that which has to do with the changing circumstances or situation as a member of the family, community and society. These may be called the sociological changes.
5. **Functional age:** Functional age can be grouped by the individual level of capacity relative to others of the same age or functioning in a given human society. The term functional is a two fold indication of measurable characteristics in the individual, on the one hand, and of his functioning in a physical, socially or otherwise determine environment on the other.

Adjustment Problems at Elderly

Human adjustment has, being distinguish from adaptation, a concept essentially applied to biological process of gaining adaptation wherein the sense organs adjusted to the incoming stimuli, to the structural changes in an organism in order to meet environmental condition, and to gain mastery in reality by means of innate productive mechanism (Hazarus, 1976). Adjustment connate the psychological process emphasizing the individual struggle to get along or survive in his social and physical environment.

Adjustment is a universal and continuous process. Life is also continuous process of overcoming differences, or of making adjustments. In making these adjustments, habits are formed that become the patterns for making future adjustments. Individuals become identified by their habits adjustment. There are a number of factors about an adjustment situation that have psychological significance.

First, a want must exist. If there is no want there is need for adjustment.

Second, adjustment is the satisfaction of a want. When a want is satisfied an adjustment has been made. Even the sudden cessation of a want constitutes an adjustment.

Third, difficulties that interfere with the satisfaction of wants constitute adjustment problem.

Causes of Adjustment Problems

1. Adolescence itself, which is a particularly difficult period in our culture and for which many children are not adequately prepaid. At this time, there are certain basic needs that must be met satisfactory if the individual is to make good adjustment.
2. The environment is which the individual lives especially that of home.
3. Whaling of impulses and desire, this leads of feeling or inferiority and inadequacy, perhaps with the feeling of guilty because of failure in school or because of sex delinquencies.
4. Undue emotional stimulation, such as some terrible emotional shock or continued over excitement over a long period of time.
5. The personality pattern of the individual. Some individuals are adaptable and thus are able to adjust to new condition and demands without under stress.

Services for the aged

The family, community, government and the elderly themselves have to contribute in providing basic services to the elderly.

Sl.No.	Types	Services
1.	Social services	1. Medical services in (hospital) nursing homes. 2. In the home for aged. 3. In families, a. Services for the in-capacitated such home visits home services, escorting, etc. b. Recreational activities, consumer education and legal aid for persons with physical capacity and social contacts. c. Housing and environments. d. Continuing/adult education.
2.	Social welfare services	1. Day care services. 2. Institutional services. 3. Infirmaries. 4. Poor homes. 5. Information and referral services. 6. Services for old persons with special needs such as physically handicapped who are unable to look after their interest, etc.
3.	Sociopsychological services	1. Community education and awareness. 2. Family support including respite care. 3. Leisure time activities. 4. Religious and spiritual activities. 5. Preparation of retirement. 6. Counseling services.
4.	Economic services	1. He belongs to a family below poverty line. 2. He is ailing or infirm, requiring long hospitalization. 3. He has some family responsibility such as education or marriage of his sons or daughters. 4. Social employment

Services provided to an elderly

1. Medical care is provided for the chronologically ill people through mobile dispensaries and access to health centers.
2. Supplementary human through on wheels.
3. Providing of aids such as spectacles, crutches, sticks, transportation, etc.
4. Organizing social and religious activities in temples and spiritual gathering.
5. Providing recreational activities such as low cost motives, holidays centers, day centers, library and reading rooms, etc.
6. Better living condition in healthy environment.
7. Providing opportunities for community services.
8. Helping the elderly in managing investments and tax exemptions.
9. Counseling service for over coming isolation.

Conclusion

The problems and needs of the elderly are different in different society because the aged suffer from multiple problems, economic, social and psychological in nature. Social work has to take into consideration the complexity of inter-relationship of several factors such as physical health, economic resources, social status, etc. The old age who has completed their duty in life with expects a peaceful life and the affection from their children and grand children. Personal interest in old age include interest in self, interest in appearance, interest in cloths and interest in money. People become increasingly more preoccupied with themselves as they grow older. They may become egocentric and self-centered to the point where they think more about themselves than about others and have little regards for others their interests and wishes.

Handicapped

Introduction

Handicapped are those who are physically and mentally impaired. They are generally called disabled persons. The difficulties of disabilities are experienced by the person's themselves. The handicapped person has to become dependents for longer period and hence considered as a burden to the society. It is estimated more than 400 million disabled in the world.

Physical handicapped is not one problem, but a wide range of problems of different kinds. It includes people who have lost limbs, who are blind or deaf, who have difficulty moving or walking, who are unable to sustain physical effort for any length of time, and so on. The treatment of disability as if it was a single problem may mean that disabled people receive insufficient or inappropriate assistance. The problems that disabled people have common are not so much their physical capacities, which are often very different, but limitations on their lifestyles.

Concept of Handicapped

The concept of handicapped is used in a broader sense in our constitution, to refer to weaker sections and so they deserve specific welfare and rehabilitation measures. Human with disabilities can take charge of their own health when they have information that affirms their own experience of their bodies and health needs. Physically and mentally handicapped persons are a social problem today. They need our cooperation. If proper training is given they can also work like normal persons. The World Health Organization identifies three elements in disability: Problems in bodily function and structure, which they used to call impairment; problems relating to activities or disability; and problems related to social participation which they called handicapped.

Causes of Handicapped

1. Congenital (inborn) defects.
2. Physical and mental disability due to accidents.
3. Decrease in morbidity from communicable diseases.
4. Malnutrition.
5. Industrialization and urbanization.
6. Poverty and ignorance.
7. Low sanitary standards.
8. Over crowding and insufficient resources of medical care and preventive measures.
9. High prevalence of infectious diseases.

Types of handicapped persons

Sl.No.	Types	Description
1.	Blindness	Those persons who have lost total insight, visual activity and those with partially sighted.
2.	Deaf and dumb	The non-function of the sense of hearing. They do not hear and so cannot understand sounds. Partially hearing, mild impairment, serious and severe impairment.
3.	Orthopedically handicapped	Persons with physical defect or deformity of bones, muscles or joints, crippled, polio affected persons.
4.	Mentally deficient or retarded	Below average function of the brain and impairment in adaptive behavior.
5.	Epileptic and the chronically sick	Like TB, leprosy, liver and renal diseases, etc.
6.	The speech impaired	Defective speech that influences with communication.

Services given to handicapped:

The services for the handicapped rendered by the government with the assistance of WHO and other foreign assistance are as follows:

1. **Medical and health services:** It includes physiotherapy, occupational therapy and prosthetic and orthotics.
2. **Training of personnel:** Training given for nurses, physiotherapists, vocational counselors, teachers for the blind, deaf, mentally deficient and speech therapist.
3. **Vocational and formal education:** It includes,
   a. Special vocational training for the disabled.
   b. Special school for the deaf and blind.
   c. Special school for the orthopedically handicapped—training in carpentry, electric work, tailoring, telephone operation, cane work, etc.
4. **Economic assistance to:**
   a. Students
   b. Government employees
   c. Patients for treatment

    d. Postal concession for braile material
    e. Income tax concession.
5. **Legislative support:** Those who suffer injury during the course of work, such worker and other physically injured persons are protected by Workmen's Compensation Act; Employees State Insurance, etc. efforts must be made to provide compensation, security and insurance.

Rehabilitation measures for handicapped

1. Government providing grant to private agencies to maintain disabled persons and other concessions. Free treatment given in hospitals to rehabilitate them physically and mentally.
2. In an attempt to meet challenges of serving the disabled person's education, preventive, diagnostic and vocational services have been taken.
3. Under preventive services National Preventive Program such as special nutritional program, maternity and child health programme. Programme of immunization (polio) national blindness eradication, malaria and TB eradication, prevention of deafness, retardation, leprosy and other program have been taken by the government.

Conclusion

Nurses who are in charge of these handicapped children should behave in such a way that they do not feel they are handicapped and incapable of doing anything. The nurses should instill confidence in them and encourage them to do things better. The nurse should see that these children do not develop any inferiority complex. They should be made to feel that by a little effort they can also become useful citizen and not a burden on society. It is the duty of the government to provide special schools, teachers and nurses, with necessary equipment to train this handicapped person in the fields of their choice and never consider them as a burden to society.

CHILD LABOR AND ABUSE

Child Labor

Introduction

Child labor is any work by children that interferes with their full physical development, their needed recreation. In most of the underdeveloped and developing countries, children of inappropriate age are forced to take part in productive activities due to economic distress. Parents of poor class send their children for work to increase family income while the employers of various business establishments employ children to maximize their profits. The results are economic exploitation of children. This economic exploitation continues both in organized and unorganized sectors—*Home folks*.

Nature of Child Labor

1. **Domestic work:** It includes cleaning, cooking, child care and other chores in the child's own household undertaken by children in almost all societies.
2. **Nondomestic but nonmonetary work:** It includes activities like farm work, fuel and water collection and hunting. Even in the urban sector many urban household production units engaged in trades and services.
3. **Bonded labor:** It is illegal; it arises as one of the obligations to landlords whereby the provision of child labor is part of the family's rent or in a situation where children are given in settlement of debts.

4. **Wage labor:** They may work on a piece rate or time rate basis, as regular or casual worker, in jobs that may or maintop involve something training.
5. **Marginal work:** They may be regular or of a short-time nature such as selling newspapers, shoe shining, looking after cars, garbage collection or sorting out objects from garbage.

Statistics of Child Labor

The finding of the operations research group, Baroda (published in 1983) came up with an estimate of 4 million working children in India. This figure is based on an All India child sample survey conducted by the operations research group in 1980-81. In 1983, the Planning Commission had projected the number of child workers at 17.36 million. More than 80% of working children belong to the rural areas work in the primary sector of the economy. According to 1981 census about 86.4 of child work force is employed in agricultural and allied activities in the rural sector. India with 44 million child laborers has the highest incidence of child labor in the world. While 10% of them are engaged in various industries, the rest 90% are bonded (child labor, Parachi Jaiswal, 1996). Large number of children is in the unorganized informal sector in which most of them are engaged as domestic helps.

Causes of Child Labor

Sl.No.	Causes	Description
1.	Economic poverty	1. India is a country in which more than 26% of the people are living below the conditions of poverty as per 2001 estimate. Many families with extreme poverty are compelled to send their children for work who contribute something for the family income. 2. Child laborers neither have a labor union of their own, nor the bargaining power to be employed in mining, glass making, carpet-weaving nor leather industries mainly with this intention. 3. To secure more profit for factories, some industrialists believe that their units are able to maximize profits because of the appointment of child laborers whose labor is very cheap.
2.	Familial factors	Family disorganization often leads to child labor. Extreme poverty and economic necessity of the family as it is already mentioned, is one of the factors favoring child labor. Divorce, desertion, rigid family relations, cruelty at home, parent too run away from the unpleasant family environment.
3.	Other factors	1. *Temptation of bad habits:* Children belong to the poor families often become the victims of certain bad and costly habits such as smoking, gambling, purchasing lottery tickets, when they do not get enough pocket money from home they often resort to outside work to earn money to satisfy their bad habits. 2. *Justification of employers of child laborers:* Some employers justify their act of employing little children for work. They argue that work keeps poor children away from starvation. 3. Failure of government machinery and legislative system. 4. *Lack of public awareness:* Public awareness is not there regarding the social evils such as child abuse and child labor.

Child Labor in India

India has the largest number of child labor in the world who is engaged in both organized and unorganized sectors. In March 1995, the number of employed children below 14 years of age and engaged in various economic activities constituted 17 million (9.5 million males and 7.5 million females). A large majority of these child laborers are engaged in agriculture and allied sectors, while others are found in urban and industrial areas.

Child Labor in Unorganized Sectors

1. **Child labor in rural areas:** A large number of children are found to be working in rural areas. It is estimated that more than 60% of them are below the age of 10 years.
2. **Working children in rural areas:** It is difficult to estimate the number of children struggling to live in urban areas as child laborers. Sizable number of them works in city canteens, petty shops, restaurants, garages, workshops, etc.
3. **Child laborers working as bonded laborers:** Child labor is also associated with bonded labor. It is said that out of the total number of bonded labor of Karnataka, 10.3% are found to be children. The figure stands at 8.7% for Tamil Nadu and 21% for Andhra Pradesh.

Child Labor in Organized Sectors

Due to poor economic conditions of the child labors are such that they are found even in the so-called organized sector in factories and various industrial units.

Working Children in Industrial Units

The most pitiable working children are those employed in hazardous industries like glass industry, brassware industry, firework and match box units, carpet-weaving industries, diamond- cutting and baci-breaking carpet weaving industry, etc.

Karnataka's five point perspective:
1. As responsible citizens of Karnataka, do we have the moral right to exploit the difficult situation of the child family and environment?
2. Child labor is not a welfare issue but a development issue.
3. Legislation alone cannot solve the issue of child labor.
4. Why it is that in India, 11 crore children are employed while 3.40 crore adults are unemployed?
5. There is no alternative to childhood.

Child Labor and Health Problems

Sl.No.	Occupation	Health and injury hazards
1.	Bidi industry	Chronic bronchitis, tuberculosis.
2.	Glass industry	Asthma, chronic bronchitis, tuberculosis, eye defects, burns.
3.	Handloom industry	Asthma, tuberculosis, bronchitis.
4.	Carpet industry	Posture related spine problems.
5.	Zart and embroidery	Eye defects.
6.	Gem and diamond cutting	Eye defects and injuries.
7.	Construction	Accidents, stunted growth.

Contd...

Contd...

Sr.No	Occupation	Health and injury hazards
8.	Reg picker	Skin diseases, infectious diseases, tetanus.
9.	Pottery	Asthma, bronchitis, tuberculosis.
10.	Stone quarries, state-quarries	Silicosis.
11.	Sex-worker	Sexually transmitted diseases (STD, AIDS).
12.	Agriculture	Hazards related to farm machinery and pesticides.

Government Measures to Prevent Child Labor

1. **Legal measures against child labor:** In the constitution of India provisions are made to protect the interests of children. Article 24 of the constitution status that children below 14 years shall not be employed in any factory or in any hazardous unit.
2. **Directive principles of state policy:** It declares their commitment to safe children's interests. The legislative policies undertaken after independence to prevent child labor are:
   a. The Indian Factories Act, 1948, which forbids appointing children below 14 years for work and fixes the duration of work at four an half hours per day.
   b. The Plantations Labor Act, 1951, which forbids appointment of children below 12 years for plantation work.
   c. The Mines Act, 1952, which prevents the appointment of children below 15 years from working deep mines.
   d. The child labor (prohibition and regulation) Act, 1986: The first national level and university applicable undertaken by the Government of India to prevent the appointment of children below 14 years.

Indian's Legal Obligations Towards Trafficking

1. Kidnapping or minming a minor for the purpose of begging (section-364A).
2. Kidnapping or abducting with intent secretly and wrongful confinement (section-365).
3. Kidnapping, abducting or inducing women to compel her marriage (section-366).
4. Procreation of minor girl (section 366A).
5. Importation of girls from foreign country (section-366B).
6. Buying or disposing of any person as slave (section-370).
7. Selling/buying a minor for purpose of prostitution, etc. (section 372-373).

UN System in India on Child Labor

A common position paper on the issue of child labor, adopted by 16 UN organizations in India was launched on 23rd October, 1998 at New Delhi. The UN system in India support a wide range of activities and program directly linked to eliminating child labor in India. ILO and UNICEF have played a leading role in this understanding and other organization like UNDP, UNDCP, UNESCO, UNFPA, UNIFEM , and UNAIDS also conduct program on child labor. The UN system view child labor as violation of the child's basic right to education, to his/her full and harmonious social, physical, and mental development and in some cases a violation of child's moral and physical integrity. Therefore, the UN system in India believes that child should not be tolerated in any form and must be prevented, awareness and eliminated.

Conclusion

Child labor includes children prematurely leading adult lives, working long hours for low wages, under conditions damaging to their health and their physical and mental development sometimes separated from their families, frequently deprived of meaningful education and training opportunities that could up for them a better future.

Child Abuse

Introduction

Child abuse is the term referred to children who have received serious physical injury causes willfully. This definition has not taken into consideration, the neglect, maltreatment of children, mental and sexual harassment. The broader meaning of child abuse includes three types of abuse, physical, sexual, and emotional types. Child abuse is harm to, or neglect of, a child by another person, whether adult or child. Child abuse happens in all cultural, ethnic and income groups. Child abuse can be physical, emotional-verbal, sexual or through neglect. Abuse may cause serious injury to the child and may even result in death.

Signs of Child Abuse

Sl.No	Child abuse	Characteristics
1.	Physical abuse	1. Unexplained or repeated injuries as welts, busy, or burns. 2. Injuries that are in the shape of an object (belt buckle, electric code, etc.). 3. Injuries not likely to happen given the age or ability of the child. For example, broken bones in a child too young to walk or climb. 4. Disagreement between the child's and the parent's explanation of the injury. 5. Unreasonable explanation of the injury. 6. Obvious neglect of the child (dirty, undernourished, inappropriate cloths for the weather, lack medical or dental care).
2.	Emotional abuse	1. Aggressive or withdrawn behavior. 2. Shying away from physical contact with parents or adults. 3. Afraid to go home.

3.	Sexual abuse	1. Child tells you he/ she was sexually mistreated.
		2. Child has physical signs such as:
		  a. Difficulty in waking or sitting.
		  b. Stained or bloody underwear.
		  c. Genital or rectal pain, itching, swelling, redness, or discharge.
		  d. Bruises or other injuries in the genital or rectal area.
		3. Child has behavior and emotional signs such as:
		  a. Difficulty eating or sleeping.
		  b. Soiling of wetting pants or bed after being potty trained.
		  c. Acting like a much younger child.
		  d. Excessive crying or sadness.
		  e. Withdrawing from activities and others.
		  f. Taking about or acting out sexual acts beyond normal sex play for age.

Contd...

Contd...

Sl.No.	Child abuse	Characteristics
4.	Family characteristics	1. Families who are isolated and have no friends, relatives, church or other support systems.
		2. Parents who tell you they were abused as children.
		3. Families who are often in crisis (having money problems, move often).
		4. Parents who abuse drug or alcohol.
		5. Parents who are very critical of their child.
		6. Parents who are very rigid in disciplining their child.
		7. Parents who show too much or little concern for their child.
		8. Parents who feel they have a different child.
		9. Parents who are under a lot of stress.

Causes of Child Abuse

The causes of child abuse are generally poverty, illiteracy, adaptation failure. Family disorganization, death of parents, disobedience of parents. Lack of adequate control and defective socialization. Irritable nature and rigidness of authorities, low income, lack of effective school education and other factors lead to child abuse.

Effects of Child Abuse

1. Child abuse produces negative attitude called social devaluation. In other words it is called loss of social esteem. Further it develops deviant behavior.
2. A large number of victimized children indulge in violation of social norms. Consequent to their dependency they try to escape from such a situation. So absence from school, absence from work or runaways, stealing of money, drug addiction is some of the common deviant behavior found among abused children.
3. Child abuses also develop social and interpersonal social problems like isolation, withdrawal from interactional settings, antagonistic relations with parents/care takers.
4. There are more chance of being revictamization, it hinder the development of their personality. So a majority of them are forced to become the child labor. They are exposed to work for longer hours in hazardous work conditions. They miss the education and many of them become bonded laborers.
5. Majority of the children are found working in fire works, tea gardens, in hotels, household works, mining, etc. The children are working under inhuman conditions and unhygienic surrounding suffer from various diseases such as lung diseases, TB, eye diseases, asthma, bronchitis, etc.

Measures to Ameliorate the Problem

1. The first Factory Act to regulate the employment of children and their hours of work was introduced in 1881. Later on the Child Labor Act, 1933 and the Factory Act of 1948 provided some safeguard to child laborers.
2. The Juvenile Justice Act, 1986 was introduced in different stages and advisory boards and establishment of state children funds for preventing the abuse of children, protection and care of children, educational facilities, and training and rehabilitation facilities were provided.

3. The government has tried to improve their working conditions, reduce working hours and ensure minimum wages, health and education. But legislative measures proved to be ineffective.

4. The Union Governments set-up a National Advisory Board in 1993 to eliminate child labor in hazardous industries by 2000. The government provided Rs. 850 crore to rehabilitate the child workers and for their education. But the government was not serious in implementing the plan.

5. The Supreme Court in 1996, banned child labor and ordered to set-up a child labor rehabilitation welfare fund and aimed at safeguarding the social and humanitarian rights.

6. UNICEF has taken up various ameliorative measures for child welfare. The present need is that law must be enforced to curb this menace. People need to change their attitude towards children and they must be provided opportunities to develop their potentialities in a healthy and free social environment, and must be protected against exploitation.

Conclusion

Child abuse and child labor is a serious problem in India. A large majority of the Indian children are neglected by parents, exploited by employers, harassed and abused. They remain in distress and turmoil. It has been estimated that the child population between the ages of 5 to14 years constitute about 298 million. Millions of children from poor families are compelled to join the labor force. In India, 15% of the children are child laborers. Sexual abuse among children, refers to involvement of immature children is sexual activities, rape, prostitution. Emotional abuse is maltreatment of children. Social abuse of children includes kidnapping and forcing them to beg in street or used for sexual gratification.

JUVENILE DELINQUENCY

Introduction

Juvenile delinquency refers to the criminal offences by children and youth. Antisocial practices of this type are a serious danger to the welfare of society. Delinquency a legal term for criminal behavior carried out by a juvenile is often the result of escalating problematic behavior. Juvenile delinquency are non-adult criminals or under aged criminals. Usually the delinquents fall between 7 and 16 years. According to juvenile justice act of 1986, 16 years for boys and 18 years for girls. High rate of delinquency are more in urban areas than in rural areas. The delinquent rates are higher among boys than girls.

Definitions

1. Juvenile delinquency involves wrong-doing by a child or young person who is under an age specified by the law of the place concerned—*MJ Sethna*.

2. Juvenile delinquency defined as any behavior which a given community at a given time considers in conflict with its best interest, whether or not the offender has been brought to court—*Robinson*.

3. A delinquent is a person under age, who is guilty of Antisocial Act and whose misconduct is an infraction of law—*Newmeyer*.

Causes of Juvenile Delinquency

1. **Personal cause:** It may be included the biological and psychological conditions of a child.

2. **Environmental cause:** It may be included the geographical or ecological causes.

3. **Psychological causes:** It may be included feeblemindedness, emotional strain, love for adventure, stubborn nature and nonfulfilment of basic wishes as recognition, response and security.
4. **Sociocultural factors:** It may be considered to be more important than biological or physical ones as sociologists hold the view that man is not born criminal but made criminal.
5. **Family:** The home is the first school of the child. His socialization and personality development takes place in the family. Most sociologists have laid much stress on the condition of the family for the causation of juvenile delinquency. Broken homes, too much discipline or too less discipline, irresponsible parents, mother working outside the home, too many children, and lonely child are some of the causes.
6. According to Pauline young, the most important causes of juvenile delinquency are poverty, slums and infected areas, immigrant communities, fronties communities, lack of meaningful and satisfying relationship, family disorganization, war, comic books, bad companionship and social change.
7. According to Healy and Bronner, the main causes of Juvenile delinquency are bad company, adolescent instability and impulses, early sex experiences, mental conflicts, extreme social instability, love for adventure, motion pictures, school dissatisfaction, sudden impulses and physical conditions of all sorts.
8. **Economic condition:** Poverty at home, unemployment of parents and the instability of the parents to provide the children with adequate facilities create delinquency.
9. **Education:** Absence of education or the lack of proper education may result in juvenile delinquency. Overcrowded schools, uncommitted teachers and teaching uninteresting to the young boys and girls may lead to truancy.
10. **Religion and morals:** Religion and morals help the children in their socialization and social control. In the absences of these, the children turn delinquent.
11. **Unhealthy recreation:** Unhealthy recreation like the cinema, television, and radio, also causes delinquency. The young mind is much influenced by the modern media.
12. **Political condition:** Healthy political situation provides control and welfare of the society. But political instability, corruption and confusing leadership mislead the young people. Political conflicts like war and revolutions also affect the behavior of the young people.

Other Causes of Juvenile Delinquency

1. **Poverty:** Due to very poor standards of life, the children cannot have good homes, schools and other facilities which stand in the way of their physical, mental and spiritual development.
2. **Social change:** The Traditional Indian Society is fast changing owing to a number of reasons. Inconsistency between ideals and ambitions compared with achievements creates problem in the minds of young people. One of the causes of youth unrest in India is frustration due to unemployment or fear of unemployment. Cultural lag is also causing delinquency in Indian youth.
3. **Breakdown of joint family:** The traditional family in India that is the joint family is breaking. This affects the children much.
4. Breakdown of caste, traditional religion, morals and values.
5. Illiteracy and lack of proper education.
6. Lack of care by the government.
7. Industrialization and urbanization, together with large scale migration to the cities.

Characteristics of Juvenile Delinquency

1. The delinquency rates are much higher among boys than girls.
2. The delinquency rates tend to be highest during early adolescence (12-16 years age group).
3. Juvenile delinquency is more in urban than a rural. The metropolitan cities produce more juvenile delinquents than small cities and towns.
4. Low education background is the prime attribute for delinquency.
5. Poor economic background is another important characteristic of juvenile delinquency in India.
6. Though some delinquencies are committed in groups but the number of juvenile gangs having support of organized adult criminals is not much in our country.
7. More than four-fifths of the juvenile delinquents are first offenders and only a little more than one-tenth are recidivists past offenders.

Forms of Juvenile Delinquency

United States of America, some of the patterns of juvenile delinquency are bullying, cheating, cruelty, drinking, gambling, obscenity, sex perversion, smoking, stealing, teasing, truancy from home, and truancy from school, undesirable companions, uncleanliness and violation of traffic rules.

In India, some of the serious forms of juvenile delinquency are delinquent action against property such as stealing, damaging, etc. gambling, murder and suicide, assault, sexual offences like rape and sodomy, ticketless travel especially in trains, escape from custody.

Types of Juvenile Delinquency

1. **Truancy:** This is called kindergarten crime. The school children attempt escape from school. Generally, a truant stays out of the school. They indulge in bad company and indulge in wandering and gambling. This kind of behavior may be due to unsuitable conditions at home, and school, strictness in school.
2. **Vagrancy:** It is another type. These are generally neglected, ill cared and wondering children. These children are generally belong to poor families or disorganized families, which could not provide them the basic needs of food, education, affection, etc.

Control and Remedy of Juvenile Delinquency

While treating a juvenile delinquent, the welfare of the child is given foremost importance. Since he is a minor, he cannot be held responsible for the offensive Act he has committed. The purpose is not punishing him, but to correct his criminal tendencies and make him a useful citizen. The Children's Act of 1960 passed by our Parliament seeks to provide for the care, protection, maintenance, welfare, training, trial and rehabilitation of delinquent and neglected children. Every attempt is made to correct his deviant behavior and also to equip him for a normal adult life.

1. Proper assessment of the entire problem, in scientific and sociological manner.
2. Improvement in economic conditions.
3. Better education.
4. Training of parents to have responsible parenthood.
5. Revival in the system of religion and morals.
6. Facilities for proper treatment, and reformation of juvenile delinquents with supervision of juvenile courts, juvenile police and reformation centers.

Preventive Measures

1. Team work of private and public agencies. These include schools, church, parent-teacher associations, youth organizations like scouts and guides, social worker, police department, etc.
2. Establishment of child guidance clinics. Serious disturbed and maladjusted children can be treating by these clinics.
3. Education of the family: Family life must be strengthened and by educating the members of the family.
4. Establishment of whole some recreational facilities such as sports, drama, puppet show, other cultural activities. Youth organization must take such responsibilities.
5. Assistance to under privileged children.
6. Propaganda about causes and protection of youth.
7. Improving the environment, better schooling, housing facilities, rising income level of poor families.

Rehabilitation Measures

Today's children are tomorrow's citizens. So if the rate of delinquency increases naturally they become tomorrow's criminals. Therefore, it is the most important task of the society and the government to think of protecting, preventing and rehabilitating children from falling into social evils.

1. Before independence in 1850, Apprentice Act was introduced in which provision was made towards learning of trade and craft, so the juvenile can make an honest living.
2. Reformatory Schools Acts of 1877 can be regarded as a land mark in the treatment of delinquents. The under aged offenders were detained in reformatory schools for a period not less than three years and not more than three years, where they will be given industrial training. They will be provided with food, clothing, bedding in a good environment.
3. After independence Juvenile Justice Act 1986 was passed which has made all provisions to provide minimum standards for basic needs, living conditions, and therapeutic services to juvenile institutions.

Important juvenile institutions are:

1. **Remand homes:** The juvenile children during the pendency of their trial kept in remand homes. They will not be mixed with adult offenders in prisons. These are observational homes, where some welfare measures are taken by probation officer, health care facility is provided.
2. **Certified schools or reformatory schools:** These are called reformatory schools where the delinquents are kept for a minimum period of 3 years and maximum period of 7 years. They are meant only for boys. They are managed by voluntary bodies or by government. They provide school education, industrial training, etc.
3. **Borstal schools:** Borstal schools are established for youth offender in age group of 16-21 years. Special treatment is provided adolescent offenders, by keeping them separately from the adult offenders. The main motto behind separation is to provide correction service and to rehabilitate the youngsters.
4. **Probation hostels:** Probation hostels are the institutions, which provide residential care and treatment to offenders released under probation. They will be under the supervision of a probation officer.

Conclusion

It is a very serious social problem. It is also an educational problem because it has been found the delinquents usually show evidence of poor adjustment in schools before they get into difficulties with the juvenile courts. The problems of juvenile delinquency and crime can be remedied by creating better social institutions and environment in our society. Better homes, better economic conditions, better education, recreation and better state and government can go a long way in this connection.

CRIME

Introduction

Crime is a great social problem facing every society. It is an act forbidden by law and there is a penalty prescribed for it. Crime is the price paid for the advantage of civilization. It is a major problem in modern civilized societies. Crime is the omission of an Act which the law of the land asks to do or commission of an act which is forbids doing. The law may be written or unwritten. When the law is not written then crime is generally recognized as transgressions against the traditions more of community. Crime, therefore, may regard as behavior of individuals which group strongly disapproves.

Definitions

1. Crime is any from of conduct which is forbidden by the law, under the pain of some punishment—*Sethna*.
2. Crime is defined legally as any overt act of commission or omission that is in violation of law—*Neumeyers*.
3. Crime is an objectively evil act, a violation of social validity, an offence against the superior dignity of a collective system—*EA Ross*.
4. Crime may be defined as antisocial behavior which the group rejects and to which it attaches penalties—*Elliott and Merrill*.
5. Crime is an act forbidden by the law of the land and for which penalty is prescribed—*C Darrow*.
6. Crime is a form of antisocial behavior that has violated public sentiment to such an extent as to be forbidden by statute—*Barnes and Tecters*.

Classifications of Crime

1. **Crimes against body:** Murder, it attempt, culpable homicide not amounting to murder, kidnapping and abduction, hurt, causing death by negligence.
2. **Crimes against property:** Dacoits, its preparation and assembly, robbery, burglary, theft, extortion.
3. **Crime against public order:** Riots, arson.
4. **Economic crimes:** Criminal breach of trust, cheating, counterfeiting.
5. **Crimes against women:** Rape, dowry death, cruelty by husband and relatives, molestation, sexual harassment and importation of girls, outraging the modesty of women.
6. **Crimes against children:** Child rape, kidnapping and abduction of children, procreation of minor girls, selling/buying of girls for prostitution, abetment of suicide, exposure and abandonment, infanticide, feticide.
7. **Professional crime:** The term professional is used when offenders and high skipped and are accorded high status among criminals. Their activities have included pick-pocketing, shop lifting, burglary, passing bad cheques, extorting money from persons in illegal sex activities and operating a variety of confidence games.

Factors of Crime

According to Elliot and Merrill, the factors in relation to the whole, rather than the sum of the single isolated factors, must be considered in any satisfactory analysis.

1. Physical and mental characteristics of the individual mental defects epilepsy and mental disorder and certain emotional disturbances have a great bearing upon the making of the criminals.
2. Biological factors are insanity, physical disability, defective glandular and nervous system. The physiological causes may be neurosis, psychopathy and emotional instability.
3. **Environmental factors:** Home conditions are definitely responsible for producing criminals. When the home is immoral or when there are immoral, drunken, epileptic, instance of feeble minded parents present in the family, the child is easily led astray.
4. **Economic factors:** Economic factors often foster crime. It has been observed in the west that crimes increase with depression and unemployment and decrease with good living conditions. Crimes are also committed when individuals are not satisfied with their lawful earning and adopt unsocial conduct for satisfaction of their desires. The economic causes are economic competition, poverty, unemployment, desire for more wealth, unlimited desires, industrialization, poor natural resources, inflation, etc.
5. **Poverty includes crime:** Large scale unemployment means social disorganization which leads to crime.
6. **Urbanization and industrialization:** The growth of industries in industrial areas has lead to agglomerations of the people in large number especially from the rural areas and from different social strata.
7. **Superstition:** People are often led to believe, because of their ignorance and weak moral that spells and sacrifice can bring material advantage and these very belief cases frequent crimes such as human murders.
8. **Sociological factors:** The frequency of offence is affected by social interactional or social disintegration, social competition, social mobility, conflict, defective social institutions, and lack of education in a society.
9. **Area and regional differences in crime:** It has been observed by sociologists the crime varies in volume and form by areas and regions. The areas of high crime rates in cities provide an unstable social setting in which individuals can become unadjusted to the way of living required by the dominant moral group.
10. **Effects of class, sex, age and race:** The individuals in the lower class level of a society are suspected of displaying greater risk and liabilities owing to their sociological positions for getting involved in crime and for being acted upon officially.

Crime in India

In India, there are no dependable figures on crime. The available statistics cover only those arrested and convicted, or the crime known to the police and even these figures are not reliable. Racketeering, black marketing, tax evading, corruption, etc. are crimes committed by white-collared men in their business and professional transactions. Our moral sense is at the lowest ebb. Terrorism has become the order of the day. The social causes of crime are disorganization, social competition, social mobility and conflict, defective social institutions, lack of education, sexual literacy, etc. are also cause of crime. Reforme of the criminal is the main motive in his treatment. In India, various measures are being taken to give better treatment to the criminals in jails.

Crimes under the Special and Local Laws

Sl.No.	Special and local law
1.	Arms Act
2.	Narcotics Drugs and Psychotropic Substances Act
3.	Gambling Act
4.	Prohibition Act
5.	Explosive and Explosive Substance Act
6.	Immoral Traffics (Prevention Act)
7.	Indian Railway Act
8.	Registration of Foreigners Act
9.	Protection of Civil Rights Act
10.	Indian Passport Act
11.	Essential Commodities Act
12.	Terrorist Disruptive Act
13.	Antiquity and Art Treasure Act
14.	Dowry Prohibition Act
15.	Child Marriage Act
16.	Indecent Representation of Women (P) Act
17.	Copyright Act
18.	Sati Prevention Act
19.	SC/ST (Prevention of Atrocities) Act

Conclusion

Crime is due to maladjustment between the individual and the group and creates a critical situation. It is an act forbidden and punished by law, which is always almost immoral according to prevailing ethical standards, which it is normally feasible to repress by penal measures and whose repression in necessary or supposed to necessary. In society's attitude towards the criminal personal responsibility has been emphasized. The criminal is looked upon as depraved sort of human being.

SUBSTANCE ABUSE

Introduction

Substance abuse is a serious social problem that confronts youth of India. This problem arises mainly due to failure to internalize norms, through frustration and habit formation. Drug abuse is more serious than alcoholic abuse. The message from narcotic control bureau and other agencies is drug abuse is life abuse. It is an evident of individual's maladjustment. It considered as aberrant behavior. Drugs are intoxicating chemical substances, which affect the physical and mental condition of persons. They can also be called narcotic drugs. Psychologically, drugs are substance which affects the brain and nervous system of the individual. By using these drugs, a person can escape from tension and worries for sometime; he feels temporary peace, happiness and elation, but gradually be become addicted to these substance and turns out to be a slave of these habits.

Definition

Drug addition defined as a state of periodic or chronic intoxication determental to the individual and to society, produced by repeated consumption of a drug either natural or synthetic—*World Health Organization*.

Terms used in Substance Abuse

1. *Drug abuse:* Drug abuse is the use of such substances which are harmful to body and mind. Hence, any abuse is the use of harmful drugs and intoxicants for momentary pleasure or peace.
2. *Drug addition:* Drug addition denotes physical dependence of drugs. Addition is that state in which a person is dependent on drug for his bodily activities and in the absence of drug body functions are affected.
3. *Drug addict:* Drug addict may use any drug or substances which is suitable and available to them. They may be addict of one or more than one drugs.

Characteristics of Drug Addition

1. Strong desire to take drugs/narcotic substances.
2. Strong determination to get it at any cost.
3. Because of the ill effects of drug, physical and mental dependence is prominent.
4. Less interest in studies, games, hobbies, home, family and occupation.
5. Irresponsible behavior.
6. Irritability and immoral behavior like stealing, telling lies, etc.
7. Absence from home, school, or place of work.
8. Tremors in hands and legs and inability to drive scooter or car.
9. Loosing strength.
10. Suicidal tendencies.

Causes of Drug Addiction

1. Bad company.
2. To attain happiness and ecstasy.
3. Escapism.
4. To satisfy curiosity.
5. To feel free and elated.
6. Urbanization/industrialization.
7. Easy availability of intoxicants.
8. Unhealthily educational environment.
9. Youth unrest/student unrest.
10. Disorganized family/guardians do not care.
11. Drug addiction by other family members.
12. Worldwide network of drug mafia.

Control of Drug Abuse/Addiction

1. Strict control over drug smuggling.
2. Change in the attitude of doctors/nurses towards drug addicts.
3. Educating people regarding drug.
4. Attention towards youth's behavior by parents, teachers and elders.
5. Treatment of addicts.
6. Proper enforcement of constitutional and legal restraints.
7. De-addiction camps and special attention towards follow-up.
8. Checking supply of drugs from broader countries.
9. International cooperation and policy against drugs and narcotics.

Nature and Impact of Abusable Drugs

1. **Alcohol:** It acts as a sedative, which calms down nerves or a kind of an anesthetic which reduces the pain or living. Alcohol relives tension and lessens aggressive inhibitions. It also impairs judgment and creates confusion.
2. **Sedatives:** Sedatives or depressants relax the central nervous system, induce sleep and provide a calming effect. Tranquilizers and barbiturates fall in to this category. In small quantities, they slow down breathing and heart beating and make the user relaxed, but higher doses, their effects resemble alcohol intoxication in which the user becomes sluggish, gloomy and sometimes irritable and quarrel some. The ability to think, concentrate, and work is impaired and his emotional control is weakened.
3. **Stimulants:** Activate the central nervous system and relieve tensions, treat mild depression, include insomnia, contract fatigue and expressive drowsiness and lessen aggressive inhibitions. The most widely known stimulants are amphetamines, caffeine, and cocaine. Heavier doses cause extreme nervousness, irritability, headache, sweating, diarrhea and unclear speech.
4. **Narcotics:** Narcotics produce a depressant effect on the central nervous system. They produce feeling of pleasure, strength, and superiority, reduce hunger, lessen inhibition and increase suggestibility. Include in this category are opium, marijuana, heroin, morphine, pethedine, cocaine and cannabis.
5. **Hallucinogens:** It produces distortions of perception (seeing or hearing things in a different way than they actually are) and dream images. Their use is not advised by medical practitioners. The well-known drug is this group is LSD, which is man-made chemical.
6. **Nicotine:** Nicotine includes cigarettes, bidi, cigars, snuff and tobacco. Nicotine has no medical use. The risk of physical dependence, however, may be there. It leads to relaxation, stimulates the central nervous system, increases wakefulness, and removes boredom. But frequent or heavy use of nicotine may cause heart attack, lung cancer and bronchitis.

Preventive Measures

1. **Primary prevention:** Primary prevention is through two main methods. (a) by limiting the availability of drugs, (b) by educational measures. In all countries, there is legislative to control the production, supply, possession and export of drug. The underlying principle is that drugs should be made available for genuine medical use, but no surplus should be allowed in the market.
2. **Secondary prevention:** This is achieved through early identification of drug abusers that they can be treated promptly to prevent the development of complications. Any change in the behavior of young people should be closely watched.
3. **Tertiary prevention:** This is the treatment of the state of severe dependence. Many dedication centers, psychotherapies, social worker and social agencies are working to help the drug addicts. Help and support of family members is extremely important in overcoming the problem.

Conclusion

Drug abuse is the use of illicit drug or misuse of legitimate drug resulting in the physical or psychological harm. Drug addiction or physical dependence is a state where the body requires continued administration of the drug in order to function. Body functioning is interfered with if the drug is withdrawn, and withdrawal symptoms appear in a pattern specific for the drug. The total reaction to deprivation is known as abstinence syndrome.

HIV/AIDS

Introduction

Acquired immunodeficiency syndrome (AIDS) is a virus borne communicable disease. This fatal disease is caused by Human immunodeficiency virus (HIV). It transmitted through sexually, destroys the antibody producing white blood cells (WBC) which are called T-cells and thus cripples the immune system. The first case of AIDS was discovered at the center of disease control in Atlanta, USA, in the year 1981. The causative organism was discovered in the year 1983.

Statistics of HIV In India

1. HIV was first detected in USA in 1981. In India, the first case of AIDS was detected in 1986 in Tamilnadu. At present, there are lahk of HIV infected people in India.
2. According to the reports of United State of America, AIDS Control Program, and WHO report in the beginning of 1998, more than 3 crores of people were affected by HIV in the world. According to reports about 16,000 people are becoming infected by AIDS daily. HIV infection is spreading among children also.
3. According to reports, maximum spread of infection of HIV is in developing countries. In January 2001, there were more than 3.61 crore of people affected by HIV in the world (USAIDS & WHO-AIDS WATCH).
4. This number increased to 3.94 crore in 2004 (WHO- A report-2004) an other estimate show it 4.60 crore.
5. Many social and health problems like; loss of young human resources, loss of immunity, social disorganization and social boycott, etc. are occurring due to AIDS.
6. AIDS affects men and women equally. AIDS is found in pregnant mothers and infants also. HIV does not consider the limits of nations, religion or sex.
7. Prostitutes are the main victims and carriers of AIDS.
8. This disease is found maximum in sexually active people (20 to 50 years). Out of every 100 people of this age group, one is affected by HIV.
9. According to a report of Health Ministry and NACO (December 2000) about 37 lahk people were infected by HIV in India. About 89% of the notified people were sexually active and belong to the age group of 18-40. Out of these more than 50% of new infections were of youth below 25 years.
10. According to WHO-report (2004), India has 5.1 million HIV infected persons. 97780 AIDS cases have been reported to NACO till 31st January 2005 (annual report 2004-05 MOHFW).
11. According to NACO, since 1986 to 2004 (31st August 2004), total 91080 AIDS patients were found in India. This cumulative number includes 65828 males and 25252 females AIDS patients.

Clinical Features of HIV

Major symptoms are:
1. Weight loss.
2. Fever more than 1 month.
3. Diarrhea for more than one month.
4. Extrapulmonary TB at more than one site.

Minor symptoms are:
1. Persistent cough for more than a month.
2. Itching skin diseases.
3. Thrush in the mouth and throat.
4. Swollen glands.
5. Chronic generalized herpes simplex (a viral disease).

HIV spread by:
1. The most important reason for spread of AIDS is sexual contact. This includes homosexuality, group sex, sexual intercourse by person infected with AIDS with person of opposite sex, anal sexes, which are the main bases for spreading HIV.
2. Transmission by blood—use of infected syringes, needles or instruments. AIDS spread through the blood transfusion.
3. People who take injections of intoxicants drugs.
4. Maternal-fetal transmission—a pregnant mother can transmit infection to the fetus.
5. Using a common razor at the barber's shop or tonsuring at religious places.

HIV does not spread by:
1. Living with or caring for people with HIV or AIDS.
2. Using the same toilets are the infected people.
3. Swimming in pools used by infected persons.
4. Shaking hands hugging or kissing infected persons.
5. Drinking water from the same glass used by an infected person.
6. By bites of mosquito which has already bitten an infected person.

Diagnosis Test

Identify HIV positive people. There are two tests are done.
1. Enzyme linked immunosorbent assay (ELISA) blood test is conducted for diagnosis of HIV.
2. **Western blot:** It has to be confirmed by the western blot test. Generally, it takes 3 to 24 weeks for persons to positive after they have been infected.
3. Virus isolation.
4. Murex SUD-HIV-1test.
5. Total, T-4 cells and T-8 cells (to find out the status of T-lymphocytes).

Effects of AIDS

The AIDS victims are killed by:
1. Chronic pneumonia.
2. Chronic diarrhea.
3. Infections which block the throat, intestine and lungs.
4. Cancer of the skin and bone.
5. Swelling in the brain.
6. Distractions of brain tissues causing loss of memory and personality changes.

Management of AIDS

1. *Aims of project made for AIDS control:*
   a. To achieve zero level of infection.
   b. Blood protection and improvement in its rational use.

c. Encouraging public awareness and community support.
d. Developing capacity for observation and management.
e. Control on sexually transmitted diseases.
f. Strengthening program management capacity.
2. *Control over bloodborne transmission:*
a. Test all blood products and blood before transmission for HIV/AIDS.
b. Ensure proper sterilization process; take precaution in organ transplantation.
c. Avoid reuse of syringe, needles or other skin puncturing instruments or use them with greatest caution.
d. Use disposable syringes.
e. Take precaution in ear piercing, tattooing, acupuncture, tooth extraction, etc.
3. *Safe sexual relations:*
a. Sexual relationship only within marriage. Have sexual relation with one husband/one wife only.
b. Condom may be used for safe sex.
c. Sexual relation should be moral. Sexual partner should be faithful to each other.
d. Avoid unnatural sexual activities like anal sex, oral sex, homosexuality, group sex, etc.
e. There should be no injury or lesion on reproductive organs.
4. *Health education:*
a. Health education includes the subject of sex education in the curriculum of general education to encourage healthy sexual relations.
b. Emphasize on the restoration of moral values and character.
c. It is necessary to remove all erroneous ideas about AIDS. It should be made clear that AIDS does not spread through mosquitoes or other insects.
d. AIDS does not spread due to sitting or having contacts with the patient neither it spread through clothes.
e. The staff that works, also does not get AIDS, but the preventive measures should not be overlooked.
5. *Other measures:*
a. Surveillance and research.
b. Reduction of impact.
c. Provide health care to people attacked by HIV.
d. Provide antiviral treatment. Encourage research regarding AIDS control and eradication.
e. Save HIV/AIDS infected people and provide them psychological support.
f. Treat complications occurring due to AIDS immediately.
g. Effective implementation and evaluation of AIDS Control Program.

AIDS and Nursing Concern

World anti AIDS day is observed on December 1, every year to spread awareness on its prevention and control. International Council of Nurses (INC) declared 12 may 2003 (nurse day) them. Nurses always for families: Fighting AIDS stigma, caring for all. It is a call to all professionals to come forward and combat the AIDS by breaking the walls of stigma and silence the surrounds HIV/AIDS. INC has short listed the following approaches to enable the nurses in their fight against stigma and discrimination. It includes:

1. **Information-based approaches:** Giving factual information about HIV / AIDS.
2. **Counseling:** Providing positive reinforcement and support to family members.
3. **Coping skill acquisition:** Generating positive attitude towards people living with HIV/AIDS through a combination of information and skill acquistation.
4. **Contact with infected or affected people:** Reducing stigma and discrimination by interacting with stigmatized group.
5. Creating HIV/AIDS patient-friendly hospitals.
6. Supporting general and specialist professional association in AIDS care.
7. Provide adequate supplies and equipment for AIDS prevention and control.

Conclusion

The HIV/AIDS epidemic is a health problem in which the disease impacts not only on the physical health of individuals, but also on their social identity, making it different from most other fatal diseases. It was first associated with gagmen, drug users and sex workers, individuals, and groups already caring the burden of societal stigmatization. Awareness of HIV infection can create enormous psychological pressures and anxieties that can delay constructive change or worsen illness, especially in view of the fear, misunderstanding, and discrimination provoked by the HIV epidemic.

DOWRY SYSTEM

Introduction

Dowry is a major problem of marriage in India, especially in certain communities. With the increasing importance of money, the amount of dowry is also increasing. Even the spread of modern education and enlighten has not been able to diminish this problem. The dowry system is fought with great danger to life and honor of women and burden to poor parents. It leads to suicide by the father when he is incapable of paying the dowry demanded by the boy's parents. Sometimes, the girl herself would commit suicide. These days we hear everyday about the burning of recently married girls for not bringing enough dowries.

Definitions

1. Dowry is the property which a woman brings with her or is given to her at the marriage— *Encyclopedia Britannica Volume-VII).*
2. Dowry is the property which a man receives from his wife or her family at the time of marriage— *Max Radin.*
3. Dowry defined as any property or valuable security which might be given or agreed to be given either directly or indirectly by one party in marriage to the other party in marriage, either by themselves or through parents or through any other person which may be presented either before or at the time of marriage or even after that—*The Dowry Prohibition Act, 1961.*

Dowry System in India

1. In the Vedic age dowry system as unknown, since women enjoyed equal status with men, in those days marriage was popularly known as *kanyadana* indicated that it was far from the evil of dowry. At the time, it was of solemnization of marriage, the parents will give gift and present to the bride and groom to express their love, affection and respect.

2. Varadakshina is not a dowry. In-laws should not demand even the stridhan as a right. Stridhan refers to the gift given to women by her kith and kin or by her husband at or after wedding and the money she inherit's from her parents or earned by personal efforts.

3. Mahatma Gandhiji the father of nation believed that the dowry system is nothing but the sale of girls. In the year 1958, dowry started as an innocent custom, a symbol of love from parents to their daughters on the eve of the marriage. In the recent years it has grown into a social evil.

4. Dowry has gained social acceptance as a normal marriage procedure, throughout the country. It has become a status symbol for both the parties. Father who is quite willing to part with lot of money as dowry at the time of marriage is hesitant to give a share of his property to his daughter.

Dowry is Considered as a Social Evil

In the recent years it has grown into social evils. Dowry has gained social acceptance as a normal marriage procedure, throughout the country. Dowry is causing suffering of the people and parents. It is the corruption and bride in the society; it has deteriorated the status of women. It results in dowry, death, suicide, homicide, etc. Thus, dowry system is considered to be a prestigious issue the demands become unaffordable in certain caste and communities but practiced by all most all castes. The dowry plays a major role in marriages irrespective of their status. In our country, marriages are fixed by the elders in the elders in the family and they demand money, jewels and other household items.

Causes of Dowry

1. To find a suitable bridegroom.
2. The tradition of kanyadan.
3. Absolute necessity of marriage.
4. The social acceptance of stridhan.
5. Dowry is linked with social status.
6. Materialistic outlook.
7. Child marriage.
8. Low status of women.
9. Social tradition.

Factors Responsible for Dowry System

1. Caste system.
2. Social custom.
3. Inevitability of marriage.
4. Physical handicaps.
5. Aspiration to money in rich families.
6. False notion of social status.
7. Vicious circle.

Measures for Eraditcation of Dowry

1. Encouraging inter-caste marriages.
2. Young men and women should marry only after they become self dependent.

3. Increasing the age of marriage.
4. Creating public opinion against dowry.
5. Leaders and elite measures of the society should present the examples of marriage without dowry.
6. Young men should take oath against dowry.
7. Social boycott of dowry seekers.
8. The girl should be given equal share in father's property and wife should have legal right in husband's property.

Legal Implications of Dowry System

Dowry Prohibition Act 1961 has declared both giving and taking of dowry as illegal, the reality is that dowry is spreading like cancer. Even in case of dowry murders, the culprits often escape due to lack of evidence or longer legal procedures.

The Dowry Prohibition Act was formulated in 1961 and amended in 1984 and 1986. Section 3 imposes:

1. A minimum of 5 years of imprisonment.
2. Rs.15,000 fines or equivalent value of the dowry taken whichever is more for giving or taking dowry.
3. For demanding dowry, the punishment is imprisonment for a minimum period of 6 months and fine.
4. If the dowry is actually received by any person other than the bride, the person has to transfer it to her within 3 months after the date of receipt. Failure gives penalty of minimum 6 months imprisonment and fine not less than the value of the dowry received.
5. Every offence under the Act is made non-bailable, non-compoundable and cognizable for the purpose of investigation (section 498A of IPC).
6. Any willful conduct is likely to drive the women to commit suicide to cause grave injury or danger to life, limb or healthy (physical/mental) of the women.

Sociological Implications of Dowry System

It provides an opportunity for meritorious boys and of poor classes to go for higher education and make their future.

1. Helps in establishment of new household.
2. Increase status of women in the family.
3. Enhances the possibility of marriages of girls with handicapped.
4. Maintains harmony and unity among the family members.
5. Promotes inter-caste and inter-religious marriages.

Measures Towards Abolition of Dowry System

1. Increase public awareness and social understanding about the evil effect of dowry system and law enforcement by conducting mass education, mass media activities and IEC training program.
2. Encourage or motivate the women to improve the will to safeguard and fight for their rights.
3. Initiate youth through propaganda and public enlighten to change their ideas.
4. Encourage full freedom for the boys and girls to select their mates.

Conclusion

Dowry means the money, property or gifts given to a woman at the time of marriage. This also called streedhan. Legally dowry is the money or property received by the man from the girl's relatives or family as a reward of marriage.

Dowry is a serious problem in India. Some states are more affected. Thousands of women are burnt every year for dowry. Women are harassed by in-laws, husband or other members of husband's family in many ways. Some of them are forced even to commit suicide it was thought that education will be helpful in eradicating this problem but unfortunately dowry still remains a terrible problem.

ALCOHOLISM

Introduction

Alcoholism is a state of excessive consumption of alcohol and getting addicted to it. It is to be understood that taking alcohol once a while or using it for medicinal purposes cannot be said as a social problem, people who start using alcohol for fun or as social drinking, might end up as alcoholics. Alcoholism is a social evil. For social upliftment and community health. Every person should try to avoid alcohol. Alcohol adversely affects liver, eyes and physical and mental activities. This encourages immorality, violence against women, sexual harassment, rape, crime, murder, poverty, etc. in society. Many of the crimes are committed under the influences of alcohol.

Definition

A problem drinker is one if, as a result of drinking, his health is endangered, his peace of mind affected, his home life made unhappy, his business jeopardized and his reputation clouded and drinking has become his routine—*Durfee*.

Classification of Alcohol Drinkers

Don Cahalan has given a five-fold classification of alcohol drinker on the basis of frequency of drinking (not the quantity of alcohol taken).

Sl.No.	Type	Description
1.	Rare user	Who drink once/twice a year.
2.	Infrequent users	Who drink once or twice in 2-3 months, that is, less than once a month.
3.	Light drinkers	Who drink once or twice a month.
4.	Moderate drinker	Who drink three or four times in a month.
5.	Heavy drinker	Who drink everyday or several drinks during the day? This category of drinkers is also called as hard-core drinkers.

Causes of Alcoholism/Drinking

1. Drinking as a recreation.
2. Pressure of friends.
3. To link alcohol with social status and serve it in social functions.
4. Tensions in occupations.
5. Ignorance regarding the evil effects of alcohol.

6. Person's weak mentality, coupled with easy availability of alcohol.
7. Tension, failure of love, disappointments and frustrations.
8. Giving importance to scenes of drinking in media, as well as in films.
9. Take help of alcohol to achieve professional or occupational progress.
10. Home environment.
11. Urbanization/industrialization.

Alcoholism has been characterized by four factors:
1. Excessive intake of alcoholic beverages.
2. Individuals increasing worry over his drinking.
3. Lose of the drinking control over his drinking.
4. The disturbance in functioning in his social world.

Features of Habitual Drinkers
1. Begins to drink from morning.
2. Drinking as means to escape reality.
3. Continuous increase in the amount of alcohol.
4. Social duties affected because of alcoholism.
5. Unusual behavior.
6. Restlessness and become unconscious.
7. Weight loss, nausea, vomiting and pain in abdomen.
8. Liver diseases.
9. Beating family members, criminal tendencies.

Treatment of Alcoholics

Sl.No.	Type	Description
1.	Detoxification in hospitals	For alcoholic addiction, the first step in detoxification. Alcoholics need medical case and medical supervision. Tranquilizers are used for treating their withdrawal symptoms like convulsions and hallucinations. High potency vitamins and fluid electrolyte balance are also used in their physical rehabilitation.
2.	Role of family	Involving an alcoholic's family in his treatment and rehabilitation enhances the chances in success by 75 to 80%. The family members do not preach; nor do they blame or condemn the alcoholic.
3.	Alcoholics anonymous	It is an organization of ex-alcoholics which started is the united started in the early 1940's and today has lakhs of persons as its members. In India, the branches exists is all the metropolitan cities.
4.	Treatment centers	There centers have been developed in some cities alternative to hospital treatment. Each center has about 10-20 residents. Here, not only counseling takes place in a supportive environment but residents are made to follow certain anti-drinking rules too.
5.	Changing values through education	Voluntary organizations undertake educational and informational programmers to alter the alcoholics to the dangers of excessive drinking. Social worker help the drinkers in coping with life and changing the social values and attitudes about drinking.

Suggestions for Controlling Alcoholism

1. Large scale health education program against alcohol.
2. Improve working conditions in industrial concerns.
3. Better recreational facilities.
4. Alcohol shops should not be in the vicinity of thickly populated areas, schools, factories, religious places, bus stands or railway stations.
5. High officials and leaders should leave drinking and thus present an ideal or example before common people.
6. Restriction on serving alcohol in social functions.
7. Increase the number of dry days.
8. Start a movement against alcohol gets the cooperation of women.
9. The government should relinquish the greed of revenue of excise duty being collected from alcohol shops, clubs.
10. Any unrest and crime committed by alcoholics should be severely dealt with immediately.

Conclusion

Addiction to alcoholism and excessive drinking disastrous physiological, psychological and socio-moral effects. Repeated consumption of alcohol beverages is harmful not only for the individual, but also for his family and society. When alcohol is consumed moderately or frequently in small quantity does not constitute a social problem. It becomes a social problem only when individuals become alcoholic. Alcoholic means a drinker, who is an excessive drinking, without which he cannot live.

UNEMPLOYMENT

Introduction

Unemployment generally means, failure of a potential individual to get an opportunity to work or who refuse to work is said to be unemployed. In other words one who fails to get an opportunity to work in gainful productive activity is called unemployment. Hence, a condition or situation in which some capable individuals though willing to work but fail to get a job opportunity to get some regular income for their livelihood is called unemployment. In India, since Independence, unemployment has increased tremendously. Based on registered unemployed persons, the magnitude of unemployment was estimated to 37.2 million in 1995 so, unemployment is a serious problem in India.

Concepts of Unemployment

1. Unemployment is an important socioeconomic problem in all societies. It hinders the economic progress and it is an indication of low standard of living and inefficient utilization of man power.
2. Unemployment whether of a permanent or temporary nature has many bad consequences not only for the worker himself but for the worker's family and the community at large.
3. Unemployment is a condition of the labor marked in which the supply of labor is greater than the number of available openings.
4. Unemployment is a state of affairs when in a country there are large numbers of able-bodied persons of working age who are willing to work, but cannot find work at the current wage levels.

5. Elements of unemployment: Prof. Ram Ahuja has pointed out three elements of unemployment.
   a. An individual should be capable of working.
   b. He should be willing to work.
   c. He must make an effort to find work.

Types of Unemployment

1. **Seasonal:** This is caused by seasonal changes in production, e.g. in the case of agriculture, or work in a dockyard.
2. **Cyclical:** Caused by economic ups and downs. When there is depression, there is much unemployment.
3. **Normal:** This type of unemployment is the inevitable concomitant or any economic system based upon a free labor market, as we find in England or America or in India too. Thus, a minimum amount of unemployment is inevitable.
4. **Technological:** It is the result of certain changes in the technique of production which may not warrant much labor.
5. **Structural unemployment:** Structural unemployment is associated with the inadequacy of productive capacity to create enough job for all those able and willing to work.
6. **Frictional unemployment:** Frictional unemployment is caused due to improper adjustment between supplies of labor, seasonal nature of work, breakdown of machinery, etc.
7. **Disguised unemployment:** Disguised unemployment may be described as a situation in which excessive number of people is doing the work than actually required.
8. **Open unemployed:** Open unemployed refers to a situation wherein a large labor force does not get employment opportunities that may yield them regular income.
9. **Voluntary unemployment:** This refers to those workers who are not willing to work at the going wage rate even if they could get one.
10. **Involuntary unemployment:** It refers to that worker currently unemployed even though they are ready to join at market wages rate.

Causes of Unemployment

1. Lack of capital and lack of investment.
2. High production or over production, imbalance between demand and supply.
3. Faulty economic planning.
4. Backwardness of agriculture.
5. Rapid growth of population.
6. Lack of man power planning.
7. Defective education system which generates only educated unemployed persons.
8. Illness and disability.
9. Geographic immobility of labor.
10. Lack of vocational guidance and training.
11. Inadequate medical facilities keep the villagers sick for a longer time.
12. Festivals, sradas, pilgrimages and other traditional religious and cultural activities. These hinder the villagers from working.
13. The excessive increase in population is the main factor in unemployment.

Evil Effects of Unemployment

1. **Social effects:** Unemployment leads to personal disorganization and family disorganization.
2. He suffers from personal disorganization, his health is affected, his family and the community is also affected.
3. The youth are prone to antisocial activities and unlawful activities like smuggling, drug trafficking and terrorism.
4. Lack of jobs lead to physical illness, tension, suicide and crime. This leads to social disorganization.

Unemployment in India

The problem of unemployment and underemployment seems to have been there for long time, but no exact estimate about the magnitude of the problem in quantitative terms was available till 1951. However, it was noted by the Planning Commission that the problem has been aggravated in the last hundred years or so because of:
1. Rapid growth of population.
2. The disappearance of the old rural industries which provided part-time employment to a large number of persons in the rural areas.
3. Inadequate development of the non-agricultural sector from the point of view of employment.
4. A large displacement of population as a result of partition.
5. The population growth has reached beyond the controllable stage.

Steps Suggested

In order to meet the problem of unemployment and underemployment various measures were to be taken.
1. Removal of personal disabilities.
2. Unemployment among the masses.
3. Educated unemployed.
4. Seasonal unemployment.
5. Unemployment due to immobility of labor and technological changes.

Measures Taken to Control Unemployment

1. The Government of India has proclaimed and implemented various measures and planning strategies to solve the problem of unemployment.
2. Employment Orientation Program have been implemented under 5-year-plan in independent India. The eighth-five-year plan gave attention to employment in the rural areas.
3. The important program that are initiated by the Government of India are:
   a. Pradhanamantri Gramodya Yojana (PMGY).
   b. Prime Minister Rozgar Yojana (PMRY-1993).
   c. Self Employment Programs.
   d. National Food for Work Program (NEWP-2004).
   e. Rural Employment Generation Program (REGP-1995).
   f. Street Shakti Yojana (Empowerment of Women).
4. The other remedies suggested are recognization of vocational courses, job oriented training, software technology, poultry and dairy farming, garment industries, leather industries, art, and crafts.

Remedies of Unemployment

1. Improvement in the agricultural system.
2. Land reclamation, conservation, and improvement.
3. Development of cottage industries, animal husbandry, poultry farming, food preservation, and fisheries.
4. Population control.
5. Assessment of the problem.
6. Organization of rural labor.

Conclusion

Unemployment is one of the major problems throughout the world and particularly in India. On the basis of available data there are more than one crore unemployed and similar figure of people under employed? Most of the unemployed are educated people with degrees to their credit. The faulty system of education is responsible for it. Thousands of young boys and girls are being admitted to the institutions of higher learning without any prospect of employment for them. Even technical people like engineers and doctors remain unemployed or under employed. Without gainful employment, an individual suffers; his family and society too suffer.

BIBLIOGRAPHY

1. Anderson and Parker Society. Van Nostrand Company, New York, 1964.
2. Ann J Zwemer. Basic Psychology for Nurses in India. BI Pub, Chennai.
3. Argyle, Michael. The Scientific Study of Social Behaviour, Methuen and Co, London, 1957.
4. Arnold Matthew. Culture and Anarchy, Smith Elder, London,1889.
5. Balsara FN. Sociology: An Analysis of General Sociological Principles, Lakhani Book Depot, Mumbai, 1956.
6. Barker, Ernest. Political Thought in England, 1884-1914. Thomton Butterworth Ltd, London, 1928.
7. Barnes H Elmer. Social Institutions, Prentice-Hall, New York, 1946.
8. Barnes, H Elmer. An Introduction to the History of Sociology. The University of Chicago Press, Chicago, 1948.
9. Barnes, Tecters, New Horizons in Criminology, Prentice-Hall, 1959.
10. Bell Clive. Civilization, Penguin Books, Middlesex, 1947.
11. Benedict Ruth. Race and Racism, Routledge and Kegan Paul, London, 1951.
12. Bogardus, Emory S. The Development of Social Thought, Longmans, New York, 1950.
13. Bosanquet Helm. The Family, Macmillan, London, 1915.
14. Broom L, Selznjck P. Sociology, Peterson and Cornpany, Row, New York, 1958.
15. Brunner and Siddhartha.Medical Surgical Nursing.
16. Carr-Sawiders AM. World Population. Oxford Press, 1937.
17. Census of India, Paper I, Govt. of India Publication 1971.
18. Childe Gardon. Social Evolution, Watts and Co., London, 1951.
19. Chilman and Thomas. Understanding Nursing Care. Churchill Livingstone.
20. Cole GDH. Social Theory, Methuen and Co., London, 1920.
21. Cooley CH. Introductory Sociology.
22. Corriis Pt HD. The Hindu Joint Family, Cambridge University Press, 1915.
23. Davis Kingsley. Human Society. The Macmillan Company, 1960.
24. Davis Kingsley. The Population of India and Pakistan, Princeton University Press, Princetones, New Jersey, 1951.
25. Dcr C. "Crime: Its Causes and Punishment," 1934.
26. Deniker S. The Races of Men. Walter Scott Ltd, London, 1960.
27. Desai AR. Introduction to Rural Sociology in India, Mumbai.
28. Disease: Health Care Professional Guide, Spring House Corporation, Pennsylvania.
29. DN Shrivastav. General Psychology. Vinod Pustak Mandir, Agra.

30. Dunn LC, Dobzhansk RH. Heredity, Race, and Society, The New American Library, New York, 1952.
31. Dunn LC. Heredity and Variation, The University Society, New York 1934.
32. Encyclopedia of Social Sciences. Vol. XV.
33. Furfey, Paul H. The Scope and Methods of Sociology, Harper and Brothers, New York, 1953.
34. Ghwye GS. Caste and Class In India, Popular Book Depot, Mumbai, 1950.
35. Giddings, Fyankiin H. Principles of Sociology, The Macmillan Company, New York, 1904.
36. Gillin and Glum. "Cultural Sociology". The Macmillan Co., New York, 1950.
37. Ginsberg, Morris, The Psychology of Society, Methuen, 7th edn, London, 1949.
38. Ginsberg, Morris. Studies In Sociology, Methuen, London, 1932.
39. Ginsberg, Morris. The Idea of Progress. Methuen and Co, London, 1953.
40. Green Arnold W. Sociology, McGraw-Hill Book Co. Inc., New York, 1956.
41. Hate Charaiccija A. Hindu Woman and Her Future, New Book Company, Mumbai, 1948.
42. Henry, Jaew Bill, Joyce Edavis, CW Benedic. Mosby's Guide to Physical Examination.
43. Himes Joseph S. "Social Planning in America", Garden City, Double-day and Company, 1954.
44. HJ Eysenck. Uses and Abuses of Psychology. Penguin Books.
45. Hobhouse LT. Moral in Evolution, Chapman Hall, reprinted, London, 1951.
46. Hobhouse LT. Social Development, Henry Holt and Co, New York, 1924.
47. Horton and Hunt. Sociology, McGraw-Hill, New York, 1968.
48. Hutton JH. Caste in India. Oxford University Press, 1951.
49. India, Government of Social Welfare in India, New Delhi, 1955.
50. India, Government of The Fives Years Plans, New Delhi, 1951, 1956.
51. India, Publications Division, New Delhi. 1974.
52. Jeannec Scherer, BK Timby. Introductory Medical Surgical Nursing, 6th edn. Lippincott.
53. Jennings HS, et al. Scientific Aspect of the Race Problem, New York, Longmans, Green and Co., 1941.
54. Johnson HM. Sociology, Allied Publishers, Mumbai, 1960.
55. K Park. Textbook of Preventive and Social Medicine, Banarsidas Bhanot, Jabalpur.
56. Kapadia KM. The Hindu Code Bill, Popular Book Depot, Mumbai,1950.
57. Karve DG. Indian Population, The National Information and Publications Ltd., Mumbai, 1948.
58. Katz. David. Animals and Men, Penguin Books, London, 1953.
59. Kelserz, Huns. Society and Nature, Kegan Paul, Trench Treuhner and Co., London, 1946.
60. Kim bolt Young, RW Mack. Systematic Sociology', East-West Press, New Delhi, 1972.
61. Koenig Samuel, Hopper, RD, Gross, Feliks, "Sociology Prentice-Hall, 1958.
62. Koenig, Samuel Sociology: Man and Society, Barnes and Noble Inc., New York,1961.
63. KP Pothen, S Pothen. Sociology for Nurses. NR Brothers, Indore.
64. Ktineberg, Otto. Race Differences, Harper and Brothers, New York, 1939.
65. La Piere RT. Sociology, McGraw, New York, 1946.
66. MA Priest. Personal and Communal Health for Nurses.
67. Ogbum WF. Social Change, Calverton, B.V.edlt. The Making of Society, The Modern Library, New York, 1937.
68. Ogburn , Nimkoff . A Handbook of Soctology, Routledge and Kegari PauL, London, 1950.
69. Park, Borgess. Introduction to the Science of Sociology.
70. Prabhu, Pandhari Nalh. Hindu Social Organisation, Bombay, Popular Book Depot, 1954.
71. Reuter, FB. Handbook of Sociology, The Drydon Press, New York 1948.
72. Rine and Bennett. Community Nursing in Developing Countries. Oxford University Press.
73. Roneck Joseph S. Social Control. Nostrand Company, 1956.
74. Rose Arnold. The Roots of Prejudice, UNESCO, Paris, 1951.
75. Ross and Wilson. Anatomy and Physiology in Health and Illness.
76. Ross EJ. Fundamental Sociology, The Bruce Publishing Co., Milkwaukee, 1945.
77. Secord, Buckmart, Social Psychology, Mc Graw-Hill Book Company, New York, 1964.
78. Seligman. Encyclopaedia of the Social Sciences, Vol. II, Introduction, Macmillan, Reprint, 1949.
79. Sheaf, Sheaf . An Outline of Social Psychology, Harper & Brothers, New York, 1956.

80. Siddhantalankor S. Samaj Shastra Ke Mul Tattwa. Dehradun Vidya Vihar, Balbir AV, 1954.
81. Sinclair and Faweett Baillere. Altschul's Psychology for Nurses. Tindall.
82. Smelser, Neil J. Sociology-An Introduction Wiley Eastern Private Limited, New Delhi, 1970.
83. Smith and Duell. Clinical Nursing Skills—Basic to Advance Skills. Appleton and Lange Stamfort CT.
84. Sorensen and Luckman. Basic Nursing—A Psychological Approach, 3rd edn. WB Saunders.
85. Soro kin P. Society Culture and Personality. Harper and Brothers, Publishers, New York, 1947.
86. Spencer Herbert. Principles of Sociology, (3 VoIs.), William and Norgate, London, 1897.
87. Sprott WJH. Social Psychology, Methuen and Co.Ltd., London, 1952.
88. Sprott WJH. Sociology. Hutchinson's University Library, London, 1956.
89. Sumner W. Graham. Folkways. New York. Ginn and Company,
90. Sutherland, Woodwczrd and Maxwell. Introductory Sociology, Oxford and IBH Publishing Go. Bombay, 1961.
91. Swnnër WG, Keller AG. The Science of Society, 4 Vols., New Haven Yale University Press, 1946.
92. Taylor, Lillis and Lemone JB. Fundamental of Nursing. Lippincott Company.
93. The Society of Agricultural Economics, 1953.
94. TNAI. Community Health Nursing Manual.
95. VB Sachdeva. An Introduction to Sociology, Kitab Mahal, Delhi.

43 *Health Promotion*

The promotion of health falls firmly into the remit of nursing. That is not to say that health promotion is an exclusively nurse led activity; rather, that lies at the very heart of nursing. Nurse practitioners encompass the principles of health promotion; indeed, every consultation can be seen as a health promoting opportunity. There is much debate about definition of health promotion and health education.

DEFINITION

Health education is communication activity aimed at enhancing positive health and preventing or diminishing ill health in individuals and groups through influencing the beliefs, attitudes and behavior of those with power and of the community at large.

Health promotion is defined as efforts to enhance positive health and reduce the risk of ill health through the overlapping spheres of health education, prevention and health promotion.

HEALTH

The world health organization (WHO) in 1948 defined health as 'a state of complete physical mental and social wellbeing, Ewles and Simnett (1995) say, "Health is to do with the ability to adapt to constantly changing demands, expectations and stimuli."

Factors Affecting Health

There are many factors, which affect a person's health status. Naidoo and Wills (1994) list the main influences upon health as genetic, biological, lifestyle, environmental and social factors. It is important to remain aware of the multiplicity of factors affecting an individual's health and therefore to consider the range of influences up on the person including family, employment, learned behavior, health beliefs, politics, housing and available health services.

HEALTH PROMOTION

Health promotion, according to the WHO definition is an action, and it includes activity at an individual level as well as at a national level. Health Promotion is defined by Tones (1993) as the product of health public policy and health education, with the major function of health education being empowerment.

IMPLEMENTING HEALTH PROMOTION IN PRACTICES

Health Promotion in Acute Setting

Traditionally the focus of health promotion has been seen as an activity, which occurs in primary care. Nurse practitioners can also be located in hospital settings where time and resources are frequently cited as reasoning for not putting health promotion into practice.

In 1978 the WHO held an international conference which resulted in the alma ata declaration exhorting governments to strengthen primary health care. There is incredible potential for the practice of health promotion in each nurse practitioner consultation.

Approaches to health education: In order to work with individuals who have a wide variety of definitions of health and have numerous influences upon their health status, it is necessary to consider the variety of approaches to health promotion. Katz and Peherdy (1997) outline five approaches to health promotion: Medical, behavioral, educational client centered and social change.

Medical Approach

The medical approach to health promotion uses scientific methods to address the problems of disease and ill health. Preventive measures include immunizations and screening to allow for prevention and the early detection of medically defined illness.

Behavioral Approach

The behavioral approach seeks to encourage individuals to adopt healthy behaviors. The individual should be at a decreased risk of developing diseases, which are associated with high-risk behaviors such as smoking, consumption of alcohol, excessive consumption of fatty foods or in some cases, sexual intercourse with barrier protection. Health education is often focused on behavior change and relies heavily upon the individuals willingness to adopt a healthier lifestyle.

Educational Approach

The educational approach aims to provide individuals with the knowledge and understanding necessary to make an informed choice about their health. This approach does not set out to persuade an individual to change in a certain direction; rather, the aim is to provide the individual with the information necessary to make an appropriate decision.

Client Centered Approach

The client centered approach helps the client to identify concerns and priorities. The role of the health educator is to provide the client with the necessary tools and skills to get the agenda and to act upon the identified concerns. This approach sets the client firmly at the center of the activity; the client is an equal partner in the health education process and the health promoter simply addresses the areas of concern to the client.

Social Change

Social change is directed at the environment with in which a person lives. Political action is focused upon changing the social, physical or economic environment and thereby making it possible, or more likely, for individuals to make healthy lifestyle choices.

MODELS OF HEALTH PROMOTION

A model of the promotion helps to provide a framework to analyze and guide practice. There are many models of health promotion suits the style of activity with certain clients or client groups more than another. Tones (1996) has developed a model of empowerment and health promotion which brings together health education, self and community empowerment, health public policy, environment and social circumstances and equity.

Each of these concepts underpins the individual's ability to achieve health.

Beattie (1991) suggests that there are four strategies for health promotion: Individual persuasion, legislative action, personal counseling and community development. The strategy employed can therefore be authoritative or based on negotiation and may be an individual activity or the focus of collective activity. The health belief model (Becker 1994) focuses on the role of health beliefs in determining an individual's action. The health belief model is based on the assumption that each person will consider the cost and benefits of a particular behavior and engage in health actions accordingly in order to engage in behavior, which will prevent illness and/or promote health and well-being. The nurse practitioner could utilize the framework of the health belief model to enhance the possibility of the patient in the above scenario engaging in health promoting activities.

Theory of Reasoned Action

Ajzen and Fishbeins (1980) theory of reasoned action is another model which can help the nurse practitioner to understand the behavior of patients and the reasons why some choose to adopt health lifestyle actions and other do not.

Helping People Change

It is clearly of great concern to any health care professional involved in health promotion that if changes are made towards a healthier lifestyle, those changes should be permanent. Prochaska and Diclemente (1984) developed a stage model of behavior acquisition, which outlines the stages involved in changing behavior. The stages model of health promotion, which has been widely used in primary health care, is particularly relevant in the management and support of people who are overweight and attempting to change the dietary habits. The stages model of health promotion can help the nurse practitioner to support and understand the patient through the change process. Social support is essential to reinforce the need for behavioral change and to maintain the change.

CONCLUSION

Health promotion is defined as "efforts to enhance positive health and reduce the risk of ill health through the overlapping spheres of health education, prevention and health production". The nurse practitioners have a role to play at a variety of levels of health promotion, however during individual consultations; the activity of nursing intervention will tend to be focused upon health education at an individual level.

The Patient as Partner in Nursing Care Set-up

44

INTRODUCTION

As the boundaries between medicine and nursing become increasingly blurred, nurse practitioners must not lose sight of one of the main advantages of the delivery of health services by a nurse—the ability to work with the patient as partner.

Brearley (1990) states that patient participation can be constructed as a potential threat to the autonomy of medicine. As nurse practitioners take on many of the tasks of medicine, however, there is a risk that patients will perceive the nurse in a different way and may be less willing to enter into a partnership.

It is essential therefore to consider why we want to encourage partnerships with patients and how we might go about enhancing such a relationship. The models of nursing and the skills that can be used to enhance partnerships with a particular focus on the consultation process.

PARTNERSHIPS

A partnership is a relationship between parties working towards a joint venture. At it is most basic level, this partnership is between the nurse and an individual patient during the consultation process. The relationship is commonly more complex than this and can include any of the following:
1. The patient's family
2. Other groups of patients
3. The local community and the population of the nation.

The one to one relationship is the most frequently occurring partnership in the everyday practice of nurse practioners. Brearley (1990) states that individual patient participation can be viewed as a continuum with complete passivity at one end and complete activity at the other.

The nurse practitioner needs to increase his or her level of activity to form a dynamic active relationship with the patient. In primary health care the relationship between the nurse practitioner and the patient often develops over a period of time. The accuracy of diagnosis associated with patient participation can also have advantages at a community level.

Nurse practitioners therefore must consider the issue of partnerships whilst remaining mindful of the individuality of each patient. Taking the risk of encouraging the patient to play an active role in health care could potentially enhance patient satisfaction. In order to implement the concept of partnership in your practice you need a clear understanding of the principles, which underpin your actions. The principles, which govern the nurse practitioner's practice, can be examined from ethical, sociological, psychological and political perspectives.

AUTONOMY

Autonomy refers to individual's capacity to choose freely for them and to direct their own life. Respecting autonomy involves respecting another person's right as a human being. The rights relating to healthcare include the right to information, the right to privacy and confidentiality and the right to appropriate care and treatment.

If the nurse practitioner utilizes the ethical principle of autonomy to consider the patient as a partner then each patient has a right to information relating to his or her diagnosis and treatment and this information should be provided for the patient in an appropriate and understandable way.

PATERNALISM

Paternalism refers to an action taken by one person in the best interests of another without the latter's consent. Paternalism does not respect the rights of the human being and results in the patient a passive role in health care.

BENEFICENCE AND NON-MALEFICENCE

Beneficence and non-maleficence relate to promoting good and doing no harm. Patients should be informed that the course of action aims to promote their wellbeing and do them no harm in the process. A patient who is participating in the process of health care therefore needs to be fully informed of the consequences of treatment decisions. Possible harmful side effects should be discussed.

SOCIOLOGICAL PERSPECTIVE

A sociological perspective on the issue of patients as partners considers the issue of the roles people play in society. Illness is seen as sociologically deviant behavior- a negative and undesirable state. The effective performance of social roles is diminished by ill health. It is useful for nurse practitioners to be aware of the social meaning of the roles we adopt in each consultation with a patient.

PSYCHOLOGICAL PERSPECTIVE

The contention than an increase in patient participation in health care will prove beneficial to patients has been supported by psychological theory. A variety of personal characteristics, including hardiness, learned helplessness, self-efficacy and locus can be examined with a psychological frame work and linked to the patient's willingness or ability to participate in health care. Hardiness is described as a group of characteristics that function as a resistance to stressful life events, including commitment, control and challenge. Learned helplessness means learning one's own actions have no influence upon outcomes. Self-efficacy is a sense of self-competence or self-mastery, which leads to a sense of self-esteem or self-worth. Locus of control is the degree to which the person believes that the events, which happen to him or her, occur as a result of his or her own behavior or as a result of luck or fate.

POLITICAL CONTEXT

The political climate has helped to enhance awareness of patient's rights and the value of engaging patients as partners in care. Community health council is available to patients who wish to make comments about health services or those who wish to complain. The National Consumer Council issued a similar document in 1938, which outlined the patient's rights in relation to choice and consent, information, the rights of children and the right to complain. It has been recognized that people expect more from their health service and provision of information has been one response to that expectation. It has also been recognized that there is value on placing the patient firmly in the center of the process of health care provision. Recognizing the value of patient's involvement in their care empowers them and tends to encourage more active partnership in health care provisions.

METHODS OF ENHANCING PARTNERSHIPS

1. The skills required to promote the active involvement of patients in their health care will be employed by nurse practitioners during the consultation process with their parents.
2. Livesey (1986) suggests that we should consider the following points in consultation with patients' expectations, welcome patient's story, partners in care, physical examination, examination of the emotions, personalities and problems, simple explanations and the farewell.
3. There are several nurse theorists who have considered the value of partnerships in care. Depending upon the area of practice and own nursing philosophy may find that a nursing model can provide a framework for your work. Dorothy Orem's self-care model for nursing, the most fundamental belief, which underpins Orem's model, is that a need for self-care exists in each individual.
4. Sister Callista Roy, who made the client visible in the health care process as setting mutual goals with clients. Henderson, who identified the nursing role as complementary to and supplementing the patient's own knowledge. The individual patient plays a limited and mostly passive role within this framework. Nurse practitioners would be offering anything more than a substitute service when the whole purpose of implementing the role of the nurse practitioner should be to enhance the service we are currently offering our clients.

QUALITY ASSURANCE AND SERVICE PLANNING

Nurse practitioners can choose to research or audit their work in variety of ways. The dynamic standard setting system is one method of setting standards of care and monitoring those standards. The dynamic standard setting system is based on six key principles, which were originally developed by a group of nurse's in Oxford.
1. Ownership—the standard is written by the practitioners delivering the care.
2. Participation—the practitioners must be involved with the process.
3. Patient-focused—the patient should be at the heart of the initiative.
4. Situation-based—it must be clear whom the standards are for.
5. Setting achievable standards—the standards must be practical and realistic.
6. Multidisciplinary standards—the standards must transfer across disciples.

This process ensures that the patient is not only a partner during individual consultations at the bedside or in the consulting room but also a partner in the planning and delivery of health care services to the local population.

CONCLUSION

The concept of patient participation is the work of nurse practitioner. The nurse practitioner finds that some patients do not wish to be actively involved in the decision making process or the management of their condition and need to be flexible to adopt the appropriate approach in each situation.

45

Basic Concepts of Holistic Nursing Care

INTRODUCTION

The term holism was coined by Jan Smutus, a South American stated in his book holism and evaluation in 1926. In holistic care, the concept of Yin and Yang of the Chinese culture and the hot and cold theory of illness in many Spanish culture is examples of holistic health belief.

The goal of holistic nursing as described by the American Holistic Nurses Association by enhancing healing of the whole person from the birth to death. Holistic health practioners focus on all brain thinking, a blending of liner processes regulated by the left hemisphere and intuitive through process regulated by the right hemisphere.

DEFINITIONS

1. Holistic care means physical, mental, emotional and spiritual care of the patient. It holds the force of nature to maintain balance or harmony.
2. Holistic care is a system that considers all components of health, health promotion health maintenance, health education, illness prevention and restorative rehabilitative care. Identification of patient's needs, planning, implementation and evaluation of holistic care require sensitivity to individual, family and cultural values.
3. Holistic health care involves, the total person, the whole of the persons being and the overall quality of life style.

Holism acknowledges and respects the interaction of a reasons mind, body and spirit within the environment.

MEANING

Holism, derived from the Greek holos (Whole), was first used by South African philosopher Jan Christian Smuts (1996) in holism and evolution. Smuts saw holism as an antidote to atomistic approach of contemporary science.

An atomistic approach takes things apart, examining the person piece by piece in an attempt to understand the large picture. Holism is based on the belief that people (or even their parts) can not be fully understood if examined solely in pieces apart from their environment. Holism sees people as ever changing system of energy.

THE HOLISTIC HEALTH MODEL

The holistic health model of nursing attempts to create condition that promotes optimal health. In this model nurses using the nursing process consider clients as the ultimate experts regarding their own health and respect client's subjective experience as relevant in maintaining health and assisting in healing. Here the clients are involved in their healing process; there by assuming some responsibilities for maintaining health, thus the clients are able to gain personal control over their health and illness. Holistic are mirrors paradox of the Yin/Yang/symbol, which the mutual interdependence of two major forces.

WELLNESS AND HOLISTIC CARE

Holistic care emphasizes humanism, choices, self-care activities and a peer relationship between the health care provider and the client. These interventions focus on the interrelated needs of body, mind/emotions and spirit.

Holistic practitioners use the term psychosomatic to mean not simply that the mind and body are so interrelated that they act on each other in an intimate, direct, inseparable way. Therefore, holistic health practitioners acknowledge the interactive process of the mind, body and spirit.

HOLISTIC PRACTICE

Holistic practitioners recognize the incredible strides that traditional medicine has made toward wellness (e.g. antibiotics and surgery).They are especially mindful of the risk of iatrogenic illness or illness that results from treatment and may be traced to the over use and abuse of prescribed medications.

DIMENSIONS OF HOLISTIC CARE

1. **Self responsibility:** The first dimension of a wellness lifestyle is self-responsibility for ones own wellbeing. There are many roles that each person fulfills in his or her daily life to provide numerous opportunities for promoting health and preventing disease.
2. **Self-awareness:** It means knowing and caring for oneself. Recognizing one's strengths and limitations. Holistic health practices add to this self knowledge on all levels (Physical, Psychological, Social and spiritual), enabling the person's to identify his or her state of being and decide the priorities of service required. Self knowing is likely to be the first step toward self-caring.
3. **Informed choices:** Making informed choices, being an active participant rather than a passive recipient, can benefit ones self-concept. Changes in self-concept may facilitate fundamental changes in the person's belief system. The holistic health practitioner can use this decision to change by encouraging the person to examine his to her lifestyle and to consider moving towards high-level wellness.

NURSING IN WELLNESS AND HOLISTIC HEALTH CARE

Nursing has traditionally been a holistic profession. Nursing theorists have promoted aspects of holistic care across time. Acknowledging the wisdom of least invasive treatment and the inter-relationship of person can maintain life, health and wellbeing.

According to Martha Rogers, the primary purpose of nursing is to help achieve their maximum health potential. By promoting high-level wellness and preventing illness whenever possible, the holistic nurse uses and approach that minimizes risk and empowers the client.

Nursing is returning the its historical roots while simultaneously responding to ever — evolving technology, cost containment and consumer demands, nurses are challenged to retain the humanspects, including the spiritual aspect of nursing that values the meaning and purpose of life and death.

Holistic nurses also recognize a duty to provide the healthiest environment for themselves and generations to come. An indication of the shared purpose and mutual support among nurses active in holistic health care.

HOLISTIC HEALTH CARE MODALITIES

1. **Lifestyle modification:** Holistic practitioners advocate the use of life style modification skills such as meditation, exercise or relaxation that alleviate stress and promote a state less susceptible to disease.
2. **Medication:** It is a deep personal thought and reflection may be one of the most basic and powerful self care activities that we can incorporate into our lives. Meditation is a way to tune and train the mind that to greater efficiency in everyday' life.
3. **Imagery:** It is the internal experience of a perceptual every in the absence of the actual external stimuli. The imagery process includes seeing themselves as whole, well and full of energy.
4. **Therapeutic touch:** Therapeutic touch is a technique derived from the ancient practice of. laying on hands. According to the philosophy on therapeutic touch, the client's state of health is reflected in the vital energy field that surrounds him or her. Therapeutic touch as a healing meditation, because the centering or achieving a sense of peace and wholeness with in himself or herself.

CONCLUSION

The holistic health care was formed in, 1980 of the American Holistic Nurses Association. The holistic health model recognizes the unique interaction of a persons mind, body and spirit within the environment. Holistic health care combines he proved success of modern medicine, participation of the client and additional activities to complement medical protocol. Holistic health care interventions include lifestyle modification exercise, meditation, imagery and therapeutic touch.

46 Psychosocial Application in Nursing: A Theoretical Approach by Imogene King

INTRODUCTION

In 1971, Imogene King introduced a conceptual model consisting of three interacting systems. King's latest model of nursing incorporates three dynamic interaction systems: Personal, Interpersonal and Social that leads to development of a theory of goal attainment. According to this theory, individuals (personal system) form groups (interpersonal system) and groups compose a society (social system).

In King's view, nurses and individuals are personal system, who interacts when the individual (or group I interpersonal system) is unable to cope with an event or health problem. These personal systems enter the health care system (social system) or request services from a health professionals and goal attainment for the individual or group.

BACKGROUND OF THEORIST

1. Imogene King completed her basic nursing education in 1945, when she received her Diploma in nursing from St. John's Hospital School of Nursing, St. Louis.
2. In 1948, she received her BSc in Nursing education and in 1957, her MSc in Nursing from St Louis University.
3. In 1961, she was awarded a doctorate in education from teachers college, Columbia University, New York city. She has held positions in nursing education, administration and practice.
4. King began formulating her theory with an associate professor of nursing in Loyola University, Chicago, where she developed a master's degree programs in nursing, using a conceptual framework.
5. In 1971, she published a theory for nursing; general concepts of human behavior, in which she proposed a conceptual framework for nursing rather than a theory.
6. In 1981, she refined her ideas in a theory of nursing system, concepts and process. King bases her theory on general system theory, the behavioral sciences and deductive and inductive reasoning.

OPEN SYSTEM FRAMEWORK

General Information

1. It is based on assumption that humans are open system in constant interaction with their environment.
2. It consists of three interacting system: Personal, interpersonal and social.

Personal System

The personal system consists solely of individual and includes perception, self, growth and development, body image, space and time.

1. Perception, is the primary feature of personal system because it influences all other behaviors, refers to a person's representation of reality; it is universal, yet highly subjective and unique to each person.
2. Self refers to a person's subjective environment, which constitutes everything that makes up the person; it includes ideas, attitudes, values, and commitments.
3. Growth and development refers to all the changes (cellular, molecular and behavioral) occurring in a person; these changes are usually orderly and predictable, yet subject to individual variations.
4. Body image refers to the manner in which one perceives one's body and the reaction of others to it: Body image is highly subjective and changes-to-changes as the person changes physically territory occupied by a person and to persons behaviors.
5. Time refers to a sequence of events and their relationship to each other.

Interpersonal System

1. This system occurs when humans socialize and includes interaction, communication, transaction, role, stress and coping.
2. The greater number of interacting individuals, the more complex the interaction: Two interacting persons form a dyad, three form a triad and four or more form small or large group.
3. Interaction refers to verbal and nonverbal behavior between an individual and the environment or between two or more individuals; it involves goal directed perception and communication.
4. Transaction refers to the interaction between a person and the environment for the purpose of goal attainment.
5. Communication refers to the transmission of information from one person to another, either directly (as face-to-face meeting) or indirectly (as through a telephone call or written message); it is the information component of interaction.
6. Role refers to the expected behaviors of a person in a specific position and their relationship to each other. Rules that govern the position, it affects the interaction between two or more persons.
7. Stress refers to an exchange of energy, either positive or negative, between a person and the environment; object, persons and events can serve as stressors.
8. Coping although considered important by king, is not defined by her.

Social System

1. When interpersonal systems come together, they form larger system (called social system), which include families, religious groups, schools, workplaces and peer groups.
2. A social system comprises the social roles, behaviors and practices which developed to maintain values includes organization, authority, power, status and decision making.
3. Organization refers to a group of people with similar interest who have prescribed roles and positions and use resources to achieve personal and organizational goals.
4. King proposes four parameters of organization: Human values, behavior patterns, needs, goals and expectations.

5. Natural environment containing essential materials and resources: individuals who form group and interact for goal achievement to facilitate goal attainment.
6. Authority refers to the observable behavior of providing guidance and being responsible for action; it is active and reciprocal.
7. Power which is situational, dynamic and goal directed it is characterized by the ability to use resources for goal achievements it also means by which one or more persons can influence others.
8. Status refers to the position occupied by a person in a group or the position occupied by a group in relation to other groups in an organization; it is accompanied by certain duties, privileges and obligations.
9. Decision making results from developing and acting on perceived choices for goal attainment.

GOAL ATTAINMENT THEORY

General Information

1. Represents an expansion of King's original ideas to incorporate the concept of nurse and the patient mutually communicating information, establishing goals and taking action to attain goals.
2. Describes a situation in which two people, usually strangers, come together in a health care organization to help or to be helped to maintain a state of health.
3. It is based on the concepts of personal systems including interaction, perception, communication, transaction role, stress, growth and development, time and space.

Interaction

1. According to King, each individual brings to an interaction of different set of values, ideas, attitudes and perception to exchange.
2. Individuals come together for a purpose; each person makes a judgment, takes mental or physical. Action and reacts to the other individuals and the situation.

Perception

1. A person imports energy from the environment and transforms processes and stores it.
2. The individual then exports this energy, as demonstrated by observable behaviors.

Communication

1. A person provides information directly or indirectly to another person.
2. The other person receives this information and processes it.

Transaction

1. Two individuals mutually identify the goals and means to achieve them.
2. They reach the agreement about how to attain these goals and then set about to realize them.

Role

1. Each person occupies a position in a social system that has specific rules and obligations.
2. Roles can be congruent (resulting in transactions) or in conflict resulting in stress.

Stress

1. When an individual interacts with the environment, an energy response occurs to objects, events and persons.
2. The individual uses this energy response to maintain balance the growth and development and the performance.

Growth and Development

1. Individuals are in a constant state of molecular, cellular and behavioral change.
2. As these changes occur, transactions are made, moving the individual toward a level of maturity and self-actualization.

Space

1. Each person has a designated area or territory that extends from the individual equally in all directions.
2. Specific behaviors exist for the person occupying than the space.

FOUR CONCEPTS OF NURSING METAPARADIGM

Person

1. An individual is a social being who are rational and sentient. Human communicate, their thoughts, action, customs and beliefs through language. Persons exhibit common characteristics such as ability to perceive, to think, to feel, to choose between alterative courses of action, to set goals to select the means to achieve goals to select the means to achieve goals to make decisions.
2. According to King's person is social, sentient, rational, perceiving, controlling, purposeful, action- oriented and time oriented being. The person has a right to self- knowledge participation in decisions that affect life and health and acceptance or rejection of health care.
3. An individual has three fundamental health needs; timely and useful health information, care that prevents illnesses and help when self-care demands cannot be met.

Environment

1. Environment is not specifically defined by king, although she uses the term internal environment and external environment in her open system.
2. It could be interpreted from the general system theory as an open system with permeable boundaries that allow the exchange of matter, energy and information.

Health

1. Health is a dynamic life experience of a human being, which implies continuous adjustment to stressor in the internal and external environment through optimum use of one's resources to achieve maximum potential for daily living.
2. Health is described by King as a dynamic state in the life cycle; an illness is viewed as interference in the continuum of the life cycle.
3. Health also implies continuous adjustments to stresses in the internal and external environment, using personal resources to achieve optimal daily living.

Nursing

1. Nursing is a process of action, reaction and interaction where nurse and client share information about their perceptions in the nursing situation. The nurse and client share specific goals, problems and concerns and explore means to achieve a goal.
2. Nursing refers to observable nurse client interaction the focus of which is to help the individual maintain health and function in an appropriate role.
3. Nursing is viewed as an interpersonal process of action, reaction, interaction and transaction, a nurse's perceptions and those of the client influence the interaction. It is a service profession that meets a social need.
4. It entails planning, implementation and evaluating nursing care. It also encourages a nurse and client to share information about their perception (if perception are accurate, then goals are attained, growth and development is enhanced and a client perceive congruent role expectations and performance, transactions occur; if role conflict ensures, stress occurs.
5. Nursing uses a goal oriented directed approach in which individuals within a social system interact; the nurse brings special knowledge and skills to the nursing process and the client brings self-knowledge and perceptions.

CONCLUSION

King's model views nurses as interacting with clients who are unable to cope with environment stressors through perception and communication to achieve transactions. The nurse and client establish mutual goals and explore and agree on means to achieve goals. When transactions occur, goals are achieved. Also, the model can be applied in numerous health care settings and include the importance of collaboration among health professionals. This model can be applied to individuals, families or groups; major psychological. Sociocultural and interpersonal concepts are answered.

47 *Transcultural Nursing*

INTRODUCTION

The English word "Culture" has been used in various concepts. In common literature culture means social charm and intellectual excellence. Some sociologists have also accepted cultured people as leaders of society. According to Sorokin and MacIver, culture stands for the moral, spiritual and intellectual attainments of man. In the words of Bogardus, "culture is composed of integrated customs, behavior patterns of human groups".

The word culture has had a number of meanings. Originally it referenced to the arts and humanities. The cultured man was one who was well-versed in drama, philosophy and the arts. Nurses have always been contender with the whole person, including the physical, emotional, psychological, spiritual and developmental dimensions. The culture incorporates not only customs, but beliefs, values and attitudes shared by a group of people and passed down through generations.

DEFINITIONS

1. According to Tylor, culture is that complex whole which includes knowledge, belief, art, morals, law, customs and any other capabilities and habits acquired by man, as member of society.
2. According to AW Green, culture is the socially transmitted system of idealized ways in knowledge and practice and belief along with the artifacts that knowledge and practice produce and maintain as the change in style.
3. According to Leininger, the transcultural nursing is described as that which incorporates all aspects of a person's culture in planning and providing care, transcultural nursing encourages an appreciation of all cultures and discourages imposing your/our cultural practices and others.

HISTORICAL PERSPECTIVES

1. The transcultural nursing has its roots in the early 1900's when public health nurse cared for immigrants from Europe who came from a wide range of cultural backgrounds and had diverse health care practices.
2. During the 19th century, the words come to be used almost interchangeably with civilization. This civilization or culture was something achieved as society is evolved people who were cultured or primitive peoples of the world.
3. In the late 1940's Dr Madeleine Leininger held the belief that "Care is essence of nursing and the central dominant and unifying focus of nursing". She then began to see the importance

of nursing care that was beginning to understand the importance of nursing care that was based on the client's cultures that has unique values.

4. Beliefs practices and life ways passed down from one generation to next. The idea that culture and care are inextricably linked, led her to study other cultures and she becomes the first nurse to obtain a doctorate in anthropology.

5. Transcultural nursing is a body of knowledge and practice for caring the people from other cultures. Many nurse leader and educators have embraced the need for culture specific care, and various approaches to gaining this knowledge have been developed.

6. One such model was developed by Dr Josephacampinha — become, a cape verdean native who now lives and works in the United States. Her model involves cultural skill and cultural encounter. It will be used here as a frame work to help nurse learn the concepts necessary to gain cultural competence in working within community settings.

TRANSCULTURAL NURSING AND THEORY APPLICATIONS

1. Nursing theories and models are transited into produce is through the continuing investigation of how to individualize care to meet the needs of every patient.

2. A leader in researching an answer to this question is Madeleine M Leininger's, a nurse and an anthropologist.

3. Leininger coined the phrase transcultural nursing to describe nursing care that incorporates all aspects of a person's culture in planning and providing care.

4. Transcultural nursing encourages an appreciation of all cultures and discourages imposing your own cultural practices on others. This means respecting other cultures from cultures other than yours.

5. Transcultural nursing is indeed the application of those nursing theories that stress understanding the whole person in the context of total environment.

6. Nurse who consider their patient's value beliefs, spiritual practices and custom before planning nursing care or practice transcultural nursing.

7. Transcultural nursing is needed became of the growing diversity in the population diversity among people in the country can be attributed in part to immigration changes in social values, changes technologies and changes in economic system.

LEININGER'S SUNRISE MODEL TO DEPICT THEORY OF CULTURAL CARE DIVERSITY AND UNIVERSITY MODEL: GOALS OF TRANSCULTURAL NURSING

1. According to Leininger, the goal transcultural nursing care is to preserve accommodate or re-pattern the culture of the patient.

2. When cultural beliefs and values do not have negative effect on care, nursing must make every effort to help the patient preserve his or her culture.

3. In some situations, it may be necessary to make accommodations to preserve the culture of the patient and the family.

4. Repeating the culture of the patient requires the patient to essentially change his or her life.

Universal Characteristics of Culture

1. **Culture includes acquired qualities:** It is the manmade part of environment culture includes all the qualities, habit and ideas, etc. acquired through socialization. Because of this symbolic communication, a man can acquire culture behavior.

2. **Culture is found only in human societies:** There are societies among animals but they do not have culture. In this way man is the only cultured being. In other words, culture is found only in human societies.
3. **Culture is communicable:** Culture is mentally communicated from one generation to another. This brings about a regular expansion of culture. Because of this communication, a new generation can benefit from the experiences of old generation. In this way culture becomes stable and extinction of an individual or group does not affect it.
4. **Culture is not individualistic but social:** Every individual take some part in the expansion and continuation of culture. But culture is instead of being induced elastic.
5. **Culture is idealistic:** Culture includes ideal behavior patterns or rules according to which the members of a society behave, these ideal standards or patterns are accepted by the society.
6. **Culture satisfies certain needs:** Culture satisfies those moral and social needs of a man which are practicable in themselves, culture includes collective habits are formed for only such actions which satisfy some needs.
7. **Culture is capable of adjustment:** Culture undergoes a regular change according to environment and its adjustment with other powers, resulting from a change, goes on.
8. **Quality of integration in culture:** There is order and unity in culture, its different parts keep united among them and any new element that arrives gets united with it. Cultures which have greater outside influence are more foreign.

DISTINGUISH BETWEEN MATERIAL AND NON-MATERIAL CULTURE

1. **Material culture:** It includes material or concrete things used by man such as house, household commodities, different kinds of apparatus, instruments, weapons and means of conveyance, etc.
2. **Non-material culture:** It includes abstract things such as different customs, conventions, methods, arts, knowledge and religion of the society, etc.

Universal Factors of Culture

1. Language.
2. Concrete things like food, house, and means of conveyance, dress, weapons, arms, industries and occupations.
3. Arts.
4. Legendary and scientific knowledge.
5. Rituals and blind beliefs.
6. Family and marriage, social control, games and other social institutions of the kind.
7. Property, value, exchange and trade.
8. Government and law.
9. War.

ROLE OF CULTURE IN DETERMINING HUMAN BEHAVIOR

1. **Human behavior:** The extreme yew of cultural determinism would suggest that human behavior is entirely the product of social learning influence on and have behavior. The influence is regarded as a much more significant determinant of behavior.
2. **The dynamics of culture:** The learning process extends across the full sectarian of human beliefs and customs. Its dynamics remain a phenomenon of natural forces acting on each other.

3. **Sexual dimensions of culture:** Cultural teaming is to deeply ingrained, and so taken for guaranteed, that we regard as "normal" that sexual behavior which conforms to our cultural standards.

Domain of Culture

1. **Ethnic identity:** It deepens on country of origin ethnic, identity, reasons or immigration degree of acculturation assimilation and levels of cultural pride.
2. **Communication:** It depends on dominant language and dialect, valium, willingness to share thoughts, meaning of touch, use of eye contact.
3. **Time and space:** It includes past, present or future orientation and personal space.
4. **Social organization:** It includes family structure gender role status/roles of elderly, Extended family, decision making and networks.
5. **Health belief:** It includes religious or spiritual beliefs and practices, sick role and health seeking behavior.
6. **Sexuality:** It includes the beliefs about sexuality and reproduction, taboos and private issues.
7. **Religion:** It includes domination of religion, beliefs, rituals, prayers, meditation, and meaning of life and source of strength.
8. **Death and dying:** Meaning of death and after life, fatalism, rituals, expectations, mourning and bereavement.

CONCLUSION

In recent years, nurses have become increasingly interested in the influence that culture and religion have on their clients' perceptions of illnesses and their willingness to cooperate with medical practitioners to achieve mutually satisfying goals of health and continued wellness. In looking for an answer to how nurses could be more effective in meeting the individual needs of patients, she found that how people respond to health and illness is strongly influenced by their culture, which is defined as the knowledge, laws, customs, religion, values, beliefs and rituals the group of people practice differently from other group.

48 *Psychosocial Conceptual Models*

DEFINITIONS

1. **Concept:** A word or idea that represents a category of things with related characteristics.
2. **Active-passive model:** A model of the practitioner- patient relationship that occurs when the patient is unable, because of medical condition, to participate in his or her own care and to make decisions for his or her own welfare.
3. **Biopsychosocial:** A model that incorporates aspects of biological, psychological, and social systems for a fuller understanding of human health and functioning.
4. **Guidance-cooperation model:** A model of the practitioner-patient relationship that occurs when the physician assumes primary responsibility for diagnosis and treatment. The patient does not contribute a perspective and leaves all decisions to the physician.
5. **Mutual participation model:** A model of the practitioner-patient relationship in which practitioner and patient make joint decisions about every aspect of care. There is joint input from physician and patient, and joint responsibility in the choices made.
6. **Mutual relationship (mutuality):** A relationship in which both doctor and patient are highly invested in patient outcomes, and each is actively involved in the medical interaction.
7. **Narrowly biomedical model:** A model in which the focus is on purely biological and medical factors and the physician spends most of his or her time asking closed-ended questions.
8. **Nonverbal communication:** Communication without words.
9. **Paternalistic relationship:** A physician-patient relationship in which the physician has most of the control.
10. **Psychosocial model:** A model in which the medical interaction is primarily focused on psychosocial issues.

A model is a means of organizing a complex body of knowledge. For example, the linkage between the various concepts related to human behavior may be represented in the form of a model, which can now be referred to as a conceptual model.

The treatment of the mentally ill depends mainly on the philosophy related to mental health and mental illness. The various models or theoretical approaches influencing current practice are:

PSYCHOANALYTICAL MODEL

Psychoanalytical model has been derived from the work of Sigmund Freud and his followers. Basic assumptions of psychoanalytical model are:

1. All human behavior is caused and thus is capable of explanation. Human behavior, however insignificant or obscure, does not occur randomly or by chance. Rather, all human behavior is determined by prior life events.
2. All human behavior from birth to old age is driven by an energy called the libido. The goal of the libido is the reduction of tension through the attainment of pleasure. The libido is closely associated with physiological or instinctual drives (e.g., hunger, thirst, elimination and sex). Release of these drives results in the reduction of tension and experience of pleasure. Hence, the pleasure principle becomes operative when pleasure seeking behaviors are used.

   The personality of the human being can be understood by way of three major hypothetical structures, viz. id, ego and superego. It represents the most primitive structure of the human personality. It houses the physiological drives. Human behavior originating from the id is impulsive, pleasure-oriented, and disconnected from reality.
3. The ego represents that part of the human personality, which is in closest contact with reality. Unlike the id, ego is capable of postponing pleasure until an appropriate time, place or object is available. Unlike the superego, the ego is not driven to blind conformity with rules and regulations. Rather, the ego acting as mediator between the Id and superego, gives rise to a much more mature and adaptive behavior.
4. The superego is the personality structure containing the values, legal and moral regulations and social expectations that thwart free expression of pleasure-seeking behaviors. The superego thus functions to oppose the id.
5. Understandably, humans occasionally experience anxiety when confronted with situations that challenge the tenuous balance between the id and the superego. At these times, the ego uses defense mechanisms that include repression, denial, regression, rationalization, reaction formation, undoing, projection, displacement, sublimation, isolation, and fixation.
6. The human personality functions on three levels of awareness: Conscious, preconscious and unconscious. Consciousness refers to the perception, thoughts and feelings existing in a person's immediate awareness. Preconscious content on the other hand, is not immediately accessible to awareness. Unlike conscious and preconscious, content in the unconscious remain inaccessible for the most part.
7. The unconscious affects all the three personality structures—id, ego and the superego. Although the id's content resides totally in the unconscious, the superego and the ego have aspects in all the three levels of consciousness. The ego maintains contact with reality, the id and the superego.
8. Human personality development unfolds through five innate psychosexual stages—oral, anal, phallic, latent and genital.

   Although these stages extend throughout the lifespan, the first 6 years of life determine the individual's long-term personality characteristics.

PSYCHOANALYTICAL PROCESS

Psychoanalysis, described by Freud, makes use of free association and dream analysis to affect reconstruction of personality. Free association refers to the verbalization of thoughts as they occur, without any conscious screening. Analysis of the patient's dreams helps to gain additional insight into his problem and the resistances. Thus, dreams symbolically communicate areas of intrapsychic conflict. The therapist then attempts to assist the patient to recognize his intrapsychic conflicts through the use of interpretation.

The patient is an active participant, freely revealing all thoughts exactly as they occur and describing all dreams. By termination of therapy, the patient is able to conduct his life according to an accurate assessment of external reality and is also able to relate to others uninhibited by neurotic conflicts.

Roles of the Patient and the Psychoanalyst

The patient is to be an active participant, freely revealing all thoughts exactly as they occur and describing all dreams. The psychoanalyst is a shadow person; while the patient is expected to reveal all his thoughts and feelings, the analyst reveals nothing personal.

APPLICATION TO NURSING

This theoretical perspective has helped mental health professionals to understand psychopathology and stress related behaviors. More importantly, this theory illustrates the importance of not taking human behavior at face value. That is, it helps the psychiatric-mental health nurse to discern and explore the meaning behind human behavior.

BEHAVIORAL MODEL

Prominent theorists of behavioral theory include Ivan Pavlov, John Watson, BF Skinner, etc. Basic assumptions of behavioral model are:
1. All behavior is learnt (adaptive and maladaptive).
2. All behavior occurs in response to a stimulus.
3. Human beings are passive organisms that can be conditioned or shaped to do anything if correct responses are rewarded or reinforced.
4. Maladaptive behavior can be unlearnt and replaced by adaptive behavior if the person receives exposure to specific stimuli and reinforcement for the desired adaptive behavior.
5. Deviations from behavioral norms occur when undesirable behavior has been reinforced. This behavior is modified through application of learning theory.

Therapeutic Approaches

1. Systematic desensitization
2. Token reinforcement
3. Shaping
4. Chaining
5. Prompting
6. Flooding
7. Aversion therapy
8. Assertiveness and social skills training.

Roles of the Patient and the Behavioral Therapist

The approach is that of a learner and a teacher.

Therapist

1. The therapist is an expert in behavior therapy who helps the patient unlearn his symptoms and replace them with more satisfying behavior.

2. The therapist uses the patient's anxiety as a motivational force towards learning.
3. The therapist teaches the patient about behavioral approaches and helps him develop behavioral hierarchy.
4. The therapist reinforces desired behaviors.

Patient

1. As a learner the patient is an active participant in the therapy process.
2. Patient practices behavioral techniques.
3. Does homework and reinforcement exercises.
   Therapy is considered to be complete when the symptoms subside.

Application to Nursing

Nurses commonly use behavioral techniques in a wide variety of mental health settings. Additionally, nurses who work with clients having physical disability, chronic pain, and chemical dependency and rehabilitation centers also apply these techniques.

INTERPERSONAL MODEL

Harry S Sullivan is the originator of interpersonal relations theory.

Basic assumptions of interpersonal model are:
1. Human being is essentially social beings.
2. Human personality is determined in the context of social interactions with other human beings.
3. Anxiety plays a central role in the formation of human personality by serving as a primary motivator of human behavior. Especially, anxiety is important in building self-esteem and enabling a person to learn from their life experiences.
4. Self-esteem is an important facet of human personality that forms in reaction to the experience of anxiety. Interactions with significant others conveying disapproval or other such negative meanings contribute to self-system formation.
5. Security mechanisms are used to reduce or avoid the experience of anxiety. These security mechanisms include sublimation, selective inattention and dissociation.
6. Early life experiences with parents, especially the mother, influence an individual's development throughout life.
7. Human development proceeds through six stages of development: Infancy, childhood, juvenility, pre-adolescence, early adolescence and late adolescence. According to interpersonal theory, juvenile and preadolescent stages hold the greatest potential for correction of previous behavior and personality difficulties.

Interpersonal Therapeutic Process

The interpersonal therapist, like the psychoanalyst, explores the patient's life history. Components of self-esteem are identified, including the security operations that are used to defend the self.

The process of therapy is essentially a process of re-education as the therapist helps the patient identify interpersonal problems and then encourages him to try out more successful styles of relating.

Therapy is terminated when the patient has developed the ability to establish satisfying human relationships thereby meeting his basic needs.

Roles of the Patient and the Interpersonal Therapist

Sullivan describes the therapist as a participant observer, who should not remain detached from the therapeutic situation. The therapist's role is to actively engage the patient to establish trust and to empathize. He will create an atmosphere of uncritical acceptance to encourage the patient to speak openly.

The patient's role is to share his concerns with the therapist and participate in the relationship to the best of his ability.

The relationship itself is meant to serve as a model of interpersonal relationships. As the patient matures in his ability to relate, he can then improve and broaden his other life experiences with people outside the therapeutic situation.

Application to Nursing

Sullivan's interpersonal theory has been the cornerstone of psychiatric-mental health nursing curricula in the undergraduate and graduate levels.

Nurse-client one-to-one interaction or interpersonal process is based on Sullivan's interpersonal theory. The use of interpersonal process recordings in the clinical aspect of psychiatric- mental health nursing courses is also derived from Sullivan's interpersonal theory.

COMMUNICATION MODEL

Communication refers to the reciprocal exchange of information, ideas, beliefs, and feelings among a group of persons. The theorists who particularly emphasized the importance of communication are Eric Berne (founder of transactional analysis), Paul Watzlawick and his associates.

Basic assumptions of communication model are:
1. The understanding of the meaning of behavior is based on the clarity of communication between the sender and receiver.
2. Breakdown in successful transmission of information causes anxiety and frustration.
3. All behavior is communication, whether verbal or nonverbal.
4. Disruptions in behavior may then be viewed as a disturbance in the communication process, and as an attempt to communicate.

Communication Therapeutic Process

Therapists locate the disruptions within the communication process and also the interventions made in the patterns of communication.

This may take place in individuals, groups or families. The communication pattern is first assessed and the disruption diagnosed. The patient is then helped to recognize his own disrupted communication.

Roles of Patient and Therapist

Therapist

1. The communication therapist induces changes in the patient by intervening in the communication process. Feedback is given about the person's success at communicating.
2. The therapist demonstrates how to relate to others clearly.

3. Nonverbal communication is also emphasized, particularly in terms of congruence with verbal behavior.
4. The therapist teaches principles of good communication.

Patient

1. The patient must be willing to become involved in an analysis of his style of communicating.
2. The responsibility for changing rests with the patient. Significant others often are included in communication therapy to bring change in the patient.

Application to Nursing

This theory helps mental health nurses to understand communication process and to correct communication disturbances.

MEDICAL MODEL

The medical model dominates much of modern psychiatric care. Other health professionals may be involved in interagency referrals, family assessment and health teaching, but physicians are viewed as the leaders of the team when this model is in effect. A positive contribution of the medical model has been the continuous exploration for causes of mental illness using the scientific process.

Basic assumptions of medical model are:

1. Medical model believes that deviant behavior is a manifestation of a disorder of the central nervous system.
2. It suspects that psychiatric disorders involve an abnormality in the transmission of neural impulses, difficulty at the synaptic level, and neurochemicals such as dopamine, serotonin and norepinephrine.
3. It focuses on the diagnosis of a mental illness and subsequent treatment based on this diagnosis.
4. Environmental and social factors are also considered in the medical model. They maybe either predisposing or precipitating factors in an episode of illness.
5. Another branch of research focuses on stressors and the human response to stress. These researchers suspect that humans have a physiological stress threshold that may be genetically determined.

Medical Therapeutic Process

The physician's examination of the patient includes history of the present illness, past history, social history, medical history and review of systems, physical examination and mental status examination. Additional data may be collected from significant others, and past medical records are reviewed if available. A preliminary diagnosis is then formulated pending further diagnostic studies and observation of the patient's behavior. After the diagnosis is made treatment is instituted.

Somatic treatments including pharmacotherapy, electroconvulsive therapy and occasionally psychosurgery, are important components of the treatment process.

Roles of the Patient and the Medical Therapist

1. The physician as the healer identifies the patient's illness and institutes a treatment plan.
2. Physician admits the patient in a psychiatric institution.

3. The role of the patient involves admitting that he is ill.

4. Patient practices prescribed therapy regimen and reports the effects of therapy to the physician.

Application to Nursing

Psychiatric-mental health nurse uses this model for assessment, diagnosis, planning and implementing nursing care to the patient.

This model helps psychiatric-mental health nurses to understand the physiological changes occurring due to psychiatric disorders.

NURSING MODEL

Nursing focuses on the individual's response to potential or actual health problems. Under the nursing model, human behavior is viewed from a holistic perspective.

Nursing View of Behavioral Deviations

1. Behavior is viewed on a continuum from healthy adaptive responses to maladaptive responses that indicate illness.
2. Each individual is predisposed to respond to life events in unique ways. These predispositions are biological, psychological, sociocultural, and the sum of the person's heritage and past experiences.
3. Behavior is the result of combining the predisposing factors with precipitating stressors. Stressors are life events that the individual perceives as challenging, threatening or demanding. The nature of the behavioral response depends on the person's primary appraisal of the stressor and his secondary appraisal of the coping resources available to him.
4. A stressor that has primary impact on physiological functioning also affects the person's psychological and sociocultural behavior. For instance, a man who had a myocardial infarction may also become severely depressed, because he fears he will lose his ability to work. On the other hand, the patient who enters the psychiatric inpatient unit with major depression may be suffering from malnutrition and dehydration because of his refusal to eat or drink. The holistic nature of nursing encompasses all of these facets of behavior and incorporates them into patient care planning.

Nursing Process

Nursing intervention may take place at any point on the continuum. Nursing diagnosis may focus on behavior associated with a medical diagnosis or other health behavior that the patient wishes to change.

A nurse may practice primary prevention by intervening in a potential health problem, secondary prevention by intervening in an actual acute health problem or tertiary prevention by intervening to limit the disability caused by actual chronic health problems. The nursing assessment of the patient includes presenting complaints, past history, family history, personal history, occupational history, sexual history, physical examination and mental status examination. Additional data may be collected from significant others and by reviewing the systems. A nursing diagnosis is then formulated and based on this diagnosis; planning and interventions are carried out. Finally, evaluation will be done to find out the effectiveness of nursing interventions.

Providing nursing care is a collaborative effort, with both the nurse and the patient contributing ideas and energy to the therapeutic process.

HOLISTIC MODEL

Major Concepts

The holistic view of the patient, with the body and soul seen as inseparable, and the patient viewed as a member of a family and community was central to Nightingale's view of nursing. The primary goal of nursing is to help clients develop strategies to achieve harmony within themselves and with others, nature and the world. Integrative functioning of the client's physical, emotional, intellectual, social and spiritual dimensions is emphasized. Each person is considered as a whole, with many factors contributing to health and illness.

Five major concepts are generally accepted as premises of holistic health care philosophy: First, each person is multidimensional; one's physical, emotional, intellectual, social and spiritual dimensions are in constant interaction with each other: The physical dimension involves everything associated with one's body, both internal and external the emotional dimension consists of affective states and feelings, including motor behavior associated with emotion, the experienced aspect of emotion, and the physiological mechanisms that underlie emotion the intellectual dimension includes receptive functions; memory and learning, cognition and expressive functions the social dimension is based on social interaction and relationships, more so the global concept of culture the spiritual dimension is that aspect of a person from which meaning in life is determined through which transcendence over the ordinary is possible.

The second premise of holistic care philosophy is that the environment makes significant contributions to the nature of one's existence. Each person's environment consists of many factors that are influential in that person's quality of life. Consequently, people cannot be fully understood without consideration of environmental factors such as family relationships, culture, and physical surroundings. Individuals interact with their unique environments through all dimensions, based on subjective experience as well as external stimuli.

The third premise is that each person experiences development across his life cycle; in each stage of life, the individual experiences and confronts different issues or similar issues in different ways. One's experience of each stage of life, forms the basis for further development as one moves through the life cycle.

Fourth, the holistic health care model maintains that stress is a primary factor in health and illness. Any event or circumstance can act as a stressor. Regardless of the source, stress has an impact on the whole person. Examples of stressors directly affecting the physical dimension include stressors associated with genetic factors, physiological processes, and body image. Emotional stress may result from any experience or situation. Examples include poor physical conditions, perceived social inequities, a significant loss, intellectual incompetence, and a sense of meaninglessness. Stressors affecting the intellectual dimension may include factors that interfere with receptive functions, memory and learning, cognitive functions, and expressive functions. Social stressors may arise from interactions and relationships with other people, as well as from more general societal and cultural factors. Stressors affecting the spiritual dimension may be any factors that interfere with one's ability to meet spiritual needs.

Fifth, people are ultimately responsible for the directions their lives take and the lifestyles they choose. Within a holistic framework, people are viewed as active participants in and contributors to their health status; they are willing to learn from illness and strive towards healthier choices.

HUMANISTIC MODEL

In contrast to the pessimism of the psychodynamic perspective, the humanistic approach optimistically argues that people have enormous potential for personal growth. When personality development focuses upon the development of self, it is called humanism. Humanists like Carl Rogers and Abraham Maslow reject the internal conflicts of Freud's view and the mechanistic nature of behaviorism. They believe that each person is creative and responsible, free to choose and each strives for fulfillment or self actualization.

Humanistic theories emphasize the importance of people's subjective attitudes, feelings, and beliefs, especially with regard to the self. Carl Rogers's theory focuses on the impact of disparity between a person's ideals, self and perceived real self. Maslow focuses on the significance of self actualization.

Rogers' Person-Centered Approach

Rogers' emphasized that each of us interprets the same set of stimuli differently, so there are as many different 'real worlds' as there are people on this planet (Rogers, 1980).

Self actualization: Carl Rogers used the term self-actualization to capture the natural, underlying the tendency of humans to move forward and fulfill their true potential. He argued that people strive towards growth, even in less-than favorable surroundings.

Personality development: Carl Rogers proposed that even young children need to be highly regarded by other people. Children also need positive self regard to be esteemed by self as well as others. Rogers believed that everyone should be given unconditional positive regard, which is a nonjudgmental and genuine love, without any strings attached.

Maslow's Hierarchy of Needs

1. Maslow proposed that our human motives are arranged in a hierarchy, with the most basic needs at the bottom. At the top are the more highly developed needs like self-esteem needs and finally self-actualization.
2. Maslow's hierarchy proposes that our needs must be fulfilled in a specified order, from physiological, safety, and love to the higher needs of esteem and self-actualization; Maslow also specified a list of characteristics descriptive of self-actualized people.
3. One of the basic themes underlying Maslow's theory is that motivation affects the person as a whole, rather than just in part. Maslow believed that people are motivated to seek personal goals which make their lives rewarding and meaningful.
4. Abraham Maslow suggested that 5 basic classes of needs or motives influence human behavior. According to Maslow, needs at the lowest level of the hierarchy must be satisfied before people can be motivated by higher-level goals.

Hierarchy of Human Needs

Physiological Needs

The physiological needs are most basic, powerful and urgent of all human needs that are essential to physical survival. Even if one of these needs remains unsatisfied the individual rapidly becomes dominated by it, so all other needs become secondary. Included in this group are the need for food, water, oxygen, sex, activity and sleep.

Safety and Security Needs

Once the physiological needs are fairly well-satisfied, safety and security needs predominate. Included here are the needs for structure, stability, law and order, and freedom from such threatening forces as illness and fear.

Love and Belongingness Needs

These needs become prominent when the physiological and safety/security needs have been met. The person at this level longs for affectionate relationship with others, for a place in his family and social groups. Accordingly a person experiences feelings of loneliness, friendlessness and rejection, especially when caused by the absence of friends and loved ones.

Self-Esteem Needs

Maslow divided these needs into two types:
Self respect and respect from others. Self-respect includes a person's desire for competence, confidence, achievement and independence. Respect from others includes his desire for prestige, reputation, status, recognition, appreciation and acceptance from others. Satisfaction of self-esteem needs generates feelings of self-confidence, self-worth and a sense of being useful and necessary in the world. Dissatisfaction of self-esteem needs in contrast, generate such feelings as inferiority, weakness, passivity and dependency.

Self-actualization

According to Maslow self-actualization is the person's desire to become everything, he is capable of the person who has achieved this highest level, presses toward the full use of his talents, capacities and potentialities. In short, the self-actualized person is someone who has reached the peak of his potential.

BIBLIOGRAPHY

1. Ahuja N. A Short Text Book of Psychiatry, 3rd edn. Jaypee Brothers Medical Publishers, New Delhi, 1999.
2. Bhatia BD. Craig Margaretta. Elements of Psychology and Mental Hygiene for Nurses in India. Orient Longman: Chennai, 2005.
3. Bhatia MS. A Concised Textbook on Psychiatric Nursing, 1st edn. CBS Publishers: New Delhi, 1997.
4. Bimla Kapoor. Textbook of Psychiatry Nursing, 1st edn. Kumar Publishing House: New Delhi, 1998.
5. Boyd AM. Psychiatric Nursing Contemporary Practice. Lippincott-Raven Publishers: New York, 1998.
6. Das G. Educational Psychology, Kind Books: New Delhi.
7. Dollard J, Miller NE. Personality and Psychotherapy, McGraw-Hill, New York, 1950.
8. Eysenck HJ. Dimensions of Personality, Kegan Paul, London, 1994.
9. Eysenck HJ. The Structure of Human Personality (3rd edn) Methuen, New York, 1971.
10. Fordham F. An Introduction to Jung's Psychology, Penguin Books, London, 1953.
11. Freud S. An Outline of Psychoanalysis, London: Hogart, 1953.
12. Good and Hatt, Methods of Social Research, McGraw Hill, New York, 1952.
13. Freud S. An Outline of Psychoanalysis, Norton, New York, 1939.

14. Gross Richard, Kinnison Nancy. Psychology for Nurses and Allied Health Professionals, Hodder Arnold: London, 2007.
15. Hogan R. Personality Theory-Englewood Cliffs, Prentice Hall, New Jersey, 1976.
16. Janis IL, Mahi O, FKagan J, Holt RR. Personality Dynamics, Development and Assessment, Harcourt Brace, New York, 1969.
17. Jones E. The Life and Work of Sigmund Freud (Lionel Trilling and Steven Marcus, Eds.) Garden City, Anchor, New York, 1963.
18. Klopfer B, Kelley D. The Rorschach Technique, World Book Co., Yonkers, 1946.
19. Mischel, Walter, Personality and Assessment, John Wiley, New York, 1976.

49 Social Psychology

INTRODUCTION

Social psychology is one of the latest extensions of the great movement of scientific thought that achieved its most striking results in the investigation of physical phenomena. The advances of natural science were the indispensable conditions for a study of psychology. In the study of man, psychology occupies a unique and commanding position. We may say that what physics is to the natural sciences, psychology is to the sciences of man. All activities in society—economic, political, artistic have their center in individuals, in their strings, needs, and understanding. The individual is the point of intersection of nearly all that is of consequence in the social sphere. For purpose of convenience we may divide our interest and concentrate on a particular phase of social process.

With the increasing variety of courses offered in psychology and education, it is inevitable that social psychology will trespass upon related fields. Inspite of possible overlapping, it has been decided that social psychology as an independent discipline that is required today, because of several transformations, with the growth of mass industrialization, the concentration of great populations in cities, and spread of rapid communication have altered the human situation in definite ways.

MEANING AND NATURE OF SOCIAL PSYCHOLOGY

Psychology and sociology each often claims the whole domain of human behavior as its individual bailiwick. The history of these two disciplines reveals basic differences in their approaches to the understanding of human behavior. These differences have generally been the result of varying approaches to the types of problems posed for different levels of behavior being analyzed by the two disciplines. One has emphasized one level of obstruction and the other, another. Some differences have stemmed from differing definitions in describing the significant problems. For example, in the early psychology, psychologists tended to emphasize the physiological bases of behavior and minimized social and cultural experience, while sociology tends to minimize the physical bases and emphasized social processes and conditions.

DEFINITIONS OF SOCIAL PSYCHOLOGY

Our glance at representative topics of social psychology, its ground rules, and the converging trends in the present state of its development was preparation for definition of social psychology. The definition of any class of objects or events requires specification of what it is and what it is not. This is not an easy matter in our complex subject matter.

Major generalizations are implied in defining a discipline-such as the claim that we know its scope and how to go about studying its problems. There has been disagreement on these matters since the first two books appeared under the label of "Social Psychology" in 1908. One was written by the psychologist William McDougall and the other by the sociologist EA Ross. Since then, several textbooks on Social Psychology have appeared.

The definition of Social Psychology offered here is suggested by three converging trends in contemporary Social Psychology that were noted above, namely:

1. Increased adherence to the ground rules of the scientific approach and utilization of scientific methods and techniques.
2. Awareness of the need for checks to guard against ethnocentric conclusions.
3. Conception of behavior within its appropriate frame of reference as a product of interacting influences coming both from the individual and his social surroundings.

Social psychology is, "The scientific study of the experience and behavior of the individual in relation to social stimulus situations."

Let us take the terms in the definition one by one as an orientation to the principal theoretical issues in social psychology and its relation to the social sciences.

PRINCIPLES OF SOCIAL PSYCHOLOGY

1. **Scientific study:** Specifying that social psychology is a scientific study underscores the task of adhering closely to the ground rules of science and their ramifications in the actual operations of research. Policy makers, religious leaders, novelists, and commentators on the social science cannot be held accountable for adhering to the ground rules of communicability and reproducibility of methods that permit verification, but social psychologists are. In this book, the scientific ground rules, their associated methods, and the techniques are presented, on the whole, through the summaries of significant research studies that exemplify their use.
2. **Of the individual:** The phrase of the individual specifies that the unit of analysis in social psychology is the individual. Because the field is social psychology and not psychological sociology, its concepts refer to the individual's perception.

   The individual is the unit of analysis for social psychology whether the investigator happens to be stationed in a university's department of psychology or sociology (the field's twin parents). Social psychologists today do not use concepts such as "group mind". A group cannot perceive, or feel, or think. The designation social in our label refers to the fact that our particular task is to study the individual's behavior in relation to those aspects of his surroundings that are interpersonal or sociocultural. When the individual has traffic first with these aspects of his environment, they are external to him—that is, on the stimulus side of the familiar S-O-R (stimulus-organism-response) scheme for analysis.
3. **Experience and behavior:** Experience is a general term that refers to the awareness of the individual, and not just to past experiences as conveyed in expressions such as "My experience has shown that....". What a person perceives, feels, learns, or remembers—in a word, his experience is inferred from his behavior, i.e. his deeds and words as well as subtle expressions and movements. For this reason, some psychologists refer to all psychological phenomena as behavior. The terms consciousness and mind and "awareness" were for a time almost banished from academic psychology.
4. **In relation to:** In any definition the choice of words is important. The importance of these particular words reflects controversies during the earlier development of social psychology.

The phrase "determined by" was deliberately avoided in our definition. The individual is not merely a passive recipient, a tabula rasa, reflecting the imprints of his environment, whether social or not. Anything that impinges on the individual from the social world around him is processed and his motives, desires, attitudes, and ideas enter into processing. The processing reflects selectivity in what he reacts to and whom he transacts with. The processing is also affected by what he confronts. Hence, experience and behavior that count for the individual and in the social process are always a joint product of influences in the social environment and those from within himself, whatever he may be at a given time with all of his past learning, his enduring and momentary motives, and his viewpoints toward the issue at hand.

Social life is the natural habitat of the human individual. It is not alien to his nature. Therefore, how an individual learns the requirements and values of his group and culture, how he responds to pressures from them, and the molding of his behavior within these requirements are not the sole problems of social psychology.

5. **Social stimulus situations:** The final phrase in the definition of social psychology is social stimulus situations. The phrase seems self-explanatory. To show that it is not, we shall consider more seriously what constitutes a social situation for the individual at a given time. This analysis will enable us to indicate the scope and variety of social stimuli that an individual may encounter in his surroundings.

RELATIONSHIP BETWEEN SOCIAL PSYCHOLOGY AND EDUCATION

Social psychology is an attempt to understand and explain how the thought, feeling and behavior of individuals are influenced by the actual, implied or imagined presence of others — *YK Allport*.

There is an increasing complexity in social life and also personal life of an individual in the society, because of explosion of population, explosion of knowledge and industrialization. This has greater impact on the education field. Because of this the educationists, administrators, parents, teachers and the persons involved in the educational activities are confronting many problems in the execution of educational programs in spite of their knowledge of psychology and sociology. This might have happened because psychology deals with individual behavior as a separate entity apart from the society, whereas sociology deals with society group behavior without emphasizing the individual. It is from this angle it is very significant to deal with social psychology in relation to education, because social psychology studies the behavior of the individual in a social context.

Social psychology begins with the individual and looks at political, social and cultural systems through the eyes of the individual, whereas political science, sociology and cultural anthropology begin as the larger systems and look at the individual through the eyes of this system in all.

Scope of Social Psychology

It is very difficult to restrict the scope of social psychology. It is inclusive of many of the aspects as its subject matter for the study. This idea becomes more clear by Krech and Crutch fields' saying that social psychology is concerned with every aspect of the individuals behavior in the society; therefore, we can define social psychology as the science of behavior of the individual in the society.

Newcomb's (1900) contention is that interaction constitutes subject matter of social psychology. Therefore, we can say that it encompasses all types of interaction processes for its study.

The subject matter of social psychology is composed of two psychologically important aspects of the individual. One is directly observable, the overt behavior—what the individual does and the second one is not directly observable, but determines behavior—psychological dynamics, what the individual experiences. The first is referred to as the phenotypic self and the second as genotypic self.

It deals with mass communication and the social structure, intergroup attitudes, interpersonal attraction,, interpersonal perception, social power, prejudice and stereotypes, group norms and social control, social roles, leadership, group productivity and satisfaction, self and personality, social motivation, social interaction, socialization, affiliation, social organization, attitudes, etc. which are social psychological approaches to the problem of human nature.

SCOPE OF EDUCATION

It is once again difficult to explain the scope of education because it is an open system and a very comprehensive discipline. In the real sense of the term, it is a process, which goes on from birth to death encompassing each and every aspect of human life.

Pestallozzi's conception of education is that "it reforms and elevates society. It involves a natural and harmonious development of all the faculties of the individual; it requires an active cooperation between home and school".

Therefore, we can say that education is joint endeavor of home, school and society to bring about a desirable behavioral change among children so that they become contributing citizens of the society.

Education as a discipline is concerned biological, physical, mental, intellectual, emotional, cultural and spiritual development of the individual.

Scope of education is very broader because it stretches its hands towards different directions as vocational education, technical education, adult education, nonformal education, guidance and with social counseling, etc. Its scope ranges from teaching three R's, through development of values, attitudes, etc. to the all round development and self-realization of the individual.

By observing the scope of social psychology and of education we can say that both of them concentrate, emphasize and deal with the individual for his harmonious development and in turn make the society a place suitable for human existence. As such it is very significant to study the relationship between social psychology and education.

Social psychology deals with the behavior of the individual in a 'social context'. School is a miniature 'society' where deliberately planned educational programs are executed. Therefore, education and social psychology are inter-related.

Formulation of social objectives for education, incorporation of social objectives into curricular or design of classroom social process as a means of achieving social goals, etc. require the helping from social psychologists to educationists.

Educators often face a series of social problems such as prejudice, pupil's dislike of school, and conflicts among students and also among staff members, that can be solved easily with the help of social psychology.

Education refers to school-related behavior and related variables. Education is fundamentally an interpersonal process, carried out through the interdependent cooperation of two roles-educator and learner, requires for its elucidation precisely the kinds of analytical tools and data provided by social psychology.

The knowledge of social psychology provides the knowledge about individual and group differences, which provide a basis for developing alternative educational treatment of different individuals or groups that would benefit all, more than teaching everyone the same way would.

Schools are complex social environments, wherein addition to learning, social interaction takes place. Therefore, social psychology, which focuses its attention and discusses elaborately on "Social Interaction" helps the education field, particularly school program to a large extent. In the same way education also helps in social interaction, understanding the group norms, which leads to minimizing group conflicts, developing right types of attitudes, inculcation of values, better interpersonal relationship, etc.

Therefore, in conclusion educational problems provide sophisticated and complex issues to challenge social psychologists to utilize the best available theory and methods and to challenge the field to develop new approaches. In a parallel way the social psychological perspective is important for educators and significantly improves educational practice.

From the above discussion we can see how intimately social psychology and education are related. Discussing this, Eradsick and High shall argue that educational psychology must be fundamentally not cognition or a developmental or a personality psychology, but a social psychology.

Though this much of intimate relationship is there between social psychology and education, educational issues were ignored by social psychologists previously say up to 1954-55. Only after this period the educational issues drew attention of social psychologists and led to the development of social psychology of education. If is from this points of view, we shall discuss largely the development of social psychology of education.

DEVELOPMENT OF SOCIAL PSYCHOLOGY OF EDUCATION

There were many reports and textbooks, containing laboratory experiments, mainly in psychology and educational psychology, up to 1935. Among them, very few of them contained about social factors. Pressay's (1933) text included a chapter Social Psychology of Childhood and Adolescence. Enrich and Garrol (1935) text included "Measurement of Personality Attitudes and Interests in Learning and Instructions".

In 1941, Trow complained that most of the educational psychologists were limiting their investigation to the psychology of the individual neglecting the social aspects of individual behavior.

In 1954, Geizels complained, in his book "The Handbook of Social Psychology" that usually textbooks contain chapters on the Social Psychology of Industry and Politics. Social psychologists have tended to ignore educational issues.

From the views of the above two authors, we can observe that though there was a change in the attention from educational psychology to social psychology emphasizing on the social aspects of the individuals behavior, there was very little or no attention of social psychologists towards the educational issues. At the same time, it reveals that initiation and awareness about the necessity of knowledge of social psychology to the educational field. Because of this, there was initiation to the development of social psychology of education. Some of the more successful texts by Bichies (1981), Jrander (1957), and Perkins (1969) contained some of the aspects of educational issues viewed from the social psychological perspective.

Though the work started in social psychology of education since 1959 to bridge the gap between social psychology and education the work was geared up in 1970s, and then social psychology of education became a sub-discipline finding clearly its scope.

Social psychology for education merely uses social psychological principles to explain educational problems. Here mostly the researches are carried out in laboratory setting (not educational settings).

In contrast, the social psychology of education defines its scope according to a problem focus on educational issues. The topics in social psychology of education are those social psychological issues that concern the social functioning of individuals and groups in educational systems, i.e. the topics of social psychology of education does not necessarily correspond to the standard topics of social psychology. Here researches are carried out on the education setting itself.

CONCLUSION

The scope of social psychology and education are vast and inclusive of many of the aspects. And they are intimately related to a larger extent. The knowledge of social psychology helps to a greater extent in solving the educational problems. This intimate relationship of mutual contribution led to the development of a new discipline, namely social psychology of education. This deals mainly with the educational issues from the social psychology perspective, which helps in achieving educational goals.

BIBLIOGRAPHY

1. Abram Kardiner. The Psychological Frontier of Society, Columbia University Press, New York 1915.
2. Alfred R Lindesmith, Anseim L Strauss. Readings in Social Psychology, Rinehart and Winston, Chicago Hort, 1969.
3. Aliport GW. Personality A Psychological Interpretation, New York Holt, 1937.
4. Allport FH. Social Psychology, Boston Houghton Mifflin, 1924.
5. Allport GW, Kramer BM. Some Roots of Prejudice, J. of Psychol., 1946; 22, 9-39.
6. Allport GW. The Nature of Prejudice, Reading, Mass. Addison Wesley Publishing Co., Inc, (1954a).
7. Argyris C. Interpersonal Competence and Organizational Effectiveness, Home-wood, III IrwinDorsey, 1962.
8. Argyris C. Personality and Organization, New York Harper,1957.
9. Asch SE. Social Psychology Englewood Cliffs, Prentice-Hall, Inc. NJ, 1952.
10. Bass BA. Leadership, Psychology and Organizational Behavior, New York Harper, 1960.
11. Baveles A. Morale and the Training of Leaders. In Watson, GB (Ed), Civilian Morale, Boston Houghton Mifflin Co, 1942.
12. Benedict R. Patterns of Culture, Boston Houghton Mifflin Co, 1934.
13. Berlyne DE. Conflict, Arousal and Curiosity, McGraw- Hill Book Co., Inc., New York, 1960
14. Bird C. Social Psychology, D. Appleton Century Co., Inc., New York, 1940,
15. Boulding K. The Organizational Revolution, New York Harper, 1953.
16. Brown JF. Psychology and the Social Order, McGraw-Hill Book Co., Inc New York 1936 .
17. Cartwright D, A Zander (Eds). Group Dynamics Research and Theory, 2nd edn. Evanston, Ill Row, Peterson, 1960.
18. Myris C. Integrating the Individual and the Organization, Wiley, New York, 1964.

Complementary and Alternative Therapies on Health

INTRODUCTION

Changes in science and medicine have provided the knowledge and technology that have successfully altered the course of many illnesses. Despite the success of allopathic medicine, many conditions such as arthritis, chronic backache, gastrointestinal problems, allergies, headache, insomnia, etc. have been difficult to treat and more clients are exploring alternative methods to relieve their symptoms. It is estimated that 75% clients referred to practitioners due to health problems such as stress, pain and other health conditions have no known etiology. While allopathic medicine is quite effective in treating numerous physical ailments such as bacterial infections, structural abnormalities, acute emergencies. It is in general less effective in preventing diseases, decreasing stress induced illnesses, managing chronic disease, and caring for the emotional and spiritual needs of individuals.

The use of complementary and alternative medicine is not new to health care, but the last two decades have seen a huge rise in its popularity, both among the public and health care professionals. One in ten people in UK have used some form of complementary therapy and research issued by the Pronce's foundation for integrated health in May 2006 found that 74% of people are in favor of integrating complementary therapies into mainstream health care. This may be due to:

1. The perception that the treatment offered by medical profession does not provide relief for a variety of common illnesses.
2. The increasing interest of clients in becoming more educated about their health and need to take a more active role in their treatment.
3. The increased number of articles in journals related to alternative medicines.
4. Programs seen on television.
5. The attraction of holistic approach to the health care that incorporates the mind, body and spirit.

Unconventional therapies are frequently referred to as either complementary or alternative medicine therapies. Complementary therapies include: Relaxation, exercise, massage, prayer, biofeedback, hypnotherapy, creative therapies such as art, music, laughter and dance therapy, acupuncture, Chinese medicine, ayurveda, unani medicine, meditation, osteopathy, herbalism and homeopathy. Complementary therapies complement the conventional treatment. For example, acupuncture contained diagnostic and therapeutic methods specific to their field.

Because of this increased interest and use of complementary and alternative medicine, many institutions including some mainstream medical school, are establishing training programs that incorporate complementary alternative medicine philosophy and content into the curriculum. Integrative medical programs are being developed that allow health care consumer the opportunity to be treated by a team of providers consisting of both allopathic and complementary practitioners.

Interest in complementary alternative medicine is also evident from the increased number of articles in medical journals and the development of several journals that specifically focus on complementary and alternative medicines.

Nurses Role in Complementary Therapies

The increased interest in complementary therapies has gone up significantly in the last 15 years. This increased interest comes not only from health care consumers, but also from allopathic physicians who have increased concern that allopathic medicine is not meeting the needs of clients. It is also seen that many allopathic practitioners are reserved about these therapies because of the lack of evidence. There is a group of people who think is just for pampering and cannot see the medical benefit.

Although many professionals are exploring the use of complementary therapies and monitoring research being conducted in this area. Proposals put forth by theses groups include assessing the need of the public for complementary therapies, incorporating complementary alternative medicine (CAM) therapies educational components in the curriculum for all health care programs, providing appropriate information to the public, encouraging and facilitating the communication between CAM practitioners and allopathic practitioners so each can be opened to the other's approaches and values.

Integrative medicine, a health care strategy that is gaining popularity, involves a multiple-practitioner treatment group in which a client seeks care simultaneously from more than one type of practitioner. The clients are given option to choose the kind of practitioner they feel would benefit their particular health problem. Most often clients suffering from chronic heath problems get benefit from CAM therapies where traditional allopathic medicine is not treating their problem completely. In Indian scenario, this is not practiced in reality, but this approach of open communication and practice between CAM practitioners and allopathic practitioner could potentially benefit a large number of patients.

As integrative medicine approach is consistent with the holistic approach, nurses have the potential of becoming essential participants in this type of health care philosophy. Nurses should be knowledgeable of complementary therapies to make recommendations. Nurses should also be able to provide advice to clients regarding when to seek conventional therapy. As nurses work very closely with their clients and are in unique position of becoming familiar with the client's religious and cultural viewpoints and existential issues. They may be able to determine which CAM therapy would be more appropriately aligned with their beliefs and offer recommendations accordingly. It is also important to obtain specific consent from a patient before carrying out any complementary procedure. As it is not part of our mainstream treatment yet, it should never be used on unconscious patients.

Client's interest and participation in complementary therapies is increasing. Therefore it is important for nurses to be knowledgeable of these complementary therapies. It is also important for nurses to keep abreast of the current research being done in this area to provide accurate information not only to the clients, but to other health care professionals also. Many studies related to complementary therapies have involved small number of subjects and were not well controlled. More research studies are needed to validate the effectiveness of Complementary therapies.

BIOFEEDBACK

Biofeedback is a rapidly developing scientific field that has grown in physiology, psychology and electronics. Ordinarily, we are unaware of the subtle internal body activities that are part of our everyday lives. Biofeedback uses sensitive electronics to detect and amplify these activities in order to bring them to be aware. By allowing us to observe these activities, biofeedback also allows us to learn to modify them. Since we are immediately aware to the outcome of our attempts, we can gradually learn to produce the results we desire.

Types of Biofeedback

Electromyography (EMG) muscle biofeedback: Electromyography Biofeedback measures electrical activity created by muscle contractions. Often use for relaxation training and performance training, stress and pain management.

Thermal or temperature biofeedback: Thermal biofeedback is used to train people to quiet the nervous system arousal mechanisms which produce hand and feet cooling. This is often used for relaxation, stress and pain management and anxiety.

EEG biofeedback of neurofeedback: It trains the central nervous system, feedback brain electrical activity, called brainwaves. This is the fastest growing field in biofeedback. Mainly used in depression, anxiety, insomnia, head injury, obsessive compulsive disorder, anger, autism.

Skin conductance level/galvanic skin response electrodermal response (SCL/GSR/EDR): These are all measures of physiological activity in skin. Part of it is based on sweat gland activity. This measure is very useful for relaxation and stress management. It is very much useful with, attention deficit disorders hyperactivity disorder.

Mechanism of Action

Biofeedback self awareness and regulation techniques teach people to develop greater awareness of their physical and mental behavior. People learn to take greater control and responsibility for their health and as they become more aware of unhealthy symptom perpetuating behaviors, such as tensed muscles, constricted blood vessels (Hypertension), over-reactive nervous system activity, rapid heart rate, respiration or sweat gland activity or upsetting thought.

Biofeedback devices magnify or zoom in on body behaviors, therefore people get more information than their normal sensory awareness provides. The feedback information is combined with coaching, training and sometimes therapeutic interventions aimed at producing more healthy, normalized or more effective functioning.

AROMATHERAPY

Aromatherapy can be defined as the art and science of utilizing naturally extracted aromatic essences from plants to balance, harmonize and promote the health of body, mind and spirit.

It is an art and science which seeks to explore the physiological, psychological and spiritual realm of the individual's response to aromatic extracts as well as to observe and enhance the individual's inmate healing process. As a holistic medicine, aromatherapy is both a preventative approach as well as an active treatment during acute and chronic stages of illness or disease.

In Nursing

A new trend among nurses has been the incorporation of Aromatherapy into their practice. This was first truly seen among nursing home works but is now blossoming into other forms of nursing and patient care. As a result, many interesting studies were conducted and published concerning the validity and usefulness of certain essential oils. Conditions studied included high blood pressure, insomnia and Alzheimer's. One study by a nurse found that different species of lavender had varying effects on blood pressure; some were found more effective compared to others.

Since 1990s nurses have considered that the increased technology of health care threatens their ability to practice holistic care, which is positively entrenched in the philosophy of nursing (Keegan et al, 1994)

Aromatherapy is used in a wide range of settings from health spas to hospitals—to treat a variety of conditions. It has proven to have therapeutic benefits for a variety of conditions.

Practical Application of Aromatherapy

Pharmacokinetics and Physiological Effects of Essential Oils

Essentials oils are lipid soluble and rapidly absorbed into the bloodstream when applied externally inhaled or ingested and are excreted via the urinary system and expired carbon dioxide. There is, however, limited understanding of the pharmacokinetics of many essential oils and their potential for interaction with conventional pharmaceuticals. Although the use of essential oils are generally not known by nurses.

The main practical issues for nurses are correct storage and handling of essential oils to prevent oxidation, bacterial, contamination or accidental overdose.

Collectively, the range of experimental work that has been undertaken to explore the therapeutic potential of essential oils contributes to greater knowledge and understating of their actions. It is unclear at this stage, however, what the implication are for human clinical situations, particularly through the dermal application mainly used by nurses.

Effects of Aroma on Health

1. **Maternal and child health:** The main concerns for maternal and child health are whether essential oils have a hormone like effect on the mother, or whether they are abortifacient or whether they cause malformation to the developing fetus. While claims exist that aromatherapy may also help with some of the minor symptoms associated with pregnancy such as morning sickness, stretchmarks, varicose veins, heartburn, hemorrhoids, backache and exhaustion, none are supported by empirical evidence. A number of studies have explored the value of aromatherapy in labor and found that women who used a range of essential oils often coped better and required less analgesia. However, it was found that massage was more effective than deep breathing exercises in reducing pain and anxiety levels. Clearly, more research is needed in this area to ascertain the effectiveness of massage and also to study other ways of using essential oils. The evidence remains inconclusive as to whether lavender oil in low doses is more effective than conventional treatment in assisting perineal repair; however women who use it, report it to be comforting.

2. **Pain relief/analgesia:** Massage has been demonstrated to stimulate endorphin production. For people who are in pain it acts as a pain relieving tool, especially in chronic or muscular pain. Whether the addition of essential oils increases the pain relieving benefits beyond an anxiety

reduction value has yet to be demonstrated. Lavender and its main constituents, linalyl acetate and linalool, have been identified as having local anesthetic effect. The effects of linalool also include anticonvulsant activities due to inhibition of several chemical pathways.

Aromatherapy is one of the form of arthritis treatment, using a variety of essential oils. They can be added to bath, massaged into the skin, inhaled or applied as compresses. The right mixture and proportion of essentials will help to promote pain relief, relaxation and alleviate fatigue. Essential oils can also provide psychological benefits like improving the mood and reducing anxiety.

3. **Cancer care:** Several studies support the ongoing use of aromatherapy as part of an integrated approach to cancer and palliative care (Cooper 1995). Aromatherapy is primarily used to help to cope with anxiety and fear and to support symptoms control, rather than as an alternative to conventional treatment. For example, patients who are diagnosed with a brain tumor often have a poorer diagnosis and more debilitating symptoms than those with other forms of cancer. Aromatherapy and massage may help sufferers to deal with such serious issues and cope with the emotional effects of the high dose of steroids. While specialized lymph massage has been well accepted to reduce lymphedema, but there is no evidence that adding essential oils improve the physical effects of the massage.

Patients may experience uncomfortable side effects related to cancer therapy and the treatment for these side effects can be quite unpleasant. Various essential oils have been explored as possible alternatives in treating some side effects, but have had mixed effects. Although a blend of tea tree and bergamot oil was just as effective as a conventional mouthwash for mucositis as it had higher patient compliance due to the pleasant taste and aroma. However, aromatherapy is not useful in relieving skin rashes, infections or nausea associated with high dose of chemotherapy.

4. **Medical conditions:** While there are numerous case studies presented in many literatures involving the use of essential oils to treat various medical conditions, these alone are insufficient to guide-evidence based practice. The potential gain seems to be in reduction of stress, especially in chronic conditions such as fibromyalgia, GBS and AIDS.

5. **Neurological conditions:** Study of Betts (1995) highlighted the potential to use essential oils in seizure control as part of a conditioned response for people who know their triggers. *In vitro* animal studies have also shown that camphor, which is a major constituent of rosemary essential oil, lowers sodium and potassium concentrations in cerebral cortex tissue, which affects oxygen consumption by the brain and thus increases the risk of convulsions. Accidental ingestion of camphor in various forms has been implicated in seizures particularly in children. Peppermint and eucalyptus oil have been shown to have muscle relaxing effects as well as analgesic effects for the relief of headaches. They are most effective when used in combination. Both oils also have the ability to improve cognitive functioning.

6. **Respiratory conditions:** Essential oils are frequently used to alleviate respiratory conditions and there is some evidence that a number of them have broncholytic and secretolytic properties. There are many articles present as evidence which have concluded that eucalyptus has great therapeutic potential for the external use. It has also been seen that it has the ability to improve surfactant function.

Aromatherapy appears to be very effective for easing respiratory complaints, especially complaints adaptable to a quick intervention like infections and some acute problems. In addition, aromatherapy shows a remarkable effectiveness in building a good functioning immune system. This is one of the strongest points of aromatherapy. For example, regular use of immunity stimulating oils can help prevent or at least reduce the gravity of the symptoms for a common cold. Recurrence of the complaint may also be avoided by the improvement of the immune system.

7. **Digestive Disorders:** Peppermint essential oil has been widely researched for its potential in gastrointestinal disorders including reducing colonic spasm during colonoscopy and for the symptoms of irritable bowel syndrome.

NON-PHARMACOLOGIC THERAPIES

1. **Distraction:** It is a useful tool for helping alleviate both acute and chronic pain. These techniques work equally well with adults and children. It simply involves diverting the patient's attention away from the sensation of pain towards other thoughts. Some examples of specific techniques involve the following:
   - Encourage the patient to recount a recent exciting or pleasant experience. Encourage the patient to relate information from all the senses, i.e. touch, taste, smell, hearing, and sight. Children can be encouraged to recite rhymes or participate in a game.
   - Music is an excellent distracter and relaxant. The patient need to select music based on personal preferences. Encourage the patient to actively listen. Have the patient close the eyes, concentrate on the music and tap out the rhythm of the music. A study conducted by Ishii et al (1993) demonstrated that music is effective to relieve a pain associated with a compulsory posture and also play a significant role on pain management in palliative therapy.
   - Participate in rhythmic singing. Chants, hymns, or simple songs with the strong beat are good to use with both adults and children. Tapping the foot or fingers for emphasis is an additional distracter.
   - Rhythmic breathing exercises are another distracter. The patient may do these exercises with eyes closed or focusing on an object. The patient focuses on the breath and silently repeats "In, 2, 3, and 4-Out, 2, 3, and 4". Breathing is to be deep and slow, preferably from the abdomen.
   - Laughter therapy for 5-10 minutes enhances the comfort of clients suffering from pain. Cousin 1974, experienced relief from pain for 1 hour following 10 minutes belly laughter.
2. **Visualization:** It is a form of distraction that uses images to modify the perception of pain and decrease the intensity of the pain experience. This is a useful strategy with all age groups, practicing it for approximately 20 minutes, 2 to 3 times a day, will improve the effectiveness of the images. One common method of visualization is guided imagery. An imaginary "magic glove" or "magic blanket" may be put in place before a painful procedure such as an intravenous injection.
3. **Hypnosis:** The clinical application of hypnosis is usually executed by a registered hypnotherapist. This technique works with all age groups. This technique involves achieving deep relaxation and then listening to or giving oneself positive suggestions. From review of literature, many studies have shown relationship of hypnosis in pain reduction.
4. **Massage:** It had a long history of use in the treatment of muscular pain. The effect of massage is similar to heat in that circulation and removal of cellular waste products is enhanced. It is a valuable technique for reducing anxiety and promoting relaxation. Many studies have shown positive effect of massage in promoting relaxation and decreasing pain perception.
5. **Relaxation techniques:** Successful reduction of anxiety and fear assists the individual to feel more comfortable and experience a decreased perception of pain.

6. **Biofeedback technique:** It is useful for individuals with chronic pain. The individuals learn to control non-conscious physiological responses such as blood pressure and muscle tension through the use of mental images and thought processes.

7. **Meditation:** This is a useful relaxation technique for patients with acute and chronic pain. Prior to beginning the meditation the patient selects a soothing word, relax or calm. The patient may close or leave them open to focus on the object. With every breath in, the patient silently says the word that was chosen.

   Miller and Perry in quasi-experimental study found that cardiac surgery patients who were taught simple deep breathing relaxation techniques preoperatively had decreased pain perception, decreased vital signs at statistically significant level.

8. **Therapeutic touch:** It is a method of directing the energy through the hands. The technique produces a relaxation response and a perception of pain relief. A study conducted in hospital has shown a positive effect of therapeutic touch on the pain perception of patients after the surgery.

Turner (1994) studied the effect of therapeutic touch on reducing the pain and infection among hospitalized patients.

Nurses Role

The pain perception is multifaceted in that it encompasses an individual's physical, emotional, cognitive and experiential realm. The uniqueness of each patient explains the distinctiveness each one's response to pain and provides the rationale for customized care plan. As nurses are the persons who are providing care to patients round the clock. They are using different approaches for promoting the health and early recovery. As pharmacologic and surgical methods of pain management are not free from side effects/complications, nurses should use non-pharmacologic methods. While using these non-pharmacologic methods, nurses not only relieves the pain perception of client but also promotes psychological wellbeing. With this, patient feels energetic and also feels emotionally satisfied. As many studies conducted in the hospital has shown the positive effect of these methods on promoting the health, nurses should participate actively in using these non-pharmacological methods. Along with this research studies can be conducted.

CONCLUSION

Nurses are supposed to think and act best for the patients and are striving hard to achieve it. Nurse is one who takes care of patient's environment and his treatment plan. Due to the evolution of aroma therapist, the aesthetic side of ward and hospitals are now looked by them. Earlier the massages and therapies were done by nurses, may be due to specialization and load of work on nurses, this area is handled by them. So now this therapy is gaining momentum as a complementary therapy.

It is necessary for nurses to keep abreast of the recent advancements and developments in the field of science. Nurses should acquire the basic understanding of the chemical structure and physical properties of essential oils as well as knowledge of the safe application of a few commonly available oils and plan to use them in their practice. Ideally, if nurses plan

BIBLIOGRAPHY

1. Banjamine V John. Biofeedback Principles and Practice for Clinicians. 3rd edn, Williams & Wikins, Baltimore, 1981.
2. Dugas BW, Knor ER. Nursing foundations. Ontario. 1995; 843-46.
3. Jess Feist, Brannon Linda. Health Psychology an Introduction to Behavior and Health. 4th edn, International Headquarters, USA, 2000.
4. Labbe EE, et al. Skin temperature biofeedback training: Cognitive developmental factors in nonclinical children. Perception Motor Skills April 1995; 80 (2): 466.
5. Miller KM, Perry PA. Relaxation technique and postoperation pain in patients undergoing cardiac surgery. Heart Lung 1990; 19:36-46.
6. Newton-John TR, et al. Cognitive behavior therapy versus EMG biofeedback in the treatment of low back pain. Behavioral Research Therapy July 1995; 33 (6); 691-97.
7. Potter PA, Perry AG. Fundamentals of Nursing. 5th edn. Harcourt Health Sciences Company, St. Louis, 2001; 1305-08.
8. Sharma S, Kaur J. Hypnosis and pain management. Indian Journal of Nursing, 2006.
9. Turner LA. The effect of therapeutic touch on pain and infection. Journal of Advanced Nursing 1994:18.

Appendices

HEALTH DAYS

Sl. No.	Date	Month	Day
1.	30th	January	Anti-leprosy day
2.	7th	April	World health day
3.	22nd	April	World habitat day
4.	31st	May	World no tobacco day
5.	12th	May	International nurses day
6.	17th	May	World hypertension day
7.	5th	June	World environmental day
8.	1st	July	Doctor's day
9.	11th	July	World population day
10.	5th	September	Teacher's day
11.	2nd	October	Anti-drug addition day
12.	12th	October	World sight day
13.	13th	October	Anti-natural disaster day
14.	1st	December	Anti-AIDS day
15.	11th	December	UNICEF day

APPENDIX 2

THEMES OF WORLD HEALTH ORGANIZATION (WHO)

Sl.No.	Year	Themes
1.	1983	Health for all by 2000 AD
2.	1984	Children's health–tomorrow's wealth
3.	1985	Healthy youth—our best resources
4.	1986	Healthy living—every one a winner
5.	1987	Immunization—a choice for every one
6.	1990	Our planet-our-health—think globally, act locally
7.	1991	Should disaster strike—be prepared
8.	1992	Heartbeat—the rhythm of life
9.	1993	Handle life with care—prevent violence and negligence
10.	1994	Oral health for a health life
11.	1995	Target 2000—a world without polio
12.	1996	Healthy cities for health life
13.	1997	Emerging infectious diseases
14.	1998	Safe motherhood
15.	2000	Safe blood starts with me
16.	2001	Mental health—stop exclusion, dare to care
17.	2002	Move to health
18.	2003	Shape the future life
19.	2004	Road safety
20.	2005	Make every mother and child count

APPENDIX 3

MENTAL HEALTH

Meaning

1. Mental health includes a sound, efficient mind controlled emotions.
2. Good adjustment is the basic component of mental health.

Definitions

1. Mental health is defined as the capacity of an individual to form harmonious relationship with others.
2. The adjustability of human being to the world and to each other with a maximum of effectiveness and happiness—*Meninger*.

Characteristics of Mentally Healthy Individual

Sl.No.	Term	Description
1.	Adjustability	A well-adjusted person has some insight into and understanding of his motives, desire, his weaknesses and strong points.
2.	Sense of personal worth	He has a sense of personal worth, feels worthwhile and important. He has self-respect and feels secure in a group.
3.	Sense of personal security	The person feels that he is wanted and loved. In other words, he has a sense of personal security.
4.	Sense of responsibility	He has faith in his ability to succeed, he believes that he will do reasonably well whatever he undertakes.
5.	Acceptability	He appreciates the many differences that he finds in people. Moreover, he gives and accept love, can form friendships.
6.	Understandability	A person has some understanding of his environment and of the forces which he must deal equipped with his understanding.
7.	Philosophical oriented	He has developed a philosophy of life that gives meaning and purpose to his daily activities.
8.	Reality oriented	A person lives in a world of reality rather than fantasy.
9.	Tolerance	He has developed a capacity to tolerate frustrations and disappointment in his daily life.
10.	Emotional maturity	He shows emotional maturity in his behavior. This means that he is able to regulate such emotions as fear, love, jealousy and expresses them in a socially desirable manner.
11.	Rational attitude	He has a rational attitude towards problems of his physical health. He maintains a daily routine of health practices which promote healthful living.
12.	Good health practices	He practices good health habits with regard to nutrition, sleep, rest, relaxation, physical activity, personal cleanliness and protection from disease.
13.	Positive thinking	He is able to think for himself and can make his own decisions. He thinks clearly and constructively in solving his problems.
14.	Well-balanced personality	He has varity of interests and generally lives a well-balanced life of work, rest, and recreation. He has ability to get enjoyment and satisfaction out of his daily routine job.

APPENDIX 4

DEFENSE MECHANISMS

Sl. No.	Term	Description
I	NARCISSISTC	Borderline or image distorting defenses.
1.	Delusional projections	Perception of one's own feelings in another person and acting on the perception.
2.	Projective identification	The projection of unconscious material on to another person.
3.	Psychotic denial	Denial of extreme reality.
4.	Distortion	Gross re-shaping of external reality to suit inner needs.
5.	Splitting	Perception of complex or contradictory elements of self or others as separate, avoiding ambivalence or conflict.
II	IMMATURE	Common in healthy individuals of 3-16 years.
1.	Projection	Attributing one's own conscious feeling to others.
2.	Schizoid fantasy	Gratify unmet needs is intimacy.
3.	Hypochondriasis	
4.	Passive aggression	Aggression towards others is expressed indirectly and turning against self.
5.	Acting out	Direct expression of wishes via impulsive action in order to avoid being conscious.
III	NEUROTIC	
1.	Intellectualization	Rationalization magical thinking.
2.	Repression	1. Unconscious inhibition of wishes or desires, resulting in their temporary or permanent loss. 2. It is process of unconscious forgetfulness of unpleasant and conflict producing emotions.
3.	Displacement	1. Redirection of feeling from significant to less emotionally significant people or circumstances. 2. Unconscious shifting of emotions usually aroused by perceived threat from an unconscious impulse, to a less threatening external object which is then felt to be the source of threat.
4.	Reaction formation	1. Replacement of unacceptable desires or action with other opposites. 2. Unconscious transformation of unacceptable impulses into exactly opposite attitude, impulses, feelings, or behavior, i.e. unacceptable real feeling are repressed and acceptable opposite feelings are expressed.
5.	Dissociation/ neurotic denial	Temporary change of character or sense of personal identity to avoid emotional distress.
IV	MATURE DEFENCE	
1.	Altruism	Partial gratification through genuine services to other (constructive reaction formation).

Contd...

Contd...

Sl. No.	Term	Description
2.	Humor	Overexpression of feeling, directly acknowledging painful or difficult emotions.
3.	Suppression	Conscious or semiconscious postponement of attending to a conscious impulse of conflict (looking on the bright side).
4.	Anticipation	Anticipation or planning for future inner discomfort before it becomes necessary to face it.
5.	Sublimation	1. Rechannelizing of instincts into productive endeavor, allowing the instincts to be an extent satisfied. 2. Unconscious gradual channelization of unacceptable impulse into personally satisfying and socially valuable behavioral pattern.
V	OTHERS	
1.	Rationalization	It is a defense mechanism in which an individual justifies his failures and socially unacceptable behavior by giving socially approved reasons.
2.	Intellectualization	Focusing of attention on technical or logical aspects of a threatening situation.
3.	Compensation	Attempting to overcome feelings of inferiority or make up for a deficiency.
4.	Subsituation	A mechanism in which originally goals are substituted by others.
5.	Suppression	Suppression is an intentional pushing away from awareness of certain unwelcome ideas, memories or feelings.
6.	Denial	Refusal to accept or believe in the existence of something that is very unpleasant.
7.	Isolation	Separation of the idea of an unconscious impulse from its appropriate affect.
8.	Regression	Coping with present conflict or stress by returning to earlier, more secure stage of life.
9.	Conversion	A mental mechanism in which an emotional conflict is expressed as a physical symptom for which there is no demons ratable organic basis.
10.	Undoing	Unconsciously motivated acts, which magically or symbolically counteract unacceptable thoughts, impulses or acts.

APPENDIX 5

SECRETS OF HEALTH (A TO Z)

FOOD FACT

The longer that fruits or vegetables sit around waiting to be sold or eaten, the more nutrients they lose. But fruits and vegetables grown for freezing are usually frozen right after they are picked. Therefore, they have less time to lose their nutrients.

A.	Apple	As basic as it may sound, an apple provides you with 13 minerals that you require daily. A sample mix of apple, walnuts and yoghurt makes for a great breakfast to start your day.
B.	Broccoli	The vilayati version of cauliflower is now readily available all over our city. Make good use of it, in a recent survey of greens, broccoli was found to be healthiest, since it is a powerful anti-carcinogen.
C.	Cucumber	As chilly as winter is.
D.	Dudhi (melon)	Melon is known to reduce blood pressure. In cooperative dudhi as part of your cuisine to lower your blood pressure, for a healthier heart in general, to lower cholesterol, and many other benefits.
E.	Egg (egg white)	Make it a habit to remove the yolk, since egg whites are a great source of protein.
F.	Fish	Omega-3 in some fish prevents cardiovascular disease. Also, good source of protein. However, avoid canned varied and over-salted, smoked dishes. Also shell fish, crab and all forms of mussels need to be strictly eaten in moderation.
G.	Garlic	There are way too many health benefits.
H.	Home grown sprouts	Sprouts while available in the local grocery are a much healthier option to grow at home. It is easy to make these at home (soak them overnight), and they makes for a quiet tasty snack either in chaats, or raitas, or salads of your choice.
I.	Iceberg lettuce	An other designer food item that is becoming readily available. This one is great to make salads with at home. Mix with tofu, spourts, tomatoes, chicken and fat-free yoghurt to get you through the day.
J.	Juice blender	Choose a juice of choice for the year. It could be anything you want. But make sure you make it home. Most bottled juice come with lots of sugar and preservatives.
K.	Karela	As bitter and unappetizing as it may sound. The health benefits of this desiveggie far outweigh its sharp taste. It regularizes blood sugar. Aside from a range of other ailments.
L.	Lemon	Sprinkle your food with lots of lemon. It is got lots of vitamin C that you need to boost your immune system. Besides, by replacing lemon with salt as it condiment for your meals, you are helping your heart in more ways than one.
M.	Milk (skimmed)	Milk (but skimmed), there is no way we have been able to escape milk; it is too ingrained in our culture. So go for it, enjoy your milk, but get a bottle of skimmed milk.

Contd...

Contd...

N.	Nuts	Nuts reduce coronary heart disease. Almonds and walnuts lower serum LDL cholesterol levels. Dieticians frequently recommended nuts to diabetes patients with insulin resistance. And those who eat nuts live two to three years longer than those who do not.
O.	Olive oil	Is clearly the healthiest option to the necessary evil that is oil. Its high content of monounsaturated fatty acids and its high content of anti-oxidants make it the best alternative.
P.	Peas	Green peas provide good amount of eight vitamins, seven minerals, dietary fiber and protein. In addition, they are a good source of vitamin K_1, which activates osteocalcin, the major non-collagen protein in bone.
Q.	Quality fruit	The price of fruits has gone over the top. However, fruits are known to be some of the best anti-oxidants, are a great source of fiber and nutrients. Up to your fridge with quality fruits. Berries, apples, bananas, even the tomato.
R.	Red cabbage	Your kids may cringe at sight of regular cabbage. But the flamboyant red cabbage might convince them. Also a source of indole-3-carinole (13C), which reducing the risk of breast cancer by 50%.
S.	Strawberries	It helps to prevent cancer. They also bring out flavor in champagne.
T.	Tea	Another desi habit we cannot give up. So why not substitute chai with green tea or black tea. Regular use is known to strengthen bone and cure osteoporosis.
U.	Ud-ruck	Sorry but G was taken by garlic. But ginger (adrak) is essential to your health.
V.	Varan-bhat (dhal-rice)	Simplicity is a virtue. Amidst your hectic socializing and gourmet fantasies, normal ghar ka khana once a day will do wonders for your health.
W.	Walnuts	Walnuts reduce the risk of prostrate cancer in men.
Y.	Yoghurt	Again is a great source of calcium, aid in digestion and can be merged with a range of salads, health food items, marinades. Always keep a bowl of fresh, home made yoghurt handy in your fridge.
Z.	Zucchini	This Italian kakadi is low in calories and contains a high amount of folate, potassium, vitamin A and manganese. Z though is also for zinc. So do not forget to stack up on your spinach, lentils and salmon.

APPENDIX 6

PERSONALITY DISORDERS

Sl. No.	Terms	Description
1.	Personality disorder	Deviate from the characteristic trait which goes beyond normal.
2.	Meaning	Personality disorders are recognized in early adolescence.
3.	Definition	An abnormal personality is one in which there are deeply ingrained maladaptive patterns of behavior recognizable by the time of adolescence or earlier and continuing through most of adult life (ICD-9).
4.	Classification–DSM-IV	Cluster-A: Schizoid, paranoid, schizotypic. Cluster-B: Histrionic, antisocial and borderline, narcissistic Cluster-C: Avoidant, dependent, obsessive compulsive, aggressive and passive.
5.	Etiology	Hereditary—chromosomal abnormality or genetic predisposition. Biological factors—brain dysfunction and changes in neurotransmitters. Developmental factors—emotional, physical and sexual abuse. Sociocultural factors—involuntary isolation, long-term psychiatric diseases. Precipitating stressors—instability in the family or divorce. Psychological stressors—high anxiety.
6.	Group psychotherapy	Widely used in antisocial personality.
7.	Individual psychotherapy	Effective in antisocial, dependent and inhibited personality disorder.
8.	Behavior therapy	It is useful in anger control and social skills training of some valve.
9.	Cognitive behavior therapy	Effective in antisocial personality disorder.

APPENDIX 7

DIFFERENCE BETWEEN PSYCHOSIS AND NEUROSIS

	Psychosis	Neurosis
Severity	It is a severe illness of the personality.	It is a mild-to-moderate illness of the personality.
Ego	It involves impairment of ego functions.	Ego function is not affected much.
Reality	Reality testing is markly impaired.	Reality testing is not affected much.
Adjustment	Signs of grave maladjustment to life.	Maladjustment to life is limited.
Causes	Organic or psychological.	Mainly due to psychological factor.
Psychodynamics	Result of weak ego.	Partial impairment of ego functioning.
Affect	Changes in terms of elation, depression, apathy, ambivalence and inappropriate affect.	The affect is appropriate to the situation.
Perception	Marked illusion and hallucination present.	Hallucination and illusion not present.
Thought changes	Delusion, flight of ideas, preservation or circumstantiality and other thought changes are present.	Not changes in thinking
Behavior	Marked behavior changes are present.	No marked changes are present.
Judgment	It is impaired and at times very poor.	Judgment is not impaired.
Memory	Markly impaired.	No effect on memory.
Attention	Markly impaired.	No effect on memory.
Intelligence	Markly impaired.	No effect on memory.
Defense mechanisms	Denial, regression, introjections and identification.	Repression, displacement, isolation, reaction, formation, undoing, substitution and conversion.
Treatment	Requires hospitalization.	Rarely requires hospitalization.
Prognosis	Psychotic patients are not very good.	Prognosis is good. Recurrence is very less.

APPENDIX 8

HEALTH STATISTICS

India's Demographic Progress and Achievements of National Family Welfare Program

Health indicator	Previous level	Current level
* Crude birth rate (CBR) per thousand population	41.7 (1951-61)	25.0 (2002)
* Crude death rate (CDR) per thousand population	22.8 (1951-61)	8.1 (2002)
* Infant mortality rate (IMR) per thousand live births	146 (1951-61)	63 (2002)
* Maternal mortality rate (MMR) (per one lakh livebirths)	437 (1992-93)	407 (1999)
* Total fertility rate (TFR) per woman	6.0 (1951)	3.2 (2000)
* Couple protection rate (CPR)	10.4 (1970-71)	48.6 (2000)
* Life expectancy at birth (in years)	54 (1951)	64.6 (RGI-2000)
Male	37.1 (1951)	63.87 (2001-06)*
Female	36.1 (1951)	66.91 (2001-06)*

* Projected.

Source: i. Office of Registrar General of India (RGI).
ii. Annual report 2002-2003, 2004-05, Ministry of Health and Family Welfare, Government of India.
iii. SRS Bulletin, April 2004, Registrar General of India.

APPENDIX 9

HEALTH STATISTICS

Some Other Basic Health Indicators

Health indicator	Present level	Remarks
Total population	1,02,70,15,247 *Male:* 53,12,77,078 *Female:* 49,57,38,169	As on 1st March, 2001
Density of population (Per sq. km)	324 (2001)	Highest in Delhi Lowest in Arunachal
Sex ratio (Females per 1000 males)	933 (2001)	
Literacy rate	65.4 (2001)	Male literacy, 75.85% Female literacy, 54.16%
Population (0-6 age group)	15.78 crores (2001)	
Rural population	72.22% (2001)	
Family size (average)	4 (1998)	
Child death rate (0-4 age group)	23.7 (1993)	HFA Target 10
Perinatal mortality	44.2 (1993)	HFA Target 35
Birth weight of infant less than 2500 gm (%)	30% (1992)	HFA Target 10
Delivery % (By trained workers)	47.3% (1992)	HFA Target 100
Average annual growth rate of population (%)	1.93 % (2001)	Projected in 2025—1.2%

Source: 1. WHO Report, 1997-98.
2. Annual Report, 2001-2002, Ministry of Health and Family Welfare, Government of India.
3. RCH News, MOHFW, Government of India.
4. Census, 2001.

APPENDIX 10

HEALTH STATISTICS

Outlays Under the Family Welfare Programs From the First-Five-Year Plan

Plan	Duration	Outlays in Crores
First plan	1951-56	0.65
Second plan	1956-61	5.00
Third plan	1961-66	27.00
Annual plan	1966-69	82.90
Fourth plan	1969-74	285.80
Fifth plan	1974-78	285.60
Annual plan	1978-80	228.00
Sixth plan	1980-85	1309.00
Seventh plan	1985-90	2868.00
Annual plan	1990-92	1424.00
Eighth plan	1992-97	6195.00
Ninth plan	1997-2002	14968.70
Tenth plan	2002-2007	26126.00 *
Annual plan	2002-2003	4930.00
Annual plan	2003-2004	4930.00
Annual plan	2004-2005	5500.00

* The figures according to allotment of five-year plans. The approved outlay was Rs 27125.00 crores. However, due to establishing six AIIMS-type institutions in the country. Rs 999.00 crores were given to Department of Health, so the Xth plan allocation is Rs 26126.00 crores.

Source: 1. Annual Report, 2000-01 and 2001-02, 2002-03, 2004-2005, Ministry of Health and Family Welfare. Government of India.

2. Expenditure Budget, 2002-2003, 2004-2005, Government of India.

APPENDIX 11

NUTRITIONAL ASSESSMENT FORMAT

1. **General Particulars**
   Name   :
   Age   :
   Sex   :
   Household No   :
   Address   :
   Family income per year   :
   Name of the village   :

2. **Feeding Particulars: (If under - 3 Children)**
   Breastfed   :   Yes/No
   Adequacy   :   Yes/No
   Specify the period of being breastfed   :
   Whether colostrums given   :   Yes/No
   If not on breastfeed now, specify the type
   of feeding given now:
   Is the child on breastfeeding + weaning foods: Yes/No.

3. **Anthropometric Measurements**
   Weight (kg)
   Height (cm)
   Head circumference (cm)
   Chest circumference (cm)
   Mid-upper arm circumference
   Degree of malnutrition

4. **Clinical Examination**

a.	General impression	: Normal built/thin built/apathy/pallor/ irritability.
b.	Hair	: a. Sparse/brownish/brittle/easily pluckable/ normal
		b. Louse infestation/dandruff
c.	Face	: Moon face/nasolabial dyssebacea/normal
d.	Eyes	: Conjunctival xerosis/corneal xerosis/Bitot's spot/keratomalacia/corneal opacity/night blindness/photophobia/normal.
e.	Lips	: Anagular stomatitis/cheilosis
f.	Tongue	: Pale/flabby/red and row/fissured/glossitis
g.	Gums	: Spongy bleeding/normal
h.	Teeth	: Mottled enamel/caries/flurosis
i.	Glands	: Thyroid enlargement/parotid enlargement
j.	Neck	: Cervical node enlargement
k.	Throat	: Enlarged tonsils
l.	Skin	: Follicular hyperkertosis (Phyrynodenna) pellagrous/dermatosis/crazy Pavement dermatosis.
m.	Nails	: Koilonychia
n.	Chest	: Pigeon chest/beading of the ribs

o. Abdomen : Potbelly
p. Edema : In dependent parts
q. Gastrointestinal system : Enlargement of spleen/enlargement of liver.
r. Extremities : Epiphyseal enlargement/knock knee/bow legs/edema
s. Nervous system : Numbness and tingling of extremities/burning feet/tenderness of calf muscles/loss of knee/ankle jerks.

Nutritional Survey

Time	Cooked food	Uncooked food	Measurement kg/ml	Nutritive value						
				CHO	PRO	F	Ca	VIT-A	KCAL	Iron
			Total							

Total :
Recommended :
Deficiency :
Note :

Nutrition
Nutrition may be defined as the science of food and its relationship to health.

Meaning of Nutritional Survey
It has been defined as "Keeping watch over nutrition, in order to make decisions that will ead to improvement in nutrition in population.

Formulas for Assessing Malnutrition

$$Malnutrition = \frac{Actual\ weight}{Expected\ weight} \times 100$$

80 and above—Normal
70 to 80—1st degrees Malnutrition
60 to 70—2nd degrees Malnutrition
50 to 60—3rd degrees Malnutrition
40 to 50—4th degrees Malnutrition

Gomez classification:

$$Weight\ for\ age = \frac{Weight\ of\ the\ child}{Weight\ of\ the\ normal\ child\ of\ same\ age} \times 100$$

Water Low's classification

$$Wt/Ht = \frac{\text{Weight of the child}}{\text{Weight of the normal child of same height}} \times 100$$

$$Ht/Wt = \frac{\text{Weight of the child}}{\text{Weight of the normal child of same age}} \times 100$$

Rules for Safe Food Supply (Personal Hygiene)
1. Do not permit people with diarrhea, sorethroat, and cold to handle food till they are well.
2. Do not allow people with boils, pimple, and carbuncles on hand to food silverware.
3. Avoid sneezing, coughing, near food.
4. Always wash hands after (defecation) use of toilets; combing the head or doing any procedures or duties.
5. Avoid indiscriminate handling of foods with fingers.
6. Do not return tasting spoon, to food without washing.

Food Processing
1. Select foods from plants or markets which maintain high standards of sanitation.
2. Purchase only pasteurized milk, fresh meal. Use it within 24 hours.
3. Protect food at home or in market from flies, insects, rodents, contamination by unnecessary handling.
4. Wash all fruits before refrigeration, use pressure cooker for caning all not-acid vegetables, meat.
5. Discard without tasting all food from can which bulge or form gas.
6. Use frozen after thawing.
7. Carefully label insect powders, do not keep them near food supply.

APPENDIX 12

AVERAGE HEIGHT AND WEIGHT OF BOYS AND GIRLS AT A GIVEN AGE

(As per ICMR)

Age	Boys		Girls	
	Standing height in cm	Weight (kg)	Standing height in cm	Weight (kg)
At birth	50.0	3.0	50.0	3.0
Up to 3 months	56.0	4.5	55.0	4.0
4-6 months	62.5	6.5	61.5	6.5
7-9 months	65.0	7.0	64.0	6.0
10-12 months	69.5	7.5	66.5	6.5
1 year	74.0	8.5	72.5	8.0
2 years	81.5	10.0	80.0	9.5
3 years	89.0	12.0	87.0	11.0
4 years	96.0	13.5	94.5	13.0
5 years	102.0	15.0	101.5	15.5
6 years	108.5	16.5	107.5	16.0
7 years	114.0	18.0	113.0	17.5
8 years	119.5	19.5	118.0	19.5
9 years	123.5	21.5	123.0	21.5
10 years	128.5	23.5	128.5	23.5
11 years	133.5	26.0	133.5	26.5
12 years	138.5	28.5	139.0	30.0
13 years	144.5	32.0	144.0	33.5
14 years	150.0	35.5	147.5	37.0
15 years	155.5	39.5	149.5	39.0

Source: Growth and physical development of Indian infants and children: Technical report series ICMR 20,8,1972.

APPENDIX 13

ESTIMATES FROM DEMOGRAPHIC PROFILE

1.	A N registration	= Population × BR of the area (District) + 10% of the above
2.	Referral of high-risk pregnancies	= 15% of the ANCs
3.	IFA tablets for therapeutic treatment	= 50% of the ANCs
4.	No. of live births	= Population of the area × Birth rate of the area
5.	Referral of high-risk newborn	= 10% of liver births
6.	Infant immunization (polio, DPT, BCG, Measles)	= 100% of infants alive at 1 year = No. of the live births, No. of IDs (or IMR of the area)
7.	Institutional delivery	= 75% of the expected delivery
8.	Skilled attention at delivery	= 95% of the expected delivery
9.	Newborn growth monitoring	= 95% of the expected delivery
10.	0-5 year children	= 10.3% of the total population (State) or under 5 population as per the VS syrvey of the district
11.	Anemia in children	= 50% of 1 to 5 years children

11. Anemia in children

$$= \frac{8.3\% \text{ of total population} \times 50\% \text{ or 1 to 5 years children\% as per the VS survey of the district}}{2}$$

12.	Vit. A-0.5 years children	= No. of under 5 years children × 2 lakh IU/dose
13.	ADD cases	= No. of 0-5 years children × 3 episodes
14.	ARI cases	= No. of 0-5 years children × 2 episodes

15. Requirement of ORS (10% of AD will require ORS)

$$= \frac{\text{No. of 0-5 years children} \times 3 \times 3}{10}$$

16.	Requirement of cotrimoxazole	= (No. of 2-12 months children × 15% × 20 tab) + (No. of 1-5 years children × 15% × 30 tab)
17.	Requirement of FST (L)	= (No. of AN cases × 100) (prophylactic) + (50% of AN cases × 100) Therapeutic + (No. of PN cases × 42 days)
18.	Children at 5 years	= 1.76% of the total population
19.	Children at 10 years	= 1.97% of the total population
20.	Children at 16 years	= 1.92% of the total population

APPENDIX 14

FORMULAE FOR CALCULATION SOME IMPORTANT VITAL RATES

1. Crude Birth Rate (CBR)

$$= \frac{\text{No. of live births during the year}}{\text{Mid-year population}} \times 1000$$

2. Crude Death Rate (CDR)

$$= \frac{\text{No. of deaths during the year}}{\text{Mid-year population}} \times 1000$$

3. Infant Mortality Rate (IMR)

$$= \frac{\text{No. of infant deaths during the year}}{\text{No. of live births during the year}} \times 1000$$

4. Stillbirth Rate (SBR)

$$= \frac{\text{No. of stillbirths during the year}}{\text{No. of live births and stillbirths during the year}} \times 1000$$

5. Perinatal Mortality Rate (PMR)

$$= \frac{\text{No. of stillbirths and infant deaths}}{\text{No. of live births and stillbirths during the year}} \times 1000$$

6. Early Neonatal Mortality Rate

$$= \frac{\text{No. of infant deaths of less than 7 days during the year}}{\text{No. of live births during the year}} \times 1000$$

7. Neonatal Mortality Rate (NMR)

$$= \frac{\text{No. of infant deaths of less than 28 days during the year}}{\text{No. of live births during the year}} \times 1000$$

8. Postneonatal Mortality Rate (PMR)

$$= \frac{\text{No. of infant deaths of over 28 days during the year}}{\text{No. of live births during the year}} \times 1000$$

9. Age Specific Mortality Rate (ASMR)

$$= \frac{\text{No. of deaths in particular age group}}{\text{Mid-year population of the same age group}} \times 1000$$

10. Maternal Mortality Rate (MMR)

$$= \frac{\text{No. of maternal deaths during the year}}{\text{No. of live births during the year}} \times 1000$$

11. Couple Protection Rate (CPR)

$$= \frac{\text{No. of ECs protected either by permanent rate or Temporary Method (RU)}}{\text{Total No. of ECs}} \times 1000$$

Glossary

1. **Accommodation:** A process of adjustment in the social relations among essentially antagonistic groups whereby certain mutually tolerable working arrangements arise which diminish for overt expressions of the underlying antagonisms among them.

2. **Acculturation:** The process whereby new traits are adopted and incorporated into an existing culture. The process of mutual modification of two or more different cultures which are in contact with each other without much sign of their fusing into a single homogeneous culture.

3. **Activities of daily living:** All the activities an individual carries out to maintain physical integrity(ADL).

4. **Acute phase of illness:** Time when therapy and nursing care are directed toward assisting the patient to recover from disabling disease or injury with a minimum of superimposed impairment-social, psychological, or physical.

5. **Adaptation:** The work expended by the body in attempting to maintain homeostasis and to ward off the effects of stressors. Adaptive behaviors are those that promote adaptation.

6. **Addiction:** Strong dependence, both physical and emotional, on alcohol or some other material.

7. **Affect:** A person's emotional feeling and its outward manifestations.

8. **Agitation:** Presence of anxiety with severe motor restlessness.

9. **Agnation:** The practice of reckoning descent and kinship exclusively through the male line.

10. **Agnosticism:** The point of view that the existence of god cannot be scientifically proved.

11. **Agrarian movement:** A social movement in which the farmers of a country seek not only to recognize the agricultural economy but to recognize the agricultural economy but to change the relative importance of agriculture in the total economy of the country and to improve their own, social, economic, educational and political status.

12. **Agrarian socialism:** The political and economic ideology, which justifies collectivization in agriculture.

13. **Ahimsa:** In politics it refers to non-violent opposition to civil authority. In Jainism, the religious doctrine which considers all life sacred.

14. **Alien:** A person living in a given country who was born elsewhere and who is not a citizen of his country of residence.

15. **Alimony:** The support payments made to a divorced spouse, as ordered by a court of law.

16. **Amalgamation:** The process of the genetic mixing of races.

17. **Amnesia:** Pathological impairment of memory.

18. **Amulet:** A small portable object, which is believed to contain supernatural power, which is worn for protection against evil.

19. **Ancestor worship:** The religious ritual that is based on the belief that the ghosts of decreased can mystically intercede on behalf of their living descendants.

20. **Animistic theory of religion:** The view that preliterate men personified every thing and therefore spirits were elevated to status of powerful gods. At that point religion as a human culture.

21. **Applied sociology:** The use of sociological knowledge in solving or reducing social problems.

22. **Aptitude:** Specific ability indicative of one's potentiality to get desired future success.

23. **Assessment:** A dynamic, on going process that uses observations and interactions to collect information, recognize changes, analyze needs and plan care.

24. **Assessments:** The evaluation and interpretation of short- and long-term measurements to provide a basis for decisio- making and to enhance public health officials' ability to monitor disaster situations.

25. **Assimilation:** The process by which the people of two or more cultures who have come into contact with each other lose their unique cultural identities, and become fused into a single homogeneous cultural unit which is different from any of the original component cultural units.

26. **Association:** The process of interaction. The process where new groups are formed or group cohesion is strengthened. A number of formally organized people who are bound together by the fact they are seeking some objectives.

27. **Atheism:** The point of view, which denies the existence of god.

28. **Attention:** The ability to focus on ability.

29. **Auscultation:** Observation by listening with the stethoscope to organ sounds within the body.

30. **Autonomy:** The governing of one's self-according to one's own system of morals and beliefs or life plan.

31. **Bacteriostasis:** The process of preventing the growth and reproduction of microorganisms by the use of chemicals or heat.

32. **Baseline data:** Information gathered about pre-illness states from initial contact used to measure changes in the patient's condition.

33. **Basic human needs:** Physical and psychological needs common to all people that create tension and anxiety if not met.

34. **Basic life support:** It includes noninvasive measures used to treat unstable patients, such as extraction of airway obstructions, cardiopulmonary resuscitation, care of wounds and hemorrhages, and immobilization of fractures.

35. **Basis four food groups:** One pattern for devising a balanced diet including milk group, meat group, vegetable-fruit group, and bread-cereal group.

36. **Beena marriage:** A matrilocal and matriarchal type of family life practiced among certain tribes of the sahara.

37. **Benedict's cultural pattern:** Ruth Benedict's dichotomous division of preliterate cultures into two ideal types. The Apollonian, or calm, restrained type of culture. The Dionysian or frenzied, emotional type of culture.

38. **Biological Determinist Vie of culture change:** The view that cultural differences among ethnic groups are caused by innate physical difference among them, and that culture change is dependent on changes in the physical characteristics of ethnic groups.

39. **Biological factor in social change:** The inherited capacity for intelligence, which would underline the creation of culture.

40. **Biological sociology:** The analysis and interpretation of society and social processes in terms of analogies to biological processes.

41. **Bladder training:** Program to assist the incontinent patient to control urination without catheter and without retention.

42. **Bland diet:** Similar to a general diet but excludes highly seasoned, fried, and fatty foods and foods high in roughage. Also called light diet.

43. **Body alignment:** The position in which the various parts of the body are held while sitting, standing, walking, and lying.

44. **Body intimacy theory of family origin:** The hypothesis that human families originated because of the fact an infant is physically dependent on its mother or on other adults in order to live.

45. **Body mechanics:** Efficient use of the body as a machine and as a means of locomotion, balance, and stability.

46. **Bogardus law of social tension:** Emory S Bogardus statement that the greater the social distance between two groups of people who live in close proximity, the greater is the likelihood of overt tension occurring between them.

47. **Bowel training:** Program to assist incontinent patient in achieving bowel control, allowing controlled bowel movement every 1 to 3 days.

48. **Broken family:** A family which once consisted of a husband and wife (with or without children) from which one parent is permanently absented either because of divorce, death or desertion. (1) A society that is controlled by codified laws, which are enforced by civil authority. (2) Any given society, no matter how simple or complex. (3) The super organic. (4) A complex, literate society, which uses metals, has a machine technology and a money economy.

49. **Bronchial drainage:** Treatment to assist removal of retained bronchial secretions. Usually follows intermittent positive pressure or nebulizer treatment. Includes special positioning and use of percussion and vibration techniques.

50. **Case definition:** Standardized criteria for deciding whether a person has a particular disease or health-related condition; often used in investigations and for comparing potential cases; case definitions help decide which disaster-specific conditions should be monitored with emergency information surveillance systems.

51. **Case finding:** A set of activities used by the nurse working in community settings that identifies clients who are not currently receiving health care, but who could benefit from such care.

52. **Case management:** A systematic process used by nurses to ensure that client's multiple health and service needs are met. These include assessing client needs, planning and coordination services, referring to other appropriate providers and monitoring and monitoring and evaluating process.

53. **Case management:** Case management is the collaborative process that assesses, plans, implements, coordinates, monitors, and evaluates the options and services required to meet an individual's health needs.

54. **Casualty:** Any person suffering physical and/or psychological damage that leads to death, injury, or material loss.

55. **Celsius:** Metric temperature measurement with 0°C being the freezing point of water and 100° being the boiling point. Normal body temperature is 37°C.

56. **Class conflict interpretation:** The view, that all social institutions, forms of social control, ideas of right and wrong forms of government and religion status system as well as the process of change as such are the outward manifestation of a basic conflict among economic classes. In this view, any given society would derived its peculiar institutions from the fact that one class had subdued and dominated all others.

57. **Clean wound:** One that has not been invaded by pathogenic microorganisms; one that heals without infection.

58. **Clear liquid diet:** Includes only broth, tea, clear or strained juices, and gelatin.

59. **Clinical nurse specialist:** A master' prepared nurse with a specific clinical expertise who assumes accountability for quality nursing care including leadership and management.

60. **Closed wound:** Has no break in the continuity of the overlying skin or mucous membrane.

61. **Cognition:** The experience of knowing. The mental process of comprehension, judgment, memory and reasoning.

62. **Collaborative nursing function:** Those activities carried out as a health team member, giving and receiving assistance to and from other health team members in the care of the patient.

63. **Communal society:** An ideal type society in which most of the everyday life is regulated by tradition, custom and the mores and in which there is relatively little emphasis on individual responsibility.

64. **Communication:** A verbal and nonverbal process for exchanging messages between individuals in person-to-person relationships.

65. **Community:** An area of common living which is defined according to the interests or characteristics of the people living in it and in which the people have the sense of being a unit. An aggregate of people living in an area among whom the relations are impersonal and formal, and who are defined ecologically and symbiotically rather than socially.

66. **Community assessment:** The process of determining the real perceived needs of defined community of people.

67. **Community health problem:** The health need identified in community assessment.

68. **Community organization:** The high degree of mutual interdependence among the institutions and groups in a community, in addition a well-developed sense of community cohesion among the people, and a willingness on their part to cooperatively achieve common interest.

69. **Community profile:** The characteristics of the local environment that are prone to a chemical or nuclear accident (these characteristics can include population density; age distribution; number of buildings; and local relief agencies).

70. **Community resources:** A collection of health care providers or supportive care providers who share common interest or a sense of unity.

71. **Community-based nursing:** Nursing care within the context of the clients family and community with a prevention focus that enhances the client's ability for self-care, a collaborative effort to maintain continuity of care.

72. **Complementary therapies:** Interventions that focus on body, mind and spirit integration, may be used in addition to conventional therapies.

73. **Concentration:** The ability to sustain attention.

74. **Concept:** A view or idea we hold about something, ranging from something highly concrete to something highly abstract.

75. **Conduction:** Means of heat transfer in which molecular collision produces transmission; direct contact between warmer and cooler object required.

76. **Conflict:** (1) The social process of opposition among antagonistic groups in which each deliberately seeks to destroy subdues or thwarts the others whether such opposition is violent or not. (2) Violent opposition among groups. (3) Relations between two individuals who seek to thwart to subdue each other.

77. **Conflict:** A mental struggle that arises from the simultaneous operation of opposing emotions.

78. **Conjungal family:** A biological family; the parents and their offspring.

79. **Consanguine family:** A type of family group, which is, organized around the brother and sister relationship. Though the siblings do not marry each other, they live together as a household group, their spouses live in other households.

80. **Constructed survey:** A time-consuming and expensive method of collecting information about a community with a valid and reliable survey, using a random sample of a targeted population where the data collected are analyzed for patterns and trends.

81. **Consultation:** An interaction problem solving process between the nurse and the client.

82. **Contaminated wound:** One in which the potential for infection is relatively great, such as in a wound occurring under accidental conditions without the benefit of aseptic technique.

83. **Contamination:** An accidental release of hazardous chemicals or nuclear materials that pollute the environment and place humans at risk of contamination.

84. **Contingency plan:** An emergency plan developed in expectation of a disaster; often based on risk assessments, the availability of human and material resources, community preparedness, and local and international response capabilities.

85. **Continuity of care:** Coordination of services provided to clients before they enter a health care setting, during the time they are in the setting, and after they leave the setting.

86. **Contract society:** A society in which social control is exerted primarily by means of formal law, rather than by custom alone.

87. **Contract theory:** The hypothesis that human societies originated in a deliberate contract decided of social origin. Upon by savages who were living in a state of nature, whereby everyone assumed a certain status in the society with its rights and obligations.

88. **Contract:** A term sometimes used to describe the fiduciary relationship in professional ethics grounded in promises or pledges.

89. **Coordinate care:** The coordination of interdisciplinary sources of care and support to provide successful continuity of care.

90. **Coordination:** A systematic exchange of information among principal participants in order to carry out a unified response in the event of an emergency.

91. **Covenant:** A solemn agreement between two or more parties that, as related to health care, emphasizes the moral and social character of the bond between professional and patient.

92. **Creed:** A body of fundamental belief, which guide ethical contact.

93. **Cretinism:** A type of mental retardation caused by thyroid deficiency.

94. **Crisis management:** Administrative measures that identify, acquire, and plan the use of resources needed to anticipate, prevent, and/or resolve a threat to public health and safety (e.g. terrorism).

95. **Crowd:** An impermanent assemblage of interacting persons who lack leadership and internal organization, and who are without a group tradition or unique cultural background which would provide them with ready responses for acting as a group; this makes them, suggestible, impulsive, irrational, fickle, and unpredictable in their behavior in new situations.

96. **Cultural anthropology:** The study of the cultures of simple and primitive societies, of cultural origins, cultural variability and the process of diffusion.

97. **Cultural area:** The geographic area in which a relatively homogeneous culture is located.

98. **Cultural assessment:** Considers the cultural beliefs, values and practices of an individual, group or community to determine needs and interventions within a specific cultural context.

99. **Cultural base:** The cultural of a people seen as consisting of the materials and techniques from which interventions may be made.

100. **Cultural care:** Health care in a cultural context, acknowledging the client's cultural beliefs about disease and treatment.

101. **Cultural center:** The place or area in which a given culture trait originated and from which it was diffused.

102. **Cultural change:** Any modification, addition or loss of ideas, cultural objects of the techniques and practices that are associated with them.

103. **Cultural conditioning:** The process of learning the valves, norms, points of view and social practices of a given society by participating in its activities.

104. **Cultural contract:** The initial state of mutual awareness between cultural groups.

105. **Cultural imperatives:** The social norms which are found in all societies, which presumably express the basic social needs of all people.

106. **Cultural integration:** The degree of consistency among the major values or ideas of a society.

107. **Cultural island:** A cultural group which lives in the midst of a large society of a different culture.

108. **Cultural knowledge:** Familiarity with a culturally or ethnically diverse group's world view, beliefs, values, practices, life styles and problem solving strategies.

109. **Cultural lag:** The discrepancy between two related parts of a culture because of different rates of change in the parts of a particular culture, which changes more slowly than the parts, which are related to it.

110. **Cultural minority:** A Group of aggregate of people who have unique culture in a society which is dominated by a group having another culture. The minority usually has a lower political, economical and social status than the dominated cultural group in the society. It may be a small cultural island in a city or it may be an entire nationality in a multinational states.

111. **Cultural myth:** A mythological explanation of the origin of a society, social practice, or culture object, which relies on the action of a cultural deity or cultural hero.

112. **Cultural orthogenesis:** The over development of a certain aspects of a culture compressed to its other aspects. This concept assumes that there is such a thing as a culture that is equally developed in all its aspects.

113. **Cultural pluralism:** The co-existence of several different culture group in a multi-national state.

114. **Cultural skill:** The ability to collect relevant cultural data regarding the client's health history.

115. **Cultural sociology:** The study of the origin and change in the social practices and norms of a given society.

116. **Cultural typology:** A logical classification of cultures which purports to characterize the similarities and differences among them.

117. **Culture complex:** A construct of a meaningful configuration of culture traits which comprise an aspect of major importance in the way of life of people.

118. **Culture determinism:** The view that the culture of a particular people is a self-contained extra-human entity which operates under its own laws and shapes the human personality, while the human initiative or will is seen as merely an appendage of culture.

119. **Culture evolution:** The gradual change in the number, variety and complexity of culture objects as well as in their meanings and functions.

120. **Culture object:** A man-made material object which is used for socially defined purpose; technically the concept would also include things which were not actually made by men, but which nevertheless would have a social meaning as for example, a sacred lake or a sacred mountain.

121. **Culture pattern:** A contract which refers to logical interpretations of all the culture into a meaningful whole; it is intended as a general characterization of an entire culture for the purpose of comparing it with other cultures.

122. **Culture triad:** A construct which refers to the simplest element in a culture; a way of using a culture object, a social norm, a social attitude and so on.

123. **Culture type:** (1) A type of personality which is either produced by a given culture or which gets its meaning from the way that the person regularly acts with references to a given culture. It is the same as a social type. (2) A type of cultural pattern.

124. **Culture:** (1) All the learned socially-meaningful conduct which is practiced in a given society including customs, norms, language, the religious, economic and political belief and practices, art and so on. This definition excludes all the man made socially meaningful objects (the cultural objects). (2) All that is learned and shared by a particular society plus all their man made material goods that have a social meaning. (3) The term also refers to super organic, or all the learned conduct and artifacts of man as a genius of animal as distinct from all that is biologically inherited by men.

125. **Culturology:** The study of the origins and development of cultures.

126. **Decontamination:** The removal of hazardous chemicals or nuclear substances from the skin and/or mucous membranes by showering or washing the affected area with water, or by rinsing with a sterile solution.

127. **Delegation:** A management principle used to obtain desired results through the work of others, and a legal concept used to empower on person to act for another.

128. **Delinquency:** The term is usually used to refer to any undesirable conduct on the part of a juvenile which is serious enough to compel the attention of persons of authority outside the family. It includes truancy, incorrigibility in school, petty offences and sometimes fairly serious crimes. The term is also used as a softer synonym for adult crimes.

129. **Dementia:** A chronic organic mental disorder. An irreversible global deterioration of mental functions. Organic or global determination of intellectual functioning without clouding of consciousness.

130. **Deprivation:** Condition under which needs are unfulfilled.

131. **Development task:** The usual and expected psychosocial, cognitive or psychomotor skill at certain periods in life, failure to master the developmental task can lead to unhappiness and difficulty with later tasks.

132. **Developmental tasks:** Identified physical, psychological and social changes occurring at various stages from the prenatal stage through the older years.

133. **Dharma:** The Hindu code of righteous conduct; a set of ritual duties.

134. **Disaster epidemiology:** The study of disaster related deaths, illnesses, and injuries in humans; also includes the study of the factors and determinants that affect death, illness, and injury following a disaster (Methodology involves identifying and comparing risk factors among disaster victims to those who were left unharmed. Epidemiologic investigations provide public health professionals with information on the probable public health consequences of disasters).

135. **Disease:** Any condition that actually or potentially hinders individual function.

136. **Divorce:** The legal dissolution of a legal marriage.

137. **Documentation:** The process of obtaining and recording information used for communication, references and legal issues.

138. **Down syndrome:** A mentally retarded condition due to chromosomal abnormalities.

139. **Dowry:** The bonus paid to groom by the family by bride.

140. **Dumont's theory of population:** A dumont's statement that as individuals rises in the social status system, they are less likely to reproduce because they lose interest in family life and race perpetuation.

141. **Durkheim's stages of social; development:** Emil's durkhim's statement that there are two ideal type stages. (1) Mechanical solidarity and (2) The organic and voluntary solidarity; which is associated with the functional organization of society.

142. **Ecology:** (1) The study of the reciprocal influences between humans and their physical; or geographic environment; (2) The study of the spatial distribution and interrelations among human being, and institutional functions which are in competition with each other for the most advantageous location in acommunity; (3) The study of the effects of the spatial distribution of human being on their social relations and the influence of their spatial distribution; (4) The study of the development and composition of a community people.

143. **Egalitarianism:** (1) The point of view that all people, regardless of wealth, social status, race, nationality or sex should have the same, political rights; (2) The view which assumes that each social economic class in a given society and each race or ethnic group in the world, has the same proportion of person in the various intelligence levels.

144. **Ego:** It is a part of mental apparatus that serves between ID and super ego.

145. **Elective surgery:** Surgery needed by the patient but in which scheduling can be performed when it is convenient and beneficial to the patient, contrasting with emergency surgery.

146. **Elimination:** One means by which the body, through the integumentary, respiratory, urinary, and gastrointestinal systems, maintains homeostasis related to temperature, chemical composition, and osmotic pressure.

147. **Employee wellness programs:** Plans that focus on keeping employees healthy and preventing illness and accidents.

148. **Enculturation:** The process by which the personality of a newborn infant in shaped by the culture of the groups in which he participate.

149. **Endogamy:** The social norm which hold that proper marriages should occur only among the members of racial, religious, tribal or other in group.

150. **Environment:** The sum of people, things, conditions, or influences surrounding persons.

151. **Environmental assessment:** Evaluation of the client's home and neighborhood environment.

152. **Environmentalism:** (1) The view that the geographic environment is the primary casual factor in social or cultural change; (2) The view which seeks to explain human social; behavior by emphasizing the importance of the economic, cultural or ecological conditions under which men live, while minimizing the factors of human initiative.

153. **Epidemic:** The occurrence of any known or suspected contagion that occurs in clear 'excess of normal expectancy' (a threatened epidemic occurs when the circumstances are such that a disease may reasonably be anticipated to occur in excess of normal expectancy).

154. **Epidemiology:** The study of the various factors and conditions that determines the occurrence and distribution of health, disease, defect, disability, and death among group of individuals.

155. **Extrapyramidal syndrome (EPS):** Commonly caused by anti-psychotic medications.

156. **Ethical:** An evaluation of actions, rules, or the character of persons, especially as it refers to the examination of a systematic theory of rightness or wrongness at the ultimate level.

157. **Ethnocentrism:** (1) Evaluating other peoples and their ways of life in terms of the norms and beliefs of the in-group; (2) An intolerance of the ways of behaving which differs from those of the group.

158. **Ethnology:** The systematic study of cultural variability for the purpose of describing generations about cultural origins, development and variability.

159. **Ethnos:** An ethnic group; a tribal society.

160. **Ethos:** The basic character of pattern, of an ethnic group which makes it distinct from all other ethnic groups.

161. **Evaluation research:** The application of scientific methods to assess the effectiveness of programs, services, or organizations established to improve a patient's health or prevent illness.

162. **Evaluation:** A detailed review of a disaster relief program designed to determine whether program objectives were met, to assess the program's impact on the community, and to generate "lessons learned" for the design of future projects (evaluations are most often conducted at the completion of important milestones, or at the end of a specified period).

163. **Exogamy:** A large family unit of three or more generations who related along the male or female lines, who live in a cluster of houses.

164. **Exposure surveillance:** To look for exposure to risk (in a disaster setting, exposure may be based on the physical or environmental properties of the disaster event; also known as a risk factor variable; predictor variable, or independent variable).

165. **Extended family:** The custom which holds the proper marriages should occur only between members of two racial, tribal, village or other groups.

166. **Extrovert:** A type of personality whose chief social and personal interests are satisfied in the company of others.

167. **Family:** A group which comes into being to establish or regularize the sexual or procreative function. Primary group which is made up of two parents (biological or legal) and at least one dependent child, all of whom are bound by a feeling of familism.

168. **Family culture:** The traditions, customs, group, habits, attitudes and understanding which are peculiar to members of a given family.

169. **Family health:** How well the family functions together as a unit, the family's ability to carry out usual and desired daily activities.

170. **Family structure:** The characteristics of individuals (age, gender, number) who make up the family unit.

171. **Fertility:** The actual number of births in a given population during a given period of time.

172. **Feudal society:** An ideal type society which is the make up of closed status categories or estates; it is made up of a large peasant labor force a small number of privileged land ower's artisan's and merchants, warriors and a scholarly or priestly estate. Each status category would be obliged to observe its own laws.

173. **Fidelity:** The state of being faithful, which includes obligations of loyalty and the keeping of promises and commitments. Also the principles that actions are right insofar as they demonstrate such loyalty.

174. **First responder:** Local police, fire, and emergency medical personnel who arrive first on the scene of an incident and take action to save lives, protect property, and meet basic human needs.

175. **Folk culture:** The way of life of the mass of the people making up a particular ethnic group.

176. **Folk society:** A small, isolated society which has a homogeneous population and culture, an elementary division of labor, an uncodified and inexplicit value system, a simple technology, a stable traditionalistic leadership, strong blood and totemic kinship ties, a high reverence for tradition, and one in which magic and religion are of great importance.

177. **Folkways:** The more or less compulsory group habits and beliefs which meet the recurring social situations.

178. **Formalism:** The view that actions are right or wrong based on their formal characteristics rather than their consequences (often a synonym for deontologist).

179. **Fraternal polyandry:** The marriage of several brothers to one woman.

180. **Functional assessment:** Determination of level of health defined by one's ability to carry out usual and desired daily activities.

181. **Functional inspired oxygen (FIO2):** The measure of oxygen concentration being taken into the respiratory system (especially in supplemental oxygen therapy).

182. **Functional:** Having a psychological rather than organic pathology.

183. **Functionalism:** (1) The interpretation of any part of a culture with reference to its meaning in a large social system, group or cultural complex. (2) The view that all the parts of a culture (or way of life) an functionally related and contribute to the welfare and survival of the society. (3) The view that a culture functions to meet the recurring requirements, of human as biological organism in a given environmental setting.

184. **Gandarva marriage:** A tribal society or one based on kinship rather on law.

185. **Gastric lavage:** Irrigation of the stomach, usually by means of a tube inserted through the nose or mouth, to remove poisons or irritating matter from stomach, to prepare for surgery, or to relieve nausea and vomiting.

186. **General adaptation syndrome:** Three stages of physiologic changes in response to stress identified by Selye; the alarm reaction, stage of resistance, and state of exhaustion.

187. **Geriatric psychiatric:** It deals with mental health problems of the elderly.

188. **Gerontology nursing:** The nursing care of older adults, particularly those older than 65 years.

189. **Gesellschaft:** The ideal-type large urban group which is characterized by impersonal and contractual relations among the people and which can be controlled only by formal laws and other institutional means.

190. **Great man theory in culture change:** A explanation of social and cultural change which emphasize the importance of talented and extraordinary individuals in bringing about such changes.

191. **Grief:** The emotional response to loss. Definite stages of typical reactions have been identified as panic, emotional response, negotiation, commitment, and completion.

192. **Group acceptance:** The act of recognizing a person as a member of a particular group, and thereby assigning him a certain role and status in the group.

193. **Group demoralization:** The sudden and drastic reeducation in group morale, and the concomitant growth of the feeling that continued group efforts is not worthwhile.

194. **Group disintegration:** The dissolution of a permanent group because of a reduced in morale and cohesiveness, and the loss of a sense of purposes.

195. **Group feeling:** The awareness among the members of a group that they constitute a distinct social unit which is different in certain ways from all other groups.

196. **Group integration:** A high degree of organization, unity of purpose and morale in a group.

197. **Group marriage:** The marriage of two or more men to two or more women. This was very rare and co-exists, the husbands were invariably bothers and the wives were sisters.

198. **Group:** (1) A number of interacting persons who are aware of being members of a more or less permanent social unit which has some organization and division of functions, something of a status system recognized norms to control their conduct and some similarity of interests or purposes. (2) And number of people who interact, even though there may be no organization, division of functions, status system norms or sense of performance among them; a crowd. (3) All the people holding allegiance to certain ideals or purposes, whether they are organized or not whether they are aware of each other or not or whether they actually interact directly or not for example, a labor union, ethnic group nationality or nation. (4) Human interaction as such.

199. **Hallucination:** It is a false perception occurring without any true sensory stimulus.

200. **Hazard:** The probability that a disaster will occur [hazards can be caused by a natural phenomenon (e.g. earthquake, tropical cyclone), by an uncontrolled human activity (e.g. conflict, overgrazing)].

201. **Head hunting:** A custom of collecting the heads of enemies as trophies to enhance prestige or to fulfill a ceremonial purpose.

202. **Health behavior:** Activities of a person engages in when feeling healthy; to take measures to prevent disease and illness or to detect them before symptoms occur.

203. **Health care system:** Made up of all services that provide promotion of health, prevention of disease, detection and treatment of disease, follow-up service, and rehabilitation.

204. **Health indicator:** Reflects the major public health concerns and illuminates factors that affect the health of individuals and communities.

205. **Health promotion:** Activities that enhance the well being of an already healthy individual.

206. **Health protection:** Environmental or regulatory measures that confer protection on large population groups.

207. **Health:** A State of complete mental, physical, and social well-being, which maximizes the individual's ability to function in a normal manner.

208. **Health:** State of physical, mental and social well being and not merely the absence of disease or infirmity.

209. **Health-illness continuum:** A complex, dynamic process that includes physical, psychological, and social components that affects the level of wellness or illness at a given point in time.

210. **Health-illness continuum:** Health described in a range of degrees from optimal health at one end to total disability or death at the other.

211. **Herd:** (1) An emotional, uncritical, and unorganized, collection of people who passively follow a leader. (2) A collection of animals of the same kind.

212. **Hereditary:** The transmission of physical characteristics from one generation to the next by means of germ cells.

213. **Hereditary-environment controversy:** The dispute as to whether a person's inherited capacities or the social groups to which he belongs are made important in shaping his personality.

214. **Historical sociology:** The study and description of the origins and development of societies, groups, ideologies, institutions and other social phenomena. It is essentially the science of culture which seeks laws and principles of development which are intrinsic to social phenomena.

215. **Holism:** A way of viewing the person as an integrated whole of mind, body and spirit, reflects the interactive process that occurs in all of us.

216. **Holistic assessment:** Considers not only physical and psychosocial factors, but also cultural, functional, nutritional, environmental and spiritual aspects of the client.

217. **Home health care:** Components of comprehensive health care whereby health services are provided to individuals and families in their places of residence for the purpose promoting, maintaining or restoring health.

218. **Home visit:** Assessment, diagnosis, planning and evaluation of nursing care in the client's home.

219. **Horde:** (1) A hypothetical concept used by some of the early social scientists to refer to an undifferentiated collection of people who lived as a unit, but within which there was no social organization into families or other kinship units. The hordes was supported to have practiced sex communism; private property among them was supported to have been unknown. There is no record of such a society among humans; (2) The word is also used as a condescending references to the mass of untutored and defined people.

220. **Hospice care:** Holistic service provided to dying persons and their loved ones to proved a more dignified and comfortable death.

221. **Human nature:** The group habits, norms, cultural attitudes, sentiments and values that persons in a given society learn through association with each other.

222. **Human relations:** The field of applied sociology which seeks to reduce tensions and antagonism that might already exist of that might arise among various groups and categories of people in a community.

223. **Hygienic care:** Those nursing measures affording personal cleanliness, comfort, rest, and exercise.

224. **Hypnosis:** An altered state of consciousness induced by suggestion.

225. **ID:** An unconscious part of mind, it acts upon the pleasurable principle.

226. **Idealistic society:** A society in which the cultural represents a compromise between the ideation and sensate types of cultures.

227. **Ideational sociology:** A society which exalts spiritual values over material value.

228. **Illness behavior:** Activities a person engages in when feeling ill that will lead to the defining of the state of health and gain help.

229. **Illusion:** Misperception of external stimuli.

230. **Incontinence:** The involuntary voiding of urine or the involuntary defecation of feces or both.

231. **Industrial society:** A society in which an industrial economic crucially affects the social relations among the people. It is one in which large masses of people who form the labor force live in large urban areas. They are differentiated into numerous status levels based on differences in wealth, political, power, occupational status and specialization because of the use of mass production techniques. A wide variety of goods is produced and the living standards are high. It is a society in which because of its size much of the social interaction is formal; government is distant and mechanical and mass communication methods have to be used to reach the people.

232. **Industrial sociology:** The study of the effects of work in industry on the way of life of workmen; it includes the study of work groups as social units and the social relations in these groups as social units and the social relations in these groups, it views workman not as faceless cogs in an impersonal enterprise, but as human being with hopes, fears, shortcoming. Aspirations and self-esteem, who carry on a particular tradition observe a work oriented status system and live a certain ways of life which is largely affected by the occupations.

233. **Infected wound:** Also called septic wound, one in which the invasion of pathogens is too great for the resistance of the first line of internal body defenses, causing clinical symptoms of infection to develop.

234. **Infection control:** Utilization of standards established to monitor infections, trace sources and patterns of disease spread. And institute measures to control spread.

235. **Initiation rites:** A ceremony commemorating the admission of a person into a new status level of group.

236. **Insight:** Ability of the patient to understand the true causes and meaning of a situation.

237. **Insight:** Understanding one's own condition.

238. **Inspection:** Observation with the eye.

239. **Institution:** (1) The social norms and standardized practices which are performed by special functionaries in meeting continuous or recurring human requirements; (2) The term is often loosely applied to a public building.

240. **Institutionalization:** The process of formalizing and standing the social practices which serve to maintain the important social values and establish regular procedures of control in a society.

241. **Intake:** Measure of fluid taken into the body. Includes liquids taken orally, intravenous fluids or tube feedings, and in special situations may include estimates of water from solid foods, injections, and so on.

242. **Integrated communications:** A system that uses a common communications plan, standard operating procedures, clear text, common frequencies, and common terminology.

243. **Integration:** In the social science, the term is used in various contexts to refer to the act of process of unifying things which were previously discrete and separate, into a composite whole.

244. **Intelligence:** (1) The capacity for learning new habits and insights, to retain learned ones, to adapt to new situations adequately, to see relationships among phenomena, to solve problems, to anticipate the actions among phenomena, to solve problems, to anticipate actions of others and so on. (2) The measurable abilities to solve problems, analyze logical fallacies, to learn new knowledge and to retain learned knowledge.

245. **Interview:** A purposeful, goal-directed conversation with patient or family.

246. **IQ:** Intelligence quotient, measured through psychological testing. Normal IQ is 90-110.

247. **Justice:** A moral principle that holds that actions (or rules) are morally right insofar as they reflect a specified pattern of distribution of benefits and harms. A synonym for moral rightness; right taking into account all moral principles.

248. **Kinship:** The relationship among people that exists because of genetic descent, or marriage.

249. **Latrines:** A pit designed to capture and contain excreta; most often trenches with multiple platforms across them, or solitary pits surrounded by a structure.

250. **Law of social migration:** Franz oppenheimer's statement that men tend to move from a place of greater socio-economic pressure to a place of less socio-economic pressure.

251. **Law of social motion:** Herbert Spenser's view that social change, or social tends, tend to follow the . direction of least observation.

252. **Law of stratification:** Vilfredo pareto's statement that a privileged aristocracy in a country can survive only so long as it uses force to perpetuate itself.

253. **Legalism:** The position that ethical action consists in strict conformity to law or rules; cf. antinomianism, rules of practice, situationalism.

254. **Liaison:** An agency official who works with individual agencies or agency officials to coordinated interagency communications.

255. **Libido:** A term used in psychoanalytical theory for sexual drive.

256. **Life cycle analogy in sociology:** The attempt to explain the development of social groups and institutional practices in terms of life-cycle stages of a biological organism; for example, the birth, growth, maturation, decline and death of an animal was considered analogus to the development of a group.

257. **Listening:** Detection of the speaker's meaning by using clues about emotional state and nonverbal cues as well as speech content.

258. **Local government:** Any country, city, village, town, district, political subdivision of any state, Indian tribe or authorized tribal organization, or Alaska native village or organization, including rural communities, unincorporated towns and villages, or any other public entity.

259. **Long-term illness:** Chronic illness. An illness of 3 or more months' duration.

260. **Loss:** A range of adverse consequences that can impact communities and individuals (e.g. damage, loss of economic value, loss of function, loss of natural resources, loss of ecological systems, environmental impact, health deterioration, mortality, morbidity).

261. **Macro-sociology:** The study of large communities and entire societies.

262. **Malthusian doctrine:** (After Thomas malthus) The view that human reproduction increases by geometric progression, and thus eventually outstrips the available food supply which increase by arithmetic progression. Famines, therefore, would be an inevitable necessity from time to time; the only way of retarding famines are either to voluntarily reproduction or to kill off people in wars.

263. **Managerial sociology:** The sociological analysis of the methods and purposes of management in industry.

264. **Marriage:** (1) The ceremony which unites a man and women into a family. (2) The legal partnership of a man and a woman. (3) The person-to-person relationship between a husband and wife, which is made up of their respective roles involving the duties and privileges of each toward the other.

265. **Marxian theory of population:** The view that capitalistic countries must necessarily have problems of population surplus because low wages make it difficult for workman to support their families. On the other hand according to the theory, the socialistic countries cannot possibly have problems of the population surplus because compensation for labor would be on the basis of need; this would allow energetic proletarians to have large families since full employment and adequate income were guaranteed.

266. **Material culture:** Culture object; anything tangible that is man-made.

267. **Matriarchal family:** A family group in which the wife has the highest status, controls the other family members, and makes important decisions affecting the family group.

268. **Matriarchate:** A society, a social group, or organization which is dominated by women.

269. **Matrilineal descent:** Tracing descent through the female line only.

270. **Medical asepsis:** The prevention of the transfer of pathogenic organisms to clean areas.

271. **Medical coordination:** The coordination between health care providers during the transition from the pre-hospital to the hospital phase of patient care; simplification and standardization of materials and methods is a prerequisite.

272. **Medical sociology:** The study of the social aspects of public health problems and conditions.

273. **Mental health:** The capacity of an individual to form harmonious relationship with others.

274. **Mentally ill:** A person who is in need of treatment by reason of any mental disorders other than mental retardation.

275. **Micro-sociology:** The study of the behavior and organization of small communities and small groups.

276. **Mitigation:** Measures taken to reduce the harmful effects of a disaster by attempting to limit the disaster's impact on human health and economic infrastructure.

277. **Mobility:** (1) A change in social status. (2) The process of changing residence.

278. **Monitoring:** A process of evaluating the performance of response and recovery programs by measuring a program's outcomes against stated objectives (monitoring is used to identify bottlenecks and obstacles that cause delays or programmatic shortfalls that require assessment).

279. **Monogamy:** A form of marriage in which there is only one spouse to each sex, as distinguished from polygamy in which a person may have two or more spouses of the other sex.

280. **Monotheism:** Worship of only one god. Monotheism preludes the existence of any plural number of gods.

281. **Mood:** An internal emotional state of an individual.

282. **Moral restraint:** Pre-marital chastity and the postponement of marriage as a means of keeping at a minimum the number of births in a population.

283. **Mortality data:** Information about the number of deaths used to assess the magnitude of a disaster, evaluate the effectiveness of disaster preparedness, evaluate the adequacy of warning systems, and to aid contingency planning by identifying high-risk groups.

284. **Natural disasters:** Natural phenomena with acute onset and profound effects (e.g. earthquakes, floods, cyclones, tornadoes).

285. **Nebulization:** A method of administering water or liquid drugs in which a mist like spray is produced, breaking the substances into minute particles for inhalation.

286. **Neurosis:** Psychiatric disorder in which the patient has insight into the illness.

287. **Neutralism:** A characteristics of moral or ethical evaluations in which there is general application not favoring one party.

288. **Non-fraternal polyandry:** A form of polyandry in which several men who are married to a given women are not brothers.

289. **Non-material culture:** The folkways, occupational techniques, norms for conduct languages habits and the religions, economic and political practices of a group of people.

290. **Nonverbal communication:** Exchanging information by using gestures, facial expressions, posture and body movements, not necessarily intentional.

291. **Normative:** The branch of ethics having to do with which actions are right or wrong, which states are valuable, or which character traits of persons are praiseworthy, e.g. metaethics.

292. **Nuclear family:** The husband, wife and their offspring. It is the same as conjugal family.

293. **Nursing assessment:** The first step of the nursing process. The sum total of data collection, observation, communication, and the physical examination.

294. **Nursing audit:** A retrospective review of patient records to evaluate written documentation of nursing care action.

295. **Nursing care plan:** The individualized written guide for nursing care actions.

296. **Nursing diagnosis:** The process of recognizing patient's needs, and identifying and stating the nature and extent of the related nursing problems.

297. **Nursing history:** Interview gathering data, focusing on the meaning of health and illness care to the patient and family; a basis for planning care.

298. **Nursing process:** A problem solving approach to providing nursing care using four essential steps; assessment, planning, implementation, and evaluation.

299. **Objective symptoms or signs:** Those that the nurse can see, hear, feel, smell, or measure.

300. **Ordering:** A characteristic of moral or ethical evaluations on which a set of principles, rules, or character assessments provides a basis for ranking conflicting claims.

301. **Orgasm:** Peak reaction to sexual stimulation.

302. **Outcome variable:** A health event, usually encompassing illness, injury or death; also known as a response variable.

303. **Output:** Measure of fluid lost by body. Includes urine, emesis, drainage, and in special situations, estimates of respiratory, gastrointestinal, and perspiration amounts.

304. **Over-population:** The existence of two many people in a given area to allow them to maintain a given plan of living.

305. **Paganism:** The polytheistic worship of idols.

306. **Paleolithic age:** The old stone age, the period of cultural development which was characterized by the use of crudely chipped stone tools which were made into almond-shaped flake tools. The men or near-men, of the Paleolithic secured their food by gathering, vegetation, by hunting wild animals. They live in the open or in natural shelters such as caves.

307. **Palpation:** Observation by touch, to feel a part with the fingers.

308. **Paranoid:** An adjective applied to individuals who are over-suspicious.

309. **Parenteral:** Literally outside the intestinal tract. Generally any of the ways by which suitable liquid preparations of drugs are injected by needle into the tissues or directly into the bloodstream.

310. **Parochialism:** A point of view which is concerned primarily with town or neighborhood conditions with only secondary regard for conditions elsewhere.

311. **Pastoral culture:** A way of life which develops out of the fact that a group of people are dependent on herds of domesticated animals for a food supply. Because of the necessary of constant migration, their culture is limited largely to portable goods and their social organization is influenced by the arduous character of migration.

312. **Patriarchal family:** A monogamous family in which the oldest male, has extensive authority over the other members of the family or the household.

313. **Pay surgery centers:** Ambulatory services that provide preoperative, operative and postoperative care on an outpatient basis.

314. **Perception:** A process of organizing environmental stimuli into some meaningful patterns of whole.

315. **Percussion:** Observation by hearing, elicitation of sound determined by tapping surfaces with fingers.

316. **Perineal care:** Cleansing of the vulvar and anal region in the female; the penis, scrotum, and anal region in the male.

317. **Personality:** The characteristic way in which a person believes. The total qualities of an individual.

318. **Phobia:** Intense and irrational fear of some specific objects or situation.

319. **Physical environment:** The total of nonliving things surrounding persons such as air, water, and land.

320. **Political sociology:** A study of the political state as a social phenomenon and the social and cultural factors influencing political organization and change.

321. **Polyandry:** A form of polygamy where is a women may legally have two or more husbands at the same time.

322. **Polygamy:** Plural marriage of one man to two or more women or the marriage of one woman to two or more men at the same time.

323. **Polytheism:** The belief in many gods of equal status.

324. **Population density:** The number of people living in each unit of area.

325. **Population problems:** The problems associated with an unwanted increase or decrease in the number of people, a change in the sex ratio, age structure, or in population quality.

326. **Preparedness:** All measures and policies taken before an event occurs that allow for prevention, mitigation, and readiness (preparedness includes designing warning systems, planning for evacuation and relocation, storing food and water, building temporary shelter, devising management strategies, and holding disaster drills and exercises. Contingency planning is also included in preparedness as well as planning for post-impact response and recovery).

327. **Prescriptivism:** The view that ethical utterances function to prescribe conduct rather than make cognitive claims.

328. **Prevention:** Primary, secondary, and tertiary efforts that help avert an emergency; these activities are commonly referred to as "mitigation" in the emergency management model (for example, prevention activities include cloud seeding to stimulate rain in a fire; in public health terms, prevention refers to actions that prevent the onset or deterioration of disease, disability and injury).

329. **Preventive rehabilitative processes:** Processes that minimize the ill effects of bed rest, inactivity, and disruption of normal patterns of activities of daily living.

330. **Primary nurse practitioner:** Nurses with advanced preparation in data gathering and assessment, who provide services in the patient's first contact with the health care system; generally in ambulatory care settings. Responsible for referral and/or collaborative follow-up care.

331. **Primary prevention:** Preventing the occurrence of death, injury, or illness in a disaster (e.g. evacuation of a community in a flood prone area, sensitizing warning systems for tornadoes and severe storms).

332. **Primitive society:** (1) A society that has not developed a system or writing. (2) A non-literate society that has a rudimentary culture, with no knowledge of metallurgy, machine manufactures, agriculture, or any systematic science, philosophy or theology.

333. **Prognosis:** Outlook of present illness, whether patient can be expected to return to normal daily routine; whether there will be a physical handicap; whether there must be continuous medical therapy; whether death is near.

334. **Prostitute:** A women who sells sex favors to practically anyone wiling to pay her. She is unbounded by the sex mores of a community, and is not affected by the normal sanctions concerning sex conduct.

335. **Protective isolation:** Sometimes called reverse isolation; seeks to protect the patient from microorganisms in the environment.

336. **Pseudodementia:** Clinical features resembling a dementia not caused by an organic mental dysfunction; most often caused by depression.

337. **PSRO:** Professional Standards Review Organization. A method of patient record evaluation to determine the effectiveness of medical diagnosis and treatment in relation to federally financed health care.

338. **Psychiatrist:** A medical practitioner possessing a postgraduate degree or diploma in psychiatry recognized by the Medical Council of India.

339. **Psychological sociology:** The body of knowledge and interpretive point of view which seeks to explain sociological phenomena primarily in terms of individual psychological factors such as desires, motives, interests, wishes, needs, feelings and impulses.

340. **Psychology:** The science investigating the behavior of mental and emotional life.

341. **Psychometery:** The science of testing and measuring mental and psychological ability, efficiency, potentials and functioning.

342. **Psychopathology:** The study of significant causes and processes in the development of mental disorders.

343. **Psychosis:** A psychotic disorder in which the patient does not have insight and his personality is distorted.

344. **Psychosurgery:** Surgical intervention to modify or alter disturbances of behavior or thought content.

345. **Puberty rites:** In preliterate societies, a ceremony which common morates the social recognition of a young person transition from the status of childhood into the status of adulthood.

346. **Publicity:** A characteristic of moral or ethical evaluations in which one must be willing to state the evaluation and the basis on which it is made publicity.

347. **Punaluan family:** A family in which a number of husbands are shared by group of sisters, or one in which a number of wives an shared by a group of brothers. This was hypothesized by Lewis H Morgan.

348. **Purdah:** The custom of secluding woman from public view.

349. **Race relations:** The relations among members of different races who are conscious of their racial differences.

350. **Race:** A major subdivision of the species home sapiens, consisting of a large number of people who form a distinct genetic entity because they have similar physical ancestors. Though such a definition has the value of precision, it has the important disadvantages of being undemonstrable with present techniques of anthropological analysis and research. Nonetheless, the term is generally used to refer to a biologically defined category of people which is to be distinguished from all culturally-defined categories of people.

351. **Racial minority:** (1) A racial aggregate that is discriminated against in a society that is dominated by members of another race. (2) A race that is numerically smaller than another race in a given society.

352. **Radiation:** Energy emitted by atoms that are unstable—radiation with enough energy to create ion pairs in matter.

353. **Radiation:** Transfer of heat or energy through space as with light, infrared, or ultrasound rays.

354. **Range-of-motion exercises:** Exercises whose action takes a limb c-joint through all angles of movement of which it is capable.

355. **Rapport:** Establishing a meaningful conversation.

356. **Readiness:** Links preparedness to relief; an assessment of readiness reflects the current capacity and capabilities of the organization involved in relief activities.

357. **Recovery:** Actions of responders, government, and the victims that help return an affected community to normal by stimulating community cohesiveness and government involvement (One type of recovery involves repairing infrastructure, damaged buildings, and critical facilities. The recovery period falls between the onset of the emergency and the reconstruction period).

358. **Referred pain:** Pain (usually from a visceral lesion) felt in a part of the body distant from the actual lesion, usually in a surface area.

359. **Regional sociology:** The study of regions as unique societies having their own peculiar culture, language dialects, political outlooks and traditions.

360. **Rehabilitation or reconstruction:** A long-term development project that follows a disaster or emergency that reconstructs a community's infrastructure to preexisting levels; is often associated with an opportunity to improve a community rather than to simply "reconstruct" a preexisting system.

361. **Rehabilitation:** Process of assisting a disabled person who is acutely or chronically ill or convalescent to realize particular goals in living and working to the utmost potential.

362. **Relief:** Action focused on saving lives (Relief activities often include search and rescue missions, first aid, and restoration of emergency communications and transportation systems. Relief also included attention to the immediate care of survivors by providing food, clothing, medical treatment, and emotional care).

363. **Religion:** A system of conduct that is based on beliefs which outline the ethical and proper relations among men, as well as the proper relationship between men and god (or gods), which often embodies worshipful and reverent ceremony.

364. **Religious conception of society:** The view that all social institutions, such as the family, economic and political practices, religious organizations, as well as the ideas of morality, derive their justifications from a divine source and that all social process as well as the direction of change are the inscrutable manifestations of a divine will.

365. **Reporting unit for surveillance:** The data source that provides information for the surveillance system (Reporting units often include hospitals, clinics, health posts, and mobile health units. Epidemiologists select reporting units after they define "what a case is" because the source of data is dependent on that definition).

366. **Representativeness:** The accuracy of the data when measuring the occurrence of a health event over time and its distribution by person and place.

367. **Resource management:** A management style that maximizes the use of and control over assets; this management style reduces the need for unnecessary communications, provides for strict accountability, and ensures the safety of personnel.

368. **Respiration:** The physical and chemical process by which oxygen and carbon dioxide are exchanged in the body. Breathing is the mechanical part of respiration.

369. **Respiratory isolation:** Isolation used for diseases that are commonly spread by droplet infection and those in which the organism is present in the respiratory system.

370. **Response:** The phase in a disaster when relief, recovery, and rehabilitation occur; also includes the delivery of services, the management of activities and programs designed to address the immediate and short-term effects of an emergency or disaster.

371. **Restorative phase:** Following acute stage of illness. Long-term considerations are examined so that appropriate actions geared toward realistic goals for the patient may be instituted.

372. **Retention:** Inability to empty the bladder voluntarily and completely.

373. **Richter scale:** A scale that indicates the magnitude of an earthquake by providing a measure of the total energy released from the source of the quake; the source of an earthquake of the quake; the source of an earthquake is the segment of the fault that has slipped.

374. **Rigorism:** The view that moral rules should be applied relatively rigidly.

375. **Rorschach test:** A projective test to identify ego function and personality conflicts which consists of 10 ink blots.

376. **Roy adaptation model:** Based on the idea that human responses fall into four broad areas of adaptation; physiologic needs, self-concept, role—function, and interdependence relations.

377. **Rural sociology:** The study of the influence of rural living on the organization and functions of social groups.

378. **Sadism:** Pleasure derived from inflicting physical or psychological pain on others.

379. **Scientific principles:** Comprehensive and fundamental laws, doctrines, truths, or sets of facts that form the basis for established rules of action.

380. **Sex ratio:** The number of male per 100 females in a given population.

381. **Sib:** A social unit made up of persons who are or who believe themselves to be, united by families or hereditary descent. The sib always has a name, as well as certain symbols towards which the sib members have feelings or reverence and respect. In addition, the sib holds various forms of poverty, such as the ceremonies and ceremonial equipment.

382. **Sick-role behavior:** Activities a person engages in, believing himself or herself ill.

383. **Situationalism:** The position that ethical action must be judged in each situation guided by, but not directly determined by, rules; cf. antinomianism, rules of practice.

384. **Six fundamental interests:** Albino W Small's statement that the six basic mainsprings of human behavior are: (1) Health, (2) Wealth, (3) Sociability, (4) Knowledge, (5) Beauty, (6) Righteousness.

385. **Six service standards:** A list of six basic services which may be provided by a village for the rural population in the vicinity, economic, education, religious, social communication and professional services. The list is used as certain for making comparisons among villages.

386. **Snellen test:** Commonly used test of gross visual acuity; used as a screening test for visual defects.

387. **Social action:** (1) Conduct that is oriented toward other people. (2) Any cooperative effort on the part of a group of people to achieve some goal.

388. **Social behavior:** Human activity which occurs in response to the meaning of the conduct of others or that which is intended to stimulate meaningful responses in others.

389. **Social cause:** Any action or situation which elict conduct in people.

390. **Social change:** The term social change usually refers to any change in the ideas, norms, values social roles and social habits of the people or in the composition or organization of their society. The precise definition depends on exactly how the word social is defined: If social and cultural are identical, then social change would be cultural change.

391. **Social control:** (1) The deliberate institutional means of making individuals and groups in a society observes and conform to the avowed social norms; (2) The informal pressure exerted by a group over an individual by means of certain techniques such as gossip, ridicule and praise; (3) The group interaction itself which functions to channel behavior into certain paths is also a kind of social control, quite apart is also a kind of social control, quite apart of any deliberate methods.

392. **Social Darwinism:** The point of view that cultural groups and races are subject to the same laws of natural selection as plants and animals in nature. Thus the weak groups are numerically diminished and their cultures delimited, while the strong groups grow in numbers as well as in their cultural influence over the week.

393. **Social differentiation:** (1) The development of status difference in a society. (2) The development of social and cultural distinctions in a society.

394. **Social disintegration:** (1) A drastic breakdown in the social control of social relations and sense of in group solidarity in a society. (2) The process by which people participate in over fewer social activities, so that the amount of interaction among them decreases and group controls over them diminish in effectiveness.

395. **Social distance:** The degree to which groups of people treat each other with reserve because of cultural, racial, religious, economic, or other differences.

396. **Social environment:** The interpersonal relationship that exist for persons.

397. **Social organization:** (1) A social group or society. (2) The organization of society into interrelated hierarchy of groups and status levels. (3) The process whereby all the groups and persons in a society cooperate in their willingness to give allegiance to their value system. (4) The condition in which there is a high degree of order and integration (singleness of purpose) in the social practices, values, and

ideologies in a society, with a minimum of ambiguity and conflict among them. (5) The customary and regular relationships among peoples; the regular ways that people usually behave toward each other.

398. **Social ossification:** (1) The process by which status levels become more distinct. (2) The process of standardization in social practices.

399. **Social parasite:** A kind of person who makes a living at the expense of others, without even trying to return anything to his supporters. For example, beggars, racketeers, paid officials who do nothing for their organizations and so no.

400. **Social pathology:** The systematic study of the development of the human personality in a group context; also the study of collective movements of crowds, masses and publics and the way in which their behavior influenced, directed and controlled.

401. **Social problems:** (1) Any social condition or practice which deviates from a given state of ideals; (2) Social practices or conditions which deviate from the values of society, and which seriously thwart the achievement or maintains of these values by serving to disorganize individual personalities or by reducing the degree of social integration and respect for order.

402. **Social process:** (1) Social integration among persons; (2) Any sequence of acts by a group of people; (3) Any way in which groups of people act toward each other as they seek to achieve certain goals; (4) Any development or evolution of society.

403. **Social relativism:** The view that moral judgments are grounded only in each society's collective opinion (cf. cultural relativism).

404. **Social revolution:** A sudden and drastic change in the social practices or in the status structure in a society.

405. **Social science:** Any of the several related sciences that objectively study and analyses the significant aspects of human social behavior. They would essentially include sociology, political science, economics, cultural anthropology, social geography, population studies and social psychology. Many social scientists would also include physical anthropology and psychology as well as historiography and archaeology.

406. **Social stratification:** (1) The process whereby clean and definite status levels are formed. (2) The organization of society into status levels.

407. **Social structure:** (1) Orderly organization of the social roles and statutes in a society. (2) Any degree of regularity in the way that people act toward each other in a given group.

408. **Social system:** (1) The whole range of habits and symbols that people use in communicating with each other; (2) The regular relationship among the people of a society.

409. **Social theories of population growth:** Theories which explain population change in terms of the social and economic conditions which are peculiar to a particular people, including such factors as their cultural level, their religious ideals and their occupational structure.

410. **Social work:** The professional attempt to help people meet their personal and family problems more effectively.

411. **Socialization:** (1) The process of developing a personality; it refers the way that people learn the habits, attitudes, social roles of self-conceptions, group norms, and uni-verses of discourse that enable to interact with other people in their society. (2) The transfer of the ownership of property from private individuals to government ownership.

412. **Society:** The largest social grouping having performance through generations of people who adhere to common culture, tradition and value system, who have a status system and a division of social functions who have modes of control over their social conduct and who are conscious of being a unique society distinct from all others.

413. **Socio-economic status:** The status or amount of prestige in society, which is associated with the amount of income, wealth or type of occupation.

414. **Sociological fact:** A verifiable statement or observation about a social phenomenon which has relevance to a sociological hypothesis or generalization.

415. **Sociological family life:** The study of the types of families in terms of the relations among the family in term of the relations among the family members; it also usually includes the study of dating and courtship behavior; the factors associated with marital happiness, the influence on urban and rural living on family and the effects of such crisis as migration, divorce, desertion. Death and war on family life.

416. **Sociology of religion:** The study of the social, economic and political factors which are associated with the establishment, maintenance and change in a religious institution or its ideology; it is also the study of the significance of religion in human conduct.

417. **Soft diet:** Made of pureed foods or those with fine texture and less cellulose or fiber content than a general diet.

418. **Spencer's stages of sociology:** Herbert Spencer's statement that society development from (1) A society organized primarily for war. (2) A society organized primarily for industry.

419. **Spiritual needs:** Those needs relating to religious and ethical/moral issues.

420. **Standards of consent:** The frame of reference upon which consent may be evaluated (see reasonable person standard, professional standard, subjective standard).

421. **Stationary population:** A population in which the birth and death rates are constant and approximate each other, so that the size of the age and sex categories remains relatively consultant.

422. **Status symbol:** Any object, skill, experience or action on which members of a group or society place a value and which they use as a criterion for determining status.

423. **Status:** The privileges, rights and duties which are associated with a higher or lower social rank in a group or society.

424. **Sterilization:** The process of destroying all microorganisms.

425. **Stimulus:** An occurrence or event that produces some effect on some organism.

426. **Strict isolation:** Isolation used to prevent spread of highly communicable disease by contact and airborne routes of transmission.

427. **Subcutaneous:** Loose areolar tissue just beneath the layers of the skin.

428. **Subjective symptoms:** Those symptoms that the patient tells about (the patient's perspective).

429. **Superstitions:** An unsystematic body of irrational and fearful beliefs in various unreasonable phenomena having a supernatural character.

430. **Support systems:** Resources the patient has available to provide caring and concern; helpful in meeting needs for warmth and reassurance.

431. **Supportive nursing measures:** Nursing measures that have as their objective the meeting of physiologic and psychological needs of the patient rising from the stresses imposed by illness or injury.

432. **Surgical asepsis:** The methods employed to maintain sterility of an area.

433. **Surveillance:** The ongoing and systematic collection, analysis, and interpretation of health data essential to the planning implementation, and evaluation of public health practice; systems are designed to disseminate data in a timely manner and often include both data collection and disease monitoring.

434. **Technological hazard:** A potential threat to human welfare caused by technological factors (e.g. chemical release, nuclear accident, dam failure) (Earthquakes and other natural hazards can trigger technological hazards as well).

435. **Tension:** An unpleasant increase in psychomotor activity.

436. **Terminal:** Used to designate patient for whom death is inevitable though dying may not have begun.

437. **Theory of family origin:** The hypothesis that human families originated because of the fact the children are dependent on adults for their biological needs.

438. **Theory:** A set of interrelated constructs (concepts), definitions, and propositions that present a systematic view of phenomena by specifying relations among variables, with the purpose of explaining and predicting the phenomena.

439. **Total communications:** Method for teaching hearing handicapped people involving maximum use of residual hearing with aids, learning of special listening techniques, use of speech reading and sign language.

440. **Totem:** (1) An animal which a group of people believe to be their sacred ancestor and protector. (2) The group that reverse a totem, and whose members believe themselves to be mystically related to it.

441. **Totemic kinship:** The symbolic relationship among the members of a sib who worships the same totem.

442. **Totemism:** (1) The belief in a totem; (2) The organization of a society into totems.

443. **Toxicological disaster:** A serious environmental pollutant that causes illness by a massive, accidental escape of toxic substances into the air, soil, or water; these disasters affect humans, animals, and plants.

444. **Trait:** Particular feature of an individual's personality the seems to stand out and endure over wide varity of situations.

445. **Tribe:** A type of large social unit which is usually made up of several clans or sib who are politically bound together by a chief or common council and who may also have a common language and culture, although it is not invariably so.

446. **Under population:** An insufficient number of residents compared to the number who could live in a given area and maintain a given plane of living.

447. **Universal culture pattern:** A construct composed of the culture elements social organizations, and type of social conduct can be found in every human society.

448. **Universality:** A characteristic of moral or ethical evaluations in which an action or character trait should be evaluated the same by all people.

449. **Urban sociology:** The study of the implications of urban living for social relations.

450. **Victim distribution:** A victim distribution plan defines the transport distribution of victims among neighboring hospital according to their hospital treatment capacity; these plans often avoid taking victims to the nearest hospital since walking victims will overcrowd hospitals closest to the disaster site.

451. **Village community:** A small number of families engaged in agriculture who live in a compact settlement and who collectively control the use and the ownership of the land they till.

452. **Village:** A single definition which would embody the great variety of legal definitions that are to be found in the various state constitutions is impossible. Generally, a village is larger than a hamlet but smaller than a town.

453. **Voluntary agency (VOLAG):** A nonprofit, non-governmental, private association maintained and supported by voluntary contributions that provides assistance in emergencies and disasters.

454. **Vulnerability analysis:** The assessment of an exposed population's susceptibility to the adverse health effects of a particular hazard.

455. **Vulnerability:** The susceptibility of a population to a specific type of event; it is also associated with the degree of possible or potential loss from a risk that results from a hazard at a given intensity (the factors that influence vulnerability include demographics, the age and resilience of the environment, technology, social differentiation, and diversity as well as regional and global economics politics)

456. **We-felling:** The recognition by a number of people that they form a unique group which is worthy of inspiring their loyalty in preference to all other similar groups.

457. **White collar worker:** Professional, business managers and proprietors and clerks.

458. **White men's burden:** The view that because white men have highest culture in the world they are obliged to assume the responsibility to uplift and civilize the preliterate non- white ethnic groups.

459. **Witch:** A person, most often a women, who is believed to have inherent powers to work magic for good or evil.

460. **Witch-craft:** (1) The belief that a witch has the inherent power to harm or help a person or his soul, by using supernatural techniques, (2) The magical techniques associated with such a belief.

461. **Withdrawal state:** Physical and mental effects withdrawing drugs from patients who have become habituated to them.

Index